Neurotransmitters and Cortical Function
From Molecules to Mind

Edited by

Massimo Avoli
McGill University and
Montreal Neurological Institute
Montreal, Quebec, Canada

Tomás A. Reader
University of Montreal
Montreal, Quebec, Canada

Robert W. Dykes
McGill University and
Royal Victoria Hospital
Montreal, Quebec, Canada

and

Pierre Gloor
McGill University and
Montreal Neurological Institute
Montreal, Quebec, Canada

PLENUM PRESS • *NEW YORK AND LONDON*

Library of Congress Cataloging in Publication Data

Neurotransmitters and cortical function: from molecules to mind / edited by Massimo
Avoli... [et al.].
     p. cm.
  Based on a symposium honoring Herbert Henri Jasper, held July 21-23, 1986, in
Montreal.
  Includes bibliographies and index.
  ISBN 0-306-42729-X
  1. Cerebral cortex—Congresses. 2. Neurotransmitters—Congresses. 3. Jasper,
Herbert H. (Herbert Henri), 1906–   —Congresses. I. Avoli, Massimo. II. Jasper,
Herbert H. (Herbert Henri), 1906–
QP383.N483 1988   87-37401
612'.825—dc19   CIP

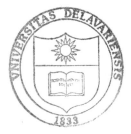

QP
383
.N483
1988

Based on a symposium on Neurotransmitters and Cortical Function: From Molecules
to Mind, held July 21-23, 1986, in Montreal, Quebec, Canada

© 1988 Plenum Press, New York
A Division of Plenum Publishing Corporation
233 Spring Street, New York, N.Y. 10013

Printed in the United States of America

Preface

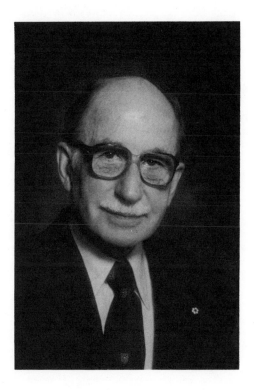

Herbert Henri Jasper is a scientist whose research activities have initiated and encompassed many of the major themes of neuroscience. He has pioneered in single unit recording, chronic neuronal studies, neurochemistry, electroencephalography, and many other disciplines. His students now hold important positions in universities and hospitals around the world.

From July 21 to 23, 1986, a symposium entitled Neurotransmitters and Cortical Function: From Molecules to Mind was held in Montreal to honor Professor Jasper and to continue his pioneering efforts. The following chapters originated in that meeting. They summarize the current status of our knowledge in some of the fields influenced by Professor Jasper. They share a focus on neurotransmitters in cortical function, where we presume higher mental events originate. Professor Jasper has made contributions to the understanding of three different classes of neurotransmitters: GABA, acetylcholine, and catecholamines. It is an interest in trying to link neurochemical events to some aspects of complex brain function and behavior that has characterized his work, and it is this philosophy that led to the present symposium to honor him. We dedicate this volume to Professor Jasper and the integrative approach that he has fostered.

The Editors

Montreal

Contents

1

H. H. Jasper, Neuroscientist of Our Century

P. Gloor

In our century we have witnessed a phenomenal growth in all the sciences. Where this growth has been most spectacular has been in nuclear physics, molecular biology, and last but not least in neuroscience, the one branch of learning which more than any other may ultimately contribute to a more profound understanding of our humanity and render human existence less subject to the ravages of neurological diseases which strike at the core of our distinctiveness as a species, the human mind.

Functional neuroscience, in particular as represented by neurophysiology, neurochemistry. and neuropsychology, has undergone its most significant growth in the 20th century. Many scientists have contributed to this unfolding story, but there are few among them whose careers reflect as faithfully this gradual coming of age of functional neuroscience in our time as does that of the man to whom this Symposium volume is dedicated, Herbert H. Jasper.

In this introductory chapter I shall attempt to sketch the scientific odyssey of this outstanding scientist whose interests and influence have been far ranging. In the final analysis, the motive force that propelled his many research activities was the quest to better understand the working of the human mind. This desire has propelled many brilliant men and women into the study of neuroscience, while in others it prompted a search for answers in philosophy or psychology, the path initially chosen by Herbert Jasper. Indeed his own personal quest began when as a college student in his native Oregon somewhat impatiently, as is the prerogative of youth, he sought answers to some of the most complex questions concerning the human psyche. His first publication reflects this orientation; it was entitled "Optimism and Pessimism in College Environments," and was published in *The American Journal of Sociology* in its 1928–29 volume. There followed two publications in 1930 and 1931 reporting on research along similar lines. It would be difficult to detect in these early papers signs of a budding experimental neuroscientist.

Not surprisingly this approach soon proved unsatisfying to his logical and inquiring mind, for it furnished no true explanations of how the human mind works. He thus reoriented his interest toward more fundamental physiological questions. This coincided with his move from Oregon to the University of Iowa. The first of his publications which testify to this new orientation is one which appeared in *Science* in 1931 where, together with R. Y. Walker, he described an eye movement camera. To a cynic, this new departure may appear like turning from the sublime to the

P. Gloor • Montreal Neurological Institute and Department of Neurology and Neurosurgery, McGill University, Montreal, Quebec, H3A 2B4, Canada.

trivial. I suspect that for Herbert Jasper, nurtured in philosophy and psychology, it must have been a difficult step to take, but it testifies to his courageous acceptance of the belief that we shall never be able to understand the human mind unless we are willing to deal first with very fundamental, measurable processes, starting with paradigms which may appear simplistic, but provide objectively verifiable and measurable data.

In 1932, a new horizon opened for Herbert Jasper. With the help of a Rockefeller Fellowship he went to Paris to study peripheral nerve physiology with Alexandre Marcel Monnier at the Sorbonne. Through collaboration with this gifted biophysicist, Jasper became an expert electrophysiologist. Much of his work in Paris was based on Lapicque's concept of chronaxie. In that period it was hoped that the study of this phenomenon in peripheral nerves could illuminate basic principles of neuronal function which might also be applicable to central mechanisms. In fact in 1932, in the *Comptes Rendus de la Société de Biologie,* Jasper reported on an attempt to extrapolate from chronaxie measurements in peripheral nerves to mechanisms present in the central nervous system. This was the first electrophysiological paper for which Jasper was the sole author.

After returning to North America in 1934, central mechanisms became the focus of his scientific interests. This evolved, undoubtedly, from the discovery he made with Leonard Carmichael at the Emma Bradley Home in Providence, Rhode Island. They observed that what Berger in Germany had reported for the first time 5 years earlier in 1929, namely that one could record the electrical activity of the human brain through the unopened skull, was in fact true. Jasper's first paper on the electroencephalogram (EEG) with Carmichael, published in *Science* in January 1935, was the first publication on the EEG on the North American continent. Figure 1 is a reproduction of the first EEG record published in North America as it appeared in this paper. It shows the normal resting EEG of a human adult and its changes in response to light stimulation. Thus started Jasper's intense interest in the human EEG which preoccupied him for many years. From the very beginning his aim has always been to use the EEG as a means to investigate fundamental aspects of brain function, rather than to merely employ it as a diagnostic test. Implied in this approach was the conviction that the effective use of the EEG for diagnostic purposes requires a knowledge of the physiological fundamentals of the normal and abnormal EEG, an attitude which unfortunately today has been allowed to become dormant to the detriment of the clinical science of electroencephalography. This outlook was the inspiration for many experimental studies that sought to clarify the physiological basis of the normal and abnormal EEG, particularly the abnormalities appearing in epilepsy.

This first paper on the EEG initiated a long and fertile period of investigations particularly on electroencephalography and in general CNS electrophysiology which firmly established Jasper's reputation as a leader in neuroscience. His first important contribution was to recognize that the EEG not only was abnormal in epilepsy, as Gibbs, Davis, and Lennox had reported in 1935, a few months after the publication of Jasper and Carmichael's paper on the EEG, but that in many instances the localization of the epileptogenic disturbance in the brain could be established by

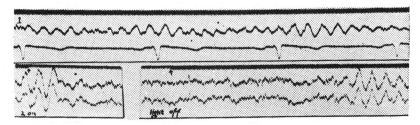

Figure 1. First illustration of a human EEG published in North America. Normal EEG from a ''relaxed cooperative subject.'' Upper record, upper line: alpha waves; lower line: control record taken from the left leg; lower record: effect of light stimulation on the alpha waves (blocking of the alpha rhythm). (From Jasper and Carmichael, 1935.)

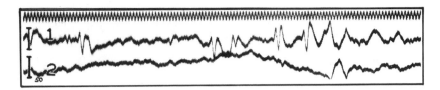

Figure 2. Interictal EEG from a patient with posttraumatic Jacksonian seizures showing characteristic spikes or sharp waves in the left precentral region (1) but not from the homologous area (2). (From Jasper and Hawke, 1938.)

surface EEG recordings (Jasper, 1936). Jasper defined the morphological characteristics of localized interictal EEG discharges. In Fig. 2 there is an example of one of his early recordings of interictal epileptiform spikes taken from his 1938 paper with William Hawke. This work led, after a chance encounter with Wilder Penfield in 1937 who was then visiting the Bradley Home in Providence, to a fruitful and long collaboration with Penfield in Montreal. Penfield (1972) described the beginning of this remarkable collaboration as follows: ". . . he [Jasper] and I . . . instituted [an] almost unthinkable commuters' research project. It was as though far-away Rhode Island were a suburb of Montreal. He would arrive each week, ordinarily late Monday night, with his electrograph on the front seat of his car, and went to bed in a resident's room at the Institute. I would operate on a focal epileptic patient Tuesday morning and possibly another on Wednesday and Thursday. Friday, he was somehow back in Providence where he carried out a full week's work, discharging his responsibilities at the Bradley Home over the weekend." Jasper was able to convince Penfield that it was indeed possible to identify the site of origin of a patient's seizures, even between attacks, by recording the EEG through the unopened skull. The location of the random interictal epileptiform discharges appearing in such records indicated the region of the brain from which the seizures originated (Jasper and Kershman, 1941). Furthermore, Jasper found that it was possible to refine this localization by recording the brain's electrical activity directly from its exposed surface during neurosurgical procedures (Figs. 3 and 4) (Jasper 1949a,b;

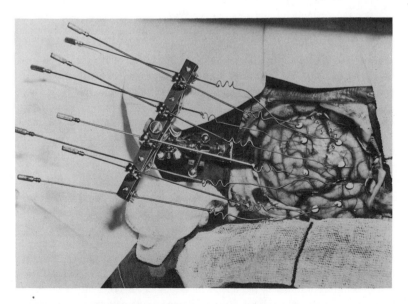

Figure 3. Technique of recording the electrocorticogram from the exposed cortex during a neurosurgical procedure for the relief of seizures. Eight electrodes made of silver with chlorided tips covered by cotton wicks were placed on the cortex. Paper tickets with numbers indicate points from which responses to localized electrical stimulations were obtained. (From Penfield and Jasper, 1954.)

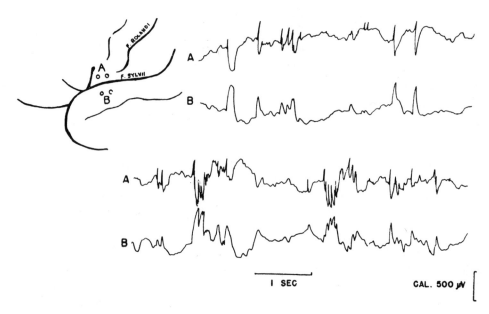

Figure 4. Random spike discharges appearing spontaneously in the electrocorticogram of a patient with focal seizures arising on the border of an epidermoid tumor. (From Jasper, 1949a.)

Jasper and Penfield, 1949). A Rockefeller Foundation grant and donations by J. W. McConnell, Sir Herbert Holt, and C. H. Duccan made it possible to convert this "commuters' project" into a more conventional setup: in January 1939 a Laboratory of Electroencephalography and Neurophysiology was opened at the Montreal Neurological Institute under the directorship of Herbert Jasper. It was dedicated to "research on the physiology of the brain with special reference to epilepsy and dementia."

Shortly after the opening of the laboratory, World War II broke out, and much of the research was reoriented to problems related to the war effort. Problems arising from the numerous cases of peripheral nerve injury were studied using the new electrophysiological techniques and Jasper became one of the initiators of another new branch of clinical neurophysiology: electromyography (Jasper, 1946). Figure 5 is an illustration from a paper he wrote with Gwen Ballem which appeared in the *Journal of Neurophysiology* in 1949 showing normal motor unit potentials from various human muscles.

As soon as the war was over, Jasper and Penfield focused their interest again on epilepsy and on what it could reveal about the functional anatomy of the human brain (Penfield and Jasper, 1954). New and exciting insights into the role played by the temporal lobe in memory mechanisms were obtained. It became possible to put on a secure foundation the various electrophysiological aspects of human epileptic discharge as they were revealed by the extracranial EEG and as they appeared in recordings taken directly from the exposed human brain (Jasper, 1949a,b). Jasper's ideas on thalamocortical relationships were another important contribution arising from these studies. Together with Penfield (Penfield and Jasper, 1946) and Jan Droogleever-Fortuyn, a visiting neurologist from Holland, he formulated some new concepts on the organization of thalamocortical projection systems and on how they operate under both normal and pathological conditions such as generalized epilepsy (Jasper and Droogleever-Fortuyn, 1946). Figure 6 is an illustration from his 1946 paper with Droogleever-Fortuyn, in which they demonstrated that the characteristic generalized 3/sec spike and wave pattern seen in human petit mal epilepsy can be elicited in the cat by midline thalamic stimulation. Jasper's views of the central role thalamocortical relationships play in generalized epilepsy have been seminal to the further

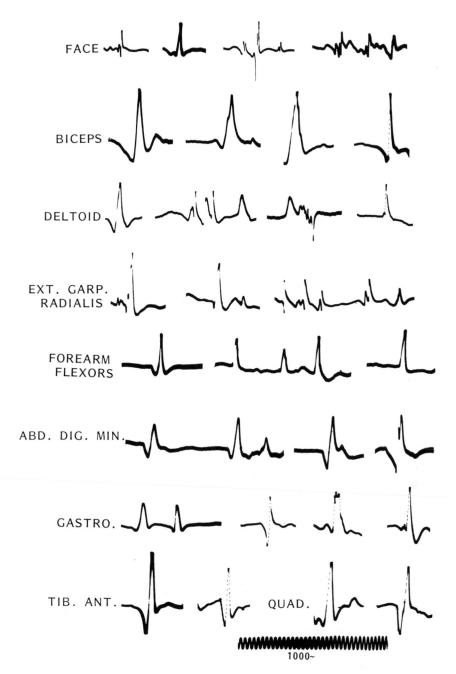

Figure 5. Varieties of motor units recorded from normal human muscles. (From Jasper and Ballem, 1949.)

development of important concepts and experimental work in this area. His views on the physiology of thalamocortical relationships were a departure from older and more simplistic concepts of how these systems worked. He proposed that a distinction be made between "specific" and "unspecific" thalamocortical systems, each having its distinctive anatomical organization and physiological significance (Jasper and Droogleever-Fortuyn, 1946; Jasper, 1948, 1949c). Figure 7

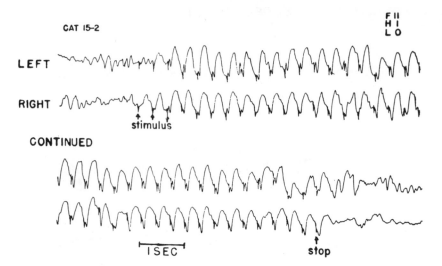

Figure 6. Bilaterally synchronous wave and spike responses of the cortex produced by repetitive stimulation of the massa intermedia of a cat at a frequency of 3 per second. (From Jasper and Droogleever-Fortuyn, 1946.)

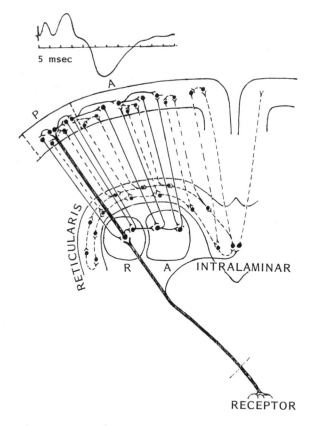

Figure 7. Diagrammatic representation of the hypothetical organization of thalamocortical systems showing the direct specific relay system (R) as related to the specific association of elaborative system (A) and the superimposed multineuronal thalamic reticular system (intralaminar nuclei and nucleus reticularis). In the sketch above are illustrated three responses. The first two represent the primary and secondary responses in the specific systems and the third the delayed response from the reticulocortical system. (Drawn by Dr. Robert Knighton; from Jasper, 1949c.)

is a beautiful diagrammatic illustration of the thalamocortical relationships proposed by him in 1949. In this organization, may be located, as he put it in 1948, "the specific controlling mechanisms for processes of attention . . . involved in the momentary limelight directed here and there in the central stream of consciousness."

In the early 1950s Jasper's restless mind was ready to push on to new frontiers. He was no longer satisfied with studying the rather gross features of the EEG. He wanted to know what was hidden behind the facade of these relatively slow potential oscillations. Could they be explained in terms of activities generated by single neurons? He tackled this problem head on in the early 1950s in collaboration with Choh-Lu Li, Hugh McLennan, and Chester Cullen, and also a few years later with Costas Stefanis (Li *et al.*, 1952, 1956a,b; Li and Jasper, 1953; Stefanis and Jasper, 1964a,b; Jasper and Stefanis, 1965). They were the first to record the activity of single neurons in the cerebral neocortex both extra- and intracellularly (Figs. 8 and 9). This work was not only a pioneering effort; it helped to clarify the complex relationships between gross surface EEG phenomena and cortical single-unit discharges. Even though Jasper at that time was preoccupied with gaining a better understanding of the fundamental mechanisms of single neuronal activity, he never lost sight of his old interest in the problem of how the mind works. Indeed, soon after he succeeded in recording from single units in the cerebral cortex, he turned his attention again to more psychological dimensions of brain physiology and with Gian Franco Ricci and Ben Doane he studied the involvement of single cortical nerve cells in conditioning (Jasper *et al.*,

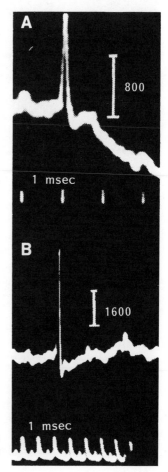

Figure 8. Action potentials of single cortical cells in the post-sigmoid gyrus of the cat recorded by means of glass microelectrodes 1 μm or less in diameter. (From Li *et al.*, 1952.)

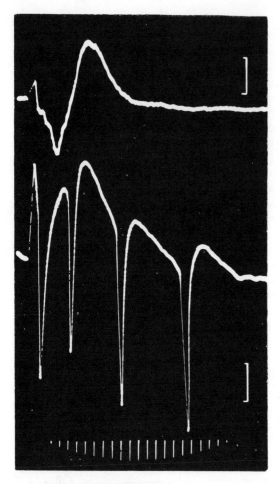

Figure 9. Response to single stimulation of thalamic sensory nucleus (n. ventralis posterolateralis) recorded in the somatosensory cortex of a cat. The upper tracing shows the surface EEG response, the lower tracing the intracellularly recorded response from a neuron in the somatosensory cortex. (From Li *et al.*, 1956a.)

1958, 1960). This was the first time anyone had attempted to employ single-unit recording techniques in the investigation of behavior (Fig. 10). The methodology Jasper developed in the course of these experiments is now widely used in many neurobehavioral studies. Jasper, in collaboration with Gilles Bertrand, extended this technique to the study of human brain physiology (Jasper and Bertrand, 1966a,b). Taking advantage of the opportunities offered by stereotaxic thalamotomies carried out for the relief of parkinsonian tremor, he recorded from single neurons in the human thalamus. The discharge of a single human thalamic neuron upon tactile stimulation applied to its receptive field localized on the patient's right middle finger is shown in Fig. 11.

The work at the Montreal Neurological Institute gave Jasper the opportunity to collaborate not only with Wilder Penfield, one of the giants of clinical neurology and neurosurgery of the century, but also with another neuroscientist whose influence was seminal in the development of modern neuroscience, K. A. C. Elliott, probably the first neurochemist to have that title. Jasper and Elliott worked closely together. The highlight of their collaboration was the elucidation of the properties of an inhibitory factor that could be extracted from brain, initially known as factor I. Painstaking chemical studies performed in Elliott's laboratory demonstrated that factor I was none other than γ-aminobutyric acid (GABA). Thus, through the collaboration of Elliott and Jasper (Iwama and Jasper, 1957; Elliott and Jasper, 1959; Jasper, 1960) the foundations of the enor-

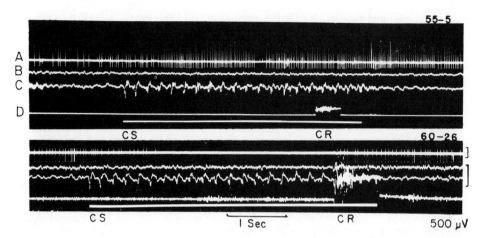

Figure 10. Unitary discharges in motor cortex (A), electrocorticogram from the motor (B) and visual cortex (C), and motor and electromyographic response (D) recorded in a monkey during a conditioned response. CS, conditioned stimulus (flashing light); CR, conditioned response. Upper tracing: response of motor cortex unit accelerating its discharge rate prior to the conditioned response; lower tracing: the response of another cell showing inhibition of discharge. (From Jasper *et al.*, 1960.)

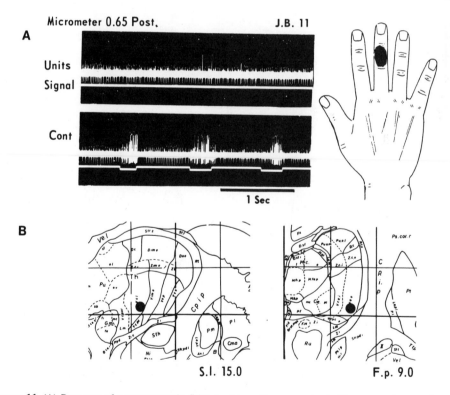

Figure 11. (A) Response of a spontaneously firing touch receptor neuron to stroking across the receptive zone outlined on the dorsum of the second phalanx of the middle finger of the contralateral hand. (B) Localization of the tip of the microelectrode as projected upon the thalamic nuclear outlines in the sagittal plane 15.0 and frontal plane 9.0 of an atlas of the human thalamus. (From Jasper and Bertrand, 1966b.)

mously successful and far-reaching GABA story were laid. This area is one of the very active areas in the neurosciences today and is covered in this symposium.

Undoubtedly through his intimate collaboration with Elliott, Jasper became increasingly aware of the importance of biochemistry for the understanding of brain function, and particularly of the importance of correlating electrophysiological with biochemical data. Rapidly this became his foremost interest, particularly during the years he worked at the Centre de Recherche en Sciences Neurologiques de l'Université de Montréal. This story began at the Montreal Neurological Institute with the study cf the effects of GABA. It was followed by the recognition that certain functional states of the brain, such as arousal mediated by the reticular formation of the brain stem, were associated with changes in the release of amino acids and with an increased release of acetylcholine from the cerebral cortex (Jasper et al., 1965; Celesia and Jasper, 1966). Pursuing these lines of research during his years at the University of Montreal, Jasper discovered that certain functional states of the brain, as revealed by changes in the electrical activity of the cerebral cortex, were associated with very specific patterns of release of a whole gamut of amino acids. These patterns could almost serve as biochemical fingerprints for certain activity states of the cerebral cortex, as is shown in Fig. 12 from Jasper and Koyama (1969), which contrasts the patterns of amino acid release from the cerebral cortex during a state of activation produced by electrical stimulation of the midbrain reticular formation with that seen at a period when the EEG indicated that the animal was asleep. An offshoot of these studies were the investigations with

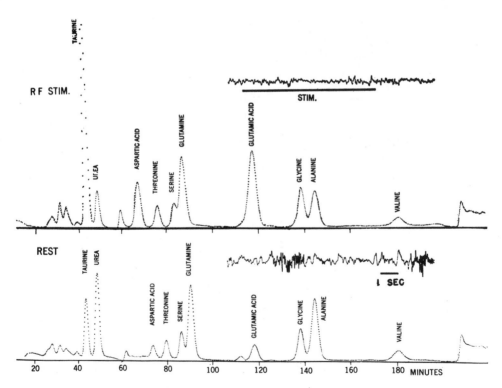

Figure 12. Profile of amino acid release from the cerebral cortex of a cat as measured in the perfusate of a chamber placed on the surface of the cortex. The upper series of chromatograms shows the profile obtained during a state of arousal (desynchronized EEG) maintained by intermittent repetitive stimulations of the midbrain reticular formation. The lower series shows the profile obtained in the same animal during a period of rest, while the EEG showed a pattern characteristic for sleep. (From Jasper and Koyama, 1969.)

Ikuko Koyama and Nico van Gelder on the importance of certain amino acids in epileptogenesis (Koyama and Jasper, 1977; van Gelder *et al.*, 1977).

There finally followed, with Tomás Reader, Jacques de Champlain, and Laurent Descarries, important work on catecholaminergic mechanisms in the cerebral cortex. This work was initiated at a time when the presence of dopaminergic terminals in regions of the cerebral cortex other than the frontal lobe had not yet been established (Reader *et al.*, 1976, 1979a,b). It became evident that there was some kind of reciprocal relationship between acetylcholine release and both noradrenaline and dopamine release with regard to activation of the cerebral cortex by sensory inputs, the former showing an increase and the catecholamines a decrease under these conditions. Certainly at this stage of his career Jasper's search for the mind had become a search for molecules. He had traveled a long road since his early college days when he had attempted to understand why some people approached life in an optimistic frame of mind, while others were subject to a gloomy pessimism.

In spite of the fact that his quest had ultimately led him to a search for molecules, Jasper never lost sight of his original goal. He always hoped that research directed at fundamental and even molecular mechanisms in the brain may help us to better understand the human mind. In 1975 when giving a personal account of what he called his "devious path of exploration in the neurosciences," Jasper described it as one "from philosophy to physics, and from mind to molecules." It is therefore not by chance that we have chosen as a title of this symposium that of *Neurotransmitters and Cortical Function: From Molecules to Mind.* Why, one may ask, have we reversed the direction of this path in describing it as one "from molecules to mind"? I think Herbert Jasper will understand. Neuroscience has now progressed to the point where we can measure, with unheard-of precision, many processes at the molecular level which are related to certain functions of the nervous system, not only simple, but even complex ones. We are now standing on an exciting threshold of scientific history, where we can hope that at least some aspects of how the human mind works can be understood, not necessarily in the traditional terms of biophysics and biochemistry—because such a hope would betray a too naively reductionist point of view—but in terms of mechanisms that involve organizational levels of which biophysical and biochemical processes are the indispensable building blocks. In this sense fundamental biophysical and biochemical principles can be brought to bear on the study of the mind. If the topics of the present symposium seem to be related more to the basic molecular aspects of these problems, to the building blocks, rather than to the study of the mind as such, it is because at the present time we are still only able to make precise scientific measurements at that level. The higher organizational principles which emerge when these mechanisms act in a complex information-handling system such as the brain are yet to be studied. How far this quest can lead us and whether we will ever reach the point where we really can fully account for the functioning of the human mind is of course impossible to say at this juncture. I believe we all secretly hope that this point will never be reached, for then what else would there be left to be investigated scientifically?

References

Berger, H., 1929, Über das Elektrenkephalogramm des Menschen, *Arch. Psychiatr. Nervenkr.* **87:**527–570. (Translated into English in Gloor, P., 1969, Hans Berger on the electroencephalogram of man, *Electroencephalogr. Clin. Neurophysiol. Suppl.* **28:**37–73.)

Celesia, G. G., and Jasper, H. H., 1966, Acetylcholine released from cerebral cortex in relation to state of activation, *Neurology* **16:**1053–1064.

Elliott, K. A. C., and Jasper, H. H., 1959, Gamma-aminobutyric acid, *Physiol. Rev.* **39:**383–406.

Gibbs, F. A., Davis, H.. and Lennox, W. C., 1935, The electroencephalogram in epilepsy and in conditions of impaired consciousness, *Arch. Neurol. Psychiatry* **34:**1133–1148.

Iwama, K., and Jasper, H. H., 1957, The action of gamma aminobutyric acid upon cortical electrical activity in the cat, *J. Physiol. (London)* **138:**365–380.

Jasper, H. H., 1928–29, Optimism and pessimism in college environments, *Am. J. Sociol.* **34:**856–873.

Jasper, H. H., 1930. The measurement of depression–elation and its relation to a measure of extraversion–introversion, *J. Abnorm. Soc. Psychol.* **25:**307–318.

Jasper, H. H., 1931, Is perseveration a functional unit participating in all behavior processes? *J. Soc. Psychol.* **2:**28–51.

Jasper, H. H., 1932, L'action asymmétrique des centres sur la chronaxie des nerfs symmétriques droit et gauche chez la grenouille, *C. R. Soc. Biol.* **110:**376–378.

Jasper, H. H., 1936, Localized analysis of the function of the human brain by the electroencephalogram, *Arch. Neurol. Psychiatry* **36:**1131–1134.

Jasper, H. H., 1946, The rate of re-innervation of muscle following nerve injuries in man as determined by the electromyogram, *Trans. R. Soc. Can. Sect. 5* **40:** 81–92.

Jasper, H. H., 1948, Charting the sea of brain waves, *Science* **108:**343–347.

Jasper. H. H., 1949a, Electrical signs of epileptic discharge, *Electroencephalogr. Clin. Neurophysiol.* **1:**11–18.

Jasper, H. H., 1949b, Electrocorticogram in man, *Electroencephalogr. Clin. Neurophysiol. Suppl.* **2:**16–29.

Jasper, H. H., 1949c, Diffuse projection systems: The integrative action of the thalamic reticular system, *Electroencephalogr. Clin. Neurophysiol.* **1:**405–420.

Jasper, H. H., 1960, The physiological significance of gamma-aminobutyric acid in the central nervous system, in: *Actualités neurophysiologiques* (A. M. Monnier, ed.), Masson. Paris, pp. 33–47.

Jasper, H. H., 1975, Philosophy or physics—Mind or molecules, in: *The Neurosciences: Paths of Discovery* (F. G. Worden, J. P. Swazey, and G. Adelman, eds.), MIT Press, Cambridge, Mass., pp. 403–422.

Jasper, H. H., and Ballem, G., 1949, Unipolar electromyograms of normal and denervated muscle, *J. Neurophysiol.* **12:**231–244.

Jasper, H. H., and Bertrand, G., 1966a, Recording from microelectrodes in stereotactic surgery for Parkinson's disease, *J. Neurosurg.* **24:**219–227.

Jasper, H. H., and Bertrand, G., 1966b, Thalamic unit involved in somatic sensation and voluntary and involuntary movements in man, in: *The Thalamus* (D. P. Purpura and M. D. Yahr, eds.), Columbia University Press, New York, pp. 365–390.

Jasper, H. H., and Carmichael, L., 1935, Electrical potentials from the intact human brain, *Science* **81:**51–53.

Jasper, H. H., and Droogleever-Fortuyn, Experimental studies on the functional anatomy of petit mal epilepsy, *Proc. Assoc. Res. Nerv. Ment. Dis.* **26:**272–298.

Jasper, H. H., and Hawke, W. A., 1938, Electroencephalography. IV. Localization of seizure waves in epilepsy, *Arch. Neurol. Psychiatry* **39:**885–901.

Jasper, H. H., and Kershman, J., 1941, Electroencephalographic classification of the epilepsies, *Arch. Neurol. Psychiatry* **45:**903–943.

Jasper, H. H., and Koyama, I., 1969, Rate of release of amino acids from the cerebral cortex in the cat as affected by brain stem and thalamic stimulation. *Can. J. Physiol. Pharmacol.* **47:**889–905.

Jasper, H. H., and Penfield, W., 1949, Zur Deutung des normalen Elektrenkephalogramms und seiner Veränderungen. Electrocorticograms in man: Effect of voluntary movement upon electrical activity of the precentral gyrus, *Arch. Psychiatr. Z. Neurol.* **183Z:**163–174.

Jasper, H. H., and Stefanis, C., 1965, Intracellular oscillatory rhythms in pyramidal tract neurons in the cat, *Electroencephalogr. Clin. Neurophysiol.* **18:**541–553.

Jasper, H. H., and Walker, R. Y., 1931, The Iowa eye-movement camera, *Science* **74:**291–294.

Jasper, H. H., Ricci, G. F., and Doane, B., 1958, Patterns of cortical neuronal discharge during conditioned responses in monkey, *Ciba Foundation Symposium on the Neurological Basis of Behavior* pp. 277–290.

Jasper, H. H., Ricci, G. F., and Doane, B., 1960, Microelectrode analysis of cortical cell discharge during avoidance conditioning in the monkey. in: *Moscow Colloquium on Electroencephalography of Higher Nervous Activity* (H. H. Jasper and G. D. Smirnov. eds.), *Electroencephalogr. Clin. Neurophysiol. Suppl.* **13:**137–155.

Jasper, H. H., Kahn, R. T., and Elliott, K. A. C., 1965, Amino acids released from the cerebral cortex in relation to its state of activation, *Science* **147:**1448–1449.

Koyama, I., and Jasper, H. H., 1977, Amino acid content of chronic undercut cortex of the cat in relation to electrical afterdischarge: Comparison with cobalt epileptogenic lesions. *Can. J. Physiol. Pharmacol.* **55:**523–536.

Li, C.-L., and Jasper, H. H., 1953, Microelectrode studies of the electrical activity of the cerebral cortex in the cat, *J. Physiol. (London)* **121:**117–140.

Li, C.-L., McLennan, H., and Jasper, H. H., 1952, Brain waves and unit discharge in cerebral cortex, *Science* **116:**656–657.

Li, C.-L., Cullen, C., and Jasper, H. H., 1956a, Laminar microelectrode studies of specific somatosensory cortical potentials, *J. Neurophysiol.* **19:**111–130.

Li, C.-L., Cullen, C., and Jasper, H. H., 1956b, Laminar microelectrode analysis of cortical unspecific recruiting responses and spontaneous rhythms, *J. Neurophysiol.* **19:**1311–143.

Penfield, W., 1972, Herbert Jasper, in: *Recent Contributions to Neurophysiology: International Symposium in Neurosciences in Honor of Herbert H. Jasper* (J. P. Cordeau and P. Gloor, eds.), *Electroencephalogr. Clin. Neurophysiol. Suppl.* **31:**9–12.

Penfield, W., and Jasper, H., 1946, Highest level seizures, *Proc. Assoc. Res. Nerv. Ment. Dis.* **26:**252–271.

Penfield, W., and Jasper, H., 1954, *Epilepsy and the Functional Anatomy of the Human Brain,* Little, Brown, Boston.

Reader, T. A., de Champlain, J., and Jasper, H. H., 1976, Catecholamines released from cerebral cortex in the cat decrease during sensory stimulation, *Brain Res.* **111:**95–108.

Reader, T. A., de Champlain, J., and Jasper, H. H., 1979a, Interactions between biogenic amines and acetylcholine in the cerebral cortex. in: *Catecholamines: Basic and Clinical Frontiers,* Vol. 2 (E. Usdin, E. J. Kopin, and J. Barchas, eds.), Pergamon Press, New York, pp. 1074–1076.

Reader, T. A., Ferron, A., Descarries, L., and Jasper, H. H., 1979b, Modulatory role for biogenic amines in the cerebral cortex: Microiontophoretic studies, *Brain Res.* **160:**217–229.

Stefanis, C., and Jasper, H. H., 1964a, Intracellular microelectrode studies of antidromic responses in cortical pyramidal tract neurons, *J. Neurophysiol.* **27:**828–854.

Stefanis, C., and Jasper, H. H., 1964b, Recurrent collateral inhibition in pyramidal tract neurons, *J. Neurophysiol.* **27:**855–877.

van Gelder, N., Koyama, I., and Jasper, H. H., 1977, Taurine treatment of spontaneous chronic epilepsy in a cat, *Epilepsia* **18:**45–54.

2

H. H. Jasper: Modern Concepts of Epilepsy

N. M. van Gelder

1. Dedication

In any generation of scientists, a few become recognized as leaders in their field. Such leadership is often difficult to define, yet appears universally acknowledged. To include the name of Herbert H. Jasper among the neurobiologists so designated seems most natural. Not only has he served as a scientific role model for numerous neuroscientists now as eminent as himself but, in addition, many of his studies represent basic contributions to our understanding of brain function. These studies have covered subjects ranging from the single synapse, the electrophysiology of the isolated neuron and assemblies of neurons, to the electrophysiology and pharmacology of the neurotransmitter systems (Jasper, 1975). However, no matter how lofty the ideals of basic research may be, to incorporate such research into the everyday practice of clinical medicine, and to improve the treatment and the quality of life of neurological patients, must be even more satisfying.

The name Herbert Jasper is almost synonymous with epilepsy research, with respect to both investigations on the electrophysiological and electroencephalographic behavior of the epileptic brain, as well as the role of neurotransmitter systems in this cerebral disorder. Patients and his colleagues can only express their appreciation and admiration for Jasper's lifelong efforts to reach a greater understanding of this ancient affliction of mankind. His dogged, untiring attitude and determination in the laboratory to master any new experimental approach which might be helpful in his search for greater scientific knowledge, are legendary. As a lifelong student, "junior" colleague, and admirer of H. H. Jasper, this is my personal tribute to him. It is my hope that he may long continue to guide and teach the next generation of neurobiologists now engaged in gaining a better understanding of that most mysterious and unpredictable characteristic of human existence: the mind and its infinite combinations of uniqueness and versatility.

2. Epilepsy and Consciousness

To observe a grand mal seizure with its uncontrollable motor expression of autonomous cerebral neuronal activity and loss of consciousness, is a dramatic event. To subsequently see

---

N. M. van Gelder • Centre de Recherche en Sciences Neurologiques, Faculté de Médecine, Université de Montréal, Montreal, Quebec H3C 3J7, Canada.

such an individual, upon recovery, carry out normal daily activities with keen intelligence is even more startling. What type of brain disorder can temporarily so disturb the entire expression of brain functions, and yet leave only minimal aftereffects? What is more, why do such episodes reoccur intermittently with little predictability or advance warning and, yet, with stereotypic and most consistent repetition of symptoms? What stops a seizure and why does one lose consciousness? Indeed, what does it mean to be conscious?

If such questions appear overly dramatic and philosophical, inappropriate in a scientific discussion of epilepsy, it is necessary only to retrace the history of epilepsy to understand why this cerebral dysfunction has loomed so large in the medical treatises on neurological disorders (Temkin, 1971). Aristotle and Plato discussed epilepsy, as did the ancient Chinese practitioners of medicine, and artists too (Akimoto, 1982). Myths and mystics were occupied with the epileptic phenomenon, as were great religious scholars (Melville, 1974; Hansen, 1986). Even today, although epilepsy by now seems to represent a well-defined clinical entity, explicable in terms of strict and logical neurobiological parameters, studies on epilepsy continue to raise philosophical questions regarding the nature of human consciousness. One has only to read the titles of publications by two renowned epileptologists of our time: "Philosophy or Physics—Mind or Molecules" by Jasper (1975) and *The Mystery of the Mind* by Penfield (1975). The fact is of course that epilepsy research has always touched on many areas of neurobiology, encompassing investigations on unicellular phenomena, such as the epileptic neuron, its synaptic input and dendritic configuration, as well as on the synchronous high-frequency discharges of entire neuronal assemblies and their propagation to other brain regions.

The development of the concept that centrencephalic mechanisms participate in the spread of epileptic discharges, had far wider implications than for epilepsy alone (Jasper, 1965). It provided a further impetus for more accurate and functionally meaningful interpretations of the electroencephalogram (EEG) and the electrocorticogram, the correlation between unicellular discharges and the EEG, and stimulated the search for more precisely defined anatomical pathways and their chemical signal carriers (Jasper, 1969). The remarkable recuperative powers of the human brain following surgical excision of epileptic foci inevitably had to touch on the neurobiological mechanisms of memory, and differences between the awake and sleeping brain. Thus, the search for a precise mechanistic explanation of epilepsy, by definition, has forced frequent reappraisal of the existing concepts of normal brain function as well as of the origin of the disruptive effects of an epileptic attack on these functions. It is no coincidence therefore that epilepsy research has contributed so much to current scientific explanations of the conscious brain and the mind.

2.1. Epilepsy as an Excitatory Phenomenon

The two major improvements after the turn of the century in epilepsy management, namely the discovery of human brain wave patterns (Berger, 1933; Jasper and Carmichael, 1935) and antiseizure treatment with potassium bromide, luminal, and phenylhydantoin, have strongly ingrained the concept that epilepsy is a problem of hyperexcitable neurons (Temkin, 1971). The epileptic EEG is a reflection of the synchronous discharges of neurons at unusually high frequencies. Furthermore, the efficacy of phenylhydantoin as an anticonvulsant was established in an experimental model of a persistent seizure state, analogous to status epilepticus (Putman and Merritt, 1937). Ever since, the suppression of convulsions has been the goal of all epilepsy treatment, while most research into this disorder has been aimed at investigating the possible implication in seizure phenomena of attenuated inhibitory processes, or the reinforcement of facilitating excitatory systems. In the absence of convincing evidence for the existence of a well-defined inhibitory system in the CNS until the late 1950s, and the then rapidly growing microelectrode studies demonstrating highly excitable neurons in epileptic foci (see Ward, 1972), few scientists or clinicians doubted that the cellular substrate of the epileptic brain was a diseased neuron caused by a "morbid nutrition" of such cells (H. Jackson, cited in Temkin, 1971).

The discovery of GABA as the principal inhibitory substance in brain by Elliott's laboratory

(Elliott, 1965) certainly did little to contradict the existing concepts regarding the origin of epilepsy and, in fact, strongly seemed to support such hypothesis. Roberts *et al.* (1958), in a series of articles, detailed the metabolism of GABA in the CNS and even indicated how the GABA shunt could contribute to the overall energy metabolism of neurons. This neatly dovetailed with persisting convictions that, despite proof to the contrary, a defective energy metabolism was an important factor in the development of a seizure state. In rapid succession, Kuffler and Edwards (1958) established, in studies on the crustacean nervous system, not only that the actions of GABA mimicked the effect of stimulating peripheral inhibitory nerves, but also that its effects were mediated by enhanced Cl^- permeability, and that the amino acid had a selective distribution in these nerves (Kravitz *et al.*, 1962).

Other investigations demonstrated that application of GABA to the mammalian cortex had a powerful (inhibitory) influence on the evoked cortical surface potential (Iwama and Jasper, 1957), could antagonize epileptic discharges in experimental foci (Berl *et al.*, 1961), and that it was released under conditions of reduced cortical alertness (Jasper *et al.*, 1965). An important debate at that time was whether GABA acted primarily by inhibiting excitatory synaptic functions, or whether it functioned as the predominant inhibitory system in the CNS (see Elliott and Jasper, 1959). This argument of a modulator role as opposed to that of a classical inhibitory neurotransmitter, while even today not totally resolved, has nevertheless been adopted in favor of the latter, following the demonstration of precisely circumscribed GABAergic pathways in the CNS. The recent work of Fromm *et al.* (1985) showing that anticonvulsant GABA mimetics act via inhibitory pathways impinging upon the reticular formation, moreover fits in nicely with the postulated participation of centrencephalic influences on the propagation of epileptic discharges. Finally, the essential role of GABA in preventing a seizure condition was early accentuated by the action of convulsant hydrazides and vitamin B_6 deficiency, where the resulting convulsions closely paralleled the lowering of cerebral GABA levels, while their reversal was accomplished by returning these levels to normal (see Elliott and Jasper, 1959; Elliott, 1965).

Findings of this type thus established that lack of inhibition as such, or an attenuation of inhibition on excitatory influences, was a cause of seizures. While the two concepts are not mutually exclusive, it should be noted that they are not identical. Lack of inhibition implies excitatory processes remaining unaltered whereas a decreased inhibition of excitation suggests enhanced excitability in neural tissue. Furthermore, neither denotes an increased excitation in the presence of an intact inhibitory system. This third concept as a possible cause for epilepsy only slowly gained a measure of credibility, and then only when evidence suggested that seizures may occur in the presence of elevated GABA levels (Chapman *et al.*, 1977), or without an apparent failure of inhibition (Schwartzkroin, 1983).

2.2. Epilepsy, Glutamic Acid, and Hyperexcitation

Despite the convincing data that lack of GABA-mediated inhibition led to convulsions, certain lines of evidence did not totally support the GABA deficiency hypothesis as the sole cause for epilepsy. In the 1950s, work by Tower (1957) and Woodbury and Esplin (1959) suggested that an abnormality in glutamate metabolism might also be a frequent occurrence in epileptic tissue. In the succeeding years, Koyama and Jasper (1977) and especially the group of Bradford, Dodd, and collaborators (Dodd *et al.*, 1980) demonstrated that epileptic tissue, very characteristically, releases higher than normal amounts of glutamic acid. In view of the strong excitatory action of glutamic acid on neurons, such a release would have to increase discharge frequency in epileptic neural tissue. Moreover, the enhanced release of glutamic acid was accompanied by the disappearance of glutamate in the tissue, proportional to the incidence and severity of the seizures (van Gelder and Courtois, 1972). The combined findings suggest that in some manner the usual detoxification of glutamate by conversion to glutamine has become deficient in such tissue (Sherwin and van Gelder, 1986).

In parallel to these studies, an eminent group of neurochemists investigated the metabolism of glutamic acid in the CNS; that work eventually led to the concept of a compartmentalized metabolism for glutamic acid. Such investigations, summarized by Berl (1965), clearly indicated that the metabolism of this excitatory amino acid was intimately related to glutamine synthesis in astrocytes. The evidence obtained over the past 20 years now must be considered sufficiently strong to state unequivocally that an excessive accumulation of extracellular glutamic acid is one of the hallmarks of epileptic neural tissue. Moreover, such accumulation can only be accounted for by postulating that the glial envelope surrounding neurons appears incapable of absorbing the larger quantities of glutamate released. Whether this is the only cause for the increase in free glutamic acid which can be detected or whether, *a priori*, the glial cells in epileptic tissue are metabolically different still remains an open question (Tursky *et al.*, 1976). The answer clearly has important bearing on the future development of new therapeutic agents (Meldrum, 1983).

There exist fairly consistent data for postulating a disruption in the transfer processes which metabolically link the neuron–nerve terminal complex to its surrounding glial cover (van Gelder *et al.*, 1983). Besides the appearance of extracellular glutamic acid as a major corollary to the onset of neuronal hyperexcitability, such accumulation is not unique to brain but is also found in CSF, plasma, and urine of certain groups of epileptic subjects (Gloor *et al.*, 1982). In at least three human studies and one involving beagle dogs genetically predisposed to epilepsy, either an increase as such of glutamic acid concentration was observed in the epileptic subjects and their relatives, or this amino acid constituted a larger percentage of the total free amino acid pool in the biological fluids (van Gelder, 1981). Since glutamic acid is a very important metabolite in a host of anabolic and energy reactions, its appearance in excess in such fluids must denote an important deficiency in tissue reserves of free glutamic acid (see van Gelder and Courtois, 1972). The findings furthermore indicate that this primary defect in tissue retention for glutamic acid is in part genetically determined, since relatives exhibiting no seizures but demonstrating a lowered convulsive threshold exhibit the same high levels of glutamic acid in CSF and blood (references above). Nevertheless, the fact that epileptic tissue often also shows a loss of taurine and accumulates glycine, or amino acids related to it by either transport or metabolism, suggests as well that the retention defect is accompanied by a dissociation of neuronal–glial contiguity (Krespan *et al.*, 1982).

Taurine, like glutamic acid, is avidly taken up in glia, whereas the passage of glycine across the blood–brain barrier systems may require as a first step, uptake into the astrocytic processes which surround cerebral capillaries (see Patel and Hunt, 1985). Exogenous glutamic acid also causes neural tissue swelling (Pappius and Elliott, 1956), which itself could be a cause for a disruption of the tissue cytoarchitecture. Of course, neonatal brain damage (Drejer *et al.*, 1985; Mathewson and Berry, 1985), genetic or hormonal influences (Léjohn *et al.*, 1969; Gadeleta *et al.*, 1985), the neonatal damage of malnutrition and environmental deprivation (Ramirez *et al.*, 1983; Thoemke and Huether, 1984) might produce a similar effect, in which case the accumulation of glutamic acid beyond normal levels would represent a consequent rather than a primary metabolic disturbance.

In this context, the possible participation of catecholamines in the epileptic process also merits further considerations (Chauvel *et al.*, 1982). Throughout life these amines reflect the nutritional, metabolic, and hormonal status of an individual (Lee and Dubois, 1972). In recent years, their role as neural tissue modulators has become increasingly evident. They are implicated in the regulation of energy metabolism and, thus, in the metabolism of amino acids whose carbon skeletons derive from glucose, including glutamic acid, GABA, aspartic acid, and glutamine (Nicklas *et al.*, 1975; Ando and Nagata, 1986). A decrease in catecholamines has been observed to lower the seizure threshold (Maynert *et al.*, 1975; Papanicolaou *et al.*, 1982). In addition, certain changes in epileptic tissue concerning adrenoceptors or enzyme activities, also suggest an altered functioning of the catecholamines in such tissue (Sherwin *et al.*, 1984; Brière *et al.*, 1986). A study by Reader and Jasper (1984) reveals a strong influence of the catecholamines on the action of other transmitter substances. Moreover, the fact that these amines are released from varicosities which do not always form classical synaptic contacts with other neuronal structures must imply that, upon release, the catecholamines probably affect equally the neuronal as well as the glial metabolism (Beaudet and Descarries, 1984).

In a number of aspects these neuromodulators therefore seem to represent a continuous but varying influence on cerebral excitability and metabolism. Whether this modulation at one instance causes reinforced inhibition via GABA-mediated effects, or in another instance imposes an alteration of glutamic acid release and uptake, or energy metabolism, Ca^{2+} redistribution, phosphokinase activities, to mention only a few other mechanisms, it leaves little doubt regarding the impact catecholamines have on the overall function of the CNS. To what extent they assume importance in the specific causes of epilepsy seems to warrant further investigations (Sherwin and van Gelder, 1986). It would appear, however, in view of the strong evidence for a direct implication of GABA and glutamic acid in the epileptic process, that the aromatic amines possibly exert a more indirect action, via their effect on the metabolism of these two amino acids.

2.3. Epilepsy: Loss of Inhibition, Excessive Excitation

As opposed to experimental seizure models, in spontaneous epilepsy interictal states usually predominate. During these seizure-free periods, the EEG nevertheless still suggests that in one or more brain regions neuronal discharges tend to be synchronized. Metabolically such areas or foci exhibit a somewhat depressed glucose metabolism (Phelps and Mazziotta, 1985). Intermittently, these regions of hypersynchrony become the locus for neurons firing at unusually high frequencies. The discharges then form the trigger for whole assemblies of neurons to exhibit seizure activity which may spread in "nearest neighbor" fashion and/or may be propagated via established anatomical pathways (Sloan and Jasper, 1950; Ward, 1972).

Ideally, antiseizure management should consist of suppressing synchronous activity since without this tendency, the high-frequency discharges in a few isolated neurons do not reach critical mass distribution (Jasper, 1961). Yet, to date, most anticonvulsant therapy seems aimed at suppressing the increased neuronal excitability, no doubt because a circumscribed region of abnormal EEG activity denoting synchrony, without the occurrence of seizures, often does not give rise to clinical complaints (Cloninger *et al.*, 1982).

The somewhat decreased glucose metabolism of an interictal focus seems to suggest that, if anything, the neurons in this state fire at low frequencies, or at an endogenous fluctuating frequency which demands less energy. The synchronized assembly may either contain fewer discharging elements or within such regions the firing frequency of many cells is depressed. Traumatized epileptic regions often do indeed demonstrate a loss of GABA-containing structures (Ribak *et al.*, 1982). This does not, however, explain the enhanced synchrony since systemic convulsants, including some GABA mimetics, create a hypersynchronous condition prior to seizure activity when GABA levels are still unchanged or even increased (van Gelder *et al.*, 1983). The most consistent and earliest signs of chemical change during the preseizure period appear to be the loss of tissue glutamic acid and a redistribution or decrease of taurine (Allen *et al.*, 1986).

While the electrophysiological inhibitory function of taurine in the CNS is still very vague (Fariello *et al.*, 1982), the role of glutamate as a probable regional modulator of excitation is becoming increasingly evident (though not necessarily accepted). Aside from the fact that a release of glutamic acid is needed to generate the precursor for GABA synthesis (see van Gelder, 1978), the phenomenon may be important in regulating glutamate receptor numbers and binding parameters (Kato *et al.*, 1984; Ramirez *et al.*, 1983). It may in addition provide the basis for nonanatomical contact within cell groups which interact as functional assemblies (van Gelder, 1981). The persistent, enhanced release of glutamic acid in epileptic tissue can account for both increased regional synchronicity and also the rise in GABA levels during an approaching seizure episode. As glutamine increases due to enhanced transport of glutamic acid into astrocytes, more glutamine becomes available for GABA synthesis. If increased levels of GABA in nerve terminals are translated into an enhanced stimulated release, this may nonetheless cause failure of inhibition. By local redistribution into astrocytes, the Cl⁻ equilibrium becomes altered, which may lead to desensitization of GABA receptors (Madtes, 1984), disturbances in the Cl^-/HCO_3^- exchange controlled by carbonic anhydrase (Takano *et al.*, 1984), and swelling of glial elements due, simply, to osmotically driven water entrance as a consequence of GABA, Na^+ uptake (Erecinska *et al.*, 1986).

Both the extracellular glutamic acid accumulation (see Nadler *et al.*, 1985), and the subsequent effects of enhanced GABA release can be prevented by improving interstitial washout conditions, which in a scarred area especially, must be impeded. If, on the other hand, GABA release is not increased or even diminished, one can envisage that any condition which increases excitatory input to a cell assembly already affected by enhanced extracellular glutamic acid accumulation and threatening failure of GABA inhibition, will reinforce a chemical milieu leading to seizures. Thus, in order to effect truly adequate epilepsy management, it may be necessary to consider measures which concentrate less on electrophysiological symptomatology but, instead, are aimed at modifying the metabolic environment. This quite likely entails intervention with conditions which slowly develop during interictal periods, to prevent a critical accumulation of glutamic acid, and to reinforce glial energy and glutamine metabolism. Unfortunately, such therapy cannot be based on simplistic notions of inhibiting glutamic acid synthesis or diminishing its depolarizing action, since such measures would not be directed exclusively at epileptic epicenters.

The metabolic defects of epilepsy so far discovered, for the most part appear to represent merely subtle modifications of neurochemical processes normally required to maintain proper brain function. For that reason, attenuation of epileptic processes may require equally subtle intervention, needing a long trial period. Certain novel dietetic modifications do offer hope, however, of being directed primarily to corrections of the metabolic disturbances without much affecting normal brain metabolism. These methods are mostly intended to restore glial neurochemistry, as neuronal damage or losses are not likely in the near future to be susceptible to any restorative manipulation.

In conclusion, examination of existing neurochemical data on epilepsy which now span well over three decades, suggests that neither total loss of (GABA) inhibition nor pure increased excitation can explain the events leading to a chronic condition of intermittent seizure activity. On the contrary, rather than indicating a specific failure of one type of cell structure in an epileptic cell assembly, the information directs attention to a possible failure of metabolic interaction between elements of the synaptic complex, including its glial envelope. Certain new palliative measures can be contemplated which for practical and biological reasons are mostly aimed at modifying glial biochemistry.

It is a testimony to Jasper's scientific abilities and skills in a variety of investigative techniques that many of the key data were provided by investigations carried out during his long career in epilepsy research. I thank the organizers of the Symposium for inviting me to participate in paying tribute to him. It indeed has been my pleasure.

References

Akimoto, H., 1982, Epilepsy—East and West, in: *Advances in Epileptology: XIIIth Epilepsy International Symposium* (H. Akimoto, H. Kazamatsuri, M. Seino, and A. Ward, eds.), pp. 1–8.

Allen, I. C., Grieve, A., and Griffiths, R., 1986, Differential changes in the content of amino acid neurotransmitters in discrete regions of the rat brain prior to the onset and during the course of homocysteine-induced seizures, *J. Neurochem.* **46**:1582–1592.

Ando, M., and Nagata, Y., 1986, Stimulation of amino acid uptake and Na^+,K^+-ATPase activity by norepinephrine in superior cervical sympathetic ganglia excised from adult rat, *J. Neurochem.* **46**:1487–1492.

Beaudet, A., and Descarries, L., 1984, Fine structure of monoamine axon terminals in cerebral cortex, in: *Monoamine Innervation of Cerebral Cortex* (L. Descarries, T. A. Reader, and H. H. Jasper, eds.), Liss, New York, pp. 77–93.

Berger, H., 1933, Uber das Elektrenkephalogramm des Menschen, *Arch. Psychiatr.* **100:**301.

Berl, S., 1965, Compartmentation of glutamic acid metabolism in developing cerebral cortex, *J. Biol. Chem.* **240:**2047–2054.

Berl, S., Takagaki, G., and Purpura, D. P., 1961, Metabolic and pharmacological effects of injected amino acids and ammonia on cortical epileptogenic lesions, *J. Neurochem.* **7:**198–209.

Brière, R., Sherwin, A. L., Robitaille, Y., Olivier, A., Quesney, L. F., and Reader, T. A., 1986, Alpha-1 adrenoceptors are decreased in human epileptic foci, *Anal. Neurol.* **19:**26–30.

Chapman, A. G., Meldrum, B. S., and Siesjö, B. K., 1977, Cerebral metabolic changes during prolonged epileptic seizures in rats, *J. Neurochem.* **28:**1025–1035.

Chauvel, P., Trottier, S., Nassif, S., and Dedek, J., 1982, Une altération des afférences noradrénergiques est-elle en cause dans les épilepsies focales? *Rev. Electroencephalogr. Neurophysiol. Clin.* **12:**1–7.

Cloninger, C. R., Rice, J., Reich, T., and McGuffin, P., 1982, Genetic analysis of seizure disorders as multidimensional threshold characters, in: *Genetic Basis of the Epilepsies* (V. E. Anderson, W. A. Hauser, J. K. Penry, and C. F. Sing, eds.), Raven Press, New York, pp. 291–309.

Drejer, J., Benveniste, H., Diemer, N. H., and Schousboe, A., 1985, Cellular origin of ischemia-induced glutamate release from brain tissue in vivo and in vitro, *J. Neurochem.* **45:**145–151.

Dodd, P. R., Bradford, H. F., Abdul-Ghani, A. S., Cox. D. W. G., and Continho-Netto, J., 1980, Release of amino acids from chronic epileptic and subepileptic foci in vivo, *Brain Res.* **193:**505–517.

Elliott, K. A. C., 1965, Gamma-aminobutyric acid and other inhibitory substances, *Br. Med. Bull.* **21:**70–75.

Elliott, K. A. C., and Jasper, H. H., 1959, Gamma-aminobutyric acid, *Physiol. Rev.* **39:**383–406.

Erecinska, M., Troeger, M. B., and Alston, T. A., 1986, Amino acid neurotransmitters in the CNS: Properties of diaminobutyric acid transport, *J. Neurochem.* **46:**1452–1457.

Fariello, R. G., Golden, G. T., and Pisa, M., 1982, Homotaurine (3 aminopropanesulfonic acid; 3 APS) protects from the convulsant and cytotoxic effect of systemically administered kainic acid, *Neurology* **32:**241–245.

Fromm, G. H., Terrence, C. F., and Chattha, A. S., 1985, Differential effect of antiepileptic and non-epileptic drugs on the reticular formation, *Lfe. Sci.* **35:**2665–2673.

Gadeleta, M. N., Renis, M., Minervini, G. R., Serra, I., Bleve, T., Giovine, A., Zacheo, G., and Giuffrida, A. M., 1985, Effect of hypothyroidism on the biogenesis of free mitochondria in the cerebral hemispheres and in cerebellum of rat during development, *Neurochem. Res.* **10:**163–177.

Gloor, P., Metrakos, J., Metrakos, K., Andermann, E., and van Gelder, N. M., 1982, Neurophysiological, genetic and biochemical nature of the epileptic diathesis, in: *Henri Gastaut and the Marseilles School's Contribution to the Neurosciences,* EEG Suppl. No. 35 (R. J. Broughton, ed.), Elsevier, Amsterdam, pp. 45–46.

Hansen, B., 1986, The complementarity of science and magic before the scientific revolution, *Am. Sci.* **74:**128–136.

Iwama, K., and Jasper, H. H., 1957, The action of gamma aminobutyric acid upon cortical electrical activity in the cat, *J. Physiol. (London)* **138:**365–380.

Jasper, H. H., 1961, General summary of "Basic Mechanisms of the Epileptic Discharge," *Epilepsia* **2:**91–99.

Jasper, H. H., 1965, Pathophysiological studies of brain mechanisms in different states of consciousness, in: *Brain and Conscious Experience* (J. E. Eccles, ed.), Springer-Verlag, Berlin, pp. 256–282.

Jasper, H. H., 1969, Mechanisms of propagation: Extracellular studies, in: *Basic Mechanisms of the Epilepsies* (H. H. Jasper, A. A. Ward, and A. Pope, eds.), Little, Brown, Boston, pp. 421–438.

Jasper, H. H., 1975, Philosophy or physics—Mind or molecules, in: *The Neurosciences: Paths of Discovery* (F. G. Worden, J. P. Swazey, and G. Adelman, eds.), MIT Press, Cambridge, Mass., pp. 403–422.

Jasper, H. H., and Carmichael, L., 1935, Electrical potentials from the intact human brain. *Science* **89:**51–53.

Jasper, H. H., Khan, R. T., and Elliott, K. A. C., 1965, Amino acids released from the cerebral cortex in relation to its state of activation, *Science* **147:**1448–1449.

Kato, S., Higashida, H., Higuchi, Y., Hatabenaka, S., and Negishi, K., 1984, Sensitive and insensitive states of cultured glioma cells to glutamate damage, *Brain Res.* **303:**365–373.

Koyama, I., and Jasper, H. H., 1977, Amino acid content of chronic undercut cortex of the cat in relation to electrical after discharge: Comparison with cobalt epileptogenic lesions, *Can. J. Physiol. Pharmacol.* **55:**523–536.

Kravitz, E. A., Potter, D. D., and van Gelder, N. M., 1962, Gamma-aminobutyric acid distribution in the lobster nervous system: CNS, peripheral nerves and isolated motor and inhibitory axons, *Biochem. Biophys. Res. Commun.* **7:**231–236.

Krespan, B., Berl, S., and Nicklas, W. J., 1982, Alteration in neuronal–glial metabolism of glutamate by the neurotoxin kainic acid, *J. Neurochem.* **38:**509–518.

Kuffler, S. W., and Edwards, C., 1958, Mechanism of gamma aminobutyric acid (GABA) action and its relation to synaptic inhibition, *J. Neurophysiol.* **21**:586–616.

Lee, C. J., and Dubois, R., 1972, Effects of neonatal infection, perinatal malnutrition, and crowding on catecholamine metabolism, *J. Exp. Med.* **136**:1031–1042.

Léjohn, H. B., Jackson, S. G., Klassen. G. R., and Sawula, R. V., 1969, Regulation of mitochondrial glutamic dehydrogenase by divalent metals, nucleotides, and alpha-ketoglutarate, *J. Biol. Chem.* **244**:5346–5356.

Madtes, P., 1984, Chloride ions preferentially mask high-affinity GABA binding sites, *J. Neurochem.* **43**:1434–1437.

Mathewson, A. J., and Berry, M., 1985, Observations on the astrocyte response to cerebral stab wound in adult rat, *Brain Res.* **327**:61–69.

Maynert, E. W., Marczynski, T. J., and Browning, R. A., 1975, The role of neurotransmitters in the epilepsies, *Adv. Neurol.* **13**:79–147.

Meldrum, B. S., 1983, Pharmacological considerations in the search for new anticonvulsant drugs, in: *Recent Advances in Epilepsy* (T. A. Pedley and B. S. Meldrum, eds.), Churchill Livingstone, Edinburgh, pp. 75–92.

Melville, I. D., 1974, The medical treatment of epilepsy: A historical review, in: *Historical Aspects of the Neurosciences* (F. C. Rose and W. F. Byrum, eds.), Raven Press, New York, pp. 127–136.

Nadler, J. V., Wang, A., and Werling, L. L., 1985, Binding sites for L-[³H]glutamate on hippocampal synaptic membranes: Three populations differentially affected by chloride and calcium ions, *J. Neurochem.* **44**:1791–1798.

Nicklas, W. J., Berl, S., and Clarke, D. D., 1975, Relationship between amino acid and catecholamine metabolism in brain, in: *Metabolic Compartmentation and Neurotransmission: Relation to Brain Structure and Function* (S. Berl, D. D. Clark, and D. Schneider, eds.), Plenum Press, New York, pp. 497–513.

Papanicolaou, J., Sumers, R. J., Vajda, F. J. E., and Louis, W. J., 1982, The relationship between alpha-2 adrenoceptor selectivity and anticonvulsant effect in a series of clonidine-like drugs, *Brain Res.* **241**:393–397.

Pappius, H. M., and Elliott, K. A. C., 1956, Water distribution in incubated slices of brain and other tissue, *Can. J. Physiol. Pharmacol.* **34**:1007–1022.

Patel, A. J., and Hunt, A., 1985, Concentration of free amino acids in primary cultures of neurons and astrocytes, *J. Neurochem.* **44**:1816–1821.

Penfield, W., 1975, *The Mystery of the Mind,* Princeton University Press, Princeton, N.J., pp. 1–123.

Phelps, M. E., and Mazziotta, J. C., 1985. Positron emission tomography: Human brain function and biochemistry, *Science* **228**:799–809.

Putnam, I. J., and Merritt, H. H., 1937, Experimental determination of anticonvulsant properties of some phenyl derivatives, *Science* **85**:525.

Ramirez, G., Barat, A., Gomez-Barriocanal, J., Manrique, E., and Batuecas, A., 1983, Development of specific binding sites for [³H]kainic acid and [³H]mucimol in the chick optic tectum: Modulation by early changes in visual input, in: *CNS Receptors—From Molecular Pharmacology to Behavior* (P. Mandel and F. V. DeFeudis, eds.), Raven Press, New York, pp. 187–198.

Reader, T. A., and Jasper, H. H., 1984, Interactions between monoamines and other transmitters in cerebral cortex, in: *Monoamine Innervation of Cerebral Cortex* (L. Descarries, T. A. Reader, and H. H. Jasper, eds.), Liss, New York, pp. 195–225.

Ribak, C. E., Bradburne, R. M., and Harris, A. B., 1982, A preferential loss of GABAergic, symmetric synapses in epileptic foci: A quantitative ultrastructural analysis of monkey neocortex, *J. Neurol. Sci.* **2**:1725–1735.

Roberts, E., Rothstein, M., and Baxter, C. F., 1958, Some metabolic studies of gamma-aminobutyric acid, *Proc. Soc. Exp. Biol. Med.* **97**:796–802.

Schwartzkroin, P. A., 1983, Local circuit considerations and intrinsic neuronal properties involved in hyperexcitability and cell synchronization, in: *Basic Mechanisms of Neuronal Hyperexcitability* (H. H. Jasper and N. M. van Gelder, eds.), Liss, New York, pp. 75–108.

Sherwin, A. L., and van Gelder, N. M., 1986, Amino acid and catecholamine markers of metabolic abnormalities in human focal epilepsy, in: *Basic Mechanisms of the Epilepsies* (A. V. Delgado-Escueta, A. A. Ward, D. M. Woodbury, and A. J. Porter, eds.), Raven Press, New York, pp. 1011–1033.

Sherwin, A., Quesney, F., Gauthier, S., Olivier, A., Robitaille, Y., McQuaid, P., Harvey, C., and van Gelder, N. M., 1984, Enzyme changes in actively spiking areas of human epileptic cerebral cortex, *Neurology* **34**:927–933.

Sloan, N., and Jasper, H. H., 1950, The identity of spreading depression and "suppression," *Electroencephalogr. Clin. Neurophysiol.* **2**:59–78.

Takano, T., Kancko, Y., Kumashiro, H., Sugai, N., and Oosaki, T., 1984, Kainate seizure and carbonic anhydrase (CAH) reaction in the hippocampal structures, *Neuroscience* **10**:309–312.

Temkin, O. (ed.), 1971, *The Falling Sickness,* Johns Hopkins Press, Baltimore, pp. 3–65.

Thoemke, F., and Huether, G., 1984, Breeding rats on amino acid imbalanced diets for three consecutive generations affects the concentrations of putative amino acid transmitters in developing brain, *Int. J. Dev. Neurosci.*
2:567–574.

Tower, D. B., 1957, Glutamic acid and gamma-aminobutyric acid in seizures, *Clin. Chim. Acta* **2:**397–402.

Tursky, T., Lassanova, M., Sramka, M., and Nadvornik, P., 1976, Formation of glutamate and GABA in
epileptogenic tissue from human hippocampus in vitro, *Acta Neurochir. Suppl.* **23:**111–118.

van Gelder, N. M., 1981, The role of taurine and glutamic acid in the epileptic process: A genetic predisposition,
Rev. Pure Appl. Pharmacol. Sci. **2:**293–316.

van Gelder, N. M., 1978, Taurine, the compartmentalized metabolism of glutamic acid, and the epilepsies, *Can. J.
Physiol. Pharm.* **56:**362–374.

van Gelder, N. M., and Courtois, A., 1972, Close correlation between changing content of specific amino acids in
epileptic cortex of cats, and severity of epilepsy, *Brain Res.* **43:**477–484.

van Gelder, N. M., Siatitsas, I., Menini, C., and Gloor, P., 1983, Feline generalized penicillin epilepsy: Changes
of glutamic acid and taurine parallel the progressive increase in excitability of the cortex, *Epilepsia* **24:**200–
213.

Ward, A. A., 1972, Mechanisms of neuronal hyperexcitability, *Electroencephalogr. Clin. Neurophysiol. Suppl.*
31:75–86.

Woodbury, D. M., and Esplin, D. W., 1959, Neuropharmacology and neurochemistry of anticonvulsant drugs, in:
The Effect of Pharmacological Agents on the Nervous System (F. J. Braceland, ed.), Williams & Wilkins,
Baltimore, pp. 24–56.

3

Functional Organization of Glutamatergic Synapses

E. Puil and A. M. Benjamin

1. Introduction

For more than 50 years, S-glutamate* has generated specialized interests within the wide domain of the neurological sciences. In 1932, biochemists drew attention to this "nonessential" amino acid by suggesting its importance in cerebral metabolism (Quastel and Wheatley, 1932). In the ensuing years, the neurochemical importance of glutamate was traced mainly to several metabolic processes: (1) oxidative deamination to α-oxoglutarate, (2) transamination to S-aspartate, (3) incorporation into peptides and proteins, (4) amidation to glutamine, and especially, (5) decarboxylation to GABA. Inevitably, glutamate therapy was initiated by practising neurologists for patients with muscular dystrophy (Tripoli and Beard, 1934), corticoreticular epilepsy of the petit mal type, or complex partial seizures (Price *et al.*, 1943), and even recently, for patients with Huntington's disease (Barr *et al.*, 1978). The reports of increased alertness as a side effect in humans and of better maze learning in rats after glutamate administration (Zimmerman and Ross, 1944), also could not be ignored, and glutamate was used in the treatment of mental retardation with brief popularity (Zimmerman *et al.*, 1946). Physiologists and pharmacologists became seriously interested after 1954 when Hayashi had demonstrated that clonic convulsions were evoked in dogs in which Na^+-glutamate was applied directly to the brain surface (see review by Puil, 1981). In 1963, Krnjević and Phillis observed the quick and powerful excitatory effects of glutamate upon its microiontophoretic application to cerebral cortical neurons and suggested that glutamate could be a major excitatory transmitter. This hypothesis was questioned by previous and subsequent workers because of demonstrable actions of glutamate on virtually all neurons, as well as by its universal presence in the CNS (see Puil, 1981). In 1969, Herbert Jasper and Ikuko Koyama indeed had demonstrated the release of glutamate from the surface of the brain during cortical activation by stimulation of the midbrain reticular formation (Jasper and Koyama, 1969). The elusive transmitter role and certain difficulties in interpreting the voltage responses of

*Here, the S-chirality is identical to that of the L-isomer. S-glutamic acid with its three functional groups is ionized at physiological pH and will be referred to simply as glutamate in this chapter.

E. Puil and A. M. Benjamin • Department of Pharmacology and Therapeutics, Faculty of Medicine, The University of British Columbia, Vancouver, British Columbia V6T 1W5, Canada.

neurons to glutamate in studies with microelectrodes during the 1970s did not deter the neuroanatomists who were able to map out specific glutamatergic pathways in the brain. Similarly, the demonstrations of "recycling mechanisms" (Benjamin and Quastel, 1972), and of excessive release of glutamate in certain pathological conditions such as epilepsy, as well as implications of a role in other degenerative disorders (e.g., ammonia detoxification in hepatic coma, olivopontocerebellar disease), have provided impetus for further studies of glutamate as a major putative transmitter in the vertebrate CNS. Hence, an understanding of glutamatergic transmission could yield insight into more complex aspects of brain function (e.g., long-term potentiation, memory) and further the development of therapeutic agents for neurological disorders.

To guide future investigations, the relationships between the known biochemical functions of glutamate and its putative transmitter role should be clarified. To this end, this review summarizes (1) how the glutamate molecule is synthesized and released from nerve terminals into the synaptic cleft, (2) postsynaptic actions of glutamate, (3) subsequent inactivation by uptake, (4) conversion of glutamate to glutamine by the surrounding glia, and (5) the return of glutamine to glutamatergic neurons.

2. Formation and Release

2.1. Glutamate-Forming Processes in the Brain

Glucose is ultimately the principal source of the carbon skeleton of cerebral glutamate. Its catabolism via the glycolytic pathway yields pyruvate which forms α-oxoglutarate within the citric acid cycle. The nitrogen atom appears in the glutamate molecule following ammonia fixation to α-oxoglutarate by a reductive amination process involving glutamate dehydrogenase and its cofactor, NAD(P)H. Glutamate is formed also from α-oxoglutarate and amino acids, particularly aspartate, by specific pyridoxal-requiring α-aminotransferases, from ornithine and α-oxoglutarate by ornithine δ-aminotransferase, from GSH-derived 5-oxoproline by 5-oxoprolinase, and most importantly, from glutamine by action of phosphate-activated glutaminase.

2.2. Synthesis and Concentrations in Nerve Terminals

Although glutamate is present in the brain in high concentrations ($\sim$ 11–12 μmole/g wet wt in rat brain or $\sim$ 115 nmole/mg protein), only a portion of this comprises the transmitter pool. Isolated nerve terminals (synaptosomes) contain only about half the glutamate concentration ($\sim$ 55 nmole/mg protein) of intact brain tissue (Benjamin and Quastel, 1975). However, the level in the glutamatergic terminal actually could be quite high because a synaptosomal preparation is a heterogeneous collection of nerve endings and additionally some loss of glutamate may occur during the preparation procedure.

In any case, glutamate can be formed rapidly from glutamine in incubating synaptosomes which apparently use this amino acid as a major substrate (Bradford et al., 1978). The organelles themselves do not synthesize glutamine from glucose or glutamate, but obtain their supply from extraneuronal sources. Glutamine is plentiful extracellularly ($\sim$ 0.5 mM) and enters nerve terminals by a low-affinity uptake system (K_m = 0.25 mM; see Benjamin et al., 1980). The extracellular pool of glutamine may be replenished periodically from an intracellular pool which is at least ten times larger (brain glutamine, $\sim$ 5 mM). It is quite likely that glia serve partly as reservoirs for neuronal glutamate because the major pool of glutamine and loci of synthesis are in glia (see Benjamin, 1983).

Glutamine entering the nerve terminals is hydrolyzed by phosphate-activated glutaminase. This enzyme has an external orientation within the inner mitochondrial membrane (Kvamme, 1983) such that synthesized glutamate is easily accessible to the synaptoplasm.

Glutamate also may be formed in synaptosomes from glucose or from α-oxoglutarate by transamination or reductive amination processes, but much less rapidly than from glutamine (see Shank and Campbell, 1983). This cannot be due to a paucity of ammonia in the system because synaptosomes readily liberate ammonia during incubation (Benjamin and Quastel, 1975). Investigations on brain slices and synaptosomes (Hamberger *et al.*, 1979a,b; Bradford *et al.*, 1978) have shown that the evoked release of glutamate derived from glutamine is four times greater than that derived from glucose. However, it is not certain if glutamine is better than glucose as a precursor of glutamate *in vivo* (see Bradford *et al.*, 1983). It is clear that the synthesis of glutamate from ornithine metabolism occurs much too slowly in synaptosomes to be of major importance (see Shank and Campbell, 1983).

2.3. Location within Nerve Terminals

An important question is whether or not synaptoplasmic glutamate is packaged into vesicles before it is released into the synaptic cleft. Early investigations demonstrated that isolated synaptic vesicles are not enriched in glutamate when compared with other subcellular fractions (Magnam and Whittaker, 1966; Rassin, 1972) nor do they take up the amino acid avidly (De Belleroche and Bradford, 1973; Rassin, 1972). These observations led to the proposal that glutamate may be released directly from the synaptoplasm (De Belleroche and Bradford, 1977). Recently, however, synaptic vesicles have been shown to accumulate glutamate if ATP is present (Naito and Ueda, 1983), which is consistent with the immunocytochemical elucidation of the amino acid in synaptic vesicles (Storm-Mathisen *et al.*, 1983). These findings imply that some tissue glutamate may be packaged into specific synaptic vesicles for release by an exocytotic process (Naito and Ueda, 1985).

2.4. Release from Nerve Terminals

Regardless of its source or location within the nerve terminals, the stimulus-evoked release of glutamate at synapses is highly dependent on external Ca^{2+}; this contrasts with the release of glutamate from glia which is apparently Ca^{2+} independent (De Belleroche and Bradford, 1972; Blaustein, 1975; Potashner, 1978). High extracellular $[K^+]$ enhances the influx of $^{22}Na^+$ and $^{45}Ca^{2+}$ into synaptosomes (Goddard and Robinson, 1976). The increased synaptoplasmic Ca^{2+} appears to be a prerequisite for transmitter release because a high external $[Mg^{2+}]$ blocks the Ca^{2+}-mediated, stimulus-coupled release of glutamate (see Potashner, 1978).

Since glutamate is a feedback inhibitor of glutaminase, a diminution of its concentration following release would result in activation of the enzyme and the formation of more glutamate (Benjamin, 1981). This would necessitate an enhanced inflow of precursor glutamine which apparently occurs following Ca^{2+}-dependent, K^+-evoked release of glutamate that is newly synthesized from glutamine (Hamberger *et al.*, 1979b).

Glutamate released from the nerve terminals diffuses across the synaptic cleft to postsynaptic sites of action. A release from glutamatergic terminals onto other nerve impingements has yet to be described, although there are some indications for presynaptic actions of glutamate (see Puil, 1981).

3. Postsynaptic Actions

3.1. Interactions with Receptors

The physiological effects of glutamate are the result of its interaction with chemical groups (receptors) on the external surface of neurons. Despite a high cytosolic concentration, glutamate does not appear to be involved directly in an internal regulation of neuronal excitability because intracellular injections of glutamate produce no response (Coombs *et al.*, 1955). Receptors for glutamate are widely distributed over the perikaryon and its dendrites. Although the nerve terminal membranes of primary afferent neurons and of cultured spinal neurons presumably have such receptors, very large applications of the amino acid to nerve axons do not produce responses during their intraaxonal recording (see Puil, 1983). Similarly, perfusion with high concentrations (10^{-2} M) of glutamate in isolated craniospinal ganglia does not affect neuronal excitability (see Puil, 1981). However, virtually all neurons within the CNS possess receptors for glutamate as judged by their excitation upon local applications of the amino acid. A *single* receptor which might mediate this response has yet to be defined in pharmacological terms.

The existence of two or three receptor types for glutamate is inferred from the differential antagonism by selective antagonists, of the excitations elicited by N-methyl-R-aspartate, S-α-kainate, or S-quisqualate, as well as by other conformational analogues (see Puil, 1981, 1983). The characteristics of a given interaction of one of these agonists with its receptor are believed to result in particular changes in ionic conductance. The interactions of glutamate with at least two such receptors produce an excitation which presumably is the result of the ionic fluxes associated with these interactions. Therefore, the concept of specific antagonism of glutamate actions has come to rest heavily on the demonstrations that the neuronal excitation caused by glutamate is partly blocked by antagonists of the actions of either N-methylaspartate, kainate, or quisqualate in a particular range of doses which do not affect the responses to one or two of the other agonists. The clearest distinction between the presumed receptor classes has been achieved for N-methylaspartate responses which can be antagonized selectively by 2-amino-5-phosphonovalerate and other conformational analogues, and reduced by Mg^{2+}. The order of potency of such blockers for antagonizing the responses of neurons to N-methylaspartate, glutamate, or other excitatory amino acids suggests the existence of a distinct receptor subtype for N-methylaspartate which also can be activated by glutamate. Since glutamate, N-methylaspartate, kainate, and quisqualate responses can be antagonized to varying degrees by γ-R-glutamylglycine, the possibility of another receptor subtype has been invoked to explain the actions of glutamate on neurons. The existence of a second type of receptor which selectively mediates quisqualate excitation is considered by some investigators to be less certain than one for kainate excitation (see Mayer and Westbrook, 1984). Unlike the actions of agonists at the kainate or quisqualate receptors, the responses attributable to actions at the N-methylaspartate receptor show a strong dependence on membrane voltage. This contingency, which appears to be a function of the extracellular $[Mg^{2+}]$, does not allow straightforward interpretations of the conductance changes subsequent to glutamate interactions with N-methylaspartate receptors and with the nearly voltage-independent receptor–ionophore complexes for kainate or quisqualate. The difficulties in interpreting the pharmacology of these three receptor classes for glutamate have been reviewed extensively and the various conductance changes (states) induced by an agonist may be attributed to actions at a single type of receptor, depending on the agonist's conformational presentation (Puil, 1981).

3.2. Effects on Neuronal Excitability and Membrane Properties

The characteristic effects of glutamate on neurons in the CNS are remarkable. The excitation leading to a brisk discharge has a fast onset and an almost equally prompt termination upon discontinuation of a microiontophoretic application. An outstanding feature of glutamate is its ability to act very transiently on postsynaptic receptors so as to provide a fast transfer of phasic information across synaptic gaps. The action has been considered unlike those of other excitatory amino acids because even with large applications, glutamate usually does not elicit burst discharges in most "normal" neurons of the CNS. However, epileptiform behavior can be evoked by direct application of Na^{+}-glutamate to the surface of the mammalian brain (Hayashi, 1959), or by systemic injection (Johnston, 1973). Also, there is a tendency for glutamate to produce regenerative burst responses in neurons under certain conditions (MacDonald and Wojtowicz, 1982; Nistri *et al.,* 1985; Connors, 1984).

Glutamate excitation is a direct consequence of the depolarization of the neuron to the threshold for voltage-dependent activation. Early investigations revealed an accompanying increase in membrane conductance (Krnjević and Schwartz, 1967; Martin *et al.,* 1970; Zieglgänsberger and Puil, 1973). The time course of this increase is similar to that of the concurrent depolarization. However, glutamate-induced depolarization often may be evoked with no accompanying change, or even with a decrease in membrane conductance (Engberg *et al.,* 1979; see Puil, 1981). In some cases, the glutamate-induced changes may be biphasic, i.e., an initial decrease in conductance slowly subsides and is replaced by an increase. The variability in the conductance changes depends partly on the dose applied and also may be attributed to several other factors: (1) indirect activation (or deactivation) of voltage-dependent conductances (e.g., time-dependent rectifying properties of the membrane), (2) differences in the degree of activation by glutamate of dendritic versus somatic areas of a neuron, (3) the extent of electrogenic uptake of glutamate by neurons, and (4) an involvement of a voltage-dependent process within the receptor-coupled ionophores which contributes to the net conductance change measured during glutamate action. The latter recently has been found to be a very important consideration.

3.3. Voltage-Dependence and Extracellular [Mg^{2+}]

A strong voltage-dependence of glutamate responses has been described (see Puil, 1981; Mayer and Westbrook, 1987). The nonlinear behavior is apparent in the relationship of membrane voltage to input current at various (displaced) levels of the resting membrane potential (MacDonald and Wojtowicz, 1982). Furthermore, recent investigations suggest that the glutamate-induced conductance changes represent a composite of both voltage-dependent and voltage-independent behavior of the ion channels activated by the interactions of glutamate at presumed receptors for *N*-methylaspartate, and for quisqualate or kainate, respectively (MacDonald and Wojtowicz, 1982). The voltage-dependent response to glutamate initially was attributed to the sensitivity of receptor-coupled conductance mechanisms involving ion channels that opened or closed in response to alterations in the membrane potential.

The reason for the voltage sensitivity has since become clear from voltage-clamp investigations on the pharmacology of receptors for glutamate and other amino acids, and from studies of single channels using the whole-cell patch clamp technique. In 1982, voltage-clamp studies of cultured spinal neurons (MacDonald *et al.,* 1982) revealed that application of S-aspartate (which is believed to act preferentially at *N*-methylaspartate receptors) induced a region of negative slope conductance in the steady-state current–voltage (I–V) relationships. The unusual electrical behavior also has been seen with administration of *N*-methylaspartate and to a lesser extent with glutamate, but not with kainate or quisqualate applications (Flatman *et al.,* 1986; Mayer and Westbrook, 1984, 1985). The ability of glutamate to evoke this nonlinear membrane behavior accounts for the variability in the membrane conductance changes which had been deduced from the observed voltage responses to glutamate applications in neurons of the CNS (Mayer and Westbrook, 1987). Pharmacological evidence suggests that such responses are a consequence of a "simultaneous activation" by glutamate of both *N*-methylaspartate and non-*N*-methylaspartate receptors (Mayer and Westbrook, 1984, 1985). For example, the I–V relationship of neurons under voltage-clamp conditions becomes more linear when the antagonist, 2-amino-5-phosphonovalerate, is added to the bathing medium, presumably because the voltage-sensitive component is eliminated after blockade of *N*-methylaspartate receptors. When this I–V curve is subtracted from the I–V relationship for glutamate action in the absence of the antagonist, a curve revealing the presence of a negative slope conductance remains (Mayer and Westbrook, 1984).

This property can account for the bistable behavior of the membrane potential and such data also may provide a basis for the tendency of glutamate to evoke epileptiform activity under certain conditions (see MacDonald and Schneiderman, 1984).

The glutamate-evoked membrane potential changes depend on the presence of extracellular Mg^{2+}. High concentrations (10 mM) can eliminate completely the voltage-sensitive component of glutamate effects (MacDonald and Wojtowicz, 1982). A remarkable susceptibility to blockade by Mg^{2+} has been observed in the excitatory responses to applications of N-methylaspartate, whereas the effects of kainate or quisqualate are much less affected by Mg^{2+} (see Puil, 1981). Removal of extracellular Mg^{2+} from the bathing solution prevents the emergence of the negative slope conductance following applications of N-methylaspartate and glutamate in voltage-clamped neurons, and the I–V relationships become much more linear (Mayer and Westbrook, 1985). As a consequence, the responses of neurons to these amino acids are potentiated by the absence of Mg^{2+}.

A link between the voltage sensitivity and the sensitivity to Mg^{2+} has been found in studies of glutamate action on single-channel currents (Nowak et al., 1984). Under Mg^{2+}-free conditions, glutamate and N-methylaspartate open cation channels which have no voltage-dependent properties. However, in the presence of physiological concentrations of Mg^{2+} and at certain negative membrane potentials, glutamate-induced single-channel currents consist of intermittent bursts and the probability of channel opening is reduced. Thus, by means of a voltage-dependent Mg^{2+} blockade, it would appear that Mg^{2+} confers a voltage sensitivity on glutamate-activated cation channels which are coupled to N-methylaspartate receptors. A removal of the voltage-dependent Mg^{2+} blockade occurs with depolarization accounting for the increased conductance at membrane potentials more positive than -30 mV. This antagonism by Mg^{2+} may be uncompetitive (Mayer and Westbrook, 1985), but cannot be attributable entirely to a fast mechanism for blocking open channels (Nowak et al., 1984). Indeed, the results of these investigations suggest that the antagonism may be noncompetitive with Mg^{2+} binding to an agonist (see Mg^{2+}-methylaspartate "cage" in Puil, 1981, p. 286) or close to the unselective cation channel, and to the agonist–receptor complex being favored by the open channel configuration.

3.4. Ionic Mechanisms

It has been suggested that the permeability changes elicited by glutamate may be preceded by the displacement of Ca^{2+} from membrane sites which are part of, or contiguous to, the types of receptors that control the specific conductances. Direct removal of Ca^{2+} from the membrane by the strong chelating action of glutamate is not very likely because much stronger chelators of Ca^{2+} are less effective neuronal excitants (see Puil, 1981). However, glutamate and other excitatory amino acids do release membrane-bound Ca^{2+} from synaptic membranes (Tan, 1975). Also, there appears to be little doubt that Ca^{2+} contributes to the cationic influx following glutamate activation of receptors particularly if these involve the N-methylaspartate class of receptors (MacDermott et al., 1986; Pumain and Heinemann, 1985; Bührle and Sonnhof, 1983). It has long been known that the addition of glutamate to brain slices in vitro causes both Ca^{2+} and Na^+ influx (Ames et al., 1967). Moreover, indirect pharmacological evidence suggests the involvement of Ca^{2+} in glutamate actions (see Nicoll and Alger, 1981; Puil, 1981). There are still uncertainties about the relative contributions of Ca^{2+} and Na^+, as well as other ions, to the generation of ionic currents underlying glutamate excitation.

Some of the reasons for these difficulties may be summarized as follows: (1) glutamate activation of ionic currents involves two conductance mechanisms; (2) interpretations of the effects of divalent cations, particularly Ca^{2+} channel blockers, are doubtful; (3) secondary activation by Ca^{2+} influx of K^+ and Cl^- currents may occur; (4) there is a possibility that internal $[Ca^{2+}]$ changes may occur during prolonged exposure of neurons to Na^+-free solutions, or to pharmacological concentrations of glutamate (see Discussion by Mayer and Westbrook,

1985); and (5) Ca^{2+} influx may influence other events, e.g., inhibit Ca^{2+} currents (MacDonald and Schneiderman, 1984) or monovalent cationic fluxes (MacDermott *et al.*, 1986).

An interesting feature of glutamate action which is evident from studies of the I–V relationships in voltage-clamped neurons, is that the voltage sensitivity disappears as the membrane potential approaches 0 mV, presumably as a result of removal of the Mg^{2+} blockade. In the absence of Mg^{2+} in voltage-clamped neurons, the reversal potential for the action of glutamate or for those of the other amino acids (e.g., *N*-methylaspartate) also is close to this value (see Mayer and Westbrook, 1985). Direct observations of the changes in ionic composition of the extracellular fluids using K^+-, Na^+-, Ca^{2+}-, and Cl^--sensitive microelectrodes indicate that glutamate evokes an increase in the Na^+ and Ca^{2+} permeability of motoneurons; these changes are counterbalanced by an outward shift of K^+ and an influx of Cl^- (Bührle and Sonnhof, 1983). Also, there have been no clear indications for a primary involvement of an altered Cl^- conductance in glutamate actions on neurons. Therefore, together with such data and other considerations, the reversal potential measured with voltage-clamp techniques suggests that glutamate depolarization may involve an increase in membrane permeability to Na^+ and/or Ca^{2+}. The ratio of the Ca^{2+}/Na^+ permeability changes linked to *N*-methylaspartate receptors appears to be much greater than those linked to kainate or quisqualate receptors. However, since the reversal potential for these amino acids is close to 0 mV, a membrane conductance change to K^+ or Cl^- is inferred. A positive shift in the reversal potential subsequent to removal of K^+ ions from the external medium also suggests that a change in K^+-conductance contributes to the magnitude and time course of the depolarizing action of glutamate (Puil, 1981).

The removal of external Na^+ ions results in a marked diminution of the depolarizing response to glutamate. This is evident from investigations of the effects of total (or partial) replacement of Na^+ in the bathing fluid by Li^+, choline$^+$, sucrose, or Tris$^+$. In such cases, the attenuated response is accompanied by a negative shift in the reversal potential which would be expected if Na^+ was the primary ion involved in glutamate-induced depolarization (Hablitz and Langmoen, 1982). Although complete agreement about the contributions of Ca^{2+} relative to those of Na^+ in the glutamate-induced depolarization has not been attained, the interaction of glutamate with its kainate or quisqualate receptor appears to trigger a primary increase in Na^+ ions, as suggested by the early biochemical studies (Puil, 1981).

The influx of Na^+ which occurs upon addition of glutamate to brain slices *in vitro* is not very effectively prevented by tetrodotoxin, a specific inactivator which acts at the external sites of Na^+ channels. This neurotoxin greatly reduces the electrical excitability but fails to block the depolarizing action of locally applied glutamate on motoneurons *in vivo* (Zieglgänsberger and Puil, 1972). This has led to the suggestion that the Na^+ channels activated by glutamate–receptor interaction are not the tetrodotoxin-sensitive and voltage-dependent Na^+ channels responsible for depolarizing inward rectification or for spike genesis. Both types of Na^+ channels appear to be vulnerable to intracellular applications of QX222, a local anesthetic agent which promotes Na^+ inactivation by interacting with the gating mechanism at the inner end of Na^+ channels (Puil and Carlen, 1984). Such data suggest that some properties of the two types of Na^+ channels may overlap, both being susceptible to blockade by internal QX222 which has strong voltage-dependent actions. The actions of QX222 are similar to those of local anesthetics on the responses to acetylcholine at vertebrate neuromuscular junctions. Indeed, a similarity also exists between the Mg^{2+}-induced modifications in glutamate-activated channel activity in neurons and the effects of local anesthetics on acetylcholine-induced currents at neuromuscular junctions.

Recent whole-cell patch-clamp investigations have revealed that glutamate activation of its receptor–ionophore complexes is accompanied by a use-dependent block of the activated channels (Vyklický *et al.*, 1986). *N*-Methyl-R-aspartate and quisqualate also induced responses that exhibited two components. Although kainate did not produce this two-component response, the results presented by the authors also may be interpreted as indicating that only an inductive type of receptor for glutamate may exist (see Puil, 1981). However, it may be that two types of glutamate-receptor channels are present in CNS neurons and that only one of these is sensitive to blockade by Mg^{2+} (Cull-Candy and Ogden, 1985; Ascher and Nowak, 1986). At micromolar concentrations of glutamate, Mg^{2+}-sensitive channels corresponding to those activated by N-methylaspartate are activated. In the absence of extracellular Mg^{2+}, these channels have linear I–V relationships with a slope of 50 pS. At concentrations approaching 10 μM, glutamate activates Mg^{2+}-insensitive channels with a single-channel conductance of approximately 8 pS; these correspond to those activated by quisqualate (Ascher and Nowak, 1986).

4. Inactivation and Recycling of Transmitter

Immediately following the binding of glutamate to a cell's receptors, inactivation processes come into play. An important postsynaptic event in the termination of glutamate excitation is the decay of excitatory ionic currents resulting from the closure of the relevant ionic (Na^+, Ca^{2+}) channels. Full inactivation of glutamate effects probably is contingent on its removal from the receptor vicinity and subsynaptic space by uptake processes allowing the ionic gradients across the membrane to be restored to the conditions of the resting state.

4.1. Uptake Processes

Synaptosomes (Logan and Snyder, 1972), bulk-isolated glia (Henn et al., 1974), and cultured astrocytes (see Hertz et al., 1983) transport glutamate by high-affinity ($K_m \sim 20$ μM) and low-affinity ($K_m > 0.1$ mM) Na^+-dependent processes. Autoradiographic studies have shown that radioactive glutamate taken up by brain tissue enters glia preferentially (see Roberts et al., 1981). Also, lesioning studies of known glutamatergic pathways have revealed a diminished uptake of glutamate by the high-affinity process into isolated nerve terminals. Conceivably, a part of the glutamate released into the synaptic cleft will be recycled following uptake into the nerve terminals (see Fonnum, 1984); the portion of glutamate diffusing out of the cleft will be sequestered by uptake into surrounding glia.

Initially, some investigators argued that high-affinity uptake systems do not effectively reduce the extracellular transmitter concentration since the apparent avid uptake of labeled transmitter may be due to homo-exchange with a larger pool of unlabeled transmitter. However, the present consensus of opinion is that net uptake of transmitter does occur and, therefore, that high-affinity uptake is a major mechanism for transmitter inactivation.

It should be noted that absence of a high-affinity uptake system does not preclude a molecule from having an excitatory action. For example, R-glutamate, which excites cerebral cortical neurons (Krnjević and Phillis, 1963), is transported only by low-affinity uptake systems (Benjamin and Quastel, 1976). These results suggest that the sites for the high-affinity carrier and the glutamate receptors in the postsynaptic neuron are not the same. It is known also that neuronal excitation evoked by application of R-glutamate is very similar to that elicited by its S-isomer (see Puil, 1981). These data imply that high-affinity uptake processes are not necessary for excitatory transmission. In contrast, the low-affinity systems may be activated near the onset of spike genesis where cooperativity in glutamate–receptor interactions is essential and where the extracellular glutamate concentrations may reach saturation limits of the high-affinity uptake systems. In this situation and during certain pathological conditions (e.g., epileptic activity), the low-affinity (high-capacity) uptake system would work in concert with its high-affinity counterpart to maintain the synaptic cleft free from extracellular glutamate between periods of excitation.

4.2. Glutamine Formation in Glia

Glutamate taken up by glia following excitation is converted to glutamine (Benjamin and Quastel, 1972, 1974) by ATP-dependent glutamine synthetase. This enzyme in the brain is predominantly located within the astrocytes (Martinez-Hernandez *et al.*, 1977; see also Benjamin, 1983). Indeed, primary cultures of astrocytes convert labeled glutamate to labeled glutamine readily in the presence of glucose (Martin *et al.*, 1984; see Hertz *et al.*, 1983). When glia contain high concentrations of ammonia, glutamine is formed also from α-oxoglutarate by the actions of glutamate dehydrogenase and glutamine synthetase (see Benjamin, 1983). α-Oxoglutarate may be replenished in part from pyruvate by initial CO_2 fixation involving pyruvate carboxylase, a process occurring largely in glial cells (see Hertz *et al.*, 1983); the oxaloacetate formed in the reaction enters the citric acid cycle.

Ouabain suppresses glutamine synthesis in intact brain slices, but has no effect on isolated glutamine synthetase. Therefore, it appears that the activity of this enzyme is linked somehow to the activity of the Na^+-K^+ pump. The inhibition by ouabain is not due solely to the suppression of the glial uptake of neuronally released glutamate (Benjamin and Quastel, 1972); a diminished energy metabolism in glia may be involved as well (Benjamin, unpublished observations).

External Ca^{2+} (in the presence of high $[K^+]$) is required for the synthesis of glutamine from glucose in slices of cerebral cortex. Apparently, Ca^{2+} deprivation causes inhibition of glutamine synthesis partly owing to a diminished evoked release of neuronal glutamate; neither the tissue content nor the uptake of glutamate into brain slices is affected under these conditions. In addition, inhibition of glutamine synthesis in the absence of external Ca^{2+} may occur because the accompanying (tetrodotoxin-insensitive) changes in the Na^+ and K^+ content of the glia resemble somewhat those brought about by suppression of the Na^+-K^+ pump. This idea is supported by the observation that Ca^{2+} is essential also for glutamine synthesis from added glutamate (Benjamin, 1983), a condition of incubation employed to bypass the glutamate-releasing process of the neuron.

In contrast to its glutamate-releasing action, high $[K^+]$ in the presence of Ca^{2+} causes retention of glutamine in incubating brain cortex slices. It is possible that part of the retained glutamine represents translocation either directly from astrocytes to neurons, or by way of an extracellular compartment. In any event, glutamine is pharmacologically inert (see Puil, 1981) and safe for transport across the neuronal membrane.

4.3. Translocation of Glutamine from Glia to Neurons

In 1972, Benjamin and Quastel proposed that a fraction of released glutamate is withdrawn by the glia from the extraneuronal space during excitation (synaptic) and returned to neurons eventually in the form of glutamine. This work has stimulated further investigations as discussed earlier. These include the demonstrations that brain glutamine synthesis is located in astrocytes, that external glutamate enhances the formation and release of glutamine from the tissue, and that glutamine hydrolysis can occur readily (though not exclusively) in nerve terminals. Such observations provided the rationale for the use of radioactive glutamine to label Ca^{2+}-dependent, stimulus-coupled, releasable pools of glutamate, GABA, and aspartate in a variety of brain areas for *in vivo* and *in vitro* experimentation (for references see Benjamin, 1983; Szerb and O'Regan, 1985; Bradford *et al.*, 1983).

Recently, Rothstein and Tabakoff (1984, 1986; see also Szerb, this volume) have shown that the Ca^{2+}-dependent, K^+-evoked release of glutamate and aspartate is diminished greatly in glutamine-depleted slices of striatum prepared from brain of rats injected with methionine sulfoximine. This effect is prevented by addition of glutamine to the superperfusion medium. There are statistically significant decreases in the initial levels of aspartate (Rothstein and Tabakoff, 1986) as well as in whole brain GABA levels (Stransky, 1969) following administration of methionine sulfoximine. Although these results need confirmation (see Hamberger *et al.*, 1983), they support the concept that glutamine formed in astrocytes may be the main precursor of glutamate in the nerve terminals as well as of its metabolite transmitters, GABA and aspartate. Concurrently, glutamine could be taken up into the perikaryon (Duce and Keen, 1983) and hydrolyzed to glutamate (see Hertz *et al.*, 1983). Then, by a process analogous to the axonal transport shown to occur in experiments with R-aspartate (Storm-Mathisen, 1981), the transmitter would be ready for release from nerve terminals.

5. Conclusion

During the past 25 years a large number of investigations have brought to the forefront the possibility that glutamate has a pivotal role in excitatory neurotransmission. These experiments have revealed the presence of glutamate in glutamatergic nerve terminals, its synthesis largely though not exclusively from glutamine, possible packaging of glutamate within vesicles, and release of the amino acid into the synaptic cleft by a Ca^{2+}-dependent process following depolarizing stimuli. Although other interpretations are possible, the pendulum of opinion has returned to the view (Puil, 1981) of postsynaptic interactions of glutamate with a single, "inductive" type of receptor thereby causing rather unselective changes in the permeability of the membrane to cations. Termination of the response may occur partly by removal of glutamate from the synaptic cleft by Na^{2+}-dependent high- and low-affinity uptake into nerve terminals and surrounding glia, particularly the astrocytes. In astrocytes, glutamate is converted by glutamine synthetase to pharmacologically inert glutamine which is recycled to the glutamatergic neuron for processing and reuse.

The functioning glutamatergic synapse therefore involves an exact integration of various biochemical, transport, and electrical events. In addition to the chemical coupling of the pre- and the postsynaptic neuron, metabolic coupling of the nerve terminal to the astrocyte in the interconversion of glutamate and glutamine is required, together with the operation of transport processes that make these couplings possible. These interrelationships within glutamatergic systems have not yet been defined clearly since, at present, only a few of the numerous events may be studied at any one time in isolation from each other. Also, it appears to be of prime importance to reconcile the longer time period required for the appearance of biochemical events relative to that for electrical responses. In any event, there can be no doubt of the importance of glutamate in the metabolism and transmitter function of the CNS.

ACKNOWLEDGMENTS. The authors are grateful to Dr. James G. Foulks for his critical reading of the manuscript and to the British Columbia Health Research Foundation and the Medical Research Council of Canada for their financial support.

References

Ames, A., Tsukada, Y., and Nesbett, F. B., 1967, Intracellular Cl^-, Na^+, Ca^{2+}, Mg^{2+} and P in nervous tissue; response to glutamate and to changes in extracellular calcium, *J. Neurochem.* **14**:145–159.

Ascher, P., and Nowak, L., 1986, Mechanisms of action of excitatory amino acids, *Proc. Int. Union Physiol. Sci., XXXth Congr.*, Vancouver, p. 382.

Barr, A. N., Heinze, W., Mendoza, J. E., and Perlik, S., 1978, Long-term treatment of Huntington's disease with L-glutamate and pyridoxine, *Neurology* **28**:1280–1282.

Benjamin, A. M., 1981, Control of glutaminase activity in rat brain cortex *in vitro*: Influence of glutamate, phosphate, ammonium, calcium and hydrogen ions, *Brain Res.* **208**:363–377.

Benjamin, A. M., 1983, Ammonia in metabolic interactions between neurons and glia, in: *Glutamine, Glutamate and GABA in the Central Nervous System* (L. Hertz, E. Kvamme, E. G. McGeer, and A. Schousboe, eds.), Liss, New York, pp. 399–414.

Benjamin, A. M., and Quastel, J. H., 1972, Locations of amino acids in brain cortex slices from the rat: Tetrodotoxin-sensitive release of amino acids, *Biochem. J.* **128**:631–646.

Benjamin, A. M., and Quastel, J. H., 1974, Fate of L-glutamate in the brain, *J. Neurochem.* **23**:457–464.

Benjamin, A. M., and Quastel, J. H., 1975, Metabolism of amino acids and ammonia in rat brain cortex slices *in vitro*: A possible role of ammonia in brain function, *J. Neurochem.* **25**:197–206.

Benjamin, A. M., and Quastel, J. H., 1976, Cerebral uptakes and exchange diffusion in vitro of L- and D-glutamates, *J. Neurochem.* **26**:431–441.

Benjamin, A. M., Verjee, Z. H., and Quastel, J. H., 1980, Kinetics of cerebral uptake processes *in vitro* of L-glutamine, branched chain L-amino acids and L-phenylalanine: Effects of ouabain, *J. Neurochem.* **35**:67–77.

Blaustein, M. P., 1975, Effects of potassium, veratridine and scorpion venom on calcium accumulation and transmitter release by nerve terminals *in vitro*, *J. Physiol. (London)* **247**:617–655.

Bradford, H. F., Ward, H. K., and Thomas, A. J., 1978, Glutamine—A major substrate for nerve endings, *J. Neurochem.* **30**:1453–1459.

Bradford, H. F., Ward, H. K., and Thanki, C. M., 1983, Glutamine as a neurotransmitter precursor: Complementary studies *in vivo* and *in vitro* on the synthesis and release of transmitter glutamate and GABA, in: *Glutamate, Glutamine, and GABA in the Central Nervous System* (L. Hertz, E. Kvamme, E. G. McGeer, and A. Schousboe, eds.), Liss, New York, pp. 249–260.

Bührle, C. P., and Sonnhof, V., 1983, The ionic mechanism of the excitatory action of glutamate upon the membranes of motoneurons of the frog, *Pfluegers Arch.* **396**:154–162.

Connors, B. W., 1984, Initiation of synchronized neuronal bursting in neocortex, *Nature* **23**:685–687.

Coombs, J. S., Eccles, J. C., and Fatt, P., 1955, The specific ionic conductances and the ionic movements across the motoneuronal membrane that produce the inhibitory post-synaptic potentials, *J. Physiol. (London)* **130**:326–373.

Cull-Candy, S. G., and Ogden, D. C., 1985, Ion channels activated by L-glutamate and GABA in cultured cerebellar neurons of the rat, *Proc. R. Soc. London Ser. B* **224**:367–373.

De Belleroche, J. S., and Bradford, H. F., 1972, Metabolism of beds of mammalian cortical synaptosomes: Response to depolarising influence, *J. Neurochem.* **19**:585–602.

De Belleroche, J. S., and Bradford, H. F., 1973, Amino acids in synaptic vesicles from mammalian cerebral cortex: A reappraisal, *J. Neurochem.* **21**:441–451.

De Belleroche, J. S., and Bradford, H. F., 1977, On the site of origin of transmitter amino acids released by depolarisation of nerve terminals *in vitro*, *J. Neurochem.* **29**:335–343.

Duce, I. R., and Keen, P., 1983, Selective uptake of (H-3) labelled glutamine and H-3 labelled glutamate into nervous and satellite cells of dorsal root ganglia *in vitro*, *Neuroscience* **8**:861–866.

Engberg, I., Flatman, J. A., and Lambert, J. D. C., 1979, The actions of excitatory amino acids on motoneurons in the feline spinal cord, *J. Physiol. (London)* **288**:227–261.

Flatman, J. A., Schwindt, P. C., and Crill, W. E., 1986, The induction and modification of voltage-sensitive responses in cat neocortical neurons by N-methyl-D-aspartate, *Brain Res.* **363**:62–77.

Fonnum, F., 1984, Glutamate: A neurotransmitter in mammalian brain, *J. Neurochem.* **42**:1–11.

Goddard, G. A., and Robinson, J. D., 1976, Uptake and release of Ca^{2+} by rat brain synaptosomes, *Brain Res.* **110**:331–350.

Hablitz, J. J., and Langmoen, I. A., 1982, Excitation of hippocampal pyramidal cells by glutamate in the guinea-pig and rat, *J. Physiol. (London)* **325**:317–331.

Hamberger, A., Chiang, G., Nylan, E. S., Scheff, S. W., and Cotman, C. W., 1979a, Glutamate as CNS transmitter. I. Evaluation of glucose and glutamine as precursors of preferentially released glutamate, *Brain Res.* **168**:513–530.

Hamberger, A., Chiang, G., Sandoval, E., and Cotman, C. W., 1979b, Glutamate as CNS transmitter. II. Regulation of synthesis in the releasable pool, *Brain Res.* **168**:531–541.

Hamberger, A., Berthold C. H., Kaulsson, B., Lehman, A., and Nystron, B., 1983, Extracellular GABA, glutamate and glutamine *in vivo*—Perfusion-dialysis of the rabbit hippocampus, in: *Glutamate, Glutamine and GABA in the Central Nervous System* (L. Hertz, E. Kvamme, E. G. McGeer, and A. Schousboe, eds.), Liss, New York, pp. 473–492.

Hayashi, T., 1959, *Neurophysiology and Neurochemistry of Convulsion*, Dainikon-Tosho, Tokyo.

Henn, F. A., Goldstein, M. N., and Hamberger, A., 1974, Uptake of the neurotransmitter candidate glutamate by glia, *Nature* **249**:663–664.

Hertz, L., Kvamme, E., McGeer, E. G., and Schousboe, A. (eds.), 1983, *Glutamine, Glutamate and GABA in the Central Nervous System*, Liss, New York.

Jasper, H., and Koyama, I., 1969, Rate of release of amino acids from the cerebral cortex in the cat as affected by brain stem and thalamic stimulation, *Can. J. Physiol. Pharmacol.* **47**:889–905.

Johnston, G. A. R., 1973, Convulsons induced in 10-day-old rats by intraperitoneal injection of monosodium glutamate and related excitant amino acids, *Biochem. Pharmacol.* **22**:137–140.

Krnjević, K., and Phillis, J. W., 1963, Iontophoretic studies of neurons in the mammalian cerebral cortex, *J. Physiol. (London)* **165**:274–304.

Krnjević, K., and Schwartz, S., 1967, Some properties of unresponsive cells in the cerebral cortex, *Exp. Brain Res.* **3**:306–319.

Kvamme, E., 1983, Glutaminase (PAG), in: *Glutamine, Glutamate and GABA in the Central Nervous System* (L. Hertz, E. Kvamme, E. G. McGeer, and A. Schousboe, eds.), Liss, New York, pp. 51–67.

Logan, W. J., and Snyder, S. H., 1972, High affinity uptake systems for glycine, glutamic and aspartic acids in synaptosomes of rat central nervous tissues, *Brain Res.* **42**:413–431.

MacDermott, A. B., Mayer, M. L., Westbrook, G. L., Smith, S. J., and Barker, J. L., 1986, NMDA-receptor activation increases cytoplasmic calcium concentration in cultured spinal neurons, *Nature* 321:519–522.

MacDonald, J. F., and Schneiderman, J. H., 1984, L-Aspartic acid potentiates 'slow' inward current in cultured spinal cord neurons, *Brain Res.* **296**:350–355.

MacDonald, J. F., and Wojtowicz, J. M., 1982, The effects of L-glutamate and its analogues upon the membrane conductance of central murine neurons in culture, *Can. J. Physiol. Pharmacol.* **60**:282–296.

MacDonald, J. F., Porietis, A. V., and Wojtowicz, J. M., 1982, L-Aspartic acid induces a region of negative slope conductance in the current–voltage relationship of cultured spinal cord neurons, *Brain Res.* **237**:248–253.

Magnam, J. L., and Whittaker, V. P., 1966, The distribution of free amino acids in subcellular fractions of guinea pig brain, *Biochem. J.* **98**:128–137.

Martin, A. R., Wickelgren, W. O., and Beranek, R., 1970, Effects of iontophoretically applied drugs on spinal interneurons of the lamprey, *J. Physiol. (London)* 207:653–665.

Martin, D. L., Waniewski, R. A., and Miller, H. S., 1984, Conversion of glutamate to glutamine by cortical astrocytes, *Soc. Neurosci. Abstr.* **10**:765.

Martinez-Hernandez, A., Bell, K. P., and Norenberg, M. D., 1977, Glutamine synthetase: Glial localization in brain, *Science* 195:1356–1358.

Mayer, M. L., and Westbrook, G. L., 1984, Mixed agonist action of excitatory amino acids on mouse spinal cord neurons under voltage clamp, *J. Physiol. (London)* **354**:29–53.

Mayer, M. L., and Westbrook, G. L., 1985, The action of N-methyl-D-aspartic acid on mouse spinal neurons in culture, *J. Physiol. (London)* **361**:65–90.

Mayer, M. L., and Westbrook, G. L., 1987, The physiology of excitatory amino acids in the vertebrate central nervous system. *Prog. Neurobiology* **28**:197–276.

Naito, S., and Ueda, T., 1983, Adenosine triphosphate-dependent uptake of glutamate into protein I-associated synaptic vesicles, *J. Biol. Chem.* **258**:696–699.

Naito, S., and Ueda, T., 1985, Characterization of glutamate uptake into synaptic vesicles, *J. Neurochem.* **44**:99–109.

Nicoll, R. A., and Alger, B. E., 1981, Synaptic excitation may activate a calcium dependent K^+ conductance in hippocampal pyramidal cells, *Science* 212:957–959.

Nistri, A., Arenson, M. S., and King, A., 1985, Excitatory amino acid-induced responses of frog motoneurons bathed in low Na^+ media: An intracellular study, *Neuroscience* 14:921–927.

Nowak, L., Bregestovski, P., Ascher, P., Herbet, A., and Prochiantz, A., 1984, Magnesium gates glutamate-activated channels in mouse central neurons, *Nature* 307:462–465.

Potashner, S. J., 1978, Effects of tetrodotoxin, calcium and magnesium on the release of amino acids from slices of guinea pig cerebral cortex, *J. Neurochem.* **31**:187–195.

Price, J. C., Waelsch, H., and Putman, T. J., 1943, dl-Glutamic acid hydrochloride in treatment of petit mal and psychomotor seizures, *J. Am. Med. Assoc.* **122**:1153–1156.

Puil, E., 1981, S-Glutamate: Its interactions with spinal neurons, *Brain Res. Rev.* **3**:229–322.

Puil, E., 1983, Actions and interactions of S-glutamate in the spinal cord, in: *Handbook of the Spinal Cord* (R. A. Davidoff, ed.), Vol. 1, Dekker, New York, pp. 105–169.

Puil, E., and Carlen, P. L., 1984, Attenuation of glutamate-action, excitatory postsynaptic potentials, and spikes by intracellular QX222 in hippocampal neurons. *Neuroscience* **11**:389–398.

Pumain, R., and Heinemann, U., 1985, Stimulus and amino acid-induced calcium and potassium changes in neocortex, *J. Neurophysiol.* **53**:1–16.

Quastel, J. H., and Wheatley, A. H. M., 1932, Oxidations by the brain, *Biochem. J.* **26**:725–744.

Rassin, D. K., 1972, Amino acid as putative transmitters: Failure to bind to synaptic vesicles of guinea pig cerebral cortex, *J. Neurochem.* **19**:139–148.

Roberts, P. J., Storm-Mathisen, J., and Johnston, G. A. R. (eds.), 1981, *Glutamate: Transmitter in the Central Nervous System,* Wiley, New York.

Rothstein, J. D., and Tabakoff, B., 1984, Alteration of striatal glutamate release after glutamine synthetase inhibition, *J. Neurochem.* **43**:1438–1446.

Rothstein, J. D., and Tabakoff, B., 1986, Regulation of neurotransmitter aspartate metabolism by glial glutamine synthetase, *J. Neurochem.* **46**:1923–1928.

Shank, R. P., and Campbell, G. L., 1983, Metabolic precursors of glutamate and GABA, in: *Glutamine, Glutamate and GABA in the Central Nervous System* (L. Hertz, E. Kvamme, E. G. McGeer, and A. Schousboe, eds.), Liss, New York, pp. 355–369.

Storm-Mathisen, J., 1981, Autoradiographic and microchemical localisation of high affinity glutamate uptake, in:

Glutamate: Transmitter in the Central Nervous System (P. J. Roberts, J. Storm-Mathisen, and G. A. R. Johnston, eds.), Wiley, New York, pp. 89–115.

Storm-Mathisen, J., Leknes, A. K., Bore, A. T., Vaaland, J. L., Edminson, P., Hang, F. M. S., and Ottersen, O. P., 1983, First visualisation of glutamate and GABA in neurons by immunocytochemistry, *Nature* **301:**517–520.

Stransky, Z., 1969, Time course of rat brain GABA levels following methionine sulfoximine treatment, *Nature* **224:**612–613.

Szerb, J. C., and O'Regan, P. A., 1985, Effect of glutamine on glutamate release from hippocampal slices induced by high K^+ or by electrical stimulation: Interaction with different Ca^{2+} concentrations, *J. Neurochem.* **44:**1724–1731.

Tan, A. T., 1975, Mobilization of synaptic membrane-bound calcium by acidic amino acids, *J. Neurochem.* **24:**127–134.

Tripoli, C. F., and Beard, H. H., 1934, Muscular dystrophy and atrophy, *Arch. Intern. Med.* **53:**435–452.

Vyklický, L., Vyklický, L., Jr., Vyskočil, F., Vlachová, V., Ujec, E., and Michl, J., 1986, Evidence that excitatory amino acids not only activate the receptor channel complex but also lead to use-dependent block, *Brain Res.* **363:**148–151.

Zieglgänsberger, W., and Puil, E. A., 1972, Tetrodotoxin interference of CNS excitation by glutamic acid, *Nature New Biol.* **239:**204–205.

Zieglgänsberger, W., and Puil, E. A., 1973, Actions of glutamic acid on spinal neurons, *Exp. Brain Res.* **17:**35–49.

Zimmerman, F. T., and Ross, S., 1944, Effect of glutamic acid and other amino acids on maze learning in the white rat, *Arch. Neurol. Psychiatry* **51:**446–451.

Zimmerman, F. T., Burgemeister, B. B., and Putman, T. J., 1946, Effects of glutamic acid on mental functioning in children and in adolescents, *Arch. Neurol. Psychiatry* **56:**489–506.

4

Anatomy of Putative Glutamatergic Neurons

Jon Storm-Mathisen and Ole Petter Ottersen

1. Introduction

An important reason why the role of glutamate as a transmitter has for long remained enigmatic is the lack of suitable methods for detailed localization of glutamate in the tissue and for discriminating the putative transmitter role of glutamate from its role in general cellular metabolism. The various markers useful for studying the localization, structure, and connections of neurons likely to transmit their message by releasing glutamate are the subject of this chapter, the receptor actions and pharmacology of glutamate being dealt with in the following chapters. Other reviews discussing this subject include Fagg and Foster (1983), Fonnum (1984), and Ottersen and Storm-Mathisen (1984a, 1986).

2. Tissue Content of Glutamate

After the discovery of the powerful depolarizing actions of glutamate applied onto neurons in the CNS (see Watkins, 1986), it was still hard to accept that the substance could have a transmitter role. People were used to thinking of transmitters as substances present in minute quantities, like acetylcholine and the catecholamines, whereas glutamate was present in comparatively huge concentrations (average about 10 mM in mammalian brain) and showed a relatively uniform regional distribution (Balcom *et al.*, 1976). Today the latter observations are easier to accept, assuming that glutamate may be the major excitatory transmitter in brain, and realizing that synapses account for a major proportion of the brain volume (boutons constitute some 30% of the volume of hippocampal cortex; Nafstad and Blackstad, 1967; S. Laurberg and T. W. Blackstad, data shown in Taxt and Storm-Mathisen, 1984). Yet, lesion-induced degeneration of putative glutamatergic pathways has led to relatively modest reductions in the biochemically measured contents of glutamate in the target areas (e.g., Kim *et al.*, 1971; Fonnum *et al.*, 1981a), possibly due to the concomitant roles of glutamate in intermediary metabolism (see below) and/or a redistribution of glutamate in the denervated tissue. By the same token, detailed dissections and ultrasensitive biochemical assay methods have revealed only modest tissue gradients of glutamate concentration in mammalian brain (Berger *et al.*, 1977); however, at this level of resolution, movements of glutamate during processing could cause artifacts. On subcellular fractionation

Jon Storm-Mathisen and Ole Petter Ottersen • Anatomical Institute, University of Oslo, Karl Johansgate 47, N-0162 Oslo 1, Norway.

synaptic vesicles have repeatedly been found to be poor in glutamate and other amino acids. This may be due to leakage during the isolation procedure, and when suitably prepared, purified brain synaptic vesicles are reported to contain as much as 210 mM glutamate (Riveros *et al.*, 1986).

The possibility of demonstrating amino acids *in situ* by immunocytochemical procedures (Storm-Mathisen *et al.*, 1983) offers a promising new tool for studying endogenous contents of glutamate (see Section 8).

3. High-Affinity Uptake of Glutamate

It was a major step forward when nerve endings in brain were demonstrated to take up putative transmitters, including glutamate, by specific transport processes (Balcar and Johnston, 1972; Logan and Snyder, 1972). These transport processes are characterized by a dependence on Na$^+$ ions and a high affinity relative to less specific uptake processes. Furthermore, evidence was produced that the high-affinity Na$^+$-dependent uptake of glutamate and other putative transmitters could be localized in distinct subpopulations of nerve endings (Wofsey *et al.*, 1971). The first direct evidence that high-affinity Na$^+$-dependent glutamate uptake was preferentially localized in certain neurons was the demonstration that the uptake was heavily reduced in synaptosome preparations from the cerebellar cortex of hamsters deprived of granule cells by a neonatal viral infection (Young *et al.*, 1974). However, this study also pointed to a problem with using glutamate uptake as the marker for putative glutamatergic neurons: the uptake of aspartate was depressed in parallel with that of glutamate, whereas glutamate was the only endogenous amino acid showing a reduction along with the loss of granule cells. In fact, the glutamate transporter appears to translocate L-glutamate, L-aspartate, and D-aspartate with similar kinetics, although D-glutamate is a poor substrate (Davies and Johnston, 1976). Nonetheless, the possibility exists that different nerve endings could show differences in their relative affinities toward glutamate and aspartate (Davies and Johnston, 1976; Thangnipon *et al.*, 1983).

In spite of this imperfection, Na$^+$-dependent high-affinity uptake of glutamate has proved to be a very useful marker for studying the anatomy of putative glutamatergic neurons (see below). In particular, D-aspartate is convenient in this connection, being a good substrate that is neither metabolized to a significant extent nor incorporated into proteins (Davies and Johnston, 1976).

Biochemical determination of glutamate or aspartate uptake in synaptosome-containing brain homogenates reveals a differential regional distribution and a heavy reduction at target sites of putative glutamatergic pathways after degeneration (review: Fonnum, 1984). The losses may be as high as 80% (Taxt and Storm-Mathisen, 1984), suggesting that the degenerated nerve endings are the predominant site of uptake in the target area. The same, virtually complete, loss of glutamate and aspartate uptake is seen autoradiographically in slices of denervated brain tissue incubated *in vitro* with the radiolabeled amino acids. These studies showed that the loss was precisely restricted to the target areas of the lesioned putative glutamatergic pathways, which in normal animals had particularly high intensities of uptake. Furthermore, electron microscopic autoradiographic observations in similarly incubated slices demonstrated that some 80% of the tissue content of [^{3}H]glutamate was localized in nerve endings and preterminal axons (Storm-Mathisen and Iversen, 1979). These studies show that under given conditions (*in casu* hippocampal slices, Krebs solution, gentle agitation, room temperature, 10–30 min, low micromolar concentrations of labeled substrate) glutamate uptake is restricted to certain classes of nerve endings, which in many cases happen to be ones that are believed to be glutamatergic based on evidence from physiological and pharmacological studies.

It should be emphasized, however, that different putative glutamatergic neuronal pathways appear to differ with respect to the intensity of glutamate and aspartate uptake in their nerve endings. Thus, the perforant paths and the Schaffer collateral system of the hippocampal formation both may be glutamatergic and both account for a very large proportion of the nerve endings in their target areas. Yet the normal intensity of glutamate and D-aspartate uptake in the target area and the percentage lost following axotomy are much greater in the latter than in the former projection system (Taxt and Storm-Mathisen, 1984).

There is a body of literature demonstrating that glutamate and aspartate also can be taken up into glial cells. Many workers have found that this uptake obscures or supersedes the neuronal uptake (for references see Ottersen and Storm-Mathisen, 1984a). In tissue cultures, putative glutamatergic neurons have a lower uptake activity per protein toward glutamate than do astrocytes (Drejer et al., 1982). Undoubtedly, glial uptake of the amino acids must be important physiologically. There is strong evidence from biochemical studies that this uptake is involved in a cycling of glutamate and glutamine between nerve endings and glia which is essential for supporting glutamate synthesis in nerve endings during synaptic release (see below). This glial uptake appears to be more easily destroyed than that which occurs in nerve endings in in vitro preparations such as synaptosomes and slices incubated in relatively harsh conditions. Although "artifactual," these conditions have proved rather useful for tracing putative glutamatergic nerve endings.

The glutamate transporter protein of nerve endings will probably soon be isolated (Kanner, 1983). The possibility exists that immunocytochemical demonstration of this could provide useful information on the localization of glutamatergic pathways. However, this would presumably depend on the neuronal transporter being distinguishable from the glial transporter.

An additional uptake system for glutamate has been reported in a population of synaptic vesicles precipitable by antibodies to synapsin I (Naito and Ueda, 1983, 1985). This transporter has a low affinity for the amino acid and is independent of Na^+, but appears to be highly selective for glutamate and dependent on ATP. The isolation and subsequent immunocytochemical demonstration of this transporter might solve three of the problems in this field of research by affording the ability to distinguish (1) nerve endings storing glutamate from ones storing aspartate, (2) glutamate reserved for neurotransmission as opposed to that subserving other roles, and (3) neuronal uptake from glial uptake of glutamate.

4. Axonal Transport of D-Aspartate

The method that has been most efficient in tracing putative glutamatergic (and aspartatergic) nerve pathways is the autoradiographic demonstration of retrograde transport of D-[^{3}H]aspartate (Streit, 1980; Baughman and Gilbert, 1980, 1981; Cuénod et al., 1981, 1982; Storm-Mathisen and Wold, 1981). This approach takes advantage of the selective uptake of dicarboxylic amino acids into certain, putatively glutamatergic (or aspartatergic) neurons, and the metabolic inertia of D-aspartate (see Section 3). The latter seems important for allowing the labeled amino acid to stay in the neuron long enough to be transported along the axon. The axonal transport appears to occur by the fast component. This would suggest that the tracer is included in an organelle, and it is tempting to speculate that this is the synaptic vesicle, although it is possible to envisage that a "stirring" effect of transported organelles could cause cytosolic solutes to move quickly along the axons (see Weiss et al., 1980). The latter mechanism would solve the problem of reconciling the axonal transport of D-aspartate in neurons thought to be glutamatergic with the reported lack of D-aspartate uptake in synaptic vesicles taking up glutamate (Naito and Ueda, 1985) (see Section 3). In any case, there is evidence that the axonally transported D-[^{3}H]aspartate gains access to the synaptic release mechanism (Cuénod et al., 1981). This also supports the physiological relevance of the technique.

The tracer appears to be gradually lost as it moves along the axons, making long projections difficult to follow (Cuénod et al., 1982). Part of this loss is undoubtedly due to branching of the axons; a label injected into the target area of a pathway labels the target areas of axon collaterals, as well as the parent cell bodies (Baughman and Gilbert, 1980), showing that the label can travel along the axons in both directions. However, anterograde labeling of axon terminals after injection of D-[^{3}H]aspartate into the area of the parent cell bodies may give less reliable results than retrograde labeling (Cuénod et al., 1982).

In spite of the relatively high concentrations of labeled D-aspartate at the injection site (about 10 mM; Streit, 1980), the uptake appears to take place through the specific high-affinity mechanism, since the results can be reproduced by infusing the tracer at concentrations corresponding to the K_m of the high-affinity uptake mechanism (Wiklund *et al.*, 1984; Storm-Mathisen and Wold, 1981).

A problem with this approach has been the extensive spread of D-[^{3}H]aspartate from the tip of the micropipette used to inject the tracer. This spread can be considerably reduced by implanting micropipettes with tip chambers packed with the tracer in solid form absorbed in a porous material such as agarose particles (Fischer *et al.*, 1986a,b). This gives a gradual release of the tracer and a circumscribed site of application and allows even local neurons to be studied by the method.

Retrograde transport of D-[^{3}H]aspartate has served to identify a large number of nerve pathways as ones for which a dicarboxylic amino acid should be considered as transmitter (see Section 10). It is especially suitable for detailed mapping and for studying pathways which are relatively sparse and therefore cannot be studied by lesioning methods combined with biochemical determinations of uptake activity. However, it should be kept in mind that the uptake activity of the nerve endings, on which the method depends, may vary among glutamatergic pathways (see Section 3), and that additional factors, e.g., the incorporation of D-aspartate into vesicles and the coupling to axonal transport, as well as the architecture of the axonal tree, may cause the efficiency of the method to vary from pathway to pathway.

5. Ca²⁺-Dependent Depolarization-Induced Release of Glutamate

Demonstrability of synaptic release is the crucial criterion for identifying glutamate as the transmitter of a synapse where the action of glutamate on the postsynaptic receptors indicates such a role. The combined use of a sensitive biochemical assay with axotomy-induced degeneration of nerve endings has made it possible to demonstrate Ca²⁺-dependent depolarization-induced release of endogenous glutamate from anatomically identified axon terminals in dissected slices, such as those of the perforant path and commissural hippocampal axons (Nadler *et al.*, 1976; Hamberger *et al.*, 1978), or the corticostriatal tract (Rowlands and Roberts, 1980; Druce *et al.*, 1982).

Dissected slice preparations have also been used to study Ca²⁺-dependent release induced by electrical stimulation of specific nerve pathways of previously accumulated, ³H-labeled, amino acids (Malthe-Sørenssen *et al.*, 1979, 1980; Wieraszko and Lynch, 1979). Another refinement of these techniques is to demonstrate release of labeled glutamate synthesized *in situ* from labeled precursors, i.e., glutamine or glucose (Hamberger *et al.*, 1978). Push–pull cannulae (Bliss *et al.*, 1986) or similar collection devices (Lerma *et al.*, 1986) have been used successfully to demonstrate evoked release of glutamate from specific nerve pathways *in vivo* (review: Abdul-Gahni *et al.*, 1981).

An "on-line" system (fluorescence of reduced nicotinamide adenine dinucleotide produced via glutamate dehydrogenase) for studying synaptic release has recently yielded important new evidence on the subcellular origin of endogenous glutamate released Ca²⁺-dependently from synaptosomes (Nicholls and Sihra, 1986). The same or similar principles could probably be adapted to studying glutamate release from identified nerve pathways.

6. Studies on Metabolism and Compartmentation

The releasable stores of glutamate have to be replenished by reuptake of the released transmitter or by resynthesis. The relative importance of the two processes under physiological conditions is difficult to assess. However, under experimental conditions in which the released transmitter is washed away, the rate of release and the tissue concentration of glutamate are effectively supported by supplying glutamine in the superfusion medium, in addition to glucose (Hamberger et al., 1978; Bradford et al., 1978; Ward et al., 1983). An effective concentration is that at which glutamine normally occurs in the cerebrospinal fluid—0.4 mM. On the other hand, severe tissue deprivation of glucose in vivo (Engelsen and Fonnum, 1983) leads to a severe fall in tissue levels of glutamine and glutamate, testifying to the importance of glucose as a precursor for synaptically released glutamate. Under experimental conditions, augmentation of release of amino acids has been observed in low-glucose media (Potashner, 1978). A likely explanation for the latter phenomenon is that shortage of high-energy phosphate impairs the uptake of released transmitter into nerve endings and glia.

The "overflow" of glutamate from the synaptic cleft and subsequent uptake into glia results in the production of glutamine (see, e.g., Waniewski and Martin, 1986), the enzyme glutamine synthetase being restricted to glial cells, mainly astrocytes (Norenberg and Martinez-Hernandez, 1979). This is also the basis for the long-observed "metabolic compartmentation" of glutamate: administration of certain radiolabeled substrates (e.g., acetate, pyruvate, aspartate, glutamate) to brain tissue leads to a higher specific radioactivity in glutamine than in glutamate. Since glutamine must be formed from glutamate, this means that only a small part of the total tissue glutamate is accessible to the action of glutamine synthetase (Berl et al., 1975). This small glutamate pool appears to be turning over quickly. Glucose does not show the "metabolic compartmentation" phenomenon, suggesting that neurons can form glutamate from glucose without the participation of the glial glutamate pool.

With histological techniques, Hamberger et al. (1978) showed that incorporation into the amino acid pool of radiolabeled acetate, a substrate showing the "metabolic compartmentation" phenomenon, is greatly increased in the target zones of the perforant path in area dentata when this pathway degenerates following axotomy. The time course of the increase in acetate incorporation seemed to follow that of reactive proliferation of astrocytes. The incorporation of glucose was heavily reduced, suggesting that it mainly occurred in the lost afferents. The compartmentation of the amino acids between nerve endings and glia and changes in the latter during physiological experiments have been demonstrated more directly by immunocytochemical visualization of the amino acids (see Section 8).

The fact that administration of labeled glutamate itself shows the "metabolic compartmentation" phenomenon suggests that exogenous glutamate, rather than mixing uniformly with the total tissue glutamate, is taken up into astrocytes and rapidly converted to glutamine (Balázs et al., 1973; Benjamin and Quastel, 1974). Nerve endings have low-affinity, high-capacity uptake systems for glutamine (although glia also have; Hertz et al., 1980), and as mentioned above, can use it for formation of releasable glutamate. These observations lead to the assumption that synaptically released glutamate is (partly) taken up into glia and channeled back into nerve endings in the form of the nonexcitatory glutamine. This cycle seems an ingenious mechanism for keeping the extracellular concentration of glutamate low, yet allowing "escaping" glutamate to be recaptured.

However, the existence of this mechanism does not preclude the reuptake of a sizable proportion of the synaptically released glutamate into a rapidly releasable small transmitter pool within the nerve endings. Such a situation would be analogous to what has been hypothesized for cholinergic nerve endings, i.e., a small pool of acetylcholine that turns over rapidly (Zimmermann, 1979; Israël et al., 1984). The enzyme converting glutamine to glutamate within the nerve endings, phosphate-activated glutaminase (PAG), appears to be tightly regulated, e.g., inhibited by glutamate and activated by Ca^{2+} (Kvamme, 1983). The immediately releasable pool therefore need not necessarily contain a large amount of glutamate. Yet, a larger pool of glutamate could be kept in reserve for release in situations of high demand. Such a storage pool of glutamate could be prevented from inhibiting PAG by being sequestered in synaptic vesicles (Kvamme and Lenda, 1981). The above discussion is valid no matter whether release of transmitter actually occurs from synaptic vesicles or not (De Belleroche and Bradford, 1972; see Israël et al., 1984). A population of synaptic vesicles can take up glutamate when supplied with ATP (Naito and Ueda, 1983, 1985). It is possible to envisage synaptic vesicles immediately engaged in transmitter release as being particularly active in accumulating glutamate from the cytosol (see Zimmermann, 1979). More direct evidence that synaptically released glutamate derives from an "exocytotic pool" rather than from cytosol has recently been provided by Nicholls and Sihra (1986), who further found that the immediately releasable pool constituted a restricted part of nerve terminal glutamate stores (less than 20%).

7. Enzymes as Markers for Transmitter Glutamate

From the above discussion, PAG would seem potentially useful as a marker for nerve endings synthesizing glutamate for use as transmitter. However, the enzyme also forms glutamate in nerve endings producing GABA and can show considerable activity even in astrocytes (Hertz et al., 1983a). Furthermore, the actual concentration or assayable activity of the enzyme at a given site may not be very interesting physiologically, the in situ enzyme activity being restrained by various regulators (Kvamme, 1983). Degeneration of the alleged glutamatergic corticostriatal tract leads to a reduction of PAG in the target area (Sandberg et al., 1985), but this is modest compared to the reduction in glutamate uptake (Divac et al., 1977; McGeer et al., 1977). On the other hand, there is a reduction in PAG in substantia nigra after kainate-induced degeneration of the striatonigral tract, correlating with, but again smaller than the reduction in the GABA-synthesizing enzyme glutamate decarboxylase (McGeer and McGeer, 1979).

Immunocytochemical results with PAG have suggested some enrichment of the enzyme in certain, potentially glutamatergic neuronal pathways (Altschuler et al., 1984, 1985; Beitz et al., 1986), whereas other workers have found a more uniform distribution (Svenneby and Storm-Mathisen, 1983; and unpublished results). All of these results suggest that recording of PAG may not be suitable as a marker for tracing potentially glutamatergic neurons.

So far, there is no compelling evidence that any of the other enzymes involved in the formation of glutamate are any more useful than PAG in this capacity. Aspartate aminotransferase was once suggested as a marker (Altschuler et al., 1981, 1982; cf. Bolz et al., 1985), but this did not turn out to be generally applicable (Wenthold and Altschuler, 1983, 1986). Glutamate dehydrogenase is less active in cultured putative glutamatergic neurons than in astrocytes (Gordon et al., 1981; Patel et al., 1982), and has been shown immunocytochemically to be primarily localized in the latter type of cell in brain tissue (Kaneko et al., 1987). A moderate reduction in the histochemically demonstrable activities of this enzyme and of succinate dehydrogenase in the target zones of hippocampal, potentially glutamatergic pathways (Wolf et al., 1984) confirms that glutamate dehydrogenase is not significantly enriched in glutamatergic neurons. Ornithine aminotransferase appears to be involved in the formation of glutamate and to be sensitive to feedback inhibition by GABA (Yoneda et al., 1982), and inhibition of the enzyme has been found to impair glutamate turnover in the hippocampo-septal pathway (Wroblewski et al., 1985). However, similar to the other enzymes involved in glutamate synthesis, ornithine aminotransferase seems not to be restricted to glutamatergic neurons (McGeer et al., 1983).

8. Immunocytochemical Demonstration of Glutamate

The advent of immunocytochemical procedures for demonstrating amino acids (Storm-Mathisen et al., 1982, 1983) has opened the possibility of studying the localization of glutamate itself in situ. Various methodological aspects of this approach have been dealt with in some detail elsewhere (Ottersen and Storm-Mathisen, 1984a,b, 1985, 1986, 1987a,b; Ottersen et al., 1986b; Storm-Mathisen and Ottersen, 1986; Storm-Mathisen et al., 1986a).

8.1. Specificity

At the present stage there is little room for doubt that the immunoreactivity demonstrable in glutaraldehyde-fixed tissue by means of our purified polyclonal antibodies represents tissue glutamate. The antibodies are raised against glutamate bound to albumin by glutaraldehyde and unwanted antibodies are absorbed from the sera by a series of Sepharose columns bearing albumin treated with glutaraldehyde or with glutaraldehyde in the presence of different amino acids (GABA, glutamine). The purified antibodies do not react significantly with any of the compounds tested other than L-glutamate (except as stated below) as assessed in a model system (Ottersen and Storm-Mathisen, 1984b) mimicking the conditions in the immunocytochemical tissue preparations (see Larsson, 1983). In this test system the small molecules are fixed to brain protein by glutaraldehyde and spotted on cellulose ester disks before immunocytochemical processing by the peroxidase-antiperoxidase method (Sternberger, 1979). (A similar test system was developed by Hodgson et al., 1985.) The concentrations of amino acids (2 μmole/mg protein) chosen to prepare the conjugates are far in excess of those likely to be present in brain, in order to detect any cross-reactivity of practical importance. The compounds tested include all common amino acids, as well as other low-molecular-weight amine compounds known to be present in brain tissue at comparable concentrations (Ottersen and Storm-Mathisen, 1985; Storm-Mathisen et al., 1986a; Ottersen et al., 1986b). Glutamate residues in polyglutamate or in proteins do not interfere, including total protein and other macromolecules from rat brain, neither do those in glutathione (γ-glutamyl-cysteinyl-glycine) or in the dipeptide γ-glutamyl-glutamate, suggesting that N-terminal γ-glutamate in small peptides does not react. Recently, slight and similar reactivities were observed with fixed α-aspartyl-glutamate and with α-glutamyl-glutamate, which could be taken to indicate that C-terminal glutamate can react under certain conditions (Ottersen and Storm-Mathisen, 1987a).

Furthermore, in an attempt to identify the endogenous compound responsible for the staining in tissue sections we have extracted compounds of rat brain in HCl-acidified 80% ethanol, separated them by thin-layer chromatography, sprayed the chromatograms with a mixture of glutaraldehyde and polylysine to fix the low-molecular-weight amino compounds, and processed the sprayed chromatograms immunocytochemically with the antibodies to glutamate exactly as for immunocytochemistry. A single band was stained, which comigrated with authentic glutamate. Parallel chromatograms processed with antibodies to aspartate or to glutamine showed single stained bands that were located in other positions, aligned with authentic aspartate or glutamine, respectively (Ottersen and Storm-Mathisen, 1987a).

Immunostaining in the tissue and of the glutamate testspot can be abolished by absorption with glutamate–glutaraldehyde complexes, either immobilized on a resin (Ottersen and Storm-Mathisen, 1985) or in soluble form added to the serum (Ottersen et al., 1986b). Similar complexes of other amino acids do not have this effect. Soluble glutamate-glutaraldehyde [molar ratio 1 : 2, i.e., optimal stoichiometry for reaction (Hardy et al., 1976)], treated with ethanolamine to block free aldehyde groups inhibits immunoreactivity at low μM concentrations and blocks it completely at 200 μM (with respect to glutamate). The soluble glutaraldehyde complexes of amino acids are easy to prepare and afford a convenient specificity control. They also afford an effective and convenient means of suppressing crossreactivities in sera that have been incompletely purified.

The reaction of amino acids with glutaraldehyde leads to the formation of complexes in which several amino acid residues are held tightly together in an orderly array (Hardy et al., 1976; see also Section 8.4). That this situation could be mimicked by the free amino acid at high concentration is suggested by the observation that free glutamate inhibits immunostaining at 50–800 mM, whereas other free amino acids do not (Storm-Mathisen et al., 1986a). This is not important for immunocytochemical applications, but shows that the antibodies are also able to interact specifically with the amino acid as such, although at a low affinity.

An antiserum showing high affinity towards free glutamate has been described (Shiosaka et al., 1986). This does not appear to produce good immunocytochemical results (Wanaka et al., 1987), but such antibodies might be particularly useful for physiological experiments on glutamatergic synapses (cf. Duggan and Hendry, 1986).

The high affinity of the sera for soluble glutaraldehyde complexes of amino acids may explain why the staining intensities obtained with the present method are rather sensitive to the amount of tissue incubated in a given volume of primary serum: soluble complexes may slowly leak out of the tissue during incubation. Such leakage can apparently be inhibited by treatment with $NaBH_4$, which should stabilize the structure of the fixation complexes (see Hardy et al., 1976). However, we do not routinely use this treatment, because it reduces immunoreactivities with our sera, which have been raised against antigens not treated with $NaBH_4$. Others (Seguela et al., 1984) routinely use $NaBH_4$ treatment of immunogens as well as tissue and find that this is important for the results in the conditions used.

It is worth noting that the fixation products formed with glutaraldehyde are heterogeneous (Hardy et al., 1976, 1979) and could vary in details among different sites in the tissue depending on the chemical composition of the microenvironment. Therefore polyclonal antibodies may be more suitable than monoclonal antibodies for the present purpose.

In spite of all the specificity controls performed, it is still conceivable that some glutamate-containing oligopeptide could show sufficient crossreactivity and could be present at high enough concentration at restricted sites in the central nervous system to be stained with our antibodies, but at present it seems highly improbable that this could explain anything more than details in the distribution of glutamate-like immunoreactivity (Ottersen and Storm-Mathisen, 1984a,b, 1985).

8.2. Quantitative Aspects

The extent to which glutamate is fixed in the tissue may be about 50%, according to experiments in which hippocampal slices were incubated with [³H]glutamate and the tissue content of ³H (about 80% [³H]glutamate) determined before and after glutaraldehyde fixation (Storm-Mathisen and Iversen, 1979).

Model experiments with test conjugates of brain protein, glutaraldehyde, and amino acid have suggested that the proportion of amino acid fixed varies by no more than a factor of 2 when the concentration of amino acid is varied by a factor of 30 (0.1-3 µmol/mg protein). Furthermore, they demonstrated a roughly linear relation between the optical density of the immunocyto-chemical reaction product (peroxidase-antiperoxidase method) and the logarithm of the amino acid concentration present when preparing the conjugate (Ottersen et al., 1986b).

These experiments further suggested that the concurrent presence of other amino acids at high concentration can to some extent interfere with the fixation and immunoreactivity of a given amino acid. However, a 30-fold surplus of one amino acid over another (tested for glutamate aspartate, GABA, and taurine) during preparation of the model conjugates only moderately reduced the immunoreactivity of the amino acid (Ottersen et al., 1986b; and unpublished results). This effect might therefore to some extent affect the distribution of immunoreactivity, but is unlikely to have jeopardized the general validity of the staining results. Poor penetration of antibodies and steric hindrance of their interaction with the antigen in the fixed tissue may pose more serious problems (Section 8.4), but may be overcome in various ways (see Sections 8.3–8.5).

8.3. Brain Slices

The most compelling immunocytochemical evidence for a selective localization of glutamate in potentially glutamatergic neurons has been obtained in hippocampal slices fixed in vitro (Fig. 1c). The hippocampal formation contains a sequence of excitatory neurons all of which may use a dicarboxylic amino acid as transmitter according to physiological criteria (Cotman and Nadler, 1981), and have their nerve endings organized in characteristic laminae facilitating investigation at the light microscopic level. Among these the axons of the CA3 pyramidal cells (comprising the Schaffer collaterals) are distributed in strata oriens and radiatum of the hippocampus (CA1–CA3) with sharp delineations toward the neighboring layers and toward the adjoining cortical subfields (subiculum and hilus fasciae dentatae, i.e., CA4). These strata stand out as particularly strongly stained in hippocampal slices fixed *in vitro* with glutaraldehyde and processed immunocytochemically with the glutamate antiserum (Storm-Mathisen *et al.*, 1983; Storm-Mathisen and Ottersen, 1983). The laminar pattern of staining is identical to that of high-affinity Na^+-dependent uptake sites for glutamate and aspartate displayed autoradiographically (Taxt and Storm-Mathisen, 1984), provided the slices are incubated identically. This could be demonstrated directly by resectioning slices fixed after incubation with D-[^{3}H]aspartate and processing adjacent sections for autoradiography and immunocytochemistry (illustration in Cotman *et al.*, 1987). The zones of termination of the lateral perforant path and of the mossy fibers also stand out as rich in glutamate-like immunoreactivity under certain conditions of treatment of the slices before fixation, such as direct fixation after brief soaking in cold isotonic sucrose, or incubation in Krebs solution supplemented with glutamine at the concentration present in the cerebrospinal fluid (particularly when combined with moderate depolarizing concentrations of K^+ or veratrine). These results would suggest that the latter two fiber systems, although less rich in glutamate uptake sites than the CA3-derived axons, can still sustain high levels of glutamate under conditions approaching the *in vivo* situation. This notion gains support from studies on release and metabolism of glutamate (Hamberger *et al.*, 1978; Nadler *et al.*, 1978), particularly in the case of the perforant path (see Section 6).

Most of the immunostaining in the hippocampal slices resides in small dots, reminiscent of nerve endings. The nerve terminal localization of the immunoreactivity could be verified electron-microscopically. Under condition in which the mossy fiber layer was stained, the stained structures had the light microscopic and ultrastructural characteristics of mossy fiber boutons. The staining appeared to be concentrated in synaptic vesicles and mitochondria, as revealed by the peroxidase-antiperoxidase method in the presence of Triton X-100 (Storm-Mathisen *et al.*, 1983; Storm-Mathisen and Ottersen, 1983; and unpublished results). However, this method may not be suitable for judging localization of immunoreactivity at this level of resolution (see Section 8.5).

A virtue of the slice preparation is that it allows us to study effects of changes in the tissue environment. In order to produce long-lasting release of transmitters, hippocampal slices were incubated at depolarizing concentrations of K^+ or veratrine. This led to loss of the characteristic staining of nerve endings (Storm-Mathisen *et al.*, 1986a,b). Instead, glutamate-like immunoreactivity appeared in astroglia (Fig. 1d). The changes were prevented by lowering the Ca^{2+} concentration of the Krebs solution to 0.1 mM and increasing the Mg^{2+} concentration to 10 mM, suggesting that they were dependent on synaptic release of glutamate. The depletion of immunoreactivity from nerve endings could also be prevented by adding glutamine to the incubation medium. This conforms with results of biochemical studies (Bradford *et al.*, 1978; Hamberger *et al.*, 1978, 1979; Ward *et al.*, 1983; Szerb and O'Regan, 1985), and suggests that supply of glutamine is necessary for sustaining tissue levels and stimulation-induced release of glutamate under conditions in which the released amino acid is washed away. In agreement, supply of glutamine has been reported to enhance the electrophysiological performance of putative glutamatergic synapses in the hippocampal slice preparation (Schiff *et al.*, 1985).

In our experiments described above the slices were incubated free-floating at 30°C in phosphate-buffered Krebs solution gassed with O_2 on a metabolic shaker, the medium being changed every 10 min for 1 hr. In these slices, immunoreactivity was usually not seen in neuronal perikarya (Fig. 1c). In neurophysiological experiments on slices it is a common finding that slices must be left at rest in the superfusion chamber for about 1 hr before electrically active neurons are regularly observed (Andersen *et al.*, 1980). It was thought of interest to investigate slices that had been incubated under these conditions and actually shown to contain electrically active neurons. Experiments performed as previously described (Andersen *et al.*, 1980) were terminated by carefully removing each slice together with the piece of tissue paper on which it was resting, and

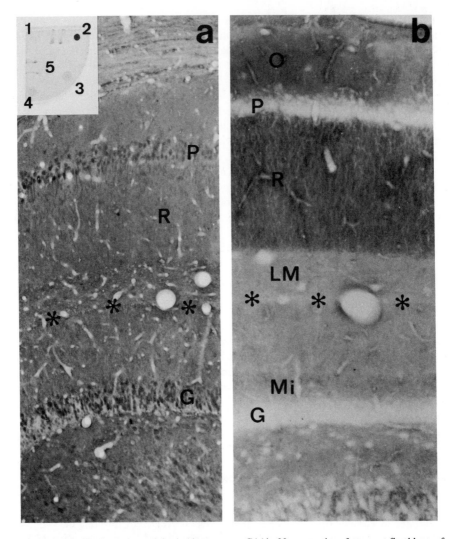

Figure 1. Glutamate-like immunoreactivity in hippocampus CA1 in 20-μm sections from a rat fixed by perfusion with 5% glutaraldehyde (a, b), and in hippocampal slices from a fresh rat brain incubated in oxygenated Krebs solution (30°C, 60 min) and subsequently fixed by immersion in the same fixative and resectioned (c, d). The section shown in (b) was digested with trypsin for 45 min (see Section 8.4) and thoroughly rinsed before immunocytochemical processing. The control section (a) was incubated in the buffer used to dissolve the trypsin. The two sections (a, b) and the test filter (inset) were processed with sera in the same vessel. Note the high specificity of staining demonstrated by the test filter with spots of amino acids fixed to rat brain protein by glutaraldehyde (a, inset: 1, L-aspartate; 2, L-glutamate; 3, GABA; 4, L-glutamine; 5, only glutaraldehyde and brain protein), and the dramatic change in staining pattern caused by trypsin treatment (b). The resulting pattern is similar to that seen after

quickly plunging it into 5% glutaraldehyde in 0.1 M sodium phosphate buffer pH 7.4 (G.-Y. Hu, Ø. Hvalby, P. O. Andersen, O. P. Ottersen, and J. Storm-Mathisen, unpublished). The slices were then resectioned at 20 μm and processed for demonstration of glutamate-like immunoreactivity. These slices showed a regular and widespread staining of perikarya and proximal dendrites of pyramidal and granular cells, although areas of unstained perikarya were still found. In the parts of the slices showing stained perikarya, the staining of the neuropil tended to be more uniform, the laminar staining pattern sometimes being obscured. A likely reason is that in these slices the staining of the neuropil is partly due to staining of fine dendritic branches, which is not

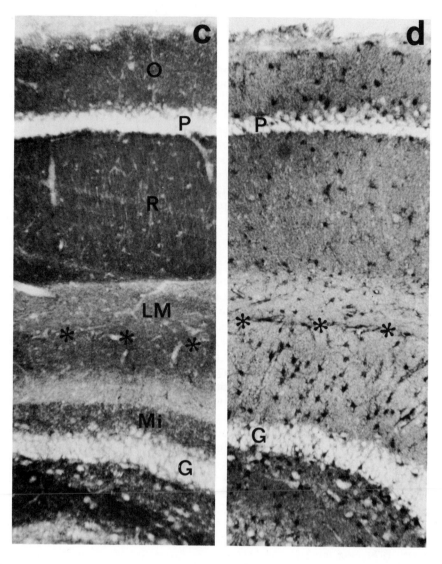

incubation in normal Krebs solution (c) and seems to represent glutamatergic nerve endings (see text). Incubation in Krebs with 40 mM K$^+$ (d) severely reduces staining of nerve endings, but causes accumulation of glutamate-like immunoreactivity in astroglia. Abbreviations: O, P, R, LM, strata oriens, pyramidale, radiatum, and lacunosum-moleculare of hippocampus; G, stratum granulare of area dentata; Mi, inner zone of dentate stratum moleculare receiving afferents from hilus (cf. Fig. 4); asterisks, fissura hippocampi. Scale: thickness of R ca. 0.3 mm [(c) and (d) from V. Gundersen, G. Nordbø, O. P. Ottersen, and J. Storm-Mathisen, unpublished.]

expected to differ between laminae. An additional possible explanation is that the network of glial lamellae surrounding the neuronal elements is ordinarily disrupted to some extent during preparation of slices and that it has been able to reseal in the parts of the slices that show uniform staining. This could then create a protected environment for the other tissue elements and allow nerve endings and dendritic branches to sustain high concentrations of internal glutamate irrespective of such factors as their uptake activity (see above). Resealing of the glial network might also create conditions of fixation mimicking the ones present *in situ* that hamper access of the antibodies to certain antigenic sites (Section 8.4).

Such a resealing of the network of glial lamellae would take some time, possibly explaining why a period of incubation in the perfusion chamber is required before electrical activity is resumed. The integrity of the glial processes and a "tight" operation of the glutamine-glutamate cycle in the stabilized hippocampal slice would also explain how it is possible to perform electrophysiological experiments with brain slices without adding glutamine to the incubation medium, which is so important in biochemical experiments (see above). The resealing would probably depend on mechanical stability of the slices. This is afforded by the suspension on a net, as used in the physiological experiments, but not by the incubation of slices free-floating in vials on a metabolic shaker as commonly used in biochemical experiments and in our experiments described above. This interpretation clearly needs more experimental confirmation, but gains support from the similarity of the distribution of glutamate-like immunoreactivity in hippocampal slices from physiological experiments (i.e., partial lack of lamination of neuropil and conspicuous staining of perikarya and dendrites) and in hippocampi from animals fixed by perfusion with glutaraldehyde.

8.4. Perfusion-Fixed Brain

In light-microscopic preparations of animals fixed by perfusion there is a conspicuous staining of perikarya and dendrites, but no lamination of the neuropil staining in the hippocampus (Fig. 1a). Furthermore, stained nerve endings are not obvious, and in the mossy fiber layer, which contains large boutons of characteristic shape, the latter are clearly less strongly stained than the intervening pyramidal cell dendrites. This distribution led us to suspect that in the "physiological" situation the arrival of the fixation could induce a profuse release of glutamate (cf. Van Harreveld and Fifkova, 1972) emptying the endogenous stores before they were fixed. To test this hypothesis, various means of inhibiting transmitter release have been tried: perfusion with ice-cold rinsing and fixing solutions, or perfusion with solutions containing Co^{2+}, Cd^{2+}, or high concentrations of Mg^{2+}, or local injections of tetrodotoxin (to inhibit depolarization through Na^+ channels), trifluoperazine (to inhibit Ca^{2+}-calmodulin-dependent mechanisms), (+) or (−) baclofen or Co^{2+} prior to perfusion with fixative. None of these measures have led to overt changes in the distribution of glutamate-like immunoreactivity, suggesting that synaptic release of glutamate evoked by the fixative is not a factor affecting the light-microscopic localization of glutamate in tissue fixed by perfusion with glutaraldehyde.

Could the apparent low staining intensity in nerve terminals be due to some artifact occurring in perfusion-fixed tissue and making the fixed glutamate inaccessible to the antibodies? Penetration of antibodies is recognized as a limiting factor in immunocytochemistry (Cuello, 1983; Sternberger, 1979). For processing of Vibratome or frozen sections for light microscopy we routinely use Triton X-100 and pretreatment with ethanol to augment penetration, but omitting these only makes the staining weaker without affecting the staining pattern. The same was observed when tissue sections were soaked in 30% sucrose and frozen in liquid N_2 to further augment penetration of antibodies, or when sections were treated with aminoethanol or $NaBH_4$ to block free aldehyde groups and reduce double bonds in cross-links prior to processing. ($NaBH_4$ reduced staining intensity.)

In histopathology proteolytic enzymes are frequently used to partially digest sections of aldehyde-fixed tissue (Huang *et al.*, 1976; Brandtzaeg, 1982). In the case of some antigens this treatment has been found useful for recovering immunoreactivity lost on fixation with aldehyde. To avoid exposing C-terminal glutamate (see Section 8.1) we selected a proteolytic enzyme (trypsin) that does not cleave polypeptide chains at the carboxyl end of glutamate residues (Lehninger, 1975). Digestion of sections of perfusion-fixed rat brain by trypsin (1 mg/ml, 25°C, 15–45 min, followed by thorough rinsing) resulted in a dramatic change in the distribution of glutamate-like immunoreactivity: staining of cell bodies and dendrites was abolished throughout the brain while staining of neuropil was increased. In the hippocampal formation the latter assumed a laminar pattern (Fig. 1b) resembling that seen in slices fixed by immersion (Fig. 1c;

see Section 8.3). However, the cytological details were somewhat less distinct than in sections not treated with proteolytic enzymes. The stained structures appeared to be mainly nerve endings. This could be ascertained in the mossy fiber layer where the characteristic giant boutons were clearly stained.

According to Hardy *et al.* (1976), glutaraldehyde and amino acids form fixation complexes in which the amino acid residues are densely packed side by side irradiating from a pyridinium core formed by the amino groups and glutaraldehyde. Participation of ϵ-amino groups of lysine residues of proteins attaches these complexes to tissue proteins. Such a structure makes it possible for several glutamate molecules to be held tightly together in a characteristic structure and in a number sufficient to fill a pocket formed by the hypervariable region of the immunoglobulin molecule (see Section 8.1). However, it is conceivable that steric hinderance could ensue at sites of high glutamate concentration or high protein density. Such hindrance could be alleviated by proteolysis making the anchored glutamate–glutaraldehyde complexes more mobile. On the other hand, proteolysis may cause loss of material which could explain the reduced staining of glutamate-like immunoreactivity in perikarya and dendrites.

From the above considerations it seems possible that the glutaraldehyde concentration routinely used (5%) could be too high. Lowering of the content of glutaraldehyde in the fixative, however, has led only to reduction in the staining intensity and to no apparent change in the distribution of glutamate-like immunoreactivity.

A paradoxical inhibition of staining with the peroxidase–antiperoxidase method can occur at sites of very high concentration of antigen (Sternberger, 1979). This is interpreted as due to both active sites of the secondary antibody being occupied by reaction with the primary antibody, and can be obviated by diluting the primary antibody. We have invariably observed that progressive dilution of the antiglutamate serum leads to progressive reduction in staining intensity without a change in the staining pattern.

In conclusion, the results obtained indicate that in tissue fixed with glutaraldehyde by perfusion, the full immunoreactivity of the neuropil is not revealed at all sites due to steric hindrance and/or poor penetration of antibodies. This could apparently be alleviated by proteolytic pretreatment of the sections, which may act by creating a more open tissue structure, and allows glutamate-like immunoreactivity to be demonstrated in putative glutamatergic nerve endings. However, at the same time immunoreactivity is lost from cell bodies and stem dendrites of putative glutamatergic neurons. Clearly, further studies are required to establish the "true" distribution of glutamate-like immunoreactivity in perfusion-fixed tissue.

8.5. Postembedding Immunogold Labeling

The problems of penetration of antibodies and steric hindrance could perhaps be overcome by postembedding immunocytochemical techniques (Sternberger, 1979; Cuello, 1983), where the antibodies gain access only to antigenic determinants exposed on the surface of the tissue sections. This approach was tried in a collaborative study with P. Somogyi, K. Halasy, and J. Somogyi (Somogyi *et al.*, 1986). Anesthetized cats were perfusion-fixed with 2.5% glutaraldehyde and 1% paraformaldehyde in 0.1 M sodium phosphate buffer, and the tissue embedded in Durcupan and further processed according to procedure I of Somogyi and Hodgson (1985) using 15-nm colloidal gold particles coated with goat anti-rabbit IgG. The cerebellum was selected for initial studies, because this region contains a limited number of neuron classes with reasonably well-known transmitter identity and ultrastructural features allowing their processes to be identified in electron microscopic sections of normal material.

There was a clear concentration of glutamate-like immunoreactivity over putative glutamatergic boutons (Fig. 2), whereas GABA-like immunoreactivity was concentrated over putative GABAergic boutons. The absolute numbers of particles per square micrometer varied somewhat between the individual preparations, but the order of particle densities between the different categories of profiles was always the same. In a representative experiment (glutamate antiserum 13, diluted 1 : 500), the following particle densities were found [particles/μm^2 expressed as percent of the highest value $\pm$ S.E.M. (numbers of profiles recorded)]: mossy fiber terminals 100 $\pm$ 4 (25), parallel fiber terminals 72 $\pm$ 2 (156), granule cell dendritic digits 61 $\pm$ 3 (110), Purkinje cell dendritic shafts and spines 42 $\pm$ 2 (171), Golgi cell terminals 40 $\pm$ 2 (48), glial cell processes in molecular layer 19 $\pm$ 1 (125). Statistical analysis (Student's t test) showed that all the differences, except that between Golgi and Purkinje cell processes, were significant at the $p < 0.005$ level. However, it should be emphasized that the quantitative relationship between the particle density and the glutamate concentration in the tissue is unknown and perhaps complex and nonlinear. The values given can therefore not be used to derive values for the ratios of glutamate concentrations in the individual compartments. Absorption controls showed that the labeling was specific for glutamate (for details, see legend of Fig. 2).

These observations suggest that, at least in the cerebellar cortex, the concentration of endogenous glutamate is highest in the boutons of putative glutamatergic neurons (parallel and mossy fiber boutons). Furthermore, the dendrites of the parent cells of the parallel fibers (granule cells) have a higher density of labeling than the dendrites of putative GABAergic cells (Purkinje cells). In GABA-producing cells the level of glutamate may be kept low by glutamate decarboxylase. The level of glutamate-like immunoreactivity in other nonglutamatergic neurons remains to be investigated at the ultra-structural level.

The particle density over glial profiles was by far the lowest. This agrees with the apparently exclusive glial localization of glutamine synthetase (Norenberg and Martinez-Hernandez, 1979), which converts glutamate to glutamine, and with measurements in cultural cerebellar cells (Patel and Hunt, 1985).

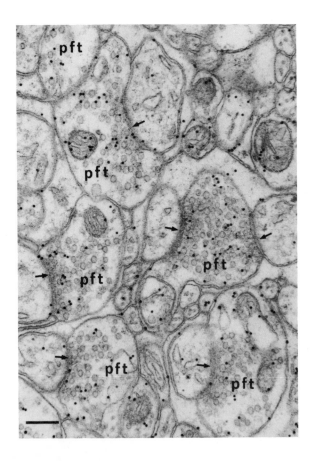

Figure 2. Glutamate-like immunoreactivity in the molecular layer of the cerebellar cortex as displayed electron microscopically by the postembedding immunogold method in a cat perfusion fixed with glutaraldehyde and paraformaldehyde. The labeling was concentrated over parallel fiber terminals (pft) compared to Purkinje cell dendritic spines (synapses marked with arrows) and glia. It was also highly concentrated over synaptic vesicles compared to cytosol (for interpretation of the latter finding, and for other details, see Section 8.5). Statistical analysis showed that the differences were significant ($p < 0.005$). The labeling was completely suppressed by solid-phase absorption of the serum with L-glutamate bound to glutaraldehyde-activated polyacrylamide gel beads, but not by absorption with similarly bound L-aspartate, L-glutamine, GABA, or glycine. Bar = 0.25 μm. (From Somogyi *et al.*, 1986.)

These quantitative results with the postembedding approach are consistent with our previous light microscopic observations in the cerebellum of perfusion-fixed rats (Storm-Mathisen and Ottersen, 1986), which showed that Purkinje cell bodies and dendritic shafts, as well as inter-neurons and glial processes in the molecular layer, were weakly stained compared to the interven-ing spaces occupied by the parallel fibers. They also agree with our light-microscopic observa-tions (unpublished) in immersion-fixed cerebellar slices showing strong glutamate-like immunoreactivity in terminals and axons of mossy fibers which was not clearly demonstrable in the perfusion-fixed material.

Recent results obtained by the postembedding immunogold method in the hippocampal formation suggest that the findings in the cerebellum have general validity: In ultrathin sections processed with the glutamate antiserum gold particles were enriched over putative glutamatergic terminals, such as the mossy fiber boutons and the smaller boutons making asymmetric contacts with dendritic spines in stratum radiatum (Ottersen O. P., in preparation; illustration in Cotman *et al.*, 1987). Various amino acids conjugated to brain macromolecules with glutaraldehyde and embedded in Durcupan together with the tissue were present in the same sections. While the glutamate conjugate was strongly labeled, the densities of gold particles over other amino acid conjugates were very low (about 2 orders of magnitude less) and similar to that over resin (Ottersen, 1987). Moreover, the labeling of test conjugates and tissue could be blocked by adding glutaraldehyde-treated (Ottersen *et al.*, 1986b) glutamate to the serum, whereas other glutaralde-hyde-treated amino acids did not have this effect. These data provide strong evidence that the labeling produced by the postembedding immunogold method in the conditions used does indeed represent tissue glutamate and indicate that this method may overcome the problems that make it difficult to fully reveal the tissue distribution of glutamate (see Sections 8.3 and 8.4).

A crucial question for the transmitter role of glutamate is the intraterminal distribution of the amino acid. We have previously reported that glutamate-like immunoreactivity may be concen-trated in synaptic vesicles (Storm-Mathisen *et al.*, 1983). These results were obtained on immer-sion-fixed hippocampal slices processed by the preembedding peroxidase–antiperoxidase meth-od. This approach is not optimal for the purpose: in spite of the use of Triton X-100, which is detrimental to the preservation of ultrastructure, penetration problems exist, and at this high level of resolution the size of the peroxidase–antiperoxidase complex and the distance between the enzyme and the site of precipitation of the final reaction product become significant. The postem-bedding immunogold method circumvents these problems (but may have others; see below).

Visual inspection strongly suggested that in preparations processed with the glutamate anti-body the immunogold particles were concentrated over areas enriched in synaptic vesicles as well as over mitochondria, rather than over other areas of the labeled boutons (Fig. 2). This notion was supported by a preliminary quantitative analysis in which the density of particles overlying synaptic vesicles was compared to that overlying the cytosol, the areas being measured by counting of grid points. Gold particles touching vesicles were recorded as belonging to vesicles. (This still may have caused underestimation, as the antibody complexes are sticking out from the surface of the particles.) Vesicles had 141 ± 20 particles/μm^2, while cytosol had 26 ± 5 (mean values $\pm$ S.E.M. for nine profiles from the preparation shown in Fig. 2, Wilcoxon signed rank test $p = 0.004$, volume ratio vesicles/cytosol 0.31 ± 0.04), suggesting that the concentration of glutamate in vesicles could be considerably higher than that in the cytosol. (No exact ratio can be given; see above about the unknown quantitative relation between particle density and glutamate concentration.)

This preliminary finding in prefusion-fixed material suggests that our previous observations on *in vitro* fixed slices processed with the peroxidase–antiperoxidase technique in the presence of Triton X-100 were valid, and supports the notion that in putative glutamatergic nerve endings, glutamate is indeed stored in synaptic vesicles *in vivo*. This notion also gains biochemical support from the demonstration that brain synaptic vesicles can accumulate glutamate in vitro (Naito and Ueda, 1983, 1985) and retain high concentrations of endogenous glutamate during purification (Riveros *et al.*, 1986). Nevertheless, when evaluating immunocytochemical results at this level of resolution, it is necessary to keep in mind that a small molecule such as glutamate could perhaps move during the process of fixation and might thereby become concentrated at sites offering favorable conditions for fixation, e.g., by virtue of the local concentration and composition of tissue protein. This problem can perhaps be approached by quick-freezing techniques and vapor-phase fixation.

8.6. Invertebrates

Some of the most compelling evidence for the transmitter role of glutamate has come from the study of excitatory motoneurons in crustacea (Freeman, 1976) and insects (Cull-Candy, 1976; Patlak *et al.*, 1979). It therefore seemed important to investigate the localization of glutamate immunoreactivity in such neurons. This has been done in locust and honeybee in collaboration with G. Bicker and S. Schäfer. Indeed, the characteristically shaped excitatory motoneurons of the locust metathoracic ganglion were strongly and selectively stained and their axons could be traced into the limb nerve, and to stained terminals in the muscles. Identified nonglutamatergic neurons were virtually unstained. The bee brain also contains putative glutamatergic neurons which are selectively immunoreactive for glutamate (Bicker *et al.*, 1987).

9. Excitatory Compounds Related to Glutamate

9.1. Aspartate

Several workers have produced antibodies to aspartate by an approach identical to (Ottersen and Storm-Mathisen, 1985; Storm-Mathisen *et al.*, 1986a; Saito *et al.*, 1986) or slightly different from (Campistron *et al.*, 1986) that introduced by us for glutamate (Storm-Mathisen *et al.*, 1983). The antibodies show high specificities and produce staining patterns partly similar to, but distinct from, that displayed by our glutamate antiserum. The possibilities exist that aspartate has a distinct transmitter role in a population of excitatory neurons (Nadler *et al.*, 1976), that it acts as a cotransmitter with glutamate in the same neurons (see Freeman, 1976), and that it has metabolic roles distinct from those of glutamate (cf. the high concentration of aspartate in apparently GABAergic neurons; Ottersen and Storm-Mathisen, 1985). The release of aspartate depends on the metabolic conditions (Chapter 10).

9.2. γ-Glutamyl-Glutamate

A monoclonal antibody has been raised against γ-glutamyl-glutamate coupled with glutaraldehyde (followed by $NaBH_4$) to hemocyanin of keyhole limpets (Madl *et al.*, 1976; Beitz *et al.*, 1986; Monaghan *et al.*, 1986). This antibody has been used to stain tissue fixed with carbodiimide and glutaraldehyde, the idea being that the former reagent causes some of the free glutamate in the tissue to form peptides, including γ-glutamyl-glutamate, and that this may occur preferentially at sites of high glutamate content. Clearly, the complexity of the reactions during fixation is no less in this case than during fixation with glutaraldehyde alone (see Section 8.1). The antibody to γ-glutamyl-glutamate yields a pattern of staining only partly overlapping with the one described by us for glutamate-like immunoreactivity in tissue perfusion-fixed with glutaraldehyde. The lack of nuclear staining is intriguing as the dipeptide, like glutamate, is expected to have access to the nucleoplasm.

9.3. N-Acetyl-Aspartyl-Glutamate

This modified dipeptide (NAAG) is present in brain at considerable concentrations and is a transmitter candidate (ffrench-Mullen *et al.*, 1985; Coyle *et al.*, 1986). Since the N-function is blocked, it cannot be fixed in the tissue by glutaraldehyde alone. Two groups have reported results with antibodies raised against carbodiimide-conjugated NAAG used in tissue fixed with carbodiimide and formaldehyde (Cangro *et al.*, 1985; Anderson *et al.*, 1986, 1987; Coyle *et al.*, 1986; Blakely *et al.*, 1987). Several other small peptides containing glutamate and/or aspartate are potential transmitter candidates (Luini *et al.*, 1984; Bernstein *et al.*, 1985) and worth localizing in brain by the immunocytochemical approach.

9.4. Sulfur-Containing Amino Acids

Cuénod *et al.* (1986) have shown that a series of sulfur-containing excitatory amino acids display Ca^{2+}-dependent depolarization-induced release from various brain regions; however, the quantities are much inferior to those of glutamate and aspartate. Monoclonal antibodies have been raised against conjugates of L-homocysteate, the most abundant of these compounds. Preliminary results indicate that it is localized, inter alia, in nerve endings in the superficial layers of the cerebral cortex and in the striatum, perhaps derived from neurons in the ''nonspecific'' thalamic nuclei (Cuénod *et al.*, 1986) which transport D-aspartate (see Section 10.4).

9.5. Quinolinic Acid

This excitatory substance is present in brain and may act as an endogenous excitotoxin. However, the glial localization of the enzymes responsible for its formation and breakdown suggests that it is not a neurotransmitter (Schwarcz *et al.*, 1986; Foster *et al.*, 1985; review: Stone and Connick, 1985).

10. Putative Glutamatergic Pathways

We have recently presented a review in tabular form of putative glutamatergic nerve pathways in the central nervous system of vertebrates (Ottersen and Storm-Mathisen, 1986). The pathways are surveyed below and depicted schematically in Figs. 3–6.

10.1. Projections from Neocortex

The most conspicuous of the brain pathways for which glutamate has been proposed as transmitter are the various corticocortical and corticofugal projections (Fig. 3). By means of

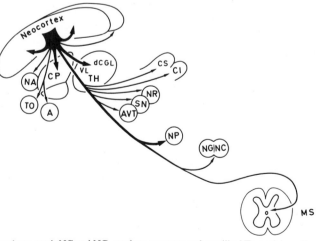

Figure 3. Efferent and intrinsic putative glutamatergic nerve pathways of neocortex. The thicknesses of arrows roughly indicate the densities of the projections. (This summary diagram and those in the following figures should not be considered complete.) For literature references see text (Section 10.1). Abbreviations: A, amygdala; AVT, area ventralis tegmenti mesencephali; CI and CS, collicus inferior and superior; CP, caudatoputamen; dCGL, dorsal part of corpus geniculatum laterale; MS, medulla spinalis; NA, nucleus accumbens septi; NC and NG, nucleus cuneatus and gracilis; NP, nuclei pontis; NR, nucleus ruber; SN, substantia nigra; TH, thalamus; TO, tuberculum olfactorium; VL, nucleus ventrolateralis of thalamus.

denervation experiments, high-affinity Na+-dependent uptake of glutamate (or aspartate; see Section 3) (Divac et al., 1977; McGeer et al., 1977; Fonnum et al., 1981a,b; Walaas, 1981; Young et al., 1981; Carter, 1982; Kerkerian et al., 1983) as well as endogenous contents of glutamate (Kim et al., 1977; Fonnum et al., 1981a; Druce et al., 1982; Hassler et al., Engelsen and Fonnum, 1983; Sandberg et al., 1985) have been localized to cortical afferents to the caudatoputamen. These results have been corroborated by retrograde tracing with D-[3H]aspartate (Streit, 1980), showing that the pyramidal cells of origin are localized mainly in layer V. The projection appears to be most dense from the frontal cortex. Depolarization-induced, Ca^{2+}-dependent release of glutamate has also been demonstrated in this pathway, endogenously present (Rowlands and Roberts, 1980; Druce et al., 1982; Roberts et al., 1982; Girault et al., 1986) or formed from precursor (Reubi and Cuénod, 1979; Godukhin et al., 1980). It should be noted that there is also some evidence for aspartate as transmitter in this pathway (Reubi et al., 1980; Fonnum et al., 1981a; Druce et al., 1982).

Evidence has been obtained by similar methods (chiefly biochemical recording of high-affinity uptake and content, and of axonal transport of D-[3H]aspartate) that glutamate is associated also with cortical projections to other target sites: nucleus accumbens (Walaas, 1981; Christie et al., 1985b), tuberculum olfactorium (Walker and Fonnum, 1983b), amygdala (Fischer et al., 1982; Walker and Fonnum, 1983a; Ottersen et al., 1986a), thalamus (Fonnum et al., 1981a,b; Walker and Fonnum, 1983a) and parts of it (dorsal subdivision of the corpus geniculatum laterale: Lund Karlsen and Fonnum, 1978; Baughman and Gilbert, 1980, 1981; Kvale and Fonnum, 1983; Fosse et al., 1984) (ventrolateral thalamic nucleus: Bromberg et al., 1981; Young et al., Kerkerian et al., 1983) (centromedian/parafascicular nuclei: Wiklund and Cuénod, 1984), superior colliculus (Lund Karlsen and Fonnum, 1978; Fonnum et al., 1979; Kvale and Fonnum, 1983; Fosse et al., 1984; Matute et al., 1984), inferior colliculus (Adams and Wenthold, 1979), ventral tegmental area (Christie et al., 1985a), red nucleus (Bromberg et al., 1981; Young et al., 1981; Kerkerian et al., 1983), substantia nigra (Streit, 1980; Fonnum et al., 1981a,b; Carter, 1982; Kerkerian et al., 1983; Kornhuber et al., 1984; Abarca and Bustos, 1985), pontine nuclei (Thangnipon and Storm-Mathisen, 1981; Young et al., 1981; Thangnipon et al., 1983), gracile and cuneate nuclei (Rustioni and Cuénod, 1982), contralateral spinal cord (Fagg et al., 1978; Young et al., 1981; Potashner and Tran, 1985), and ipsilateral and contralateral parts of the neocortex (Streit, 1980; Baughman and Gilbert, 1981; Fonnum et al., 1981a,b; Fischer et al., 1982; Ottersen et al., 1983; Hicks et al., 1985).

10.2. Projections in the Hippocampal Region

The intrinsic putative glutamatergic connections of the hippocampal formation are summarized in Fig. 4, while efferents to other regions are depicted in Fig. 5a. High-affinity glutamate

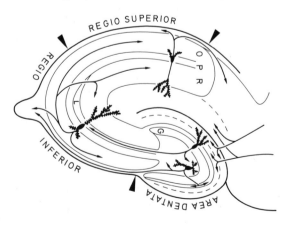

Figure 4. Afferent, intrinsic, and efferent putative glutamatergic connections of the hippocampal formation. Medial and lateral perforant path fibers project from area entorhinalis (area 28) to different laminae of area dentata and hippocampus. Granular cells (G) of area dentata project to stratum lucidum (L) of hippocampus regio inferior (= CA3). Pyramidal cells (P) of CA3 project bilaterally to hippocampus strata oriens (O) and radiatum (R) and to lateral septum. Modified pyramids of the dentate hilus (= CA4) project bilaterally to the inner zone of the dentate stratum moleculare. For references see text (Section 10.2).

uptake recorded by biochemical measurements or autoradiography after degenerations and in normal animals has been shown to be present in the perforant path from the entorhinal area to the dentate area, in the mossy fibers from dentate granule cells to CA3, in contralaterally and ipsilaterally (including Schaffer collaterals) projecting axons of CA3 and CA4 pyramidal cells, and in axons projecting from CA1 to the subiculum (Nadler et al., 1976; Storm-Mathisen, 1977, 1981, 1982; Fonnum and Walaas, 1978; Storm-Mathisen and Iversen, 1979; Heggli et al., 1981; Storm-Mathisen and Wold, 1981; Taxt and Storm-Mathisen, 1984). These connections have also been traced by axonal transport of D-[³H]aspartate (Storm-Mathisen and Wold, 1981; Fischer et al., 1982c, 1986a,b), and for some of them there is evidence from biochemical measurements in lesioned animals for enrichment of endogenous glutamate (Nadler et al., 1978; Nadler and Smith, 1981; Storm-Mathisen, 1978; Nitsch et al., 1979a,b). The terminals of the fibers are rich in glutamate-like immunoreactivity, as observed in slice preparations (see Section 8.3), and so are their parent cell bodies (see Section 8.4). Ca^{2+}-dependent release of endogenous or labeled glutamate or D-[³H]aspartate after various types of stimulation has been demonstrated for several of these systems (Crawford and Connor, 1973; Nadler et al., 1976, 1978; Hamberger et al., 1978, 1979; Malthe-Sørenssen et al., 1979; Wieraszko and Lynch, 1979; Skrede and Malthe-Sørenssen, 1981a,b; Spencer et al., 1981; Dolphin et al., 1982; Bliss et al., 1986).

Results on uptake, contents, and axonal transport also implicate glutamate in efferents (Fig. 5a) from hippocampus to the entorhinal area (Nitsch et al., 1979a), from CA1 and subiculum to the amygdala (Fischer et al., 1982a, 1986a; Ottersen et al., 1986a), from subiculum to the accumbens nucleus, the interstitial nucleus of the stria terminalis, mammillary body, and mediobasal hypothalamus and from CA3 to the lateral septum (Storm-Mathisen and Woxen Opsahl, 1978; Nitsch et al., 1979a; Zaczek et al., 1979; Walaas and Fonnum, 1979, 1980; Walaas, 1981), and from entorhinal area to the amygdala (Fischer et al., 1982a; Walker and Fonnum, 1983a; Ottersen et al., 1986a). Ca^{2+}-dependent release of D-[³H]aspartate has been demonstrated in septal slices after stimulation of fibers from hippocampus (Malthe-Sørenssen et al., 1980).

10.3. Projections from Allocortical Areas Other Than Hippocampus

The putative glutamatergic pathways of allocortical areas other than the hippocampal formation are summarized in Fig. 5b. There is a body of evidence that the centripetal fibers from the olfactory bulb are enriched in glutamate (Harvey et al., 1975; Godfrey et al., 1980; Scholfield et al., 1983; Sandberg et al., 1984) and may release this amino acid Ca^{2+}-dependently on stimulation (Bradford and Richards, 1976; Yamamoto and Matsui, 1976). There is similar evidence for aspartate (Collins et al., 1981; Collins, 1984, 1987). The parent cell bodies in the olfactory bulb

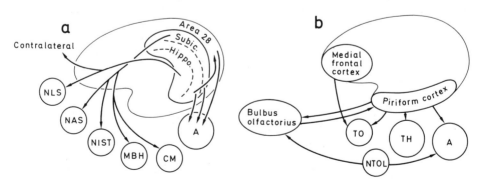

Figure 5. Putative glutamatergic projections from allocortex: (a) hippocampal formation, (b) other parts. For references see text (Section 10.2 and 10.3). Abbreviations for target areas: CM, corpus mammillare; MBH, mediobasal hypothalamus; NAS, nucleus accumbens septi; NIST, nucleus interstitialis striae terminalis; NLS, nucleus lateralis septi; NTOL, nucleus tractus olfactorii lateralis; for other abbreviations, see Fig. 3.

are rich in glutamate-like (Ottersen and Storm-Mathisen, 1984a,b) and aspartate-like (Saito *et al.*, 1986; Ottersen and Storm-Mathisen, unpublished observations) immunoreactivities. However, neither high-affinity uptake nor retrograde transport of the amino acids has been demonstrated in this system. It has recently been suggested that NAAG is the actual transmitter of the lateral olfactory tract (ffrench-Mullen *et al.*, 1985; Anderson *et al.*, 1986; Blakely *et al.*, 1987).

Axonal transport of D-[³H]aspartate has been demonstrated in efferents to the olfactory bulb from the nucleus of the lateral olfactory tract (Watanabe and Kawana, 1984) and from layer III of the latter nucleus to the amygdala (Fischer *et al.*, 1982a; Ottersen *et al.*, 1986a). There is evidence from various techniques for glutamatergic efferents from the piriform cortex to the olfactory tuberculum, olfactory bulb, thalamus, and amygdala (Fonnum *et al.*, 1981b; Fischer *et al.*, 1982a; Walker and Fonnum, 1983a; Watanabe and Kawana, 1984; Ottersen *et al.*, 1986a).

10.4. Projections from Subcortical Structures

Subcortical putative glutamatergic pathways are summarized in Fig. 6. In submammalian species there is evidence from studies on uptake (Henke *et al.*, 1976; Bondy and Purdy, 1977), axonal transport (Beaudet *et al.*, 1981), contents (Yates and Roberts, 1974; Fonnum and Henke, 1982), and release (Čanžek *et al.*, 1981) that glutamate may have a transmitter role in centripetal fibers from retina. If such fibers exist in mammals, they appear to be rare. Recent results suggest that NAAG may be a transmitter in these fibres (Anderson *et al.*, 1987).

There is evidence mainly from axonal transport studies for the association of an excitatory amino acid with fibers from the anterior olfactory nucleus to the olfactory bulb (Watanabe and Kawana, 1984), from the accumbens nucleus and caudatoputamen to the substantia nigra (Streit, 1980) (for the latter, aspartate may be involved; see Taniyama *et al.*, 1980; Korf and Venema,

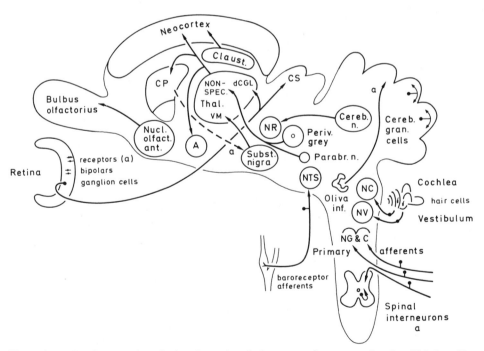

Figure 6. Putative glutamatergic projections from subcortical structures. Some connections for which the evidence is mainly in favor of aspartate are included (marked "a"). For references see text (Section 10.4). Abbreviations for target areas: NC, nuclei cochleares; NONSPEC., "nonspecific" thalamic nuclei; NTS, nucleus tractus solitarii; NV, nuclei vestibulares; VM, nucleus ventromedialis of thalamus; for other abbreviations, see Fig. 3.

1983), from "nonspecific" thalamic nuclei to the caudatoputamen (Streit, 1980), neocortex (Ottersen *et al.*, 1983), and amygdala (Fischer *et al.*, 1982a; Ottersen *et al.*, 1986a), from the claustrum to the neocortex (Fischer *et al.*, 1982b), from the substantia nigra to the ventromedial nucleus of the thalamus (Fletcher *et al.*, 1979), and from several sites in the mesencephalon and pons to the centromedian/parafascicular nuclei of the thalamus (Wiklund and Cuénod, 1984). Cerebellar mossy fibers, the main origin of which is the pontine nuclei, have recently been shown to be enriched in glutamate-like immunoreactivity (Somogyi *et al.*, 1986; see Section 8.5).

Several categories of primary afferents have been suggested to be glutamatergic based on studies on uptake and axonal transport and in some cases on endogenous contents and release: vestibular afferents (Cuénod *et al.*, 1982; Demêmes *et al.*, 1984; Raymond *et al.*, 1985), cochlear afferents (Wenthold and Gulley, 1977, 1978; Wenthold, 1978, 1979; Kane, 1979; Čanžek and Reubi, 1980; Hansson *et al.*, 1980; Oliver *et al.*, 1983; Potashner, 1983), vagal afferents (Talman *et al.*, 1980; Perrone, 1981; Reis *et al.*, 1981; Granata and Reis, 1983), and trigeminal and spinal nerve afferents (Roberts, 1974; Johnston, 1976; Roberts and Hill, 1978; Cuénod *et al.*, 1982; Hunt, 1983; Potashner and Tran, 1985; Potashner and Dymczyk, 1986; Wanaka *et al.*, 1987). For the best documented cases (auditory and baroreceptor afferents) the evidence is now rather strong. Recently NAAG has been demonstrated in a subpopulation of spinal ganglion cells (Cangro *et al.*, 1987).

In addition, there is evidence from recording of axonal transport of D-[³H]aspartate that glutamate or another dicarboxylic amino acid is associated with the granule cell/parallel fiber system in the cochlear nucleus (Oliver *et al.*, 1983). In spinal interneurons (Davidoff *et al.*, 1967; Homma *et al.*, 1979; Rustioni and Cuénod, 1982) and in the olivo-cerebellar climbing fiber system (Nadi *et al.*, 1977; McBride *et al.*, 1978; Rea *et al.*, 1980; Künzle and Wiklund, 1982; Wiklund *et al.*, 1982, 1984; Toggenburger *et al.*, 1983; Campistron *et al.*, 1986) the evidence is in favor of aspartate rather than glutamate.

Studies on uptake, contents, and release associate glutamate with the granule cell/parallel fiber system (Valcana *et al.*, 1972; Young *et al.*, 1974; McBride *et al.*, 1976a,b; Hudson *et al.*, 1976; Rea and McBride, 1978; Roffler-Tarlov and Sidman, 1978; Sandoval and Cotman, 1978; Rohde *et al.*, 1979; Nieoullon and Dusticier, 1981; Rea *et al.*, 1981; Roffler-Tarlov and Turey, 1982; Nieoullon *et al.*, 1984). Recently, these studies have been confirmed by postembedding demonstrations of glutamate-like immunoreactivity at the electron microscopic level (Somogyi *et al.*, 1986; see Section 8.5).

From uptake studies it appears that cells in the cerebellar nuclei may project glutamatergic fibers to the ventrolateral nucleus of the thalamus and to the red nucleus (Nieoullon and Dusticier, 1981; Nieoullon *et al.*, 1984).

11. Summary

Markers useful for tracing of putative glutamatergic neurons are endogenous content, Ca^{2+}-dependent release, and high-affinity Na^+-dependent uptake of the amino acid. These markers can be localized by means of biochemical micro methods, autoradiography, and immunocytochemistry, and assigned to specific neuronal pathways through axonal transport, effects of denervation or electrical stimulation, or by their characteristic positions. *In vivo* uptake and subsequent retrograde axonal transport of D-[³H]aspartate has proved particularly useful for the study of potentially glutamatergic pathways. The approach has recently been improved by implanting the tracer absorbed in agarose particles packed into the tip of a micropipette. This permits gradual release of the tracer, reduces spread, and allows even local neurons to be studied.

Endogenous glutamate and other free amino acids can be fixed in the tissue by glutaraldehyde and demonstrated by means of highly specific antibodies, which detect the fixation products. While GABA-ergic neurons are effectively traced in this way, interpretation of staining for glutamate is complicated by the metabolic role of this amino acid. Under certain conditions glutamatelike immunoreactivity can be shown to be selectively concentrated in the nerve endings of putative glutamatergic neurons. For mammalian brain this has been achieved (1) in incubated hippocampal slices where the localization of glutamatelike immunoreactivity mimics that of exogenous [^{3}H]glutamate accumulated by the high-affinity Na$^+$-dependent process, (2) in sections of perfusion-fixed brain after partial proteolysis with trypsin (which may act by reducing steric hindrance and increasing antibody permeability), (3) in ultrathin sections of Durcupan embedded perfusion-fixed brain processed for electron microscopy by the post-embedding immunogold method. Results with the latter method indicate that glutamate may indeed be concentrated in synaptic vesicles.

The methods mentioned are being used to pointing out putative glutamatergic pathways in the brain. At present these include cortico-cortical and corticofugal systems, cerebellar granular cells and major afferent systems. However, in most cases definite proof for the transmitter identity is pending. Other endogenous excitatory compounds with possible transmitter role are also being localized.

ACKNOWLEDGMENTS. This work was supported by the Norwegian Research Council for Science and the Humanities, the Norwegian Council on Cardiovascular Disease, the Norwegian Society for Fighting Cancer, and the Royal Norwegian Academy of Sciences. We are grateful to A. Holter, T. Eliassen, and I. Fridstrøm for secretarial assistance.

References

Abarca, J., and Bustos, G., 1985, Release of D-[^{3}H]aspartic acid from the rat substantia nigra: Effect of veratridine-evoked depolarization and cortical ablation, *Neurochem. Int.* **7**:229–236.

Abdul-Ghani, A.-S., Coutinho-Netto, J., and Bradford, H. F., 1981, In vivo superfusion methods and the release of glutamate, in: *Glutamate: Transmitter in the Central Nervous System* (P. J. Roberts, J. Storm-Mathisen, and G. A. R. Johnston, eds.), John Wiley & Sons, Chichester, pp. 155–203.

Adams, J. C., and Wenthold, R. J., 1979, Distribution of putative amino acid transmitters, choline acetyltransferase and glutamate decarboxylase in the inferior colliculus, *Neuroscience* **4**:1947–1951.

Altschuler, R. A., Neises, G. R., Harmison, G. G., Wenthold, R. J., and Fex, J., 1981, Immunocytochemical localization of aspartate aminotransferase immunoreactivity in cochlear nucleus of the guinea pig, *Proc. Natl. Acad. Sci. USA* **78**:6553–6557.

Altschuler, R. A., Mosinger, J. L., Harmison, G. G., Parakkal, M. H., and Wenthold, R. J., 1982, Aspartate aminotransferase-like immunoreactivity as a marker for aspartate/glutamate in guinea pig photoreceptors, *Nature* **298**:657–659.

Altschuler, R. A., Wenthold, R. J., Schwartz, A. M., Haser, W. G., Curthoys, N. P., Parakkal, M., and Fex, J., 1984, Immunocytochemical localization of glutaminase-like immunoreactivity in the auditory nerve, *Brain Res.* **291**:173–178.

Altschuler, R. A., Monaghan, D. T., Haser, W. G., Wenthold, R. J., Curthoys, N. P., and Cotman, W., 1985, Immunocytochemical localization of glutaminase-like and aspartate aminotransferase-like immunoreactivities in the rat and guinea pig hippocampus, *Brain Res.* **330**:225–233.

Andersen, P., Silfvenius, H., Sundberg, S. H., and Sveen, O., 1980, A comparison of distal and proximal dendritic synapses on CA1 pyramids in guinea-pig hippocampal slices *in vitro*, *J. Physiol. (London)* **307**:273–299.

Anderson, K. J., Monaghan, D. T., Cangro, C. B., Namboodiri, M. A. A., Neale, J. H., and Cotman, C. W., 1986, Localization of N-acetylaspartyl-glutamate-like immunoreactivity in selected areas of the brain, *Neurosci. Lett.* **72**:14–20.

Anderson, K. J., Borja, M. A., Cotman, C. W., Namboodiri, M. A. A., and Neale, J. H., 1987, N-acetylaspartylglutamate identified in the rat retinal ganglion cells and their projections in the brain, *Brain Res.* **411**:172–177.

Balázs, R., Patel, A. J., and Richter, D., 1973, Metabolic compartments in the brain: Their properties and relation to morphological structures, in: *Metabolic Compartmentation in the Brain* (R. Balázs and J. E. Cremer, eds.), Macmillan, London, pp. 167–184.

Balcar, V. J., and Johnston, G. A. R., 1972, The structural specificity of the high affinity uptake of L-glutamate and L-aspartate by rat brain slices, *J. Neurochem.* **19**:2657–2666.

Balcom, G. J., Lenox, R. H., and Meyerhoff, J. L., 1976, Regional glutamate levels in rat brain determined after microwave fixation, *J. Neurochem.* **26**:423–425.

Baughman, R. W., and Gilbert, C. D., 1980, Aspartate and glutamate as possible neurotransmitters of cells in layer 6 of the visual cortex, *Nature* **287**:848–850.

Baughman, R. W., and Gilbert, C. D., 1981, Aspartate and glutamate as possible neurotransmitters in the visual cortex, *J. Neurosci.* **1**:427–439.

Beart, P. M., 1976, An evaluation of L-glutamate as the transmitter released from optic nerve terminals of the pigeon, *Brain Res.* **110**:99–114.

Beaudet, A., Burkhalter, A., Reubi, J.-C., and Cuénod, M., 1981, Selective bidirectional transport of [3H]D-aspartate in the pigeon retinotectal pathway, *Neuroscience* **6**:2021–2034.

Beitz, A. J., Larson, A. A., Monaghan, P., Altschuler, R. A., Mullett, M. M., and Madl, J. E., 1986, Immunohistochemical localization of glutamate, glutaminase and aspartate aminotransferase in neurons of the pontine nuclei of the rat, *Neuroscience* **17**:741–753.

Benjamin, A. M., and Quastel, J. H., 1974, Fate of L-glutamate in the brain, *J. Neurochem.* **23**:457–464.

Berger, S. J., Carter, J. G., and Lowry, O. H., 1977, The distribution of glycine, GABA, glutamate and aspartate in rabbit spinal cord, cerebellum and hippocampus, *J. Neurochem.* **28**:149–158.

Berl, S., Clarke, D. D., and Schneider, D. (eds.), 1975, *Metabolic Compartmentation and Neurotransmission: Relation to Brain Structure and Function*. Plenum Press, New York.

Bernstein, J., Fisher, R. S., Zaczek, R., and Coyle, J., 1985, Dipeptides of glutamate and aspartate may be endogenous neuroexcitants in the rat hippocampal slice, *J. Neurosci.* **5**:1429–1433.

Bicker, G., Schäfer, S., Ottersen, O. P., and Storm-Mathisen, J., 1987, Glutamate-like immunoreactivity in identified neuronal populations of insect nervous systems, *J. Neurosci.* (in press).

Blakely, R. D., Ory-Lavollée, L., Grzanna, R., Koller, K. J., and Coyle, J. T., 1987, Selective immunocytochemical staining of mitral cells in rat olfactory bulb with affinity purified antibodies against N-acetyl-aspartyl-glutamate, *Brain Res.* **402**:373–378.

Bliss, T. V. P., Douglas, R. M., Errington, M. L., and Lynch, M. A., 1986, Correlation between long-term potentiation and release of endogenous amino acids from dentate gyrus of anaesthetized rats, *J. Physiol. (London)* **377**:391–408.

Bolz, J., Thier, P., and Brecha, N., 1985, Localization of aspartate aminotransferase and cytochrome oxidase in the cat retina, *Neurosci. Lett.* **53**:315–320.

Bondy, S. C., and Purdy, J. L., 1977, Putative neurotransmitters of the avian visual pathways, *Brain Res.* **119**:417–426.

Bradford, H. F., and Richards, C. D., 1976, Specific release of endogenous glutamate from piriform cortex stimulated in vitro, *Brain Res.* **105**:168–172.

Bradford, H. F., Ward, H. K., and Thomas, A. J., 1978, Glutamine—A major substrate for nerve endings, *J. Neurochem.* **30**:1453–1459.

Brandtzaeg, P., 1982, Tissue preparation methods for immunohistochemistry, in: *Techniques in Immunocytochemistry* (G. R. Bullock and P. Petrusz, eds.), Academic Press, New York, pp. 1–75.

Bromberg, M. B., Penney, J. B., Jr., Stephenson, B. S., and Young, A. B., 1981, Evidence for glutamate as the neurotransmitter of corticothalamic and corticorubral pathways, *Brain Res.* **215**:369–374.

Campistron, G., Buijs, R. M., and Geffard, M., 1986, Specific antibodies against aspartate and their immunocytochemical application in the rat brain, *Brain Res.* **365**:179–184.

Cangro, C. B., Garrison, D. E., Luongo, P. A., Truckenmiller, M. E., Namboodiri, M. A. A., and Neale, J. H., 1985, First immunohistochemical demonstration of N-acetyl-aspartyl-glutamate in specific neurons, *Soc. Neurosci. Abstr.* **11**:108.

Cangro, C. B., Namboodiri, M. A. A., Sklar, L. A., and Neale, J. H., 1987, Biosynthesis and immunohistochemistry of *N*-acetylaspartylglutamate in spinal sensory ganglia, *J. Neurosci.* (in press).

Čanžek, V., and Reubi, J. C., 1980, The effect of cochlear nerve lesion on the release of glutamate, aspartate and GABA from cat cochlear nucleus in vitro, *Exp. Brain Res.* **38**:437–441.

Čanžek, V., Wolfensberger, M., Amsler, U., and Cuénod, M., 1981, In vivo release of glutamate and aspartate following optic nerve stimulation, *Nature* **293**:572–574.

Carter, C. J., 1982, Topographical distribution of possible glutamatergic pathways from the frontal cortex to the striatum and substantia nigra in rats, *Neuropharmacology* **21**:379–383.

Christie, M. J., Bridge, S., James, L. B., and Beart, P. M., 1985a, Excitotoxin lesions suggest an aspartatergic projection from rat medial prefrontal cortex to ventral tegmental area, *Brain Res.* **333**:169–172.

Christie, M. J., James, L. B., and Beart, P. M., 1985b, An excitant amino acid projection from the medial prefrontal cortext to the anterior part of nucleus accumbens in the rat, *J. Neurochem.* **45**:477–482.

Collins, G. G. S., 1984, Amino acid transmitter candidates in various regions of the primary olfactory cortex following bulbectomy, *Brain Res.* **296**:145–147.

Collins, G. G. S., 1986, Excitatory amino acids as transmitters in the olfactory system, in: *Excitatory Amino Acids* (P. J. Roberts, J. Storm-Mathisen, and H. F. Bradford, eds.), Macmillan, London, pp. 131–142.

Collins, G. G. S., Anson, J., and Probett, G. A., 1981, Patterns of endogenous amino acid release from slices of rat and guinea-pig olfactory cortex, *Brain Res.* **204:**103–120.

Cotman, C. W., and Nadler, J. V., 1981, Glutamate and aspartate as hippocampal transmitters: Biochemical and pharmacological evidence, in: *Glutamate: Transmitter in the Central Nervous System* (P. J. Roberts, J. Storm-Mathisen, and G. A. R. Johnston, eds.), John Wiley & Sons, Chichester, pp. 117–154.

Cotman, C. W., Monaghan, D. T., Ottersen, O. P., and Storm-Mathisen, J., 1987, Anatomical organization of excitatory amino acid receptors and their pathways, *Trends Neurosci.* **10:**273–280.

Coyle, J. T., Blakely, R., Zaczek, R., Koller, K., Abreo, M., Ory-Lavollée, L., Fisher, R., ffrench-Mullen, J. M., and Carpenter, D. O., 1986, Acidic peptides in brain: Do they act at putative glutamatergic synapses? in: *Excitatory Amino Acids and Epilepsy* (R. Schwarcz and Y. Ben-Ari, eds.), Plenum Press, New York, pp. 375–384.

Crawford, I. L., and Connor, J. D., 1973, Localization and release of glutamic acid in relation to the hippocampal mossy fibre pathway, *Nature* **244:**442–443.

Cuello, A. C. (ed.), 1983, *Immunohistochemistry,* Vol. 3, Wiley, New York.

Cuénod, M., Beaudet, A., Čanžek, V., Streit, P., and Reubi, J.-C., 1981, Glutamatergic pathways in the pigeon and the rat brain, in: *Advances in Biochemical Psychopharmacology,* Vol. 27 (G. Di Chiara and G. L. Gessa, eds.), Raven Press, New York, pp. 57–68.

Cuénod, M., Bagnoli, P., Beaudet, A., Rustioni, A., Wiklund, L., and Streit, P., 1982, Transmitter specific retrograde labeling of neurons, in: *Cytochemical Methods in Neuroanatomy* (V. Chan-Palay and S. L. Palay, eds.), Liss, New York, pp. 17–44.

Cuénod, M., Do, K. Q., Herrling, P. L., Turski, W. A., Matute, C., and Streit, P., 1986, Homocysteic acid, an endogenous agonist of NMDA-receptor: Release, neuroactivity and localization, in: *Excitatory Amino Acids and Epilepsy* (R. Schwarcz and Y. Ben-Ari, eds.), Plenum Press, New York, pp. 253–262.

Cull-Candy, S. G., 1976, Two types of extrajunctional L-glutamate receptors in locust muscle fibres, *J. Physiol. (London)* **255:**449–464.

Davidoff, R. A., Graham, L. T., Jr., Shank, R. P., Werman, R., and Aprison, M. H., 1967, Changes in amino acid concentrations associated with loss of spinal interneurons, *J. Neurochem.* **14:**1025–1031.

Davies, L. P., and Johnston, G. A. R., 1976, Uptake and release of D- and L-aspartate by rat brain slices, *J. Neurochem.* **26:**1007–1014.

De Belleroche, J. S., and Bradford, H. F., 1977, On the site of origin of transmitter amino acids released by depolarization of nerve terminals in vitro, *J. Neurochem.* **29:**335–343.

Demêmes, D., Raymond, J., and Sans, A., 1984, Selective retrograde labeling of neurons of the cat vestibular ganglion with [³H]D-aspartate, *Brain Res.* **304:**188–191.

Divac, I., Fonnum, F., and Storm-Mathisen, J., 1977, High affinity uptake of glutamate in terminals of corticostriatal axons, *Nature* **266:**377–378.

Dolphin, A. C., Errington, M. L., and Bliss, T. V. P., 1982, Long-term potentiation of the perforant path in vivo is associated with increased glutamate release, *Nature* **297:**496–498.

Drejer, J., Larson, O. M., and Schousboe, A., 1982, Characterization of L-glutamate uptake into and release from astrocytes and neurones cultured from different brain regions, *Exp. Brain Res.* **47:**259–269.

Druce, D., Peterson, D., De Belleroche, J., and Bradford, H. F., 1982, Differential amino acid neurotransmitter release in rat neostriatum following lesioning of the cortico-striatal pathway, *Brain Res.* **247:**303–307.

Duggan, A. W., and Hendry, I. A., 1986, Laminar localization of the sites of release of immunoreactive substance P in the dorsal horn with antibody-coated microelectrodes, *Neurosci. Lett.* **68:**134–140.

Ehinger, B., 1981, [³H]-D-Aspartate accumulation in the retina of pigeon, guinea-pig and rabbit, *Exp. Eye Res.* **33:**381–391.

Engelsen, B., and Fonnum, F., 1983, Effects of hypoglycemia on the transmitter pool and the metabolic pool of glutamate in rat brain, *Neurosci. Lett.* **42:**317–322.

Fagg, G. E., and Foster, A. C., 1983, Amino acid neurotransmitters and their pathways in the mammalian central nervous system, *Neuroscience* **9:**701–719.

Fagg, G. E., Jordan, C. C., and Webster, R. A., 1978, Descending fibre-mediated release of endogenous glutamate from the perfused cat spinal cord *in vivo, Brain Res.* **158:**159–170.

ffrench-Mullen, J. M. H., Koller, K., Zaczek, R., Coyle, J. T., Hori, N., and Carpenter, D. O., 1985, N-Acetylaspartylglutamate: Possible role as the neurotransmitter of the lateral olfactory tract, *Proc. Natl. Acad. Sci. USA* **82:**3897–3900.

Fischer, B. O., Ottersen, O. P., and Storm-Mathisen, J., 1982a, Labelling of amygdalopetal and amygdalofugal projections after intra-amygdaloid injections of tritiated D-aspartate, *Neuroscience* **7**(Suppl.):S69.

Fischer, B. O., Ottersen, O. P., and Storm-Mathisen, J., 1982b, Axonal transport of D-[³H]aspartate in the claustro-cortical projection, *Neuroscience* **7**(Suppl.):S69.

Fischer, B. O., Ottersen, O. P., and Storm-Mathisen, J., 1982c, Anterograde and retrograde axonal transport of D-[³H]aspartate (D-Asp) in hippocampal excitatory neurones, *Neuroscience* **7**(Suppl.):S68.

Fischer, B. O., Ottersen, O. P., and Storm-Mathisen, J., 1986a, Implantation of D-[³H]aspartate loaded gel particles permits restricted uptake sites for transmitter-selective axonal transport, *Exp. Brain Res.* **63**:620–626.

Fischer, B. O., Storm-Mathisen, J., and Ottersen, O. P., 1986b, Hippocampal excitatory neurons: Anterograde and retrograde axonal transport of D-[³H]aspartate, in: *Excitatory Amino Acids* (P. J. Roberts, J. Storm-Mathisen, and H. F. Bradford, eds.), Macmillan, London, pp. 442–443.

Fletcher, A., James, T. A., Kilpatrick, I. C., MacLeod, N. K., and Starr, M. S., 1979, Neurochemical and electrophysiological evidence for GABAergic and glutamatergic nigro-thalamic neurons, *Neurosci. Lett. (Suppl.)* **3**:222.

Fonnum, F., 1984, Glutamate: A neurotransmitter in mammalian brain, *J. Neurochem.* **42**:1–11.

Fonnum, F., and Henke, H., 1982, The topographical distribution of alanine, aspartate, γ-aminobutyric acid, glutamate, glutamine, and glycine in the pigeon optic tectum and the effect of retinal ablation, *J. Neurochem.* **38**:1130–1134.

Fonnum, F., and Walaas, I., 1978, The effect of intrahippocampal kainic acid injections and surgical lesions on neurotransmitters in hippocampus and septum, *J. Neurochem.* **31**:1173–1181.

Fonnum, F., Lund Karlsen, R., Malthe-Sørenssen, D., Skrede, K. K., and Walaas, I., 1979, Localization of neurotransmitters, particularly glutamate, in hippocampus, septum, nucleus accumbens and superior colliculus, *Prog. Brain Res.* **51**:167–192.

Fonnum, F., Storm-Mathisen, J., and Divac, I., 1981a, Biochemical evidence for glutamate as neurotransmitter in the corticostriatal and corticothalamic fibres in rat brain, *Neuroscience* **6**:863–873.

Fonnum, F., Søreide, A., Kvale, I., Walker, J., and Walaas, I., 1981b, Glutamate in cortical fibers, in: *Glutamate as a Neurotransmitter* (G. Di Chiara and G. L. Gessa, eds.), Raven Press, New York, pp. 29–41.

Fosse, V. M., Heggelund, P., Iversen, E., and Fonnum, F., 1984, Effects of area 17 ablation on neurotransmitter parameters in efferents to area 18, the lateral geniculate body, pulvinar and superior colliculus in the cat, *Neurosci. Lett.* **52**:323–328.

Foster, A. C., Zinkand, W. C., and Schwarcz, R., 1985, Quinolinic acid phosphoribosyltransferase in rat brain, *J. Neurochem.* **44**:446–454.

Freeman, A. R., 1976, Polyfunctional role of glutamic acid in excitatory synaptic transmission, *Prog. Neurobiol.* **6**:137–153.

Freeman, M. E., Lane, J. D., and Smith, J. E., 1983, Turnover rates of amino acid neurotransmitters in regions of rat cerebellum, *J. Neurochem.* **40**:1441–1447.

Girault, J. A., Barbeito, L., Spampinato, U., Gozlan, H., Glowinski, J., and Besson, M.-J., 1986, In vivo release of endogenous amino acids from the rat striatum: further evidence for a role of glutamate and aspartate in corticostriatal neurotransmission, *J. Neurochem.* **47**:98–106.

Godfrey, D. A., Ross, C. D., Carter, J. A., Lowry, O. H., and Matschinsky, F. M., 1980, Effect of intervening lesions on amino acid distributions in rat olfactory cortex and olfactory bulb, *J. Histochem. Cytochem.* **28**:1157.

Godukhin, O. V., Zharikova, A. D., and Novoselov, V. I., 1980, The release of labeled L-glutamic acid from rat neostriatum in vivo following stimulation of frontal cortex, *Neuroscience* **5**:2151–2154.

Gordon, R. D., Hunt, A., and Patel, A. J., 1981, The cellular distribution of certain enzymes associated with the metabolic compartmentation of glutamate, *Biochem. Soc. Trans.* **9**:115–116.

Granata, A. R., and Reis, D. J., 1983, Release of [³H]L-glutamic acid (L-Glu) and [³H]D-aspartic acid (D-Asp) in the area of nucleus tractus solitarius in vivo produced by stimulation of the vagus nerve, *Brain Res.* **259**:77–93.

Halász, N., and Shepherd, G. M., 1983, Neurochemistry of the vertebrate olfactory bulb, *Neuroscience,* **10**:579–619.

Hamberger, A., Chiang, G., Nylén, E. S., Scheff, S. W., and Cotman, C. W., 1978, Stimulus evoked increase in the biosynthesis of the putative neurotransmitter glutamate in the hippocampus, *Brain Res.* **143**:549–555.

Hamberger, A. C., Chiang, G. H., Nylén, E. S., Scheff, S. W., and Cotman, C. W., 1979, Glutamate as a CNS transmitter. I. Evaluation of glucose and glutamine as precursors for the synthesis of preferentially released glutamate, *Brain Res.* **168**:513–530.

Hamberger, A., Jacobsson, I., Molin, S.-O., Nyström, B., Sandberg, M., and Ungerstedt, U., 1982, Metabolic and transmitter compartments for glutamate, in: *Neurotransmitter Interaction and Compartmentation,* NATO Advanced Study Institutes Series, Series A: Life Sciences, Volume A48 (H. F. Bradford, ed.), Plenum Press, New York & London, pp. 359–378.

Hansson, E., Jarlstedt, J., and Sellström, Å., 1980, Sound-stimulated ^{14}C-glutamate release from the nucleus cochlearis, *Experientia* **36**:576–577.

Hardy, P. M., Nicholls, A. C., and Rydon, H. N., 1976, The nature of the crosslinking of proteins by glutaraldehyde. Part 1. Interaction of glutaraldehyde with the amino-groups of 6-aminohexanoic acid and of alpha-N-acetyl-lysine, *J. Chem. Soc. Perkin Trans.* **I**:958–962.

Hardy, P. M., Hughes, G. J., and Rydon, H. N., 1979, The nature of the crosslinking of proteins by glutaraldehyde. II. The formation of quaternary pyridinium compounds by the action of glutaraldehyde on proteins and the identification of a 3-(2-piperidyl)-pyridinium derivative, anabilysine, as a cross-linking entity, *J. Chem. Soc. Perkin Trans.* **I**:2282–2288.

Harvey, J. A., Scholfield, C. N., Graham, L. T., Jr., and Aprison, M. H., 1975, Putative transmitters in denervated olfactory cortex, *J. Neurochem.* **24**:445.

Hassler, R., Haug, P., Nitsch, C., Kim, J. S., and Paik, K., 1982, Effect of motor and premotor cortex ablation on concentrations of amino acids, monoamines, and acetylcholine and on the ultrastructure in rat striatum: A confirmation of glutamate as the specific corticostriatal transmitter, *J. Neurochem.* **38**:1087.

Heggli, D. E., Aamodt, A., and Malthe-Sørenssen, D., 1981, Kainic acid neurotoxicity: Effect of systemic injection on neurotransmitter markers in different brain regions, *Brain Res.* **230**:253.

Henke, H., Schenker, T. M., and Cuénod, M., 1976, Effects of retinal ablation on uptake of glutamate, glycine, GABA, proline and choline in pigeon tectum, *J. Neurochem.* **26**:131.

Hertz, L., Yu, A., Svenneby, G., Kvamme, E., Fosmark, H., and Schousboe, A., 1980, Absence of preferential glutamate uptake into neurons—An indication of a *net* transfer of TCA constitutents from nerve endings to astrocytes? *Neurosci. Lett.* **16**:103–109.

Hertz, L., Yu, A. C. H., Potter, R. L., Fisher, T. E., and Schousboe, A., 1983a, Metabolic fluxes from glutamate and towards glutamate in neurons and astrocytes in primary cultures, in: *Glutamine, Glutamate, and GABA in the Central Nervous System* (L. Hertz, E. Kvamme, E. G. McGeer, and A. Schousboe, eds.), Liss, New York. pp. 327–342.

Hertz, L., Kvamme, E., McGeer, E. G., and Schousboe, A. (eds.), 1983b, *Glutamine, Glutamate, and GABA in the Central Nervous System*, Liss, New York.

Hicks, T. P., Ruwe, W. D., Veale, W. L., and Veenhuizen, J., 1985, Aspartate and glutamate as synaptic transmitters of parallel visual cortical pathways, *Exp. Brain Res.* **58**:421.

Hodgson, A. J., Penke, B., Erdei, A., Chubb, I. W., and Somogyi, P., 1985, Antisera to y-aminobutyric acid. I. Production and characterization using a new model system, *J. Histochem. Cytochem.* **33**:229–239.

Homma, S., Suzuki, T., Murayama, S., and Otsuka, M., 1979, Amino acid and substance P contents in spinal cord of cats with experimental hindlimb rigidity produced by occlusion of spinal cord blood supply, *J. Neurochem.* **32**:691.

Huang, S., Minassian, H., and More, J. D., 1976, Application of immunofluorescent staining on paraffin sections improved by trypsin digestion, *Lab. Invest.* **35**:383–390.

Hudson, D. B., Valcana, T., Bean, G., and Timiras, P. S., 1976, Glutamic acid: A strong candidate as the neurotransmitter of the cerebellar granule cell, *Neurochem. Res.* **1**:73.

Hunt, S. P., 1983, Cytochemistry of the spinal cord, in: *Chemical Neuroanatomy* (P. C. Emson, ed.), Raven Press, New York. pp. 53–84.

Israël, M., Lesbats, B., Morel, N., Manaranche, R., Gulik-Krzywicki, T., and Dedieu, J. C., 1984, Reconstitution of a functional synaptosomal membrane possessing protein constituents involved in acetylcholine translocation, *Proc. Natl. Acad. Sci. USA* **81**:277–281.

Johnston, G. A. R., 1976, Glutamate and aspartate as transmitters in the spinal cord, *Adv. Biochem. Psychopharmacol.* **15**:175.

Kane, E. S., 1979, Central transport and distribution of labelled glutamic and aspartic acids to the cochlear nucleus in cats: An autoradiographic study, *Neuroscience* **4**:729.

Kaneko, T., Akiyama, H., and Mizuno, N., 1987, Immunohistochemical demonstration of glutamate dehydrogenase in astrocytes, *Neurosci. Lett.* **77**:171–175.

Kanner, B., 1983, Bioenergetics of neurotransmitter transport, *Biochem. Biophys. Acta* **726**:293–316.

Kerkerian, L., Nieoullon, A., and Dusticier, N., 1983, Topographic changes in high-affinity glutamate uptake in the cat red nucleus, substantia nigra, thalamus and caudate nucleus after lesions of sensorimotor cortical areas, *Exp. Neurol.* **81**:598.

Kim, J. S., Bak, I. J., Hassler, R., Okada, Y., 1971, Role of γ-aminobutyric acid (GABA) in the extrapyramidal motor system. 2. Some evidence for the existence of a type of GABA-rich strio-nigral neurons, *Exp. Brain Res.* **14**:95–104.

Korf, J., and Venema, K., 1983, Amino acids in the substantia nigra of rats with striatal lesions produced by kainic acid, *J. Neurochem.* **40**:1171–1173.

Kornhuber, J., Kim, J. S., Kornhuber, M. E., and Kornhuber, H. H., 1984, The cortico-nigral projection: reduced glutamate content in the substantia nigra following frontal cortex ablation in the rat, Brain Res. 322:124–126.

Künzle, H., and Wiklund, L., 1982, Identification and distribution of neurons presumed to give rise to cerebellar climbing fibers in turtle. A retrograde axonal flow study using radioactive D-aspartate as a marker, Brain Res. 252:146–150.

Kvale, I., and Fonnum, F., 1983, The effects of unilateral removal of visual cortex on transmitter parameters in the adult superior colliculus and lateral geniculate body, Develop. Brain Res. 11:261–266.

Kvamme, E., 1983, Deaminases and aminases, in: Handbook of Neurochemistry, Volume 4, 2nd ed: (A. Lajtha, ed.), Plenum Press, New York, pp. 85–110.

Kvamme, E., and Lenda, K., 1981, Evidence for compartmentalization of glutamate in rat brain synaptosomes using the glutamate sensitivity of phosphate-activated glutaminase as a functional test, Neurosci. Lett. 25:193–198.

Larsson, L.-I., 1983, Method for immunocytochemistry of neurohormonal peptides, in: Handbook of Chemical Neuroanatomy, Vol. 1 (A. Björklund and T. Hökfelt, eds.), Elsevier/North Holland, Amsterdam, pp. 147–209.

Lehninger, A. L., 1975, The Molecular Basis of Cell Structure and Function, Worth, New York.

Lerma, J., Herranz, A. S., Herreras, O., Abraira, V., and Martin del Rio, R., 1986, In vivo determination of extracellular concentration of amino acids in the rat hippocampus. A method based on brain dialysis and computerized analysis, Brain Res. 384:145–155.

Logan, W. J., and Snyder, S. H., 1972, High affinity uptake systems for glycine, glutamic and aspartic acids in synaptosomes of rat central nervous tissues, Brain Res. 42:413–431.

Luini, A., Tal, N., Goldberg, O., and Teichberg, V. I., 1984, An evaluation of selected brain constituents as putative excitatory neurotransmitters, Brain Res. 324:271–277.

Lund Karlsen, R., Fonnum, F., 1978, Evidence for glutamate as a neurotransmitter in the corticofugal fibres to the dorsal lateral geniculate body and the superior colliculus in rats, Brain Res. 151:457–467.

Madl, J. E., Larson, A. A., and Beitz, A. J., 1986, Monoclonal antibody specific for carbodiimide-fixed glutamate: immunocytochemical localization in the rat CNS, J. Histochem. Cytochem. 34:317–326.

Malthe-Sørenssen, D., Skrede, K. K., and Fonnum, F., 1979, Calcium-dependent release of D-[^{3}H]aspartate evoked by selective electrical stimulation of excitatory afferent fibers to hippocampal pyramidal cells in vitro, Neuroscience 4:1255–1263.

Malthe-Sørenssen, D., Skrede, K. K., and Fonnum, F., 1980, Release of D-[^{3}H]aspartate from the dorsolateral septum after electrical stimulation of the fibria in vitro, Neuroscience 5:127–133.

Matute, C., Waldvogel, H. J., Streit, P., and Cuénod, M., 1984, Selective retrograde labeling following D-[^{3}H]aspartate and [^{3}H]GABA injections in the albino rat superior colliculus, Neurosci. Lett. (Suppl.) 18:S190.

McBride, W. J., Aprison, M. H., and Kusano, K., 1976a, Contents of several amino acids in the cerebellum, brain stem and cerebrum of the 'staggerer', 'weaver' and 'nervous' neurologically mutant mice, J. Neurochem. 26:867–870.

McBride, W. J., Nadi, N. S., Altman, J., and Aprison, M. H., 1976b, Effects of selective doses of X-irradiation on the levels of several amino acids in the cerebellum of the rat, Neurochem. Res. 1:141–152.

McBride, W. J., Rea, M. A., and Nadi, N. S., 1978, Effects of 3-acetylpyridine on the levels of several amino acids in different CNS regions of the rat, Neurochem. Res. 3:793–801.

McGeer, E. G., and McGeer, P. L., 1979, Localization of glutaminase in the rat neostriatum, J. Neurochem. 32:1071.

McGeer, E. G., McGeer, P. L., and Thompson, S., 1983, GABA and glutamate enzymes, in: Glutamine, Glutamate, and GABA in the Central Nervous System (L. Hertz, E. Kvamme, E. G. McGeer, and A. Schousboe, eds.), Liss, New York, pp. 3–17.

McGeer, P. L., McGeer, E. G., Scherer, U., and Singh, K., 1977, A glutamatergic corticostriatal path? Brain Res. 128:369–373.

Monaghan, P. L., Beitz, A. J., Larson, A. A., Altschuler, R. A., Madl, J. E., and Mullett, M. A., 1986, Immunocytochemical localization of glutamate-, glutaminase- and aspartate aminotransferase-like immunoreactivity in the rat deep cerebellar nuclei, Brain Res. 363:364–370.

Nadi, N. S., Kanter, D., McBride, W. J., and Aprison, M. H., 1977, Effects of 3-acetylpyridine on several putative neurotransmitter amino acids in the cerebellum and medulla of the rat, J. Neurochem. 28:661.

Nadler, J. V., and Smith, E. M., 1981, Perforant path lesion depletes glutamate content of fascia dentata synaptosomes, Neurosci. Lett. 25:275.

Nadler, J. V., Vaca, K. W., White, W. F., Lynch, G. S., and Cotman, C. W., 1976, Aspartate and glutamate as possible transmitters of excitatory hippocampal afferents, Nature 260:538–540.

Nadler, J. V., White, W. F., Vaca, K. W., Perry, B. W., and Cotman, C. W., 1978, Biochemical correlates of transmission mediated by glutamate and aspartate, *J. Neurochem.* **31**:147.

Nafstad, P. H. J., and Blackstad, T. W., 1966, Distribution of mitochondria in pyramidal cells and boutons in hippocampal cortex, *Z. Zellforsch. Mikrosk. Anat.* **73**:234–245.

Naito, S., and Ueda, T., 1983, Adenosine triphosphate-dependent uptake of glutamate into protein I-associated synaptic vesicles, *J. Biol. Chem.* **258**:696.

Naito, S., and Ueda, T., 1985, Characterization of glutamate uptake into synaptic vesicles, *J. Neurochem.* **44**: 99.

Nicholls, D. G., and Shira, T. S., 1986, Synaptosomes possess an exocytotic pool of glutamate, *Nature* **321**:772–773.

Nieoullon, A., and Dusticier, N., 1981, Decrease in choline acetyltransferase and in high affinity glutamate uptake in the red nucleus of the cat after cerebellar lesions, *Neurosci. Lett.* **24**:267.

Nieoullon, A., Kerkerian, L., and Dusticier, N., 1984, High affinity glutamate uptake in the red nucleus and ventrolateral thalamus after lesion of the cerebellum in the adult cat: Biochemical evidence for functional changes in the deafferented structures, *Exp. Brain Res.* **55**:409.

Nitsch, C., Kim, J.-K., Shimada, C., and Okada, Y., 1979a, Effect of hippocampus extirpation in the rat on glutamate levels in target structures of hippocampal efferents, *Neurosci. Lett.* **11**:295.

Nitsch, C., Kim, J.-K., and Shimada, C., 1979b, The commissural fibers in rabbit hippocampus: Synapses and their transmitter, *Prog. Brain Res.* **51**:193.

Norenberg, M. D., and Martinez-Hernandez, A., 1979, Fine structural localization of glutamine synthetase in astrocytes of rat brain, *Brain Res.* **161**:303–310.

Oliver, D. L., Potashner, S. J., Jones, D. R., and Morest, D. K., 1983, Selective labeling of spinal ganglion and granule cells with D-aspartate in the auditory system of cat and guinea pig, *J. Neurosci.* **3**:455.

Ottersen, O. P., 1987, Postembedding light- and electronmicroscopic immunocytochemistry of amino acids. Description of a new model system allowing identical conditions for specificity testing and tissue processing. *Exp. Brain Res.* (in press).

Ottersen, O. P., and Storm-Mathisen, J., 1984a, Neurons containing or accumulating transmitter amino acids, in: *Handbook of Chemical Neuroanatomy* (A. Björklund, T. Hökfelt, and M. J. Kuhar, eds.), Elsevier/North-Holland, Amsterdam, pp. 141–246.

Ottersen, O. P., and Storm-Mathisen, J., 1984b, Glutamate- and GABA-containing neurons in the mouse and rat brain, as demonstrated with a new immunocytochemical technique, *J. Comp. Neurol.* **229**:374.

Ottersen, O. P., and Storm-Mathisen, J., 1985, Different neuronal localization of aspartate-like and glutamate-like immunoreactivities in the hippocampus of rat, guinea pig, and Senegalese baboon (*Papio papio*), with a note on the distribution of gamma-aminobutyrate, *Neuroscience* **16**:589–606.

Ottersen, O. P., and Storm-Mathisen, J., 1986, Excitatory amino acid pathway in the brain, in: *Excitatory Amino Acids and Epilepsy* (R. Schwarcz and Y. Ben-Ari, eds.), Plenum Press, New York, pp. 263–284.

Ottersen, O. P., and Storm-Mathisen, J., 1987a, Immunocytochemical visualization of glutamate and aspartate, in: *Excitatory Amino Acid Transmission* (T. P. Hicks, D. Lodge, and H. McLennan, eds.), Liss, New York, pp. 131–138.

Ottersen, O. P., and Storm-Mathisen, J., 1987b, Localization of amino acid neurotransmitters by immunocytochemistry, *Trends Neurosci.* **10**:250–255.

Ottersen, O. P., Fischer, B. O., and Storm-Mathisen, J., 1983, Retrograde transport of D-[^{3}H]aspartate in thalamocortical neurons, *Neurosci. Lett.* **42**:19.

Ottersen, O. P., Fischer, B. O., Rinvik, E., and Storm-Mathisen, J., 1986a, Putative amino acid transmitters in the amygdala, in: *Excitatory Amino Acids and Epilepsy* (R. Schwarcz and Y. Ben-Ari, eds.), Plenum Press, New York, pp. 53–66.

Ottersen, O. P., Madsen, S., Storm-Mathisen, J., Skumlien, S., and Strømhaug, J., 1986b, Evaluation of the immunocytochemical method for amino acids, *Med. Biol.* **64**:147–158.

Patel, A. J., and Hunt, A., 1985, Concentration of free amino acids in primary cultures of neurones and astrocytes, *J. Neurochem.* **44**:1816.

Patel, A. J., Hunt, A., Gordon, R. D., Balázs, R., 1982, The activities in different neural cell types of certain enzymes associated with the metabolic compartmentation glutamate, *Develop. Brain Res.* **4**:3–11.

Patlak, J. B., Gration, K. A. F., and Usherwood, P. N. R., 1979, Single glutamate-activated channels in locust muscle, *Nature* **278**:643–645.

Perrone, M. H., 1981, Biochemical evidence that L-glutamate is a neurotransmitter of primary vagal afferent nerve fibers, *Brain Res.* **230**:283.

Potashner, S. J., 1978, The spontaneous and electrically evoked release, from slices of guinea pig cerebral cortex, of endogenous amino acids labelled via metabolism of D-[U-^{14}C]glucose, *J. Neurochem.* **31**:177–186.

Potashner, S. J., 1983, Uptake and release of D-aspartate in the guinea pig cochlear nucleus, *J. Neurochem.* **41**:1094.

Potashner, S. J., and Tran, P. L., 1985, Decreased uptake and release of D-aspartate in the guinea pig spinal cord after partial cordotomy, *J. Neurochem.* **44**:1511.

Potashner, S. J., and Dymczyk, L., 1986, Amino acid levels in the guinea pig spinal gray matter after axotomy of primary sensory and descending tracts, *J. Neurochem.* **47**:412–422.

Raymond, J., Nieoullon, A., Demêmes, D., and Sans, A., 1984, Evidence for glutamate as a neurotransmitter in the cat vestibular nerve: Radioautographic and biochemical studies, *Exp. Brain Res.* **56**:523.

Rea, M. A., and McBride, W. J., 1978, Effects of X-irradiation on the levels of glutamate, aspartate and GABA in different regions of the cerebellum of the rat, *Life Sci.* **23**:2355.

Rea, M. A., McBride, W. J., and Rohde, B. H., 1980, Regional and synaptosomal levels of amino acid neurotransmitters in the 3-acetylpyridine deafferentated rat cerebellum, *J. Neurochem.* **34**:1106.

Rea, M. A., McBride, W. J., and Rohde, B. H., 1981, Levels of glutamate, aspartate, GABA, and taurine in different regions of the cerebellum after X-irradiation-induced neuronal loss, *Neurochem. Res.* **6**:33.

Reis, D. J., Granata, A. R., Perrone, M. H., and Talman, W. T., 1981, Evidence that glutamic acid is the neurotransmitter of baroreceptor afferents terminating in the nucleus tractus solitarius (NTS), *J. Auton. Nerv. Syst.* **3**:321.

Reubi, J. C., and Cuénod, M., 1979, Glutamate release in vitro from cortico-striatal terminals, *Brain Res.* **176**:185.

Reubi, J. C., Toggenburger, C., and Cuénod, M., 1980, Asparagine as precursor for transmitter aspartate in corticostriatal fibres, *J. Neurochem.* **35**:1015.

Riveros, N., Fiedler, J., Lagos, N., Munoz, C., and Orrego, F., 1986, Glutamate in rat brain cortex synaptic vesicles: Influence of the vesicle isolation procedure, *Brain Res.* **386**:405–408.

Roberts, F., and Hill, R. G., 1978, The effect of dorsal column lesions on amino acid levels and glutamate uptake in rat dorsal column nuclei, *J. Neurochem.* **31**:1549.

Roberts, P. J., 1974, The release of amino acids with proposed neurotransmitter function from the cuneate and gracile nucleic of the rat in vivo, *Brain Res.* **67**:419.

Roberts, P. J., McBean, G. J., Sharif, N. A., and Thomas, E. M., 1982, Striatal glutamatergic function: Modifications following specific lesions, *Brain Res.* **235**:83.

Roffler-Tarlov, S., and Sidman, R. L., 1978, Concentrations of glutamic acid in cerebellar cortex and deep nuclei of normal mice and weaver, staggerer and nervous mutants, *Brain Res.* **142**:269.

Roffler-Tarlov, S., and Turey, M., 1982, The content of amino acids in the developing cerebellar cortex and deep cerebellar nuclei of granule cell deficient mutant mice, *Brain Res.* **247**:65.

Rohde, B. H., Rea, M. A., Simon, J. R., and McBride, W. J., 1979, Effects of X-irradiation induced loss of cerebellar granule cells on synaptosomal levels and the high affinity uptake of amino acids, *J. Neurochem.* **32**:1431.

Rowlands, G. J., and Roberts, P. J., 1980, Specific calcium-dependent release of endogenous glutamate from rat striatum is reduced by destruction of the cortico-striatal tract, *Exp. Brain Res.* **39**:239.

Rustioni, A., and Cuénod, M., 1982, Selective retrograde transport of D-aspartate in spinal interneurons and cortical neurons of rats, *Brain Res.* **236**:143.

Saito, N., Kumoi, K., and Tanaka, C., 1986, Aspartate-like immunoreactivity in mitral cells of rat olfactory bulb, *Neurosci. Lett.* **65**:89–93.

Sandberg, M., Bradford, H. F., and Richards, C. D., 1984, Effect of lesions of the olfactory bulb on the levels of amino acids and related enzymes in the olfactory cortex of the guinea pig, *J. Neurochem.* **43**:276.

Sandberg, M., Ward, H. K., and Bradford, H. F., 1985, Effect of corticostriate pathway lesion on the activities of enzymes involved in synthesis and metabolism of amino acid neurotransmitters in the striatum, *J. Neurochem.* **44**:42.

Sandoval, M. E., and Cotman, C. W., 1978, Evaluation of glutamate as a neurotransmitter of cerebellar parallel fibers, *Neuroscience* **3**:199.

Schiff, S. J., Szerb, J. C., and Somjen, G. G., 1985, Glutamine can enhance synaptic transmission in hippocampal slices, *Brain Res.* **343**:366–365.

Scholfield, C. N., Mornoi, F., Corradetti, R., and Pepeu, G., 1983, Levels and synthesis of glutamate and aspartate in the olfactory cortex following bulbectomy, *J. Neurochem.* **41**:135.

Schwarcz, R., Speciale, C., Okuno, E., French, E. D., and Köhler, C., 1986, Quinolinic acid: A pathogen in seizure disorders? in: *Excitatory Amino Acids and Epilepsy* (R. Schwarcz and Y. Ben-Ari, eds.), Plenum Press, New York, pp. 697–707.

Séguéla, P., Geffard, M., Buijs, R. M., and Le Moal, M., 1984, Antibodies against γ-aminobutyric acid: specificity studies and immunocytochemical results, *Proc. Natl. Acad. Sci. USA* **81**:3888–3892.

Shiosaka, S., Kiyama, H., Wanaka, A., and Tohyama, M., 1986, A new method for producing a specific and high titre antibody against glutamate using colloidal gold as a carrier, *Brain Res.* **382**:399–403.

Skrede, K. K., and Malthe-Sørenssen, D., 1981a, Increased resting and evoked release of transmitter following repetitive electrical tetanization in hippocampus: A biochemical correlate to longlasting synaptic potentiation, *Brain Res.* **208**:436.

Skrede, K. K., and Malthe-Sørenssen, D., 1981b, Differential release of D-[^{3}H]aspartate and [^{14}C]γ-aminobutyric acid following activation of commissural fibres in a longitudinal slice preparation of guinea pig hippocampus, *Neurosci. Lett.* **21**:71.

Somogyi, P., and Hodgson, A. J., 1985, Antiserum to γ-amino-butyric acid. III. Demonstration of GABA in Golgi-impregnated neurons and in conventional electron microscopic sections of cat striate cortex, *J. Histochem. Cytochem.* **33**:249–257.

Somogyi, P., Halasy, K., Somogyi, J., Storm-Mathisen, J., and Ottersen, O. P., 1986, Mossy and parallel fibre terminals have significantly higher levels of glutamate immunoreactivity, than glia, dendrites or GABA-immunoreactivity Golgi cell terminal in the cerebellum of cat, *Neuroscience* **19**:1045–1050.

Spencer, H. J., Tominez, G., and Halpern, B., 1981, Mass spectrographic analysis of stimulated release of endogenous amino acids from rat hippocampal slices, *Brain Res.* **212**:194.

Sternberger, L. A., 1979, *Immunocytochemistry,* 2nd ed., Wiley, New York.

Stone, T. W., and Connick, J. H., 1985, Quinolinic acid and other kynurenines in the central nervous system, *Neuroscience* **15**:597–617.

Storm-Mathisen, J., 1977, Glutamic acid and excitatory nerve endings: Reduction of glutamic acid uptake after axotomy, *Brain Res.* **120**:379.

Storm-Mathisen, J., 1978, Localization of putative transmitters in the hippocampal formation with a note on the connection to septum and hypothalamus, in: *Functions of the Septohippocampal System,* Ciba Foundation Symposium 58 (New Series), Elsevier/Excerpta Medica/North-Holland, Amsterdam.

Storm-Mathisen, J., 1981, Autoradiographic and microchemical localization of high affinity glutamate uptake, in: *Glutamate: Transmitter in the Central Nervous System* (P. J. Roberts, J. Storm-Mathisen, and G. A. R. Johnston, eds.), Wiley, New York.

Storm-Mathisen, J., 1982, Amino acid compartments in hippocampus: An autoradiographic approach, in: *Neurotransmitter Interaction and Compartmentation* (H. F. Bradford, ed.), Plenum Press, New York.

Storm-Mathisen, J., and Iversen, L. L., 1979, Uptake of [^{3}H]glutamic acid in excitatory nerve endings: Light and electronmicroscopic observations in the hippocampal formation of the rat, *Neuroscience* **4**:1237.

Storm-Mathisen, J., and Ottersen, O. P., 1983, Immunohistochemistry of glutamate and GABA, in: *Glutamine, Glutamate and GABA in the Central Nervous System* (L. Herz, E. Kvamme, E. G. McGeer, A. Schousboe, eds.), Liss, New York, pp. 185–201.

Storm-Mathisen, J., and Ottersen, O. P., 1986, Antibodies against amino acid neurotransmitters, in: *Neurohistochemistry: Modern Methods and Applications* (P. Panula, H. Päivärinta, and S. Soinila, eds.), Liss, New York, pp. 107–136.

Storm-Mathisen, J., and Wold, J. E., 1981, In vivo high-affinity uptake and axonal transport of D-[2,3-^{3}H]aspartate in excitatory neurons, *Brain Res.* **230**:427.

Storm-Mathisen, J., and Woxen Opsahl, M., 1978, Aspartate and/or glutamate may be transmitters in hippocampal efferents to septum and hypothalamus, *Neurosci. Lett.* **9**:65.

Storm-Mathisen, J., Leknes, A., and Bore, A. B., 1982, Immunohistochemical visualization of glutamate in excitatory boutons, *Neuroscience* **7**:(Suppl.) S203.

Storm-Mathisen, J., Leknes, A. K., Bore, A. T., Vaaland, J. L., Edminson, P., Haug, F.-M. S., and Ottersen, O. P., 1983, First visualisation of glutamate and GABA in neurons by immunocytochemistry, *Nature* **301**:517.

Storm-Mathisen, J., Ottersen, O. P., and Fu Long, T., 1986a, Antibodies for the localization of excitatory amino acids, in: *Excitatory Amino Acids* (P. J. Roberts, J. Storm-Mathisen, and H. F. Bradford, eds.), Macmillan, London, pp. 101–116.

Storm-Mathisen, J., Ottersen, O. P., Fu-long, T., Gundersen, V., Laake, J. H., and Nordbø, G., 1986b, Metabolism and transport of amino acids studied by immunocytochemistry, *Med. Biol.* **64**:127–132.

Streit, P., 1980, Selective retrograde labeling indicating the transmitter of neuronal pathways, *J. Comp. Neurol.* **191**:429.

Svenneby, G., and Storm-Mathisen, J., 1983, Immunological studies on phosphate activated glutaminase, in: *Glutamine, Glutamate and GABA in the Central Nervous System* (L. Hertz, E. Kvamme, E. G. McGeer, and A. Schousboe, eds.), Liss, New York, pp. 69–76.

Szerb, J. C., and O'Regan, P. A., 1985, Effect of glutamine on glutamate release from hippocampal slices induced by high K$^+$ or by electrical stimulation: Interaction with different Ca^{2+} concentrations, *J. Neurochem.* **44**:1724–1731.

Talman, W. T., Perrone, M. H., and Reis, D. J., 1980, Evidence for L-glutamate as the neurotransmitter of baroreceptor afferent nerve fibers, *Science* **209**:813.

Taniyama, K., Nitsch, C., Wagner, A., and Hassler, R., 1980, Aspartate, glutamate and GABA levels in pallidum, substantia nigra, center median and dorsal raphe nuclei after cylindric lesion of caudate nucleus in cat, *Neurosci, Lett.* **16**:155.

Taxt, T., and Storm-Mathisen, J., 1984, Uptake of D-aspartate and L-glutamate in excitatory axon terminals in hippocampus: Autoradiographic and biochemical comparison with γ-aminobutyrate and other amino acids in normal rats and in rats with lesions, *Neuroscience* **11**:79.

Thangnipon, W., and Storm-Mathisen, J., 1981, K$^+$-evoked Ca^{2+}-dependent release of D-[^{3}H]aspartate from terminals of the cortico-pontine pathway, *Neurosci Lett.* **23**:181.

Thangnipon, W., Taxt, T., Brodal, P., and Storm-Mathisen, J., 1983, The cortico-pontine projection: Axotomy-induced loss of high affinity L-glutamate and D-aspartate uptake, but not of GABA uptake, glutamate decarboxylase or choline acetyltransferase, in the pontine nuclei, *Neuroscience* **8**:449.

Toggenburger, G., Wiklund, L., Henke, H., and Cuénod, M., 1983, Release of endogenous and accumulated exogenous amino acids from slices of normal and climbing fibre-deprived rat cerebellar slices, *J. Neurochem.* **41**:1606.

Valcana, T., Hudson, D., and Timiras, P. S., 1972, Effects of X-irradiation on the content of amino acids in the developing rat cerebellum, *J. Neurochem.* **19**:2229.

Van Harreveld, A., and Fifkova, E., 1972, Release of glutamate from the retina during glutaraldehyde fixation, *J. Neurochem.* **19**:237–241.

Walaas, I., 1981, Biochemical evidence for overlapping neocortical and allocortical glutamate projections to the nucleus accumbens and rostral caudatoputamen in the rat brain, *Neuroscience* **6**:399.

Walaas, I., and Fonnum, F., 1979, The effect of surgical and chemical lesions on neurotransmitter candidates in the nucleus accumbens of the rat, *Neuroscience* **4**:209.

Walaas, I., and Fonnum, F., 1980, Biochemical evidence for glutamate as a transmitter in hippocampal efferents to the basal forebrain and hypothalamus in the rat brain, *Neuroscience* **5**:1691.

Walker, J. E., and Fonnum, F., 1983a, Regional cortical glutamergic and aspartegic projections to the amygdala and thalamus of the rat, *Brain Res.* **267**:371.

Walker, J. E., and Fonnum, F., 1983b, Effect of regional cortical ablations on high-affinity D-aspartate uptake in striatum, olfactory tubercle, and pyriform cortex of the rat, *Brain Res.* **278**:283.

Wanaka, A., Shiotani, Y., Kiyama, H., Matsuyama, T., Kamasa, T., Shiosaka, S., and Tohyama, M., 1987, Glutamate-like immunoreactive structures in primary sensory neurons in the rat detected by a specific antiserum against glutamate, *Exp. Brain Res.* **65**:691–694.

Waniewski, R. A., and Martin, D. L., 1986, Exogenous glutamate is metabolized to glutamine and exported by rat primary astrocyte cultures, *J. Neurochem.* **47**:304–313.

Ward, H. K., Thanki, C. M., Peterson, D. W., and Bradford, H. F., 1982, Brain glutaminase activity in relation to transmitter glutamate biosynthesis, *Biochem. Soc. Trans.* **10**:369.

Ward, H. K., Thanki, C. M., and Bradford, H. F., 1983, Glutamine and glucose as precursors of transmitter amino acids: Ex vivo studies, *J. Neurochem.* **40**:855–860.

Watanabe, K., and Kawana, E., 1984, Selective retrograde transport of tritiated D-aspartate from the olfactory bulb to the anterior olfactory nucleus, pyriform cortex and nucleus of the lateral olfactory tract in the rat, *Brain Res.* **296**:148–151.

Watkins, J. C., 1986, Twenty-five years of excitatory amino acid research. The end of the beginning? in: *Excitatory Amino Acids* (P. J. Roberts, J. Storm-Mathisen, and H. F. Bradford, eds.), Macmillan, London, pp. 1–39.

Weiss, D. G., Schmid, G., and Wagner, L., 1980, Influence of microtubule inhibitors on axoplasmic transport of free amino acids: Implications for the hypothetical transport mechanism, in: *Microtubules and Microtubule Inhibitors* (M. De Brabander and J. De Mey, eds.), Elsevier/North-Holland, Amsterdam, pp. 31–41.

Wenthold, R. J., 1978, Glutamic acid and aspartic acid in subdivisions of the cochlear nucleus after auditory nerve lesion, *Brain Res.* **143**:544–548.

Wenthold, R. J., 1979, Release of endogenous glutamic acid, aspartic acid and GABA from cochlear nucleus slices, *Brain Res.* **162**:338–343.

Wenthold, R. J., and Altschuler, R. A., 1983, Immunocytochemistry of aspartate aminotransferase and glutaminase, in: *Glutamine, Glutamate and GABA in the Central Nervous System* (L. Hertz, E. Kvamme, E. G. McGeer, and A. Schousboe, eds.), Liss, New York, pp. 33–50.

Wenthold, R. J., and Altschuler, R. A., 1986, Immunocytochemical localization of enzymes involved in the metabolism of excitatory amino acids, in: *Excitatory Amino Acids* (P. J. Roberts, J. Storm-Mathisen, and H. F. Bradford, eds.), Macmillan, London, pp. 85–100.

Wenthold, R. J., and Gulley, R. L., 1977, Aspartic acid and glutamic acid levels in the cochlear nucleus after auditory nerve lesion, *Brain Res.* **138**:111–123.

Wenthold, R. J., and Gulley, R. L., 1978, Glutamic and aspartic acid in the cochlear nucleus of the waltzing guinea pig, *Brain Res.* **158**:295–302.

Wieraszko, A., and Lynch, G., 1979, Stimulation-dependent release of possible transmitter substances from hippocampal slices studied with localized perfusion, *Brain Res.* **160**:372–376.

Wiklund, L., and Cuénod, M., 1984, Differential labelling of afferents to thalamic centromedian–parafascicular nuclei with [³H]choline and D-[³H]aspartate: Further evidence for transmitter specific retrograde labelling, *Neurosci. Lett.* **46:**275–281.

Wiklund, L., Toggenburger, G., and Cuénod, M., 1982, Aspartate: Possible neurotransmitter in cerebellar climbing fibers, *Science* **216:**78–79.

Wiklund, L., Toggenburger, G., and Cuénod, M., 1984, Selective retrograde labelling of the rat olivocerebellar climbing fiber system with D-[³H]aspartate, *Neuroscience* **13:**441–468.

Wofsey, A. R., Kuhar, M. J., and Snyder, S. H., 1971, A unique synaptosomal fraction which accumulates glutamic and aspartic acids in brain tissue, *Proc. Natl. Acad. Sci. USA* **68:**1102–1106.

Wolf, G., Schünzel, G., and Storm-Mathisen, J., 1984, Lesions of Schaffer's collaterals in the rat hippocampus affecting glutamate dehydrogenase and succinate dehydrogenase activity in the stratum radiation of CA 1. A study with special reference to the glutamate transmitter metabolism, *J. Hirnforsch.* **25:**249–253.

Wroblewski, J. T., Blaker, W. D., and Meek, J. L., 1985, Ornithine as a precursor of neurotransmitter glutamate: Effect of canaline on ornithine aminotransferase activity and glutamate content in the septum of rat brain, *Brain Res.* **329:**161–168.

Yamamoto, C., and Matsui, S., 1976, Effect of stimulation of excitatory nerve tract on release of glutamic acid from olfactory cortex slices in vitro, *J. Neurochem.* **26:**487–491.

Yates, R. A., and Roberts, P. J., 1974, Effects of enucleation and intraocular colchicine on the amino acids of frog optic tectum, *J. Neurochem.* **23:**891–893.

Yoneda, Y., Roberts, E., Dietz, G. W., Jr., 1982, A new synaptosomal biosynthetic pathway of glutamate and GABA from ornithine and its negative feedback inhibition by GABA, *J. Neurochem.* **36:**1686–1694.

Young, A. B., Oster-Granite, M. L., Herndon, R. M., and Snyder, S. H., 1974, Glutamic acid: Selective depletion by viral induced granule cell loss in hamster cerebellum, *Brain Res.* **73:**1–13.

Young, A. B., Bromberg, M. B., and Penney, J. B., Jr., 1981, Decreased glutamate uptake in subcortical areas deafferented by sensorimotor cortical ablation in the cat, *J. Neurosci.* **1:**241–249.

Zaczek, R., Hedreen, J. C., and Coyle, J. T., 1979, Evidence for a hippocampal–septal glutamatergic pathway in the rat, *Exp. Neurol.* **65:**145–156.

Zimmermann, H., 1979, Vesicle recycling and transmitter release, *Neuroscience* **4:**1773–1804.

5

Molecular and Functional Characterization of a Brain Neuronal Membrane Glutamate-Binding Protein

E. K. Michaelis, J.-W. Chen, T. M. Stormann, and S. Roy

1. Characteristics of Glutamate Neurotransmission and Glutamate Receptor Involvement in CNS Physiology

The dicarboxylic amino acids L-glutamic acid and L-aspartic acid play an important role as excitatory neurotransmitters or neuromodulators in both the vertebrate and invertebrate nervous systems (Curtis and Johnson, 1974; Krnjević, 1974; Nistri and Constanti, 1979). Both L-glutamate and L-aspartate are ubiquitous within the mammalian CNS and are known to have very extensive excitatory activity when applied to most CNS neurons. The excitatory responses produced in mammalian CNS neurons and in invertebrate muscles by the action of L-glutamic acid are the result of glutamate-induced increases in membrane conductance of Na^+ and K^+ (Nistri and Constanti, 1979; Takeuchi and Onodera, 1973; Anwyl, 1977) and, to a small extent, Ca^{2+} (Zanotto and Heinemann, 1983). These receptor-associated channels differ from the voltage-dependent channels of axonal or muscle membranes in their lack of sensitivity to tetrodotoxin (TTX) (Ozeki *et al.*, 1966; Curtis *et al.*, 1972).

Some crucial physiological functions in the CNS have been linked to the transmitter activity of L-glutamic acid. The region which has been studied in greatest detail is the hippocampus–dentate gyrus where much of the afferent innervation and the intrinsic excitatory transmission is believed to be mediated by L-glutamate or L-aspartate (e.g., Storm-Mathisen and Iversen, 1979). Long-term potentiation (LTP) of synaptic transmission following high-frequency stimulation was first described for the granule cells of the dentate gyrus (Bliss and Lomo, 1973) and has since been considered to be a neurophysiologic analogue of the formation of memory. The molecular mechanism for LTP, and consequently that for memory formation, may be the long-term activation of L-glutamate receptors in neurons postsynaptic to the excitatory afferents that were stimulated (Baudry *et al.*, 1980). Other researchers, however, have presented evidence that LTP is due to enhanced presynaptic L-glutamate release (Dolphin *et al.*, 1983; Sastry, 1982). Nevertheless, the possibility that L-glutamate receptor activity is altered in states of enhanced neuronal excit-

E. K. Michaelis, J.-W. Chen, T. M. Stormann, and S. Roy • Center for Biomedical Research and Departments of Human Development and Biochemistry, University of Kansas, Lawrence, Kansas 66045.

ability is worthy of further investigation. The molecular events that may bring about such L-glutamate receptor "up-regulation" need clearer definition. For example, increases in the rate of synthesis of the receptor macromolecules, the transfer to and insertion into plasma membranes, and activation through posttranslational modification need to be demonstrated.

2. Classes of Glutamate Receptors in the Vertebrate CNS and Approaches to the Study of These Receptors

At least three different types of excitatory amino acid receptors have been defined neurophysiologically and pharmacologically (Watkins and Evans, 1981). One group of receptors is highly responsive to N-methyl-D-aspartate (NMDA) and ibotenic acid and is blocked effectively by D-α-aminosuberic acid and 5-phosphonovaleric acid (2-APV). This group is referred to as the "NMDA class" of excitatory amino acid receptors. Watkins and Evans (1981) have also proposed glutamate receptor differentiation based on kainic acid and quisqualic acid excitation. These acids activate receptors that are moderately sensitive to inhibition by γ-D-glutamyl glycine and much more sensitive to inhibition by γ-D-glutamyl amino methyl sulfonate (e.g., Davies and Watkins, 1985). The difference between these two types of receptors is the insensitivity of kainate-induced excitation to L-glutamate diethyl ester as compared with this agent's relatively good inhibition of quisqualate-induced depolarization. Finally, there are responses to exogenously applied L-glutamate and L-aspartate that do not fit in any of the pharmacological categories of excitatory amino acid receptors described above since these physiologic responses persist after nearly complete blockade of NMDA, kainate, and quisqualate responses and might represent activation of a distinct class of glutamate/aspartate receptors (Luini et al., 1981; Surtees and Collins, 1985; Davies and Watkins, 1985).

Several alternative approaches have been used to identify receptor sites for the excitatory amino acids. These involve the measurement of binding interactions of agonists or antagonists with subcellular fractions of brain, stimulation of accumulation of cGMP in brain slices (Foster and Roberts, 1980, 1981), enhancement of phosphatidylinositol metabolism in slices and cultured neurons (Nicoletti et al., 1986a,b,c), and initiation of ion fluxes in neuronal membrane sacs or brain slices (Chang and Michaelis, 1980, 1981; Luini et al., 1981). It has generally been assumed that the molecular event preceding each of these signal transduction processes is the binding of L-glutamate or L-aspartate to the receptor recognition sites. It has been suggested by numerous investigators that Na^+-independent L-[^{3}H]glutamate binding to neuronal membranes at least in part labels sites which are related to physiologic glutamate receptors (e.g., Michaelis et al., 1974; Roberts, 1974; Foster and Roberts, 1978; Foster et al., 1981; Michaelis et al., 1981; Baudry and Lynch, 1981; de Barry et al., 1980; Honore et al., 1982; Werling and Nadler, 1982; Fagg et al., 1983; Foster and Fagg, 1984). Therefore, studies of ligand binding to putative receptor recognition sites, such as the interaction of L-[^{3}H]glutamate, L-[^{3}H]aspartate, [^{3}H]kainate, and L-[^{3}H]cysteine sulfinate with neuronal membrane sites, have become a common investigative approach to the topographical and molecular characterization of the receptor macromolecules. A recent review of the literature related to the use of ligand-binding studies to define putative excitatory amino acid receptors has been published (Foster and Fagg, 1984).

3. Molecular Characterization of Glutamate Recognition Sites and Glutamate-Sensitive Ion Channels in Synaptic Membranes

The study of the molecular characteristics of excitatory amino acid receptors should optimally be focused on an isolated, highly purified macromolecular complex that represents the receptor. This goal would be much easier to achieve if there were selective, high-affinity (almost irreversible) ligands for these receptor sites that might be used to label and purify the respective receptors. Ultimately, of course, it will be necessary to demonstrate that any macromolecular species so labeled and purified exhibits the functional features that define these receptors, i.e., the activation of ion channels or enzymes involved in the biochemical transduction of receptor-mediated cell stimulation, such as Na^+ channels, guanylate cyclase, or phospholipase C. Demonstration of the functional properties of such an isolated receptor macromolecular complex would probably require the reconstitution of the complex into a lipid environment, presumably lipid membrane bilayers, that would allow for the study of ligand-induced ion channel opening or receptor-mediated enzyme activation.

Unfortunately, the neuropharmacology of excitatory amino acids is not sufficiently well developed yet to afford a clear resolution of receptor subtypes through the use of highly selective, high-affinity agonists and antagonists. As has been shown by neurophysiologic experiments, none of the currently available antagonists offers complete discrimination between NMDA, kainate, and quisqualate receptors (Davies and Watkins, 1983; Peet *et al.*, 1983). Furthermore, as pointed out earlier, exogenously applied L-glutamate and L-aspartate act through some receptor sites that cannot be clearly classified into the three categories of receptors (Luini *et al.*, 1981; Surtees and Collins, 1985; Davies and Watkins, 1985). Therefore, in the investigations that were designed to probe the molecular nature of the receptor sites for L-glutamate, researchers have had to use L-glutamate as the radioactive labeling agent of the putative receptor macromolecular complexes. This approach is fraught with the difficulties of attempting to distinguish between the labeling of receptor sites and the ligand attachment to enzymes or transport carriers.

In one of the initial studies of L-[^{3}H]glutamate binding to brain homogenate and subcellular fractions, it was shown that synaptic plasma membranes isolated from whole rat brain exhibited an enrichment in L-glutamate binding activity (Michaelis *et al.*, 1974), and this observation has been confirmed by other investigators (e.g., Foster and Roberts, 1978; Foster *et al.*, 1981). L-[^{3}H]-Glutamate binding was measured at 4°C in the absence of any Na^+ in the medium, a procedure used to avoid the labeling of high-affinity glutamate transport carriers that are active at physiologic temperatures and in the presence of a transmembrane Na^+ gradient (Logan and Snyder, 1972). A crude molecular characterization of the glutamate binding sites labeled under such conditions indicated that these sites were associated with a plasma membrane glycoprotein whose activity was partially inhibited by proteolytic degradation with pronase and trypsin or by binding of concanavalin A to the membranes (Michaelis *et al.*, 1974). Furthermore, the glutamate binding activity associated with the synaptic membranes could be brought into solution by treatment of the membranes with the nonionic detergent Triton X-100 (Michaelis *et al.*, 1974). Finally, in a series of studies with invertebrate muscle and vertebrate brain homogenates, De Robertis and his colleagues (Fiszer De Plazas and De Robertis, 1974, 1977; De Robertis and Fiszer De Plazas, 1976a,b) extracted by chloroform–methanol treatment a proteolipid fraction that bound L-[^{14}C]glutamate. To the extent that the sites being labeled by the procedures described above were related to the glutamate receptor complex, these observations indicated that the recognition sites in brain membranes, and possibly those in invertebrate muscle membranes, were associated with a hydrophobic membrane glycoprotein.

These initial observations were extended in later studies from our laboratory in which we reported the purification of a glutamate-binding membrane glycoprotein from a Triton X-100-soluble extract of synaptic plasma membranes (Michaelis, 1975). This glutamate-binding protein was a low-molecular-weight (M_r 14,300) protein, an intrinsic plasma membrane acidic glycoprotein (Michaelis *et al.*, 1983, 1984a). A very similar, probably identical glutamate-binding protein has been purified by Dambinova and colleagues (Dambinova *et al.*, 1982) through the use of nearly identical procedures as those employed in our studies. The glutamate-binding protein isolated from synaptic membranes was found to be devoid of any enzymatic activity related to glutamate-metabolizing enzymes, and it differed in many of its characteristics from the high-affinity glutamate transport carriers in synaptic membranes (Michaelis, 1975; Michaelis *et al.*, 1974, 1982, 1983, 1984b).

The binding affinity and selectivity of its binding site for L-glutamic acid, other glutamate analogues, metal ligands, and amphipathic drugs, such as the local anesthetics, were very similar to those that we had determined for the glutamate binding sites in synaptic membranes (Michaelis et al.. 1981, 1982, 1984b). In general, both the isolated binding protein and the glutamate binding sites on synaptic membranes studied in our laboratory exhibited the following order of relative affinities for various glutamate analogues: L-glutamate $\geq$ L-aspartate $>$ L-cysteine sulfinate $>$ L-glutamate-monohydroxamate $>$ ibotenate $\simeq$ L-glutamate diethyl ester $>$ D-α-amino adipate. Kainic acid was found to produce inhibition of only 10–20% of glutamate binding, whereas NMDA and D-glutamate had almost no inhibitory activity on glutamate binding sites of synaptic membranes or of the isolated protein. It was also noteworthy that quisqualic acid produced very limited inhibition of glutamate binding to the protein purified from either rat or bovine brain (Michaelis et al., 1983, 1984a).

In more recent studies we have systematically examined the subcellular distribution of glutamate binding that is sensitive to inhibition by quisqualic acid in fractions obtained from rat brain homogenates. The quisqualate-sensitive glutamate binding sites are distributed in most particulate fractions such as the crude mitochondrial, synaptosomal, microsomal, and synaptic plasma membrane fractions. Quisqualic acid up to 10 μM produces a maximal inhibition of glutamate binding to synaptic membrane sites that is equal to 20% of the total glutamate binding activity and has an estimated IC_{50} for this inhibition of $\sim$ 0.2 μM (Cunningham and Michaelis, unpublished observations). At concentrations higher than 50 μM, quisqualate inhibits an additional 20% of the glutamate binding sites, but this inhibition was characterized by a much lower estimated K_i. These observations are similar to the reported quisqualate inhibition of glutamate binding sites in isolated postsynaptic densities from rat brain (Fagg and Matus, 1984). They differ, of course, from the previously described glutamate "binding" sites whose activity is measured in the presence of Cl^-- and Ca^{2+}-containing buffers and which are highly sensitive to inhibition by quisqualate (Fagg et al., 1983). The fact that this Cl^--dependent glutamate "binding" is very strongly dependent on the incubation temperature, on the presence of membrane-permeable anions such as Cl^-, Br^-, and NO_3^-, and on the presence of integral membrane vesicular structures strongly indicates that it is not likely to represent a binding process but rather an anion-activated transport of glutamate into membrane vesicles (Pin et al., 1984).

Nevertheless, there is obviously a measurable quisqualate inhibition of glutamate binding to synaptic membranes and postsynaptic densities that is distinguishable from any glutamate transport on the basis of the fact that it is not sensitive either to low temperatures (0°C) or to increasing medium osmolarity (Cunningham and Michaelis, unpublished observations) and it is not dependent on intact membrane vesicular structures (Fagg and Matus, 1984). The glutamate binding protein we have purified differs from these synaptic membrane sites in that its binding activity does not exhibit sensitivity to inhibition by quisqualic acid. Possible explanations for these differences between the glutamate binding sites in synaptic membranes and the purified glutamate binding protein are that the isolated protein did not represent the recognition site for either the glutamate/quisqualate, NMDA, or kainate receptor subtypes. Alternatively, it is possible that the purified protein may represent a component, or possibly even a fragment, of the intact protein complex that constitutes the receptor in synaptic plasma membranes and that this component has lost its capacity to bind these glutamate receptor agonists.

In a recent report, Koshiya (1985) has described a procedure of membrane solubilization with the zwitterionic detergent CHAPS in the presence of ammonium thiocyanate which apparently does not destroy the quisqualate-sensitive glutamate binding sites in crude membrane preparations from guinea pig brain. Although we have been unable to reproduce the results obtained by Koshiya with respect to the solubilization of quisqualate-sensitive glutamate binding sites from rat brain crude membrane fractions or purified synaptic membranes (Cunningham and Michaelis, unpublished observations), it is nevertheless possible that the type of membrane solubilization we have previously employed may have dissociated such receptor complexes and destroyed their activity. We are currently exploring this issue and attempting to define the molecular composition of the quisqualate-sensitive glutamate binding sites from brain synaptic membrane preparations.

4. Procedures for Determining the Functional Properties of the Purified Glutamate-Binding Protein

An important question is whether the purified glutamate-binding protein has any relationship to the macromolecular complexes of some of the glutamate receptors of brain neurons. Since this is the only nonenzyme glutamate-binding protein that has been isolated from vertebrate neuronal membranes and may be linked to the excitatory amino acid receptors, it is a potential model protein for a receptor-related function. If this protein is involved in the function of any glutamate receptors, then such function should be inhibited by specific antibodies developed against this protein and activity might be reconstituted following the purification of the protein from synaptic membranes.

4.1. Immunochemistry of the Glutamate-Binding Protein

Antibodies against the glutamate-binding protein purified from bovine brain were raised in rabbits and used to probe the function of the binding protein (Roy and Michaelis, 1984; Roy et al., 1985). These antibodies exhibited a very high degree of immune reactivity and specificity for the glutamate-binding protein purified from bovine as well as from rat brain, while having essentially no cross-reactivity against the enzymes glutamate dehydrogenase, glutamine synthetase, and γ-glutamyl transpeptidase (Roy and Michaelis, 1984). Only the enzyme glutamic acid decarboxylase from either bacteria (Roy and Michaelis, 1984) or bovine brain cortex (Michaelis et al., 1987) exhibited a moderate to low reactivity with the antibodies. Examination of the distribution of immune reactivity in rat brain subcellular fractions revealed a progressive enrichment of such reactivity in the crude mitochondrial, synaptosomal, and purified synaptic plasma membrane fraction (Michaelis et al., 1987). The absorbance readings for the synaptic membranes obtained from enzyme-linked immunoassays (ELISA) were 6.5 times higher than those measured for equal amounts of protein in the brain homogenate.

Three physiological processes in which the glutamate-binding protein might be involved were examined for their sensitivity to the antisera raised against this protein. These were the excitatory amino acid stimulation of Na^+ flux in synaptic membranes, L-glutamic acid transport across these membranes, and depolarization-induced L-glutamate release from synaptic membranes. Only the amino acid-induced changes in ion flux were affected by the antibodies raised against the binding protein (Roy et al., 1985). The characteristics of this glutamate- and related excitatory amino acid-activated ion flux processes are described below.

In the control experiments, without the antibody, micromolar and submicromolar concentrations of L-glutamate, L-aspartate, cysteine sulfinic acid, and kainic acid increased $^{22}Na^+$ influx into synaptosomes and isolated and resealed synaptic plasma membranes (Chang and Michaelis, 1980, 1981). The stimulation by L-glutamate of Na^+ influx into either the synaptosomes or synaptic membrane vesicles was not affected by exposure of these preparations to TTX and was, therefore, unrelated to the activation of voltage-sensitive Na^+ channels. Furthermore, this glutamate-stimulated ion flux process could be activated by L-glutamate in the *trans* location across the membrane with respect to the ion gradient, and the activity was not eliminated by lowering the incubation temperatures to 4°C (Chang and Michaelis, 1981). These are expected characteristics of the activation of a glutamate-sensitive ion channel-like response rather than a transport carrier. Finally, since the Na^+ flux processes that are enhanced by glutamate and other excitatory amino acids are electrogenic and cause the appearance of a transient intravesicular positive potential difference which averages between 5 and 13 mV (Chang and Michaelis, 1982; Chang et al., 1984), the appearance of a transmembrane potential following activation of Na^+ flux by the excitatory amino acids could be detected by measuring the distribution of the lipophilic ion $^{35}SCN^-$ (Chang and Michaelis, 1982; Chang et al., 1984). It is obvious, though, that the exact location of the macromolecules activated by glutamate and other excitatory amino acids to produce these ion flux responses is not known, and may represent, to a large extent, the contribution of presynaptic membrane sites.

The antibodies against the glutamate binding protein inhibited the glutamate, kainate- and quisqualate-activated SCN^- flux. The L-glutamate activation of SCN^- flux into synaptic membrane vesicles was at least 40 times more sensitive to the presence of the antibodies than was the stimulation of ion flux by kainate and 60 times more sensitive than that induced by quisqualate (Roy et al., 1985). The stimulation of SCN^- influx by NMDA was not affected, even by high concentrations of the antibodies. The specificity of the inhibition of L-glutamate-stimulated SCN^- influx into synaptic membranes was demonstrated by the fact that preimmune sera from the same animals had no effect on the activation of ion flux by L-glutamate.

Based on these results, one might conclude that the glutamate-binding protein does play a role in glutamate, kainic acid, and quisqualic acid activation of receptor-associated ion channels in synaptic membranes. The antibodies exhibited a rather surprising level of activity since there was no evidence of any strong interaction of either kainate or quisqualate with the glutamate binding site of the purified protein. One possible explanation for these observations is that the glutamate-binding protein represents a core component of glutamate/aspartate/ibotenate receptors and that kainate- or quisqualate-interaction subunits form part of the intact macromolecular complex in some neuronal membranes. There is some neurophysiologic evidence suggesting that sites maximally sensitive to quisqualate in dentate granule cell dendrites are not coincident with sites maximally sensitive to exogenously applied L-glutamate (Crunelli et al., 1984). Nevertheless, a certain degree of caution is warranted in considering the role of the glutamate-binding protein in the formation of an ion channel, since this protein has a relatively low molecular weight (M_r 14,300) in comparison with other proteins that function as receptor–ion channel complexes.

Pretreatment of synaptic membranes with the antibodies against the glutamate-binding protein produced only a limited inhibition of glutamate binding to the membranes. In addition, large amounts (5–100 μg) of the antibodies were required to bring about moderate inhibition of L-glutamate binding to the active site of the soluble, purified protein (Roy et al., 1985). The immune globulin (IgG) fraction used in these studies represented a heterogeneous population and it was likely that only a few species of IgG were directly reactive with the ligand binding site of the glutamate-binding protein. Therefore, the specific anti-glutamate-binding protein IgG was purified by immunoaffinity chromatography on a column of binding protein Affi-Gel (N-hydroxysuccinimide ester of agarose reacted with purified bovine brain glutamate binding protein) and tested for its effects on the glutamate binding activity of the purified protein. The purified IgG eluted from the Affi-Gel column with a 0.1 M glycine-HCl buffer, pH 3, represented 0.03% of the immune serum protein added to the column but exhibited very high immune reactivity toward the purified glutamate-binding protein as determined by the ELISA procedure. In addition, the maximal inhibition of glutamate binding to the protein produced by this purified IgG was somewhat greater than that observed with the serum. More important, however, is the fact that the inhibition was observed with only 5–100 ng of the purified antibodies. Half-maximal inhibition of binding was achieved at approximately 10 ng of purified IgG, which represented a concentration of 1 nM for the IgG under the conditions of the assay.

4.2. Reconstitution of the Glutamate-Binding Protein and of a Glutamate-Sensitive Ion Flux Response

The specific function we have attempted to reconstitute in liposomes is the activation of a Na^+ flux response that is produced following interaction of L-glutamate with neuronal membrane receptors, since this is the best-studied physiological action of glutamate on CNS neurons.

Purification of the glutamate-binding protein by the procedures that included solubilization with Triton X-100 under alkaline conditions, affinity batch chromatography through glutamate-loaded glass fiber, and affinity chromatography through concanavalin A (Michaelis, 1975; Michaelis *et al.*, 1983), did not yield consistently active preparations following reconstitution of the protein into phosphatidylcholine liposomes. Although the ligand-binding activity was preserved essentially unaltered, no consistent stimulation of $^{22}Na^+$ flux could be demonstrated. This lack of success in functional reconstitution may have been due to the denaturation of the protein during the solubilization and purification steps. In order to avoid the possibility of rapid protein delipidation or denaturation due to high concentrations of the detergent in the absence of any exogenously added lipids and to elevations in the pH of the medium, we have pursued a more gentle extraction of the protein from the synaptic membranes through the use of either 2% *n*-octylglucoside or Triton X-100, at 0°C, in a buffered medium (pH 7.4), and in the presence of a large excess of added phospholipids (10–20 mg/ml of asolectin lipids) (Stormann *et al.*, 1984).

Under these conditions of membrane protein solubilization and reconstitution into liposomes, a small, but consistent, glutamate stimulation of Na^+ flux could be measured (Stormann *et al.*, 1984). Furthermore, this glutamate-activated Na^+ flux was dependent on the concentration of L-glutamate introduced into the assays and was blocked by L-glutamate diethyl ester. Further processing of the solubilized synaptic membrane extract through the affinity-column chromatographic steps described above for purification of the glutamate-binding protein brought about a progressive enrichment in both the glutamate binding activity and glutamate-activated $^{22}Na^+$ flux in each succeeding fraction that was reconstituted into liposomes (Stormann *et al.*, 1984). These observations seemed to indicate that progressive purification of the glutamate-binding protein was associated with increased glutamate-sensitive ion flux following its reconstitution into liposomes. However, when the pattern resulting from SDS electrophoresis of these preparations was examined, we did not observe a progressive purification and enrichment of the 14,000-dalton (14k) protein we had previously identified as the glutamate-binding protein. In some preparations we did detect protein bands of low molecular weight (15–25k) that were labeled by our antisera following electrophoretic transfer onto nitrocellulose membranes (immunoblotting). However, the fractions producing the best ion flux activity following reconstitution, such as the partially purified fraction following affinity batch separation through glutamate-loaded glass fiber, showed a consistent enrichment of a 32k protein together with other proteins of 48–68k and some of higher molecular weight.

We interpreted these results to indicate that the 14k protein we had previously identified as the glutamate-binding protein might have been a proteolytic fragment of a higher-molecular-weight protein, possibly generated by the solubilization conditions that we have employed in our standard purification procedure (Michaelis, 1975; Michaelis *et al.*, 1983, 1984a). The few low-molecular-weight bands that were reactive with the antisera in immunoblot studies were also indicative of possible proteolytic degradation of a higher-molecular-weight protein.

5. Further Molecular Characterization of the Synaptic Membrane Glutamate-Binding Protein from Rat Brain

We have recently pursued this issue of protein degradation by purifying the glutamate-binding protein in solutions that contain five protease inhibitors in the steps from homogenization to synaptic membrane solubilization and three protease inhibitors in all subsequent steps. An additional modification of the purification procedure involves the use of a 5-mM sodium azide solution to elute the glutamate-binding protein from glutamate-loaded glass fiber, since we had previously observed that the binding activity of the glutamate-binding protein that we had purified was reversibly inhibited by millimolar concentrations of metal ligands such as sodium azide and potassium cyanide (Michaelis, 1979; Michaelis *et al.*, 1982). Elution of the glutamate-derivatized

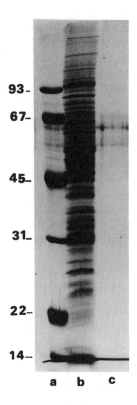

Figure 1. SDS gel electrophoresis of synaptic membranes and azide-eluted fraction from glutamate-derivatized glass fiber. Lane a, molecular weight standards; lane b, synaptic membrane fraction used to isolate the glutamate-binding protein; lane c, protein fraction obtained by affinity batch chromatography of solubilized synaptic membranes through glutamate-derivatized glass fiber and elution with 5 mM sodium azide. Gel polyacrylamide concentration was 10%; the gel was stained with silver nitrate following fixation in glutaraldehyde. The molecular weight of standards in kilodaltons is shown on the left.

glass fiber with sodium azide leads to marked enrichment of a doublet of protein bands on SDS gel electrophoresis with apparent M_r or 55–60k and 68–70k (Fig. 1). In preliminary studies, the same proteins have also been prepared in the presence of 20% glycerol plus the protease inhibitors and purified by successive chromatographic elutions through glutamate-derivatized Affi-gel and DEAE-Sephadex. When these proteins were reconstituted into liposomes, they gave good $^{22}Na^+$ flux activation in response to L-glutamate additions. Further purification of the proteins obtained from the glutamate-derivatized glass fiber by means of DEAE-Sephadex chromatography and TSK size-exclusion high-performance liquid chromatography (HPLC) yields a protein peak eluting from the TSK column which is homogeneous for the 68–70k protein as judged by SDS gel electrophoresis with silver staining (Fig. 2). This protein exhibits specific glutamate binding activity that is equivalent to or greater than that of the mixture of proteins obtained in the azide eluate from the glutamate-loaded glass fiber.

We have raised antibodies against each protein band, the 55–60k and the 68–70k band, from material transferred onto nitrocellulose filters following SDS gel electrophoresis of DEAE-Sephadex- and HPLC-purified protein. When the immune sera obtained from the immunized rabbits were used in immunoblot studies, they gave identical results regardless of the protein band used to immunize the animals. Both immune sera strongly labeled a protein band whose M_r corresponds to the 68–70 protein and weakly labeled other bands of M_r 55–66k (Fig. 3). These results suggest that the two protein bands we observed are derived from a single protein that has undergone partial proteolysis to form a lower-molecular-weight species (55–60k). It is also possible that the same protein exhibits heterogeneity because of differences in glycosylation or other posttranslational modifications.

Further indications that the 68–70k protein is related to the previously purified glutamate-binding protein are the facts that its binding affinity for glutamate has been estimated to be 0.32 μM and that the competition for the ligand binding sites by other glutamate analogues (Table I) is

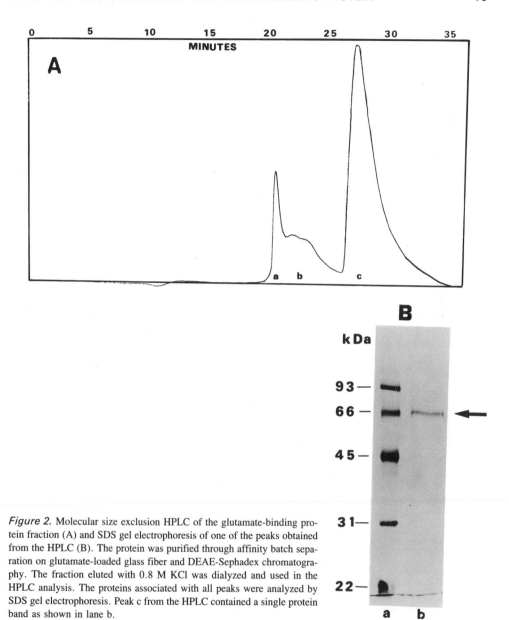

Figure 2. Molecular size exclusion HPLC of the glutamate-binding protein fraction (A) and SDS gel electrophoresis of one of the peaks obtained from the HPLC (B). The protein was purified through affinity batch separation on glutamate-loaded glass fiber and DEAE-Sephadex chromatography. The fraction eluted with 0.8 M KCl was dialyzed and used in the HPLC analysis. The proteins associated with all peaks were analyzed by SDS gel electrophoresis. Peak c from the HPLC contained a single protein band as shown in lane b.

similar to that which we had previously described for the glutamate-binding protein (Michaelis *et al.*, 1983). Also, the antibodies raised against the low-molecular-weight glutamate-binding protein (M_r 14k) label the 68–70k protein in synaptic membranes rather strongly in immunoblots and in the various fractions obtained during the purification of this protein. Finally, immunoaffinity chromatography of a solubilized synaptic membrane extract prepared under conditions to prevent proteolysis, leads to the isolation of a protein fraction enriched in the 68–70k protein species.

These observations lead us to believe that the 14k protein that we had previously identified as the glutamate-binding protein represented a proteolytic fragment containing the glutamate binding site(s) of a synaptic membrane glutamate-binding protein with an M_r of 68–70k. The present indication that a glutamate-binding macromolecule of synaptic membranes is a protein of esti-

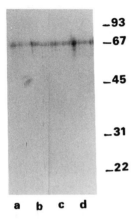

_93
—67
_45
_31
_22

a   b   c   d

Figure 3. Immunoreaction of electrotransferred samples from SDS gel electrophoresis with the antisera raised against the 55–60k and the 68–70k proteins associated with the glutamate-binding protein fraction (see Fig. 2). Lanes a and c contained proteins obtained through azide elution of material bound to glutamate-derivatized glass fiber; lanes b and d contained proteins obtained through azide elution of material bound to glutamate-derivatized polystyrene beads. Lanes a and b were reacted with antiserum against the 55–60k protein and lanes c and d with antiserum against the 68–70k protein. The immune reaction was detected by the application of a peroxidase-derivatized anti-rabbit antibody.

mated $M_r \sim$ 70k is in very good agreement with the determination of the molecular weight of glutamate binding sites in synaptic membranes obtained by radiation inactivation studies (Bardsley and Roberts, 1985). Their estimate of the subunit molecular weight of the glutamate-binding entities was 74 ± 15k.

6. Conclusions

Progress in defining the molecular entities that comprise the physiologic glutamate receptors in synaptic plasma membranes has been slow and difficult because selective probes for these receptors are lacking. The glutamate-binding protein described here is a candidate for a compo-

Table I. Displacement of L-[³H]-Glutamate Bound to the Glutamate-Binding Protein by Excitatory Amino Acids, Amino Acid Analogues, and Metal Ligands[a]

Agent	Concentration (μM)	Percent displacement
L-Glutamate	100	100
L-Aspartate	100	93.2
L-Glutamate γ-hydroxamate	100	75.9
Ibotenic acid	100	29.1
Quisqualic acid	100	25.1
L-Glutamate diethyl ester	500	30.1
D-Aminoadipate	100	6.9
D-Glutamate	100	0.0
Kainate	100	0.0
N-Methyl-D-aspartate	100	0.0
Aminooxyacetic acid	100	0.0
Sodium azide	5000	94.8
Potassium cyanide	5000	89.6

[a]The glutamate-binding protein was purified through affinity batch separation on glutamate-derivatized glass fiber and subsequent DEAE-Sephadex chromatography. The protein eluted at 0.8 M KCl was dialyzed and used in the binding assays at 0.75 μg/assay. The L-[³H]glutamate concentration was 150 nM.

nent of the excitatory amino acid receptor complex, but we must proceed cautiously until we have conclusively ruled out some other function in either glutamate metabolism or glutamate transport across neuronal membranes. The tools that we have developed for the purification of this protein, for the study of its molecular properties, and for the exploration of its immunochemical and immunohistochemical distribution in brain tissue should accelerate the acquisition of information about this neuronal membrane glutamate acceptor site.

Some of our current efforts are attempts to identify the proteins that interact with other excitatory amino acids such as quisqualate and ibotenate and to determine the protein constituents of these macromolecular complexes and their relationship to the glutamate-binding protein system that we have purified. In addition, we have begun to use our antibodies to isolate the immunoreactive protein(s) from proteins synthesized by *in vitro* translation of brain mRNA. Such techniques will be useful in studying the regulation of the synthesis and insertion of this protein into neuronal membranes, in extracting the specific mRNA and translating it in other cells such as frog oocytes, and, finally, in cloning and sequencing the DNA for this protein.

ACKNOWLEDGMENTS. We thank Linda Kunkle for her excellent assistance in typing the manuscript. This work was supported in part by grants from NIAAA (AA04732), from U.S. A.R.O. (DAAG29-83-K0065 and DAAL03-86-K0086), and from Biomedical Research Support, RR 5606. We acknowledge the support provided by the Center for Biomedical Research of the University of Kansas.

References

Anwyl, R., 1977, Permeability of the post-synaptic membrane of an excitatory glutamate synapse to sodium and potassium, *J. Physiol. (London)* **273**:367–388.

Bardsley, M. E., and Roberts, P. J., 1985, Molecular size of the high-affinity glutamate-binding sites on synaptic membranes from rat brain, *Biochem. Biophys. Res. Commun.* **126**:227–232.

Baudry, M., and Lynch, G., 1980, Hypotheses regarding the cellular mechanisms responsible for long-term synaptic potentiation in the hippocampus, *Exp. Neurol.* **68**:202–204.

Baudry, M., and Lynch, G., 1981, Characterization of two [³H]glutamate binding sites in rat hippocampal membranes, *J. Neurochem.* **36**:811–820.

Bliss, T. V. P., and Lomo, T., 1973. Long lasting potentiation of synaptic transmission in the dentate area of the anesthetized rabbit following stimulation of the perforant path, *J. Physiol. (London)* **232**:331–356.

Chang, H. H., and Michaelis, E. K., 1980, Effects of L-glutamic acid on synaptosomal and synaptic membrane Na⁺ fluxes and (Na⁺ + K⁺)-ATPase, *J. Biol. Chem.* **255**:2411–2417.

Chang, H. H., and Michaelis, E. K., 1981, L-Glutamate stimulation of Na⁺ efflux from brain synaptic membrane vesicles, *J. Biol. Chem.* **256**:10084–10087.

Chang, H. H., and Michaelis, E. K., 1982, L-Glutamate effects on electrical potentials of synaptic plasma membrane vesicles, *Biochim. Biophys. Acta* **688**:285–294.

Chang, H. H., Michaelis, E. K., and Roy, S., 1984, Functional characteristics of L-glutamate, N-methyl-D-aspartate and kainate receptors in isolated brain synaptic membranes, *Neurochem. Res.* **9**:901–913.

Crunelli, V., Forda, S., and Kelly, J. S., 1984, The reversal potential of excitatory amino acid action on granule cells of the rat dentate gyrus, *J. Physiol. (London)* **351**:327–342.

Curtis, D. R., and Johnston, G. A. R., 1974, Amino acid transmitters in the mammalian central nervous system, *Ergeb. Physiol.* **69**:94–188.

Curtis, D. R., Duggan, A. W., Felix, D., Johnston, G. A. R., Tebecis, A. K., and Watkins, J. C., 1972, Excitation of mammalian central neurones by acidic amino acids, *Brain Res.* **41**:283–301.

Dambinova, S. A., Besedin, V. I., and Demina, M. N., 1982, Molecular organization of glutamate-sensitive chemoexcitable membranes of nerve cells: Physicochemical properties of glutamate-binding proteins from synaptic membranes of rat cerebral cortex. *Neurokhimia* **1**:352–360.

Davies, J., and Watkins, J. C., 1983, Role of excitatory amino acid receptors in mono- and polysynaptic excitation in the cat spinal cord, *Exp. Brain Res.* **49**:280–290.

Davies, J., and Watkins, J. C., 1985, Depressant actions of γ-D-glutamylaminomethyl sulfonate (GAMS) on amino acid-induced and synaptic excitation in the cat spinal cord, *Brain Res.* **327**:113–120.

de Barry, J., Vincendon, G., and Gombos, G., 1980, High affinity glutamate binding during postnatal development of rat cerebellum, *FEBS Lett.* **109:**175–179.

De Robertis, E., and Fiszer De Plazas, S., 1976a, Differentiation of L-aspartate and L-glutamate high-affinity binding sites in a protein fraction isolated from rat cerebral cortex, *Nature* **260:**347–349.

De Robertis, E., and Fiszer De Plazas, S., 1976b, Isolation of hydrophobic proteins binding amino acids: Stereoselectivity of the binding of L-[^{14}C] glutamic acid in cerebral cortex, *J. Neurochem.* **26:**1237–1243.

Dolphin, A. C., Errington, M. L., and Bliss, T. V. P., 1983, Long-term potentiation of the perforant path *in vivo* is associated with increased glutamate release, *Nature* **297:**496–498.

Fagg, G. E., and Matus, A., 1984, Selective association of N-methyl aspartate and quisqualate types of L-glutamate receptor with brain postsynaptic densities, *Proc. Natl. Acad. Sci. USA* **81:**6876–6880.

Fagg, G. E., Foster, A. C., Mena, E. E., and Cotman, C. W., 1983, Chloride and calcium ions separate L-glutamate receptor populations in synaptic membranes, *Eur. J. Pharmacol.* **88:**105–110.

Fiszer De Plazas, S., and De Robertis, E., 1974, Isolation of hydrophobic proteins binding neurotransmitter amino acids: Glutamate receptor of the shrimp muscle, *J. Neurochem.* **23:**1115–1120.

Fiszer De Plazas, S., De Robertis, E., and Lunt, G. G., 1977, L-Glutamate and γ-amino butyrate binding to hydrophobic protein fractions from leg muscle of fly (*Musca domestica*), *Gen. Pharmacol.* **8:**133–137.

Foster, A. C., and Fagg, G. E., 1984, Acidic amino acid binding sites in mammalian neuronal membranes: Their characteristics and relationship to synaptic receptors, *Brain Res. Rev.* **7:**103–164.

Foster, A. C., and Roberts, P. J., 1978, High affinity L-[^{3}H]glutamate binding to postsynaptic receptor sites on rat cerebellar membranes, *J. Neurochem.* **31:**1467–1477.

Foster, A. C., Mena, E. E., Fagg, G. E., and Cotman, C. W., 1981, Glutamate and aspartate binding sites are enriched in synaptic junctions isolated from rat brain, *J. Neurosci.* **1:**620–625.

Foster, G. A., and Roberts, P. J., 1980, Pharmacology of excitatory amino acid receptors mediating the stimulation of rat cerebellar cyclic GMP levels *in vitro, Life Sci.* **27:**215–221.

Foster, G. A., and Roberts, P. J., 1981, Stimulation of rat cerebellar guanosine 3'5'-cyclic monophosphate (cyclic GMP) levels: Effects of amino acid antagonists, *Br. J. Pharmacol.* **74:**723–729.

Honore, T., Lauridsen, J., and Krogsgaard-Larsen, P., 1982, The binding of [^{3}H]AMPA, a structural analogue of glutamic acid, to rat brain membranes, *J. Neurochem.* **38:**173–178.

Koshiya, K., 1985, Solubilization of quisqualate-sensitive L-[^{3}H]glutamate binding sites from guinea pig brain membranes using a zwitterionic detergent, *Life Sci.* **31:**1373–1379.

Krnjević, K., 1974, Chemical nature of synaptic transmission in vertebrates, *Physiol. Rev.* **54:**418–540.

Logan, W. J., and Snyder, S. H., 1972, High affinity uptake systems for glycine, glutamic acid and aspartic acids in synaptosomes of rat central nervous tissues, *Brain Res.* **42:**413–431.

Luini, A., Goldberg, O., and Teichberg, V. I., 1981, Distinct pharmacological properties of excitatory amino acid receptors in the rat striatum: Study by Na$^+$ efflux assay, *Proc. Natl. Acad. Sci. USA* **78:**3250–3254.

Michaelis, E. K., 1975, Partial purification and characterization of a glutamate-binding glycoprotein from rat brain, *Biochem. Biophys. Res. Commun.* **65:**1004–1012.

Michaelis, E. K., 1979, The glutamate receptor-like protein of brain synaptic membranes is a metalloprotein, *Biochem. Biophys. Res. Commun.* **87:**106–113.

Michaelis, E. K., Michaelis, M. L., and Boyarsky. L. L., 1974, High affinity glutamic acid binding to brain synaptic membranes, *Biochim. Biophys. Acta* **367:**338–348.

Michaelis, E. K., Michaelis, M. L., Chang, H. H., Grubbs, R. D., and Kuonen, D. R., 1981, Molecular characteristics of glutamate receptors in the mammalian brain, *Mol. Cell. Biochem.* **38:**163–179.

Michaelis, E. K., Belieu, R. M., Grubbs, R. D., Michaelis, M. L., and Chang, H. H., 1982, Differential effects of metal ligands on synaptic membrane glutamate binding and uptake systems, *Neurochem. Res.* **7:**417–430.

Michaelis, E. K., Michaelis, M. L., Stormann, T. M., Chittenden, W. L., and Grubbs, R. D., 1983, Purification and molecular characterization of the brain synaptic membrane glutamate binding protein, *J. Neurochem.* **40:**1742–1753.

Michaelis, E. K., Chittenden, W. L., Johnson, B. E., Galton, N., and Decedue, C., 1984a, Purification, biochemical characterization, binding activity, and selectivity of the glutamate binding protein purified from bovine brain, *J. Neurochem.* **42:**397–406.

Michaelis, E. K., Magruder, C. D., Lampe, R. A., Galton, N., Chang, H. H., and Michaelis, M. L., 1984b, Effects of amphipathic drugs on L-[^{3}H]glutamate binding to synaptic membranes and the purified binding protein, *Neurochem. Res.* **9:**29–44.

Michaelis, E. K., Roy, S., Galton, N., Cunningham, M., LeCluyse, E., and Michaelis, M., 1987, Correlation of glutamate binding activity with glutamate-binding protein immunoreactivity in the brain of control and alcohol-treated rats, *Neurochem. Int.* **11:**209–218.

Nicoletti, F., Iadarola, M. J., Wroblewski, J. T., and Costa, E., 1986a, Excitatory amino acid recognition sites coupled with inositol phospholipids metabolism: Developmental changes and interaction with a_1-adrenoceptors, *Proc. Natl. Acad. Sci. USA* **83:**1931–1935.

Nicoletti, F., Meek, J. L., Iadarola, M. J., Chuang, D. M., Roth, B. L., and Costa, E., 1986b, Coupling of inositol phospholipid metabolism with excitatory amino acid recognition sites in rat hippocampus, *J. Neurochem.* **46:**40–46.

Nicoletti, F., Wroblewski, J. T., Novelli, A., Alho, A., Guidotti, A., and Costa, E., 1986c, The activation of inositol phospholipid metabolism as a signal-transducing system for excitatory amino acids in primary cultures of cerebellar granule cells, *J. Neurosci.* **7:**1905–1911.

Nistri, A., and Constanti, A., 1979, Pharmacological characterization of different types of GABA and glutamate receptors in vertebrates and invertebrates, *Prog. Neurobiol.* **13:**117–235.

Ozeki, M., Freeman, A. R., and Grundfest, H., 1966, The membrane components of crustacean neuro-muscular systems. II. Analysis of interactions among the electrogenic components, *J. Gen. Physiol.* **49:**1335–1349.

Peet, M. J., Leah, J. D., and Curtis, D. R., 1983, Antagonists of synaptic and amino acid excitation of neurons in the cat spinal cord, *Brain Res.* **266:**83–95.

Pin, J.-P., Bockaert, J., and Recasens, M., 1984, The Ca^{2+}/Cl^- dependent L-[^{3}H]glutamate binding: A new receptor or a particular transport process, *FEBS Lett.* **175:**31–36.

Roberts, P. J., 1974, Glutamate receptors in rat CNS, *Nature* **252:**399–401.

Roy, S., and Michaelis, E. K., 1984, Antibodies against the bovine brain glutamate binding protein, *J. Neurochem.* **42:**838–841.

Roy, S., Galton, N., and Michaelis, E. K., 1985, Effects of anti-glutamate-binding protein antibodies on synaptic membrane ion flux, glutamate transport and release, and L-glutamate binding activities, *J. Neurochem.* **44:**1809–1815.

Sastry, B. R., 1982, Presynaptic change associated with long-term potentiation in hippocampus, *Life Sci.* **25:**1179–1188.

Stormann, T. M., Chang, H. H., Johe, K., and Michaelis, E. K., 1984, Functional reconstitution of the synaptic membrane glutamate-binding protein: Glutamate receptor-like activity in liposomes, *Soc. Neurosci. Abstr.* **10:**958.

Storm-Mathisen, J., and Iversen, L. L., 1979, Uptake of [^{3}H]-glutamic acid in excitatory nerve endings: Light and electronmicroscopic observations in the hippocampal formation of the rat, *Neuroscience* **4:**1237–1253.

Surtees, L., and Collins, G. G. S., 1985, Receptor types mediating the excitatory actions of exogenous L-aspartate and L-glutamate in rat olfactory cortex, *Brain Res.* **334:**287–295.

Takeuchi, A., and Onodera, K., 1973, Reversal potentials of the excitatory transmitter and L-glutamate at the crayfish neuromuscular junction, *Nature New Biol.* **242:**124–126.

Watkins, J. C., and Evans, R. H., 1981, Excitatory amino acid transmitters, *Annu. Rev. Pharmacol. Toxicol.* **21:**165–204.

Werling, L. L., and Nadler, J. V., 1982, Complex binding of L-[^{3}H]glutamate to hippocampal synaptic membranes in the absence of sodium, *J. Neurochem.* **38:**1050–1062.

Zanotto, L., and Heinemann, U., 1983, Aspartate and glutamate induced reductions in extracellular free calcium and sodium concentration in area CAl of '*in vitro*' hippocampal slices of rats, *Neurosci. Lett.* **35:**79–84.

6

L-Glutamate and Its Agonists

Synaptic and Ionic Mechanisms in the Central Nervous System

R. Pumain, I. Kurcewicz, and J. Louvel

1. Introduction

Since the pioneering studies of Curtis *et al.* (1960) on spinal neurons, the excitatory amino acids L-glutamate (Glu) and L-aspartate (Asp) have been considered as neurotransmitter candidates in the vertebrate CNS. Both Glu and Asp are present in large quantities in brain nervous tissue (about 10 and 2 mM, respectively) (Berl and Waelsch, 1958; Perry *et al.*, 1981; Schousboe *et al.*, 1975); Glu is released from several cortical areas following stimulation of afferent pathways (Jasper and Koyama, 1969), this release being calcium dependent (see review by Fonnum, 1984); increased Glu release has been observed during electroencephalographic wakefulness (Jasper *et al.*, 1965); and studies *in vitro* have indicated that Glu is predominantly released from nerve terminals (Potashner, 1978a,b). In addition, it has been shown that Glu and Asp induce large and fast depolarizations when applied onto neurons (Curtis *et al.*, 1972) and low- and high-affinity uptake mechanisms have been demonstrated in neurons and glia for these amino acids (Logan and Snyder, 1972; Balcar and Johnston, 1972).

The neurotransmitter status of Glu and Asp was, however, questioned on the basis that they activated almost all the neurons tested in the CNS, in contrast to the specificity of action expected for a neurotransmitter. Furthermore, the lack of specific and sensitive pharmacological tools precluded a detailed analysis of the action of these amino acids. However, recent advances in the pharmacology and physiology of excitatory amino acids helped to decipher some of these issues. Extensive reviews have been devoted to amino acid actions (Curtis and Johnston, 1974; Krnjević, 1974; Puil, 1981). Some of the more recent developments will be considered in this short review, and some of our recent results using ion-selective microelectrodes will be summarized and discussed.

R. Pumain, I. Kurcewicz, and J. Louvel • Unité de Recherches sur l'Epilepsie, INSERM U 97, 75014 Paris, France.

2. Receptors for Excitatory Amino Acids

In early studies, it was tacitly assumed that the various excitatory amino acids would react with a homogeneous group of receptors. However, subsequent studies on the frog and rat spinal cord made it clear that several classes of receptors were activated by excitatory amino acids. For instance, it was shown that magnesium at low concentration (with a threshold dose of 10 μM) depressed the responses to the aspartate analogue, N-methyl-D-aspartate (NMDA), while having no effect on the responses to the other glutamate agonists, kainate (Ka) or quisqualate (Quis) (Ault et al., 1980). Several organic antagonists were described: the most potent and selective antagonist was 2-amino-5-phosphonovalerate (2APV) which, at low doses, selectively antagonized NMDA responses (Davies et al., 1981). In addition, another glutamate analogue, L-glutamate di-ethylester, antagonized Quis responses (McLennan and Lodge, 1979) while the dipeptide γ-D-glutamylglycine (DGG) depressed both NMDA and Ka responses with a greater efficacy than it depressed Quis responses in the spinal cord (Francis et al., 1980). γ-D-Glutamylaminomethyl sulfonate antagonized Ka and Quis responses, while being considerably less effective than DGG in depressing NMDA-induced responses (Davies and Watkins, 1985).

From such studies, three classes of receptors to excitatory amino acids could be distinguished (McLennan, 1981; Watkins, 1981; Watkins and Evans, 1981). The receptors activated by NMDA were the most easily characterized since the corresponding responses were selectively depressed or abolished by 2APV and by increasing the concentration of extracellular magnesium. The other classes of receptors corresponded to the agonists Quis and Ka. In this context, glutamate and aspartate were considered to have a mixed action on two or more of these classes. Similar but not identical receptors have been described in the hippocampus (Koerner and Cotman, 1982; Monaghan et al., 1983).

3. Conductance Changes Induced by Excitatory Amino Acids

The picture was further complicated because the conductance changes underlying the depolarizing action of the excitatory amino acids were not clearly defined. In early experiments the depolarizations induced by applications of Glu were shown to be accompanied by increases in input conductance (Krnjević and Schwartz, 1967; Martin et al., 1970; Zieglgänsberger and Puil, 1972) while in later studies it was reported to produce either no change in input conductance, or a decrease at small doses followed by an increase at larger doses (Bernardi et al., 1972; Altmann et al., 1976; Constanti et al., 1980; Engberg et al., 1979; Segal, 1981; Hablitz and Langmoen, 1982). It appeared that the depolarizations induced by excitatory amino acids could be attributed to two different mechanisms, one involving a decrease in input conductance, which could not be accounted for by anomalous rectification, and the other involving an increase in input conductance. The former was preferentially activated by NMDA, DL-homocysteate (DLH), and in some cases by Asp, while the latter was activated by Ka and Quis (Engberg et al., 1978, 1979; MacDonald and Wojtowicz, 1980, 1982; Hablitz, 1982; MacDonald and Porietis, 1982; Flatman et al., 1983).

Voltage- and patch-clamp experiments, however, helped clarify the underlying mechanisms. It was shown that the amino acid-induced decreases in input conductance were produced by the activation of a voltage-dependent inward current (MacDonald et al., 1982; Mayer and Westbrook, 1984). Thus, the inward current activated by NMDA, Asp, or DLH increased as the membrane potential was shifted from resting level to about -30 mV, thus producing a region of negative slope conductance and a J-shaped inflection on the I–V curve (MacDonald et al., 1982; Flatman et al., 1983; Mayer and Westbrook, 1984). Under current-clamp conditions, the hyperpolarizing current pulses used to measure the input conductance could bring the membrane potential to values which reduced the voltage-dependent depolarizing current, thereby generating an apparent conductance decrease (see Dingledine, 1983).

The unusual shape of the NMDA-induced I–V curve accounted for the peculiar bursting and bistable behavior of the depolarizations induced, in most cases, by NMDA. In contrast, the increased membrane conductance induced by Ka or Quis are nearly voltage independent, making their action similar to that of acetylcholine at the neuromuscular junction. Thus, the depolarizations induced through Quis or Ka usually give rise to a steady discharge of action potentials.

On spinal neurons in culture, glutamate was demonstrated to activate both conductance changes. I–V plots of Glu responses recorded under voltage-clamp were nonlinear, the slope of the curve decreasing and approaching zero at membrane potentials more negative than −30 mV. Subsequent application of the NMDA antagonist 2APV eliminated the decreases in conductance observed at potentials more negative than −30 mV, such that the I–V curve became more linear, similar to that obtained with Quis or Ka. Furthermore, the glutamate responses could be mimicked by concurrent applications of NMDA and Ka, showing that glutamate has a mixed effect, activating both NMDA and non-NMDA receptors (Mayer and Westbrook, 1984; Westbrook and Mayer, 1984).

The mechanism of the peculiar voltage-dependence of the responses associated with NMDA receptors has recently been elucidated. It had been shown in frog spinal cord that the depolarizations evoked by NMDA were selectively antagonized by low concentrations of magnesium (Ault *et al.*, 1980). Subsequent studies in cultured neurons demonstrated that, when magnesium was omitted from the extracellular fluid, the voltage sensitivity of the NMDA and Glu responses was largely reduced such that the resulting I–V curves were no longer associated with a region of negative slope conductance (Mayer *et al.*, 1984; Nowak *et al.*, 1984; Mayer and Westbrook, 1985). Patch-clamp studies on mouse central neurons in culture have shown that NMDA receptors activate a homogeneous population of channels, whose unitary conductance was about 48 nS. In magnesium-free solutions, the conductance changes induced by the openings of such channels were not voltage sensitive. In the presence of magnesium, the currents recorded at positive potentials remained unaltered, while the currents recorded near resting potential (−60 mV) were reduced, due to fast openings and closings of the channels (''bursts'') and to a reduction of the probability of opening of the channel (Nowak *et al.*, 1984). Both effects were increased with hyperpolarization, therefore accounting for the negative conductance slope observed in the I–V curves during NMDA applications. Thus, the voltage dependence of the responses associated with NMDA receptors appears to result not from an intrinsic property of the channel but from a voltage-dependent channel block occurring in the presence of magnesium. Such a voltage-dependent blocking action of magnesium on NMDA responses has likewise been observed in slices of hippocampus (Crunelli and Mayer, 1984) and neocortex (Thomson, 1986).

4. Ionic Mechanisms

The reversal potentials of the responses to the various excitatory amino acids had similar values between −10 and +2 mV (Langmoen and Hablitz, 1981; Crunelli *et al.*, 1984; Mayer and Westbrook, 1984; Nowak *et al.*, 1984). Such values do not correspond to the equilibrium potential of any single ion. Therefore, the excitatory amino acid-induced depolarizations are produced very probably by a mixed ionic permeability change.

4.1. Sodium Ions

In invertebrates, although at the crayfish neuromuscular junction the glutamate-induced current appeared to be carried mainly by sodium ions (Onodera and Takeuchi, 1976), a mixed ionic current was demonstrated to underlie glutamate depolarizations at insect neuromuscular junctions (Jan and Jan, 1976; Anwyl, 1977). In vertebrates an increased permeability to sodium ions is considered the likely mechanism for at least part of the depolarizing action of glutamate (see review by Puil, 1981). Recent studies in hippocampus and neocortex slices have demonstrated that the reversal potential of glutamate responses was shifted to more negative values when the extracellular sodium was decreased (Hablitz and Langmoen, 1982). In frog spinal cord *in vitro,* glutamate evoked a decrease in extracellular sodium and a concomitant increase in intracellular sodium (Bührle and Sonnhof, 1983), while a reduction in external sodium produced a strong reduction of the glutamate response (Nistri *et al.,* 1985). In cat and rat neocortex, iontophoretic applications of Glu and Asp induced decreases in the concentration of extracellular sodium (Fig. 1). These experiments, among others, demonstrated that the mechanism of action of glutamate involves an increase in sodium permeability. Moreover, the Glu-induced increase in permeability to sodium ions was found to be insensitive to tetrodotoxin (TTX) since Glu responses were not altered by this toxin (Curtis *et al.,* 1972; Zieglgänsberger and Puil, 1972). Similarly, in rat neocortex Glu- and Asp-induced reductions in the concentration of extracellular sodium were TTX insensitive (Fig. 2A) (Pumain *et al.,* 1986b).

Likewise, increased permeability to sodium ions is involved in mediating the responses to NMDA, Ka, and Quis (Flatman *et al.,* 1983, 1986; Luini *et al.,* 1983; Dingledine, 1983; Nowak *et al.,* 1984; Mayer and Westbrook, 1985). Using ion-selective microelectrodes, we observed that, during iontophoretic applications of such amino acids, large, TTX-insensitive decreases in the concentration of extracellular sodium occurred in rat motor cortex in *in vivo* (Fig. 2A) as well as in *in vitro* preparations (Pumain *et al.,* 1986b, 1987). Such decreases were dose dependent, monotonous, and reached a plateau value which was maintained until the applications stopped (Fig. 2A). The maximum values for the decreases were roughly the same for NMDA, Quis, and Ka, about 50 to 60 mM from a baseline level of 145 mM. Sodium-dependent uptake mechanisms do not appear to contribute to the sodium signals since other amino acids, like GABA, for which a powerful uptake system is present in the brain (Balcar and Johnston, 1972; Schousboe, 1981), did not produce any sizable drop in the concentration of extracellular sodium. Therefore, during prolonged applications of excitatory amino acids, there is an important influx of sodium ions into a cellular compartment, probably mainly neuronal. Such an influx should induce a negative shift in the equilibrium potential for sodium ions, which can be estimated to have a maximum value larger than 30 mV.

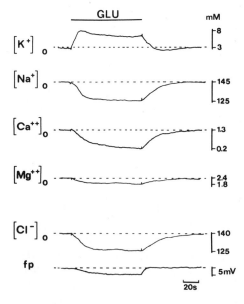

Figure 1. Schematic drawings of the simultaneous changes in the concentration of extracellular ions, measured using ion-selective microelectrodes, induced by iontophoretic applications of L-glutamate in rat cerebral cortex. The tips of the ion-selective microelectrode and of the iontophoretic pipettes were usually no more than 10 μm apart. For more details see Pumain and Heinemann (1985). The various traces were taken from different experiments, and the values given are representative of what is usually observed in the superficial cortical layers using an iontophoretic current of 100 nA. The values were obtained in *in vivo* experiments, except for magnesium, which was measured from neocortical slices.

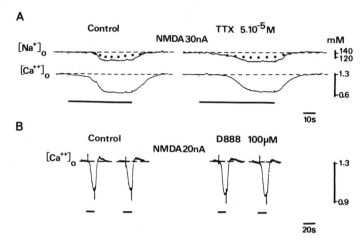

Figure 2. (A) Simultaneous recordings of changes in the concentration of extracellular calcium and sodium induced by the iontophoretic release of NMDA, before (control) and during application of tetrodotoxin (TTX) on the cortical surface at a time when the responses evoked through electrical stimulation were totally abolished. The dotted lines on the sodium traces represent the true sodium signal, corrected for the interference of calcium ions. The recordings were performed in rat sensorimotor cortex *in vivo*. (B) Effect of the organic calcium channel blocker (D-888) on the extracellular calcium signals induced by iontophoretic applications of NMDA. The recordings were performed in a slice of rat sensorimotor cortex. D-888 was introduced in the perfusing medium.

4.2. Potassium Ions

The role of potassium ions in the responses induced by glutamate has been more controversial. In view of the conductance changes induced on spinal motoneurons (see above), several authors proposed that glutamate would induce a decrease of an outward potassium current (Shapovalov *et al.*, 1978; Engberg *et al.*, 1979; MacDonald and Wojtowicz, 1982). Therefore, blockers of various potassium currents were applied or injected to determine if they are affected by excitatory amino acids. Intracellular injections of cesium were usually ineffective (Hablitz and Langmoen, 1982; Dingledine, 1983; Nowak *et al.*, 1984; Crunelli *et al.*, 1984; Mayer and Westbrook, 1985), with the exception of one study in which a nonspecific block of excitatory amino acid responses was observed (Arenson and Nistri, 1985). Tetraethylammonium and 4-aminopyridine were likewise ineffective (Arenson and Nistri, 1985), barium had a slightly potentiating effect (Dingledine, 1983), and increasing the potassium concentration did not reduce markedly the amino acid-induced responses (Dingledine, 1983). Therefore, the decreases in conductance observed during glutamate, aspartate DLH, or NMDA applications could not be accounted for by closure of the various potassium channels which have been described on central neurons, and such decreases have been ascribed to the voltage-dependent blocking effect of magnesium on NMDA channels (see above).

The data obtained using ion-selective microelectrodes have demonstrated that an accumulation of potassium ions, usually moderate, occurs in the extracellular space during applications of glutamate or aspartate (Fig. 1) (Heinemann and Pumain, 1980; Bührle and Sonnhof, 1983; Pumain and Heinemann, 1985), as well as with NMDA, Quis, or Ka (Pumain *et al.*, 1987). Therefore, it appears that the responses to excitatory amino acids are accompanied by an efflux of potassium ions, indicating that channels activated by these amino acids are permeable to potassium, in spite of the suggestion that such an efflux could be passive (Bührle and Sonnhof, 1983). For large iontophoretic doses, the amino acid-induced increases in the concentration of extracellular potassium decline, and an undershooting of the signal below the baseline level is usually observed (Fig. 1), suggesting that an uptake mechanism is activated, possibly due to intracellular accumulation of sodium ions.

4.3. Chloride Ions

Intracellular injections of chloride ions into neurons or the substitution of chloride in the extracellular fluid did not produce any significant alteration of the responses to excitatory amino acids. Therefore, chloride ions do not appear to contribute to such responses and are probably passively distributed during the amino acid-induced depolarizations (Engberg et al., 1979; Bührle and Sonnhof, 1983; Dingledine, 1983; Nowak et al., 1984). In cat and rat neocortex, iontophoretic applications of various excitatory amino acids produced dose-dependent decreases in the concentration of extracellular chloride ions, by up to 30 mM (Fig. 1). Such signals had a time course of decay and of recovery similar to those of the corresponding sodium signals (Heinemann and Pumain, 1988). These results indicate that, during amino acid applications, chloride ions enter nerve cells, contributing to the maintenance of electroneutrality.

4.4. Calcium Ions

Various experiments indicated that glutamate and aspartate responses are associated with an increase in calcium permeability (Heinemann and Pumain, 1980; Bührle and Sonnhof, 1983; Berdichevsky et al., 1983; Dingledine, 1983; Pumain and Heinemann, 1985). However, it was not clear whether the calcium ions entered through voltage-dependent calcium channels or through amino acid-operated channels. Besides, the permeability to calcium of the various conductance mechanisms activated by glutamate might differ. Thus, it has been suggested that NMDA responses have a relatively large calcium component (Dingledine, 1983; Mayer and Westbrook, 1985; MacDermott et al., 1986; Pumain et al., 1986a). Moreover, the relative contributions of sodium and calcium ions to Glu and NMDA responses were unknown.

Therefore, we recorded changes in the concentration of extracellular calcium and sometimes the corresponding change in the concentration of extracellular sodium produced by iontophoretic applications of excitatory amino acids in cat and rat neocortex. Glu and Asp induced dose-dependent and monotonous decreases in extracellular calcium maintained throughout the application (Fig. 1) (Heinemann and Pumain, 1980; Pumain and Heinemann, 1985). Such decreases were largest in the upper cortical layers. The largest changes observed were 1.15 mM (baseline level is about 1.25 mM). NMDA was even more effective in producing decreases in extracellular calcium, since passive diffusion alone from the iontophoretic pipette could produce a reduction in extracellular calcium of 80% of the baseline value. In contrast, Quis and Ka produced very small decreases or even slight increases in extracellular calcium in the upper cortical layers, and no decreases or restricted decreases in deeper layers (Fig. 3A) (Pumain et al., 1987). The calcium signals were unaffected by TTX (Heinemann and Pumain, 1981; Pumain and Heinemann, 1985) or by organic calcium antagonists such as D-888, a derivative of verapamil (Fig. 2A,B), known to abolish high-threshold voltage-dependent calcium channels (Boll and Lux, 1985). Further, the NMDA-induced calcium and sodium signals were both abolished by the selective NMDA receptor antagonist 2APV, as was the Glu-induced calcium signal; the corresponding sodium signal was only slightly reduced (Fig. 3B). These data show that the NMDA channels, besides being permeable to sodium and possibly to potassium, are permeable to calcium, and that the Glu-induced calcium signal reflects mainly the activation by Glu of NMDA receptors. In contrast, Quis and Ka channels have a reduced permeability to calcium, if any. Comparison of the values of the simultaneously recorded NMDA- or Glu-induced sodium and calcium signals provides an estimate of the relative contributions of sodium and calcium ions to the corresponding inward currents: the contribution of calcium appears to be about 8% for NMDA responses (Pumain et al., 1987) and about 2% for Glu responses. Sodium ions appear therefore to form the main charge carrier for inward currents in NMDA and Glu responses.

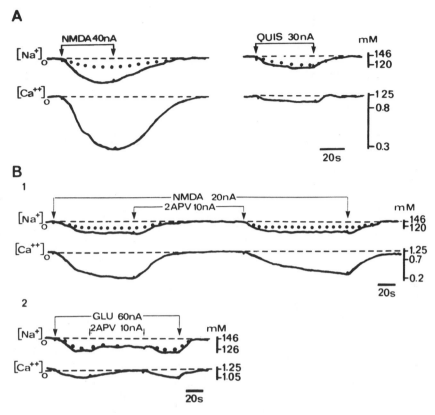

Figure 3. (A) Simultaneous recordings of changes in the concentration of extracellular calcium and sodium induced through applications of NMDA and Quis in rat sensorimotor cortex. The dotted lines on the sodium traces represent the true sodium signal. (B) Effect of the specific NMDA receptor antagonist 2APV on the sodium and calcium responses induced by NMDA and Glu.

4.5. Magnesium Ions

The contribution of magnesium to excitatory amino acid responses is largely unknown. However, in preliminary studies, using a newly developed liquid sensor for magnesium (Lanter *et al.*, 1980), we determined that the resting value of free magnesium in the interstitial space is slightly above 2 mM, and that the extracellular magnesium concentration decreases slightly during NMDA or Glu applications (Fig. 1), indicating that magnesium could enter through the corresponding channels. However, the magnesium sensor is not very selective, and quantitative data are now easily obtained.

5. Involvement of Excitatory Amino Acids in Central Synaptic Transmission

Glutamate and aspartate have been considered as the natural synaptic transmitters at a large number of sites in the CNS. However, due to their mixed agonist action, the resulting mixed conductance changes, and the lack of potent and specific antagonists, a clear-cut demonstration of their involvement in synaptic transmission has seldom been obtained. The recent development of selective antagonists for NMDA responses and the peculiar sensitivity to magnesium of such responses, have yielded a wealth of information. In the spinal cord, polysynaptic activation of single cells following stimulation of low-threshold primary afferent fibers appears to be mediated by NMDA receptors (Watkins, 1984). In rat neocortex, stimulation of the underlying white matter at certain sites evoked, in neurons located in the superficial layers, excitatory postsynaptic potentials which were sensitive to manipulations of the extracellular magnesium concentrations and blocked by the selective NMDA antagonist, 2APV (Thomson et al., 1985; Thomson, 1986). Likewise, 2APV-sensitive postsynaptic potentials have been observed in the red nucleus (Miller and Sheardown, 1986).

However, many synaptic pathways appear to be resistant to NMDA antagonists. In the hippocampus, where a high density of NMDA binding sites has been observed (Monaghan et al., 1983), fast synaptic activity elicited through stimulation of Schaffer collaterals was insensitive to 2APV (Koerner and Cotman, 1982; Collingridge et al., 1983b). However, in magnesium-free medium, there was a pronounced prolongation of the excitatory synaptic potential, which was abolished by 2APV. Thus, during low-frequency stimulation, a component of synaptic excitation mediated by NMDA receptors is hindered by the presence of interstitial magnesium (Herron et al., 1985) During high-frequency stimulation, a slow depolarizing potential developed, which was reduced when 2APV was added to the perfusion medium (Herron et al., 1986). Therefore, responses mediated by NMDA receptors may develop during high-frequency synaptic transmission. A related observation has been made in the thalamus: the responses of ventrobasal neurons to electrical stimulation of afferent fibers were not affected by 2APV, while the responses of the same cells to natural stimuli were abolished (Salt, 1986).

Also, NMDA receptor-mediated events have been implicated in long-term potentiation in the hippocampus (Collingridge et al., 1983; Harris et al., 1984) and in epilepsy (Croucher et al., 1982; Pumain et al., 1986a,b). For example, in the frontal cortex of the photosensitive baboon Papio papio, the drastic reductions in the concentration of extracellular calcium observed in all cortical layers during generalized seizures (Pumain et al., 1985) may result from widespread activation of NMDA receptors. In this context, it may be significant that NMDA receptor antagonists have antiepileptic properties in P. papio (Meldrum et al., 1983).

6. Conclusion

The recent advances in the pharmacology of excitatory amino acids have promoted a revival of interest in these substances in several fields of neuroscience. Increasingly, it has become apparent that, besides the role for which they were initially studied, i.e., the fast synaptic interactions, glutamate and aspartate may contribute to modulatory aspects of functioning of the CNS, and that they may be involved in the physiopathology of various neurological or neuropsychiatric diseases. However, the development of the new pharmacological tools, particularly to manipulate the receptors for Quis and Ka, would be very useful in efforts to understand the role of excitatory amino acids in the brain.

ACKNOWLEDGMENTS. We are grateful to Prof. Dr. R. Kretzschmar (Knoff Ag.) for kindly providing the verapamil derivatives, and to Prof. M. Lamarche for helpful and constructive discussion.

References

Altmann H., ten Bruggencate, G., Pickelmann. P., and Steinberg, R., 1976, Effects of glutamate, aspartate, and two presumed antagonists on feline rubrospinal neurons, *Pfluegers Arch.* **364**:249–255.
Anwyl, R., 1977, Permeability of the post-synaptic membrane of an excitatory glutamate synapse to sodium and potassium. *J. Physiol. (London)* **273**:367–388.

Arenson, M. S., and Nistri, A., 1985, The effect of potassium channel blocking agents on the responses of in vitro frog motoneurones to glutamate and other excitatory amino acids: An intracellular study, *Neuroscience* **14:**317–325.

Ault, B., Evans, R. H., Francis, A. A., Oakes, D. J., and Watkins, J. C., 1980, Selective depression of excitatory amino acid-induced depolarizations by magnesium ions in isolated spinal cord preparations, *J. Physiol. (London)* **307:**413–428.

Balcar, V. J., and Johnston, G. A. R., 1972, The structural specificity of the high affinity uptake of *L*-glutamate and *L*-aspartate by rat brain slices, *J. Neurochem.* **19:**2657–2666.

Berdichevsky, E., Riveros, N., Sanchez-Armass, S., and Orrego, F., 1983, Kainate, N-methylaspartate and other excitatory amino acids increase calcium influx into rat brain cortex cells in vitro, *Neurosci. Lett.* **36:**75–80.

Berl, S., and Waelsch, H., 1958, Determination of glutamic acid, glutamine gluthathione and γ-aminobutyric acid and their distribution in brain tissues, *J. Neurochem.* **3:**161–169.

Bernardi, G., Zieglgänsberger, W., Herz, A., and Puil, E., 1972, Intracellular studies on the action of *L*-glutamic acid on spinal neurones of the cat, *Brain Res.* **39:**523–525.

Boll, W., and Lux, H. D., 1985, Action of organic antagonists on neuronal calcium currents, *Neurosci. Lett.* **56:**335–339.

Bührle, C., and Sonnhof, U., 1983, The ionic mechanism of the excitatory action of glutamate upon the membranes of motoneurones of the frog, *Pfluegers Arch.* **396:**154–162.

Collingridge, G. L., Kehl, S. J., and McLennan, H., 1983a, The antagonism of amino acid-induced excitations of rat hippocampal CA1 neurones in vitro, *J. Physiol. (London)* **334:**19–31.

Collingridge, G. L., Kehl, S. J., and McLennan, H., 1983b, Excitatory amino acids in synaptic transmission in the Schaffer collateral–commissural pathway of the rat hippocampus, *J. Physiol. (London)* **334:**33–46.

Constanti, A., Connor, J. D., Galvan, M., and Nistri, A., 1980, Intracellularly-recorded effects of glutamate and aspartate on neurones in the guinea-pig olfactory cortex slice, *Brain Res.* **195:**403–422.

Croucher, M. J., Collins, J. F., and Meldrum, B. S., 1982, Anticonvulsant action of excitatory amino acid antagonists, *Science* **216:**899–901.

Crunelli, V., and Mayer, M. L., 1984, Mg^{2+} dependence of membrane resistance increases evoked by NMDA in hippocampal neurones, *Brain Res.* **311:**392–396.

Crunelli, V., Forda, S., and Kelly, J. S., 1984, The reversal potential of excitatory amino acid action on granule cells of the rat dentate gyrus, *J. Physiol. (London)* **351:**327–342.

Curtis, D. R., and Johnston, G. A. R., 1974, Amino acid transmitters in the mammalian central nervous system, *Ergeb. Physiol.* **67:**97–188.

Curtis, D. R., Phillis, J. W., and Watkins, J. C., 1960, The chemical excitation of spinal neurones by certain acidic amino acids, *J. Physiol. (London)* **150:**656–682.

Curtis, D. R., Duggan, A. W., Felix, D., Johnston, G. A. R., Tebecis, A. K., and Watkins, J. C., 1972, Excitation of mammalian central neurones by acidic amino acids, *Brain Res.* **41:**283–301.

Davies, J., and Watkins, J. C., 1985, Depressant action of gamma-D-glutamylaminomethyl sulfonate (GAMS) on amino acid induced and synaptic excitation in the cat spinal cord, *Brain Res.* **327:**113–120.

Davies, J., Francis, A. A., Jones, A. W., and Watkins, J. C., 1981, 2-Amino-5-phosphonovalerate (2APV), a potent and selective antagonist of amino-acid-induced and synaptic excitation, *Neurosci. Lett.* **21:**77–81.

Dingledine, R., 1983, N-methyl aspartate activates voltage-dependent calcium conductance in rat hippocampal pyramidal cells, *J. Physiol. (London)* **343:**385–406.

Engberg, I., Flatman, J. A., and Lambert, J. D. C., 1978, The action of N-methyl-D-aspartic and kainic acids on motoneurones with emphasis on conductance changes, *Br. J. Pharmacol.* **64:**384–385.

Engberg, I., Flatman, J. A., and Lambert, J. D. C., 1979, The actions of excitatory amino acids on motoneurones in the feline spinal cord, *J. Physiol. (London)* **288:**227–261.

Flatman, J. A., Schwindt, P. C., Crill, W. E., and Stafstrom, C. E., 1983, Multiple actions of N-methyl-D-aspartate on cat neocortical neurons in vitro, *Brain Res.* **266:**169–173.

Flatman, J. A., Schwindt, P. C., and Crill, W. E., 1986, The induction and modification of voltage-sensitive responses in cat neocortical neurons by N-methyl-D-aspartate, *Brain Res.* **363:**62–77.

Fonnum, F., 1984, Glutamate: A neurotransmitter in mammalian brain, *J. Neurochem.* **42:**1–11.

Francis, A. A., Jones, A. W., and Watkins, J. C., 1980, Dipeptide antagonists of amino acid-induced and synaptic excitation in the frog spinal cord, *J. Neurochem.* **35:**1458–1460.

Hablitz, J. J., 1982, Conductance changes induced by DL-homocysteic acid and N-methyl-DL-aspartic acid in hippocampal neurons, *Brain Res.* **247:**149–153.

Hablitz, J. J., and Langmoen, I. A., 1982, Excitation of hippocampal pyramidal cells by glutamate in the guinea-pig and rat, *J. Physiol. (London)* **325:**317–331.

Harris, E. W., Ganong, A. H., and Cotman, C. W., 1984, Long-term potentiation in the hippocampus involves activation of N-methyl-D-aspartate receptors, *Brain Res.* **323:**132–137.

Heinemann, U., and Pumain, R., 1980, Extracellular calcium activity changes in cat sensorimotor cortex induced by iontophoretic application of aminoacids, *Exp. Brain Res.* **40**:247–250.

Heinemann, U., and Pumain, R., 1981, Effects of tetrodotoxin on changes in extracellular free calcium induced by repetitive electrical stimulation and iontophoretic application of excitatory amino acids in the sensorimotor cortex of cats, *Neurosci. Lett.* **21**:87–91.

Heinemann, U., and Pumain, R., 1988, Changes in the brain cell microenvironment and their functional consequences, *Physiol. Rev.,* (in preparation).

Herron, C. E., Lester, R. A. J., Coan, E. J., and Collingridge, G. L., 1985, Intracellular demonstration of an N-methyl-D-aspartate receptor mediated component of synaptic transmission in the rat hippocampus, *Neurosci. Lett.* **60**:19–23.

Herron, C. E., Lester, R. A. J., Coan, E. J., and Collingridge, G. L., 1986, Frequency-dependent involvement of NMDA receptors in the hippocampus: A novel synaptic mechanism, *Nature* **322**:265–268.

Jan, L. Y., and Jan, Y. N., 1976, L-Glutamate as an excitatory transmitter at the "drosophila" larval neuromuscular junction, *J. Physiol. (London)* **262**:215–236.

Jasper, H. H., and Koyama, I., 1969, Rate of release of amino acids from the cerebral cortex in the cat as affected by brainstem and thalamic stimulation, *Can. J. Physiol. Pharmacol.* **47**:889–905.

Jasper, H. H., Khan, R. T., and Elliott, K. A. C., 1965, Amino acids released from cerebral cortex in relation to its state of activation, *Science* **147**:1448–1449.

Koerner, J. F., and Cotman, C. W., 1982, Response of Shaffer collateral–CA1 pyramidal cell synapses of the hippocampus to analogues of acidic amino acids, *Brain Res.* **251**:105–115.

Krnjević, K., 1974, Chemical nature of synaptic transmission in vertebrates, *Physiol. Rev.* **54**:419–540.

Krnjević, K., and Schwartz, S., 1967, Some properties of unresponsive cells in the cerebral cortex, *Exp. Brain Res.* **3**:306–319.

Langmoen, I. A., and Hablitz, J. J., 1981, Reversal potential for glutamate responses in hippocampal pyramidal cells, *Neurosci. Lett.* **23**:61–65.

Lanter, F., Erne, D., Ammann, D., and Simon W., 1980, Neutral carrier based ion-selective electrode for intracellular magnesium activities studies, *Anal. Chem.* **52**:2400–2402.

Logan, W. J., and Snyder, S. H., 1972, High affinity uptake systems for glycine, glutamic and aspartic acids in synaptosomes of rat central nervous tissues, *Brain Res.* **42**:413–431.

Luini, A., Goldberg, O., and Teichberg, V. I., 1983, Differential sensitivity of selected brain areas to excitatory amino acids, *Neurosci. Lett.* **41**:307–312.

MacDermott, A. B., Mayer, M. L., Westbrook, G. L., Smith, S. J., and Barker, J. L., 1986, NMDA-receptor activation increases cytoplasmic calcium concentration in cultured spinal cord neurones, *Nature* **321**:519–522.

MacDonald, J. F., and Porietis, A., 1982, DL-Quisqualic and L-aspartate acids activate separate excitatory conductances in cultured spinal cord neurons, *Brain Res.* **245**:175–178.

MacDonald, J. F., and Wojtowicz, J. M., 1980, Two conductance mechanisms activated by applications of L-glutamic, L-aspartic, DL-homocysteic, N-methyl-D-aspartic, and DL-kainic acids to cultured mammalian central neurones, *Can. J. Physiol. Pharmacol.* **58**:1393–1397.

MacDonald, J. F., and Wojtowicz, J. M., 1982, The effects of L-glutamate and its analogues upon the membrane conductance of central murine neurones in culture, *Can. J. Physiol. Pharmacol.* **60**:282–296.

MacDonald, J. F., Porietis, A., and Wojtowicz, J. M., 1982, L-Aspartic acid induces a region of negative slope conductance in the current–voltage relationship of cultured spinal cord neurons, *Brain Res.* **237**:248–253.

McLennan, H., 1981, On the nature of the receptors for various excitatory amino acids in the mammalian central nervous system, in: *Glutamate as a Neurotransmitter* (G. Di Chiara and G. L. Gessa, eds.), Raven Press, New York, pp. 253–262.

McLennan, H., and Lodge, D., 1979, The antagonism of amino acid-induced excitation of spinal neurones in the cat, *Brain Res.* **169**:83–90.

Martin, A. R., Wickelgren, W. O., and Beranek, R., 1970, Effect of iontophoretically applied drugs on spinal interneurons of the lamprey, *J. Physiol. (London)* **207**:653–665.

Mayer, M. L., and Westbrook, G. L., 1984, Mixed-agonist action of excitatory amino acids on mouse spinal cord neurones under voltage clamp, *J. Physiol. (London)* **354**:29–53.

Mayer, M. L., and Westbrook, G. L., 1985, The action of N-methyl-D-aspartic acid on mouse spinal neurones in culture, *J. Physiol. (London)* **361**:65–90.

Mayer, M. L., Westbrook, G. L., and Guthrie, P. B., 1984, Voltage-dependent block by Mg^{2+} of NMDA responses in spinal cord neurons, *Nature* **309**:250–263.

Meldrum, B. S., Croucher, M. J., Badman, G., and Collins, J. F., 1983, Antiepileptic action of excitatory amino acid antagonists in the photosensitive baboon, *Papio papio, Neurosci. Lett.* **39**:101–104.

Miller, D. J., and Sheardown, M. J., 1986, Amino acid receptor-mediated excitatory synaptic transmission in the rat red nucleus, *J. Physiol. (London)* **376**:14–30.

Monaghan, D. T., Holets, V. R., Toy, D. W., and Cotman, C. W., 1983, Anatomical distribution of four pharmacological distinct ³H-L-glutamate binding sites, *Nature* **306:**176–179.

Nistri, A., Arenson, M. S., and King, A., 1985, Excitatory amino acid-induced responses of frog motoneurones bathed in low Na+ media: An intracellular study, *Neuroscience* **14:**921–927.

Nowak, L., Bregestovski, P., Ascher, P., Herbert, A., and Prochiantz, A., 1984, Magnesium gates glutamate-activated channels in mouse central neurones, *Nature* **307:**462–465.

Onodera, K., and Takeuchi, A., 1976, Permeability changes produced by L-glutamate at the excitatory post-synaptic membrane of the crayfish muscle, *J. Physiol. (London)* **255:**669–685.

Perry, T. L., Hansen, S., and Gandham, S. S., 1981, Post mortem changes of amino compounds in human and rat brain, *J. Neurochem.* **36:**406–412.

Potashner, S. J., 1978a, The spontaneous and electrically evoked release, from slices of guinea-pig cerebral cortex, of endogenous amino acids labelled via metabolism of D-[U-¹⁴C]glucose, *J. Neurochem.* **31:**177–186.

Potashner, S. J., 1978b, Effects of tetrodotoxin, calcium and magnesium on the release of amino acids from slices of guinea-pig cerebral cortex, *J. Neurochem.* **31:**187–195.

Puil, E., 1981, S-Glutamate: Its interactions with spinal neurons, *Brain Res. Rev.* **3:**229–322.

Pumain, R., and Heinemann, U., 1985, Stimulus- and amino acid-induced calcium and potassium changes in rat neocortex, *J. Neurophysiol.* **53:**1–16.

Pumain, R., Menini, C., Heinemann, U., Louvel, J., and Silva-Barrat, C., 1985, Chemical synaptic transmission is not necessary for epileptic seizures to persist in the baboon *Papio papio*, *Exp. Neurol.* **89:**250–258.

Pumain, R., Kurcewicz, I., and Louvel, J., 1986a, Ionic concomitants in chronic epilepsies, in: *Epilepsy and Calcium* (E.-J. Speckmann, H. Schulze, and J. Walden, eds.), Urban & Schwarzenberg, Munich, pp. 207–226.

Pumain, R., Louvel, J., and Kurcewicz, I., 1986b, Long-term alterations in amino acid-induced ionic conductances in chronic epilepsy, in: *Amino Acids and Epilepsy* (Y. Ben Ari and R. Schwarcz, eds.), Plenum Press, New York, pp. 439–447.

Pumain, R., Kurcewicz, I., and Louvel, J., 1987, Ionic changes induced by excitatory amino acids in the rat cerebral cortex, *Can. J. Physiol. Pharmacol.* **65:**1067–1077.

Salt, T. E., 1986, Mediation of thalamic sensory inputs by both NMDA- and non-NMDA receptors, *Nature* **322:**263–265.

Schousboe, A., 1981, Transport and metabolism of glutamate and GABA in neurons and glia cells, *Int. Rev. Neurobiol.* **22:**1–45.

Schousboe, A., Fosmark, H., and Hertz, L., 1975, High content of glutamate and of ATP in astrocytes cultured from rat brain hemispheres: Effect of serum withdrawal and of cyclic AMP, *J. Neurochem.* **25:**909–911.

Segal, M., 1981, The actions of glutamic acid on neurons in the rat hippocampal slice, in: *Glutamate as a Neurotransmitter* (G. Di Chiara and G. L. Gessa, eds.), Raven Press, New York, pp. 217–225.

Shapovalov, A. I., Shiriaev, B. I., and Velumanian, A. A., 1978, Mechanisms of post-synaptic excitations in amphibian motoneurones, *J. Physiol. (London)* **279:**437–455.

Thomson, A. M., 1986, A magnesium sensitive postsynaptic potential in rat cerebral cortex resembles neuronal responses to N-methylaspartate, *J. Physiol. (London)* **370:**531–549.

Thomson, A. M., West, D. C., and Lodge, D., 1985, An N-methyl-aspartate receptor mediated synapse in rat cerebral cortex: A site of action of ketamine, *Nature* **313:**479–481.

Watkins, J. C., 1981, Pharmacology of excitatory amino acid transmitters, in: *Amino Acid Neurotransmitters* (F. V. De Feudis and P. Mandel, eds.), Raven Press, New York, pp. 205–212.

Watkins, J. C., 1984, Excitatory amino acids and central synaptic transmission, *Trends Pharmacol. Sci.* **5:**373–376.

Watkins, J. C., and Evans, R. H., 1981, Excitatory amino acids, *Annu. Rev. Pharmacol. Toxicol.* **21:**165–204.

Westbrook. G. L., and Mayer, M. L., 1984, Glutamate currents in mammalian spinal neurons: resolution of a paradox, *Brain Res.* **301:**375–379.

Zieglgänsberger, W., and Puil, E. A., 1972, Tetrodotoxin interference of CNS excitation by glutamic acid, *Nature New Biol.* **239:**204–205.

7

Effects of Excitatory Amino Acid Agonists and Antagonists on in Vitro Motoneurons

A. Nistri

1. Introduction

Since the pioneering observations by Hayashi (1954) on the convulsive action of the naturally occurring amino acid glutamate, electrophysiological work by Curtis *et al.* (1960) and by Krnjević and Phillis (1963) demonstrated an intense excitatory activity produced by this substance when applied to single neurons of the CNS. Effects very similar to those of glutamate were also induced by aspartate, another amino acid endogenous to the brain, and a series of structurally related analogues (Curtis and Watkins, 1963; Krnjević, 1965). Nevertheless, it was thought at that time that glutamate was unlikely to be a major central excitatory neurotransmitter particularly in view of its apparent lack of selectivity, i.e., it excited almost all neurons tested. The perception of the role of glutamate as a central neurotransmitter did, however, change owing to the fundamental work by Jasper *et al.* (1965), who studied the release of endogenous glutamate from the cat cerebral cortex *in vivo*. These workers found that significantly higher amounts of endogenous glutamate were released during wakefulness than during sleep; it appeared therefore that the rate of release of this amino acid was closely related to the degree of activity of cortical neurons. Subsequent neurochemical and electrophysiological work has confirmed the view that glutamate is probably an important excitatory transmitter in the vertebrate CNS (for some reviews see: Nistri and Constanti, 1979; Puil, 1981; Watkins and Evans, 1981; Fagg and Foster, 1983; Fonnum, 1984; Nistri, 1985).

Electrophysiological studies on glutamate have focused on two main issues: (1) whether glutamate, aspartate, and related analogues act via a homogeneous receptor population; and (2) whether glutamate activates neurons by increasing their permeability to Na^+ and K^+ in a fashion like the classical transmitter acetylcholine operates at the neuromuscular junction.

Regarding the nature of the glutamate receptor, it was suggested by Duggan (1974) and McCulloch *et al.* (1974) that different receptors for glutamate and aspartate may exist. Since these compounds can assume various spatial conformations owing to the flexibility of their molecules, it was thought that some receptors would accept glutamate in an extended conformation while others would preferentially accept aspartate, which has a relatively folded conformation. However, it was the systematic work by Watkins and his associates (Watkins and Evans, 1981) based on

A. Nistri • Department of Pharmacology, St. Bartholomew's Hospital Medical College, University of London, London EC1M 6BQ, United Kingdom.

extracellular recordings from spinal neurons which eventually led to a classification of excitatory amino acid receptors dependent on their sensitivity to various glutamate analogues: N-methyl-D-aspartate (NMDA)-sensitive receptors, quisqualate-sensitive receptors, and kainate-sensitive receptors. Glutamate and aspartate are considered to be "mixed agonists" able to bind more than one type of receptor, although glutamate may prefer the quisqualate receptor and aspartate may predominantly act on NMDA sites. An important validation of this classification came with the availability of selective antagonists, in particular D-aminophosphonovalerate (D-APV), which is to date the most specific and potent blocker of NMDA receptors (Evans *et al.*, 1982). The search for selective antagonists of quisqualate or kainate receptors continues and new compounds affecting these sites are eagerly awaited.

Investigations into the mechanisms responsible for the excitatory effects of glutamate have also provided an interesting insight into the regulation of neuronal excitability. While it is widely accepted that glutamate acts by depolarizing the neuronal membrane, there has been controversy about the ionic basis for depolarization. Intracellular recording from mammalian neurons unexpectedly showed little or no neuronal conductance change associated with the glutamate depolarization (e.g., see Altmann *et al.*, 1976; Engberg *et al.*, 1979). Even after corrections for membrane rectification, the action of glutamate on cell conductance was found to be small and in the case of some agonists (e.g., NMDA and homocysteate) there was an actual decrease in the recorded conductance. Several views were advanced to explain this phenomenon accompanying the glutamate depolarization: a decrease in membrane permeability to K^+, an increased permeability to Na^+ together with a decreased permeability to K^+, or a predominantly remote location of glutamate-activated channels so that their conductance responses could not be detected (these theories are discussed by Puil, 1981). More recently, it has been suggested (Nowak *et al.*, 1984; Mayer and Westbrook, 1985) that the ionic channels opened by activation of NMDA receptors display a strong voltage sensitivity in the presence of Mg^{2+}. Since Mg^{2+} blocks these channels over a fairly large range of membrane potential values, this phenomenon can account for the apparent lack of conductance increases in the presence of NMDA, glutamate, and aspartate.

Most of the studies conducted so far have used either extracellular recordings or cultured embryonic neurons. Although highly desirable from an experimental viewpoint, it is difficult to record intracellularly from *in vivo* neurons while controlling the extracellular ionic composition and drug concentrations effectively. Hence, it is advantageous to employ a slice preparation of central nervous tissue which can retain a synaptic circuitry with fully developed architectural organization while allowing manipulations of the extracellular environment and applications of drugs of known concentrations. Since a considerable number of pharmacological (Watkins and Evans, 1981) and electrophysiological (Nistri and Constanti, 1979) studies have been carried out on the frog spinal cord *in vitro*, we decided to use this preparation for intracellular recordings from motoneurons under current- and voltage-clamp conditions. Our experimental goals were essentially to clarify the amino acid receptor pharmacology on spinal motoneurons and to investigate the ionic basis of the depolarization evoked by the excitatory amino acids. We used a hemisected slice preparation of the frog spinal cord retaining pairs of spinal roots and continuously superfused with Ringer solution at 5–7°C to minimize the cellular uptake of amino acids (Davidoff and Adair, 1975). Furthermore, as motoneurons have relatively large somata (about 50 μm), it was possible to record intracellularly from them for prolonged periods of up to a few hours (the slice itself, when maintained at 5–7°C, often survived for several days). Finally, since motoneurons are functionally identified on the basis of their all-or-none antidromic spike, these cells provided a homogeneous population for the studies described herein.

2. Methods

Experiments were carried out on frogs (*Rana temporaria*) kept in an aquarium at 6°C for several days before use. After decerebration the spinal cord was removed and a parasagittal slice prepared with two pairs of lumbar roots attached. The preparation was transferred to a three-chambered Perspex bath, the center part containing the spinal slice and the two side chambers containing either ventral or dorsal roots gently drawn through silicon grease-filled grooves in the bath walls. The bath was maintained at 5–7°C and the temperature was monitored with the miniature probe of an electronic thermometer. Drug solutions were admitted via separate pre-cooled flowlines with a common entry to the bath whose small volume (0.2 ml) coupled with a relatively small dead space allowed rapid exchange of bathing solutions applied at a fast rate (5–10 ml/min). Spinal ventral and dorsal roots were gently drawn into miniature suction electrodes for electrical stimulation (0.20–0.25 Hz; 0.1 msec; variable intensity). Motoneurons were impaled with 3 M KCl-filled microelectrodes (40–80 MΩ) although 2–3 M CsCl or 1.5 M potassium citrate electrodes were occasionally used. Responses were recorded via high-impedance electrometers (WPI M-707 or Dagan 8100), monitored on a storage oscilloscope, displayed on a linear pen recorder, and stored on FM magnetic tape (DC—3 kHz) for subsequent analysis. For somatic voltage clamping, the single electrode voltage clamp (SEVC) facility of the Dagan amplifier was used with switching frequency of about 8 kHz and a 50% duty cycle. Voltage clamping required relatively low-resistance microelectrodes with consequently less prolonged periods of intracellular recording.

The composition of the standard Ringer solution was as follows (mM): NaCl 111, KCl 2.5, NaHCO$_3$ 17, NaH$_2$PO$_4$·2H$_2$O 0.1, CaCl$_2$ 2, glucose 4 and was gassed with 95% O$_2$–5% CO$_2$ (pH 7.4).

3. Results

3.1. Characteristics of Motoneuronal Electrical Responses

In over 100 motoneurons studied, resting membrane potential was found to be about −70 mV; input conductance was measured either from electrotonic potentials evoked by constant hyperpolarizing 600-msec current pulses or from the slope of I–V relations. Conductance values at rest were 70–90 nS. The antidromic spike of motoneurons had an overshooting of 15–20 mV and was followed by typical afterpotentials, namely an early afterhyperpolarization (AHP$_e$), an afterdepolarization (ADP), and a late AHP (AHP$_l$) (see also Schwindt, 1976). Motoneurons often displayed spontaneous synaptic activity mainly consisting of depolarizing postsynaptic potentials frequently large enough to trigger action potentials. Spontaneous and root-evoked electrical activities were abolished by tetrodotoxin (TTX) (1–6 μM).

3.2. Effects of Excitatory Amino Acid Agonists

Several excitatory compounds were tested including glutamate (0.7–2 mM), aspartate (2 mM), NMDA (30 μM), quisqualate (15–30 μM), DL-homocysteate (DLH) (0.1–1 mM), and DL-α-amino-3-hydroxy-5-methyl-4-isoxazole-propionate (AMPA) (25–100 μM). Figure 1 (top) shows a chart record of membrane potential changes produced by 1 mM glutamate and 1 mM DLH. Both agonists elicited a depolarization which was much larger in the case of DLH. In this experiment the cell conductance estimated by the amplitude of hyperpolarizing electrotonic potentials (monitored as downward deflections) was increased by only 7 and 14% at the peak of the depolarizations induced by glutamate and DLH, respectively. Responses a–i of Fig. 1 are oscilloscope records of antidromic action potentials taken at the corresponding times indicated in the chart record. At the peak of the depolarizing effects the spike time to peak was reduced and the amplitude of the AHP$_e$ (seen as an early undershoot of the baseline) was increased. Thus, these effects were consistent with a membrane depolarization which was gradually reversible on washout. They represent the principal response of motoneurons to these compounds. In most studies done to compare agonist activity

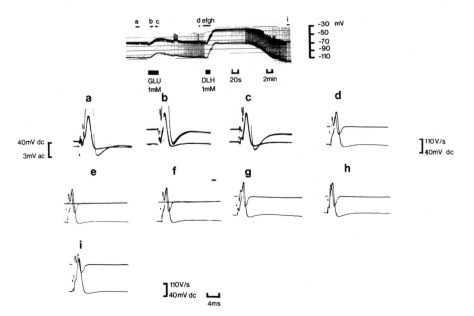

Figure 1. Effects of glutamate (GLU) and DL-homocysteate (DLH) on spinal motoneuron. (Top) Chart record of membrane potential with hyperpolarizing electrotonic potentials (downward deflections) elicited by constant-current injections and used to monitor cell input conductance. Note that DHL elicits a larger depolarization than glutamate (during both responses there is little conductance change). (Bottom) Oscilloscope records of antidromic action potentials taken during periods (a–h) shown by lines above the chart record of membrane potential. In a–c the top trace is high-gain ac and the bottom trace is low-gain dc. In d–i the top trace is the first time derivative of the spike and the bottom is low-gain dc. (A. Nistri and M. S. Arenson, unpublished.)

of these excitants, applications were adjusted to produce equipotent depolarizations (of approximately 10 mV amplitude). In this way it was possible to avoid excessive membrane depolarization and hence a shift of membrane potential values to a region of rectification (Schwindt, 1976). In some cells the depolarizations induced by the excitants were associated with large increases in the baseline thickness (e.g., see top left of Fig. 4) reflecting intense synaptic bombardment of the motoneuronal membrane. This phenomenon, which was abolished by TTX, was presumably also responsible for the measured conductance increases indirectly caused by release of unidentified neurotransmitters (compare top tracings in Fig. 4).

Responses to glutamate, NMDA, or quisqualate were also studied under SEVC conditions with the holding potential at the level of resting membrane potential. The clamp gain was adjusted to the maximum value permissible without oscillations and checks were carried out to establish that EPSPs (of up to 10 mV amplitude) could be voltage clamped. Figure 2 shows spontaneous synaptic potentials under current clamp (A) and subsequently under voltage clamp (B) where responses were observed as inward currents (displayed as downward deflections). Figure 2C shows the inward current response elicited by electrical stimulation of a lumbar dorsal root. Under these conditions, glutamate, quisqualate, and NMDA evoked responses consisting predominantly of inward currents of 100–200 pA amplitude with different time courses (see Fig. 5). In fact, glutamate currents had a consistently faster risetime and decay when compared to those activated by NMDA or quisqualate. Much larger inward currents could not be adequately clamped by the SEVC used in the present experiments.

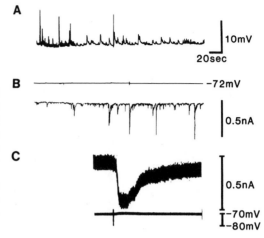

Figure 2. Current- and voltage-clamp records of synaptic activity in a motoneuron. (A) Spontaneous synaptic potential in control Ringer solution under current clamp. (B) Spontaneous inward currents (bottom) recorded from the same cell voltage clamped at membrane potential level (top). (C) Inward current elicited by dorsal root stimulation (top, current; bottom, voltage) of motoneuron clamped at resting membrane potential (−70 mV). Time calibration in C is 20 msec (bar calibration is in A). (A. Nistri and A. E. King, unpublished.)

3.3. Unusual Components of the Responses to Excitatory Amino Acid Agonists

In addition to the typical depolarization seen following the application of excitatory amino acids, two additional effects were observed. Under conventional current-clamp conditions, provided that the excitant-evoked depolarization did not develop very rapidly, a small but significant increase in the duration (and/or size) of the ADP of the antidromic spike was detected prior to measurable changes in resting membrane potential or conductance (Fig. 3). This ADP alteration was small but distinctive as the other components of the spike did not vary in parallel. Of course, when a membrane depolarization occurred, this phenomenon was fully masked by the alteration in the spike configuration imposed by the new membrane potential level (Arenson and Nistri, 1982a). The transient nature of this event prevented further systematic studies.

In about 33% of the motoneurons the depolarization was preceded by a small hyperpolarization (on average 3 mV) accompanied by a conductance increase of approximately 30% (e.g., see Fig. 4 top). This small effect manifested itself as an outward current under SEVC (Fig. 5). Interestingly, the hyperpolarizing response was sufficient to block firing and was not prevented by abolishing synaptic transmission with Mn^{2+} (2 mM) or by injecting the K^+ channel blocker Cs^+ inside motoneurons (Arenson and Nistri, 1982b).

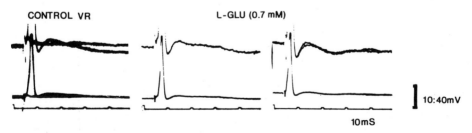

Figure 3. Oscilloscope records of antidromic action potentials (at high and low gain, top and bottom respectively) of motoneuron evoked by ventral root (VR) stimulation. (Left) Control (with intermittent failure); middle: 10 sec after starting superfusion with glutamate (note increase in amplitude and particularly in duration of ADP in top trace); right: 60 sec after starting glutamate application (note depolarization and increase in amplitude of $AHP_{e,1}$). (A. Nistri and M. S. Arenson, unpublished.)

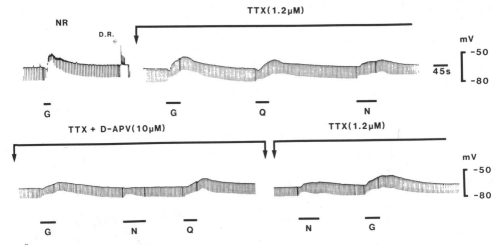

Figure 4. Membrane potential records obtained from a single motoneuron showing the effect of D-APV on responses to glutamate (G; 2 mM), quisqualate (Q; 30 μM), and NMDA (N; 30 μM); the durations of application are represented by horizontal bars. (Upper traces) NR indicates a glutamate response in control Ringer and is followed by amino acid responses after 35 min exposure to 1.2 μM tetrodotoxin (TTX); note dorsal root-evoked excitatory potentials (*D.R.) in NR. (Lower traces) Responses after superfusions with a TTX- and 10 μM D-APV-containing solution and subsequent recovery after D-APV removal. The downward deflections are hyperpolarizing electrotonic potentials evoked by intracellular current injection. (From Corradetti *et al.*, 1985.)

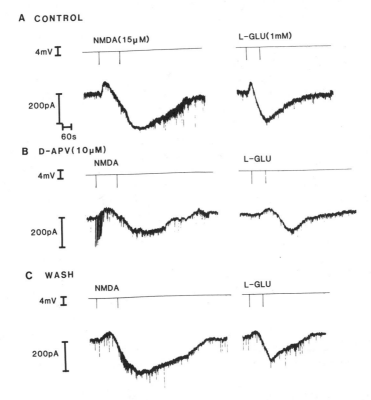

Figure 5. Chart records of responses induced by NMDA or glutamate (L-GLU) in motoneuron clamped at resting membrane potential (−70 mV). In each pair of tracings, top shows voltage record and bottom shows current. (A) Control inward currents induced by NMDA or glutamate (note also spontaneous activity). (B) In the presence of D-APV there is a strong depression of both responses with recovery on washout (C). (A. Nistri and A. E. King, unpublished.)

3.4. Pharmacological Antagonism of Excitatory Amino Acid Responses

In view of the reported selectivity of D-APV as an NMDA antagonist (Evans *et al*, 1982), we compared the responses evoked by this compound with the responses evoked by NMDA, glutamate, aspartate, quisqualate, and AMPA. Figure 4 shows one such experiment. After applying TTX to abolish indirect actions of amino acids, matched depolarizations were evoked by glutamate, quisqualate, and NMDA. In the presence of 10 μM D-APV, the depolarizing action of NMDA was fully antagonized but that of quisqualate was unaffected. The glutamate depolarization was reduced to an intermediate level (Corradetti *et al.*, 1985). Nevertheless, there was no significant change in the input conductance values observed during application of the excitants in TTX- or D-APV-containing media. Pooled data from 31 motoneurons indicated that 1 μM D-APV blocked the NMDA depolarization by 85%, the glutamate and aspartate depolarizations by 37 and 39%, respectively, with no significant effect on responses to quisqualate or AMPA (25–100 μM). Much higher doses of D-APV (up to 200 μM) failed to antagonize further the action of glutamate. Voltage-clamp data validated the conclusions about the selectivity of the D-APV antagonism (King and Nistri, 1985). As shown in Fig. 5, the NMDA current was strongly depressed by 10 μM D-APV while a comparatively smaller antagonism of the glutamate current was seen. A less potent and specific NMDA antagonist is D-aminoadipate (Watkins and Evans, 1981). This substance (50–200 μM) was also found to be a blocker of NMDA depolarizations while sparing quisqualate responses (Arenson *et al.*, 1984). Glutamate and aspartate responses were, however, more profoundly reduced than in the presence of D-APV.

Attempts to block selectively quisqualate receptors were far less successful. Glutamic acid diethylester (GDEE) has been considered to be a relatively specific antagonist for these receptors (Watkins and Evans, 1981). In our experiments (King *et al.*, 1985), GDEE (0.1–1 mM) was ineffective against quisqualate- or AMPA-evoked depolarizations and revealed only a slight (15%) antagonism of glutamate responses. Indeed, the highest concentration (1 mM) of GDEE produced some local anesthetic action seen as a depression and broadening of the antidromic action potential.

It is well known that divalent cations are antagonists of excitatory amino acid responses (e.g., see Ault *et al.*, 1980). More recently, Mg^{2+} has been shown to interact with NMDA-activated channels (Nowak *et al.*, 1984; Mayer and Westbrook, 1985). Since the frog Ringer solution is typically Mg^{2+} free, we decided to investigate the influence of this divalent cation on motoneuronal responses to excitatory amino acids. At concentrations higher than 1–2 mM, Mg^{2+} depresses neuronal excitability in the frog spinal cord (Erulkar *et al.*, 1974) in the same way it does so on mammalian brain neurons (Kelly *et al.*, 1969). In our study we used smaller Mg^{2+} concentrations (0.1–0.5 mM) in an attempt to observe a selective effect of this ion on the membrane mechanisms activated by excitatory amino acids. Mg^{2+} (0.1 mM) halved the depolarizing action of NMDA without significant effect toward glutamate or quisqualate responses (Fig. 6 top; Nistri and King, 1986). Higher Mg^{2+} concentrations were found to abolish NMDA responses and to reduce those to glutamate more than those to quisqualate. Results were essentially the same when preparations were pretreated with TTX. Analysis of the conductance changes due to excitatory amino acids during application of Mg^{2+} revealed complex and variable results. In a few cells, as shown in the example of Fig. 6 (bottom), Mg^{2+} blocked the NMDA conductance increases and depressed those evoked by glutamate. Nevertheless, in most cells bathed in a TTX solution the amino acids elicited rather small conductance changes and subsequent addition of Mg^{2+} did not significantly alter these responses.

3.5. Effects of Excitatory Amino Acid Antagonists on Motoneuronal EPSPs

By applying electrical stimuli to dorsal root fibers it was possible to elicit from motoneurons synaptic potentials which were regarded as mono- or polysynaptic EPSPs. The differentiation was based on the latency and amplitude of the responses and on the intensity of stimulation required to

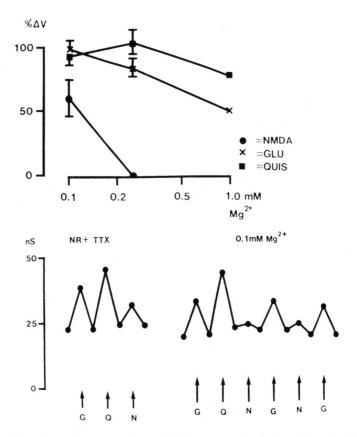

Figure 6. (Top) Plot of increasing concentrations of MG^{2+} versus amplitude of excitant-induced depolarizations (ΔV expressed as % of controls in normal Ringer solution). GLU, glutamate; QUIS, quisqualate. (Bottom) Graph of input conductance increases elicited by excitants on motoneuron bathed in TTX or TTx plus Mg^{2+} solution. G, Q, and N denote applications of glutamate, quisqualate, and NMDA. (From Nistri and King, 1986.)

generate the synaptic potentials. While GDEE (0.1–1 mM) did not block mono- or polysynaptic EPSPs, low concentrations of D-APV (0.5–10 μM) or D-aminoadipate (50–100 μM) preferentially and reversibly attenuated monosynaptic EPSPs (Arenson *et al.*, 1984; Corradetti *et al.*, 1985). Polysynaptic EPSPs had a reduced decay phase but an essentially unchanged amplitude. Table I shows that monosynaptic EPSPs were not fully antagonized by D-APV and that approximately 40% of their peak depolarization remained. Mg^{2+} was found to be a far less selective but potent blocker of EPSPs (Nistri and King, 1986). Even concentrations of Mg^{2+} as low as 0.25 mM strongly reduced both mono- and polysynaptic EPSPs with recovery after sustained washout. At 1 mM Mg^{2+} it was sometimes possible to block EPSPs fully.

Table I. Effect of D-APV on EPSP Amplitude[a]

	Control (mV)	D-APV (mV)	p	Percent change
Monosynaptic EPSP	2.3 ± 0.2	0.9 ± 0.4	<0.05	-61
Polysynaptic EPSP	15.0 ± 4.5	13.6 ± 4.5	>0.05	-10

[a]Results are mean ± S.E. from seven motoneurons; in each cell the amplitudes of mono- or polysynaptic EPSPs were averaged from a minimum of five tests in control Ringer and five in D-APV (1–10 μM) solution (at least 15 min exposure). As data with 1 and 10 μM D-APV were similar, they were pooled. (Modified from Corradetti *et al.*, 1985.)

3.6. Ionic Dependence of Motoneuronal Depolarizations on Excitatory Amino Acids

The first hypothesis to be tested was that increased permeability to Na^+ was responsible for the observed depolarizations. One way of checking this possibility was to remove extracellular Na^+ and substitute it with a presumably impermeant large cation. For this purpose we replaced Na^+ with glucosamine or choline; in the latter case 1 μM atropine was also used to prevent any muscarinic action of choline. An index of effective Na^+ removal was considered to be the disappearance of antidromic action potentials and of spikes evoked by brief intracellular depolarizing pulses. To achieve this condition it was necessary to superfuse continuously the preparation with a Na^+-free medium for 45–60 min. During such a period the motoneuronal membrane potential underwent two changes: in fact, there was an initial hyperpolarization (8–10 mV) followed by a depolarization (10–12 mV), reversible on return to control Ringer solution. When testing the amino acid effects, the resting potential of cells was reset to the initial control value by passing steady DC current through the recording microelectrode. In general, a completely Na^+-free Ringer was poorly tolerated by motoneurons. More stable and prolonged recordings were obtained when 15% of the Na^+ content of the bathing solution was retained.

Figure 7 shows the effect of Na^+-deficient media on the responses to quisqualate, glutamate, and NMDA (glucosamine was the replacing cation). The depolarizing action of the three excitants was almost completely blocked with recovery on washout. When choline was used to replace Na^+, the depolarizations elicited by glutamate or NMDA were similarly blocked (Nistri *et al.*, 1985). However, it was surprising to note that the quisqualate response was not depressed in this medium. Addition of the Ca^{2+} antagonist Mn^{2+} to the choline-containing Ringer solution did then depress the quisqualate-evoked depolarizations (Nistri *et al.*, 1985). The possible involvement of K^+ in the depolarizing actions of these amino acids (see Engberg *et al.*, 1979) was studied by applying well-established K^+ channel blockers (Arenson and Nistri, 1985). Neither tetraethylammonium (3–5 mM) nor 4-aminopyridine (0.5 mM) depressed these excitant-induced responses while greatly prolonging the spike duration and suppressing its $AHP_{e,l}$. Cs^+ was applied iontophoretically inside neurons via the recording microelectrode and produced a distinctive broadening of the antidromic action potential and a loss of its $AHP_{e,l}$. The depolarizing action of the excitants was reduced by about 60% following the application of Cs^+, which also reduced the input conductance of motoneurons.

4. Discussion

The main goal of this study was to clarify the receptor mechanisms and ionic dependence of the responses to excitatory amino acids. Frog spinal motoneurons were chosen as experimentally advantageous cells on the basis of their easy identification, somatic diameter, and prolonged survival *in vitro*. There is evidence that the amino acid pharmacology of mammalian and amphibian spinal cords is similar (Watkins and Evans, 1981) so that amphibian data may not be vitiated by species-dependent factors. By recording from frog motoneurons at low temperature, there was also the advantage of minimizing amino acid uptake processes while retaining an adult preparation with well-preserved synaptic pathways. Additionally, the relatively low temperature was useful for our voltage-clamp studies since it presumably reduced the kinetics of activated channels and raised the cell input resistance. Hence, it was possible to clamp at least the somatic responses generated by comparatively large neurons possessing extensive dendritic branches.

Our data provide direct evidence for distinct receptor classes mediating excitatory amino acid responses. One class is preferentially activated by NMDA and potently blocked by D-APV. Since, under voltage clamp, D-APV selectively antagonized the NMDA-generated inward currents which are the most direct index of receptor activation, there is little doubt about the specificity of this antagonism. Another receptor class is selectively activated by quisqualate and AMPA but its

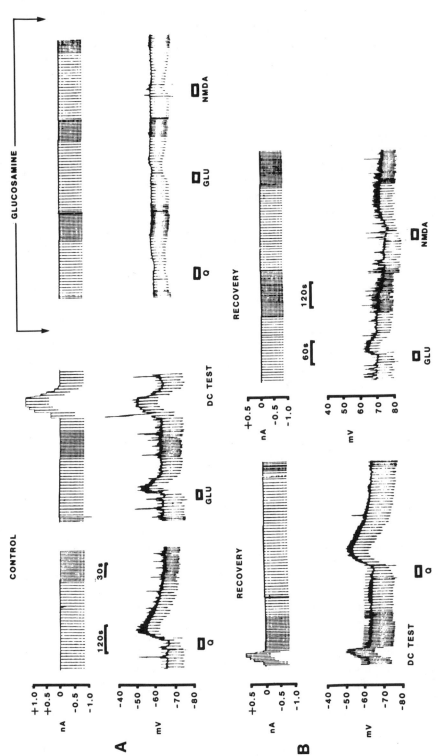

Figure 7. Chart records of motoneuronal responses to quisqualate (Q; 30 μM), glutamate (GLU; 2 mM), and NMDA (30 μM) in control Ringer (A), in glucosamine Ringer (A), and recovery (B). In each pair of tracings, top shows intracellularly injected current and bottom membrane potential. Downward deflections are electrotonic potentials used to calculate cell input conductance. Note in (A) and (B) passive depolarizations of cell membrane evoked by injecting current intracellularly to mimic the amino acid-induced depolarizations and conductance changes. NMDA response in control Ringer is not shown. All data from the same cell. (From Nistri *et al.*, 1985.)

further characterization must await the availability of specific antagonists. Our attempts based on GDEE were unsuccessful and simply confirmed earlier work (Nistri and Constanti, 1975) on the lack of antagonist activity of such a compound. For the same reason it is not yet possible to distinguish between quisqualate and kainate receptors. As initially suggested by Watkins and Evans (1981) and demonstrated with intracellular recording from cultured neurons (Mayer and Westbrook, 1984), glutamate and aspartate are "mixed agonists" in the sense that they can bind to different receptor populations.The present results which showed a saturation of D-APV antagonism to these amino acids, fully support this view. Since in the present study a preferential antagonism of the monosynaptic EPSP was observed, it is feasible that NMDA-sensitive receptors are involved in this response (Corradetti et al., 1985). It was of interest that a complete block of the monosynaptic EPSPs could not be achieved with D-APV applications, suggesting that the receptors responsible for this synaptic potential may be a heterogeneous mixture of NMDA- and quisqualate-sensitive sites. Our observations strengthen the case of the "mixed agonist" glutamate as an important excitatory neurotransmitter in the frog spinal cord (Takeuchi et al., 1983).

In a study on cultured mouse neurons it was observed that, in the presence of D-APV, glutamate elicited large conductance increases similar to those produced by quisqualate (Mayer and Westbrook, 1984). In the present experiments we found that D-APV caused no significant variation in the conductance values during the application of glutamate. Since our experiments were usually carried out in Mg^{2+}-free Ringer (unlike the work by Mayer and Westbrook, 1984), the different results can perhaps be attributed to the action of this divalent cation on amino acid channels (Nowak et al., 1984; Mayer and Westbrook, 1985). Indeed, voltage-clamp studies of cultured neurons have shown that the strong voltage dependence of the conductance changes induced by NMDA or glutamate is related to the blocking action of Mg^{2+} on the NMDA-activated channels (Nowak et al., 1984; Mayer and Westbrook, 1985). However, our work on adult frog motoneurons cannot be explained entirely on the basis of this notion. In fact, contrary to this view no significant conductance increases during NMDA or glutamate applications were found in Mg^{2+}-free TTX-containing Ringer. Although it may be argued that very low levels of Mg^{2+} might have been contaminants of "Mg^{2+}-free" solutions or that other voltage-dependent conductances were operative within the membrane potential ranges examined, we have no firm evidence to support either of these possibilities. In all frog motoneurons investigated, we observed a differential antagonism by Mg^{2+} of amino acid depolarizations (Fig. 6, top), but only in a few cells (like the one depicted in Fig. 6, bottom) was there a distinctive action of Mg^{2+} on the amino acid conductance responses. It seems likely that on frog motoneurons the blocking action of Mg^{2+} may result from a combination of effects on amino acid opened channels as well as on other voltage-dependent ionic (probably Ca^{2+}) channels (Nistri and King, 1986). It is also possible that, in addition to their effects on postsynaptic membranes, excitatory amino acids may act presynaptically to facilitate neurotransmitter release which is highly dependent on Mg^{2+} but insensitive to TTX (for a discussion see Nistri and King, 1986). This presynaptic effect of Mg^{2+} would contribute to the observed postsynaptic responses but it may be difficult to quantify it.

The demonstration of inward currents produced by excitatory amino acids on frog motoneurons is in keeping with similar recent findings on cultured spinal cells (Mayer and Westbrook, 1984) and excludes the possibility of a K^+ permeability decrease (Engberg et al., 1979) as the main mechanism underlying the observed depolarizations. Moreover, the inability of K^+ channel blockers (with the exception of Cs^+) to change amino acid responses is also consistent with the depolarizations being generated by an increased conductance to cations (Arenson and Nistri, 1985). The depressant action of Cs^+ on amino acid depolarizations was probably due to a nonspecific block of large cationic channels (Puil and Werman, 1981; Arenson and Nistri, 1985). The present work suggests that in control conditions Na^+ was the main charge carrier for the depolarizations induced by glutamate, NMDA, and quisqualate. In fact, in the absence of Na^+ these responses substantially declined (Nistri et al., 1985). As the reversal potential of the amino acid depolarizations is more negative than the Na^+ equilibrium potential

(Mayer and Westbrook, 1984), it is likely that entry of Na^+ into the cell is associated with an exit of K^+. Surprisingly, however, when choline replaced Na^+, the depolarizations evoked by quisqualate were not reduced. Since there is evidence that choline increased the motoneuronal resistance, it is possible that in this particular circumstance quisqualate might trigger an entry of Ca^{2+} which is normally obscured by large outward currents (Nistri et al., 1985). In support of this view is the finding that Mn^{2+} (a Ca^{2+} channel blocker) depressed the quisqualate responses in choline Ringer solutions (Nistri et al., 1985). Recently, it has been observed that in cultured neurons bathed in Mg^{2+}-free media, NMDA elicited a rise in intracellular Ca^{2+} apparently due to a transmembrane flux of this divalent cation (MacDermott et al., 1986). It is not yet clear whether quisqualate shares a similar action. Nevertheless, the persistence of glutamate responses following full pharmacological block of Ca^{2+} channels argues against a role of this ion as the primary charge carrier responsible for the amino acid depolarizations (Bührle and Sonnhof, 1983; Nistri and Arenson, 1983).

The mechanisms responsible for the less conventional responses to glutamate, namely an early increase in the spike ADP and a membrane hyperpolarization, are poorly understood. Since the ADP is thought to represent a depolarizing current flow from the dendrites to the cell body (Nelson and Burke, 1967), an early change in this potential may indicate a primary site of action of glutamate at the level of the dendrites. The small hyperpolarizing responses produced by glutamate and its analogues were observed as outward currents under voltage-clamp conditions. Since these responses were accompanied by a conductance increase, it is probable that the underlying mechanism is an increased ionic permeability (Arenson and Nistri, 1982b). The nature of the ionic species is still unknown but it may be of interest to note that glutamate has hyperpolarizing, Cl^--dependent effects on locust muscle fibers (Cull-Candy and Usherwood, 1973) and on cultured Xenopus neurons (Wetzel et al., 1984).

In conclusion, the present study, based on current- and voltage-clamp recordings, has provided direct evidence for distinct receptor classes for excitatory amino acids and suggests that a Na^+-dependent depolarization is the main mechanism underlying their actions on frog motoneurons. As the precise mechanism responsible for the relatively small conductance changes during amino acid applications remains unclear, it is possible only to speculate on some plausible causes. One of them would be the level of extracellular Mg^{2+}, although its concentration was likely to be very low in standard Mg^{2+}-free Ringer and the action of this exogenously applied cation on conductance responses was not always predictable. Other contributing factors might be the small changes in the Na^+/K^+ permeability ratio (Bührle and Sonnhof, 1983) and the relatively remote location of excitatory amino acid-sensitive sites with respect to the recording microelectrode which probably is located in the cell soma. Our data indicate that frog motoneurons represent an advantageous neuronal population for studying the physiological and pharmacological properties of excitatory amino acid receptors.

ACKNOWLEDGMENTS. This work was supported by grants from the National Fund for Research into Crippling Diseases (Action Research) and from the Wellcome Trust.

References

Altmann, H., ten Bruggencate, G., Pickelmann, P., and Steinberg, R., 1976, Effects of glutamate, aspartate, and two presumed antagonists on feline rubrospinal neurones, Pfluegers Arch. 364:249–255.

Arenson, M. S., and Nistri, A., 1982a, The initial effect of glutamate on frog motoneurones consists in a selective change in the spike late afterdepolarization, J. Physiol. (London) 325:26–27P.

Arenson, M. S., and Nistri, A., 1982b, A novel inhibitory–excitatory response of frog motoneurones in vitro to glutamate, J. Physiol. (London) 328:9P.

Arenson, M. S., and Nistri, A., 1985, The effects of potassium channel blocking agents on the responses of in vitro frog motoneurones to glutamate and other excitatory amino acids: an intracellular study, *Neuroscience* **14**:317–325.

Arenson, M. S., Berti, C., King, A. E., and Nistri, A., 1984, The effect of D-α-amino-adipate on excitatory amino acid responses recorded intracellularly from motoneurones of the frog spinal cord, *Neurosci. Lett.* **49**:99–104.

Ault, B., Evans, R. H., Francis, A. A., Oakes, D. J., and Watkins, J. C., 1980, Selective depression of excitatory amino acid induced depolarizations by magnesium ions in isolated spinal cord preparations, *J. Physiol. (London)* **307**:413–428.

Bührle, C. P., and Sonnhof, U., 1983, The ionic mechanism of the excitatory action of glutamate upon the membranes of motoneurones of the frog, *Pfluegers Arch.* **396**:154–162.

Corradetti, R., King, A. E., Nistri, A., Rovira, C., and Sivilotti, L., 1985, Pharmacological characterization of D-aminophosphonovaleric acid antagonism of amino acid and synaptically evoked excitations on frog motoneurones *in vitro:* an intracellular study, *Br. J. Pharmacol.* **86**:19–25.

Cull-Candy, S. G., and Usherwood, P. N. R., 1973, Two populations of L-glutamate receptors on locust muscle fibres, *Nature New Biol.* **246**:62–64.

Curtis, D. R., and Watkins, J. C., 1963, Acidic amino acids with strong excitatory actions on mammalian neurones, *J. Physiol. (London)* **166**:1–14.

Curtis, D. R., Phillis, J. W., and Watkins. J. C., 1960, The chemical excitation of spinal neurones by certain acidic amino acids, *J. Physiol. (London)* **150**:656–682.

Davidoff, R. A., and Adair, R., 1975, High affinity amino acid transport by frog spinal cord slices, *J. Neurochem.* **24**:545–552.

Duggan, A. W., 1974, The differential sensitivity to L-glutamate and L-aspartate of spinal interneurones and Renshaw cells, *Exp. Brain Res.* **19**:522–528.

Engberg, I., Flatman, J. A., and Lambert, J. D. C., 1979, The actions of excitatory amino acids on motoneurones in the feline spinal cord, *J. Physiol. (London)* **288**:227–261.

Erulkar, S. D., Dambach, G. E., and Mender, D., 1974, The effect of magnesium at motoneurones of the isolated frog spinal cord, *Brain Res.* **66**:413–424.

Evans, R. H., Francis, A. A., Jones, A. W., Smith, D. A. S., and Watkins, J. C., 1982, The effects of a series of ω-phosphonic α-carboxylic amino acids on electrically evoked and excitant amino acid-induced responses in isolated spinal cord preparations, *Br. J. Pharmacol.* **75**:65–75.

Fagg, G. E., and Foster, A. C., 1983, Amino acid neurotransmitters and their pathways in the mammalian central nervous system, *Neuroscience* **9**:701–719.

Fonnum, F., 1984, Glutamate: A neurotransmitter in mammalian brain, *J. Neurochem.* **42**:1–11.

Hayashi, T., 1954, Effects of sodium glutamate on the nervous system, *Keio J. Med.* **3**:183–192.

Jasper, H. H., Khan, R. T., and Elliott, K. A. C., 1965, Amino acids released from cerebral cortex in relation to its state of activation, *Science* **147**:1448–1449.

Kelly, J. S., Krnjević, K., and Somjen, G., 1969, Divalent cations and electrical properties of cortical cells, *J. Neurobiol.* **1**:197–208.

King, A., and Nistri, A., 1985, Current and voltage clamp studies of the mixed agonist action of L-glutamate and its antagonism by D-aminophosphonovalerate on spinal motoneurones in vitro, *Soc. Neurosci. Abstr.* **11**:822.

King, A. E., Nistri, A., and Rovira, C., 1985, The excitation of frog motoneurones in vitro by the glutamate analogue, DL-α-amino-3-hydroxy-5-methyl-4-isoxazole-propionic acid (AMPA), and the effect of amino acid antagonists, *Neurosci. Lett.* **55**:77–82.

Krnjević, K., 1965, Action of drugs on single neurones in the cerebral cortex, *Br. Med. Bull.* **21**:10–14.

Krnjević, K., and Phillis, J. W., 1963, Iontophoretic studies of neurones in the mammalian cerebral cortex, *J. Physiol. (London)* **165**:274–304.

McCulloch, R. M., Johnston, G. A. R., Game, C. J. A., and Curtis, D. R., 1974, The differential sensitivity of spinal interneurones and Renshaw cells to kainate and N-methyl-D-aspartate, *Exp. Brain Res.* **21**:515–518.

MacDermott, A. B., Mayer, M. L., Westbrook, G. L., Smith, S. J., and Barker, J. L., 1986, NMDA-receptor activation increases cytoplasmic calcium concentration in cultured spinal cord neurones, *Nature* **321**:519–522.

Mayer, M. L., and Westbrook, G. L., 1984. Mixed-agonist action of excitatory amino acids on mouse spinal cord neurones under voltage clamp, *J. Physiol. (London)* **354**:29–53.

Mayer, M. L., and Westbrook, G. L., 1985, The action of N-methyl-D-aspartic acid on mouse spinal neurones in culture, *J. Physiol. (London)* **361**:65–90.

Nelson, P. G., and Burke, R. E., 1967, Delayed depolarization in cat spinal motoneurons, *Exp. Neurol.* **17**:16–26.

Nistri, A., 1985, Glutamate, in: *Neurotransmitter Actions in the Vertebrate Nervous System* (M. A. Rogawski and J. L. Barker, eds.), Plenum Press, New York, pp. 101–123.

Nistri, A., and Arenson, M. S., 1983, Multiple postsynaptic responses evoked by glutamate on *in vitro* spinal motoneurones, in: *CNS Receptors—From Molecular Pharmacology to Behaviour* (P. Mandel and F. V. DeFeudis, eds.), Raven Press, New York, pp. 229–236.

Nistri, A., and Constanti, A., 1975, Effect of glutamate and glutamic acid diethyl ester on the lobster muscle fibre and the frog spinal cord, *Eur. J. Pharmacol.* **31:**377–379.

Nistri, A., and Constanti, A., 1979, Pharmacological characterization of different types of GABA and glutamate receptors in vertebrates and invertebrates, *Prog. Neurobiol.* **13:**117–235.

Nistri, A., and King, A. E., 1986, Blockade by D-aminophosphonovalerate or Mg^{2+} of excitatory amino acid-induced responses on spinal motoneurons *in vitro,* in: *Excitatory Amino Acids and Epilepsy* (R. Schwarcz and Y. Ben-Ari, eds.), Plenum Press, New York pp. 485–495.

Nistri, A., Arenson, M. S., and King, A. E., 1985, Excitatory amino acid-induced responses of frog motoneurones bathed in low Na^+ media: an intracellular study, *Neuroscience* **14:**921–927.

Nowak, L., Bregestovski, P., Ascher, P., Herbert, A., and Prochiantz, A., 1984, Magnesium gates glutamate-activated channels in mouse central neurones, *Nature* **307:**462–465.

Puil, E., 1981, S-Glutamate: Its interactions with spinal neurons, *Brain Res. Rev.* **3:**229–322.

Puil, E., and Werman, R., 1981, Internal cesium ions block various K conductances in spinal motoneurons, *Can. J. Physiol. Pharmacol.* **59:**1280–1284.

Schwindt, P. C., 1976, Electrical properties of motoneurons. in: *Frog Neurobiology* (R. Llinás and W. Precht, eds.), Springer, Berlin, pp. 750–764.

Takeuchi, A., Onodera, K., and Kawagoe, R., 1983, The effects of dorsal root stimulation on the release of endogenous glutamate from the frog spinal cord, *Proc. Jpn. Acad. Ser. B* **59:**88–92.

Watkins, J. C., and Evans, R. H., 1981, Excitatory amino acid transmitters, *Annu. Rev. Pharmacol. Toxicol.* **21:**165–204.

Wetzel, D. M., Erulkar, S. D., Kilgren, L., Rendt, J., Parsons, T., and Yang, S., 1984, Chloride channels activated by glutamate and GABA in patch-clamped adult *Xenopus laevis* neurons in long-term cell culture, *Soc. Neurosci. Abstr.* **10:**940.

8

Blockade of Excitatory Amino Acid Transmitters and Epilepsy

J. F. MacDonald, Z. Miljkovic, and J. H. Schneiderman

1. Introduction

The excitatory amino acids, and in particular L-glutamic acid (L-Glu), have long been considered possible transmitters in the mammalian CNS (Nistri and Constanti, 1979; Puil, 1981; Fagg and Foster, 1983). However, only recently have advances in the availability of the appropriate pharmacological tools, such as specific antagonists, stimulated a renewed interest in identification of these synapses (Jahr and Jessell, 1985; Jahr and Yoshioka, 1986; Nelson *et al.*, 1986; Thomson, 1986). Initially, the remarkable ubiquity of neuronal responsiveness to L-Glu, together with its role in intermediate metabolism, brought into question a transmitter role for this substance (Curtis *et al.*, 1960). In retrospect, it now seems that this characteristic may simply be a reflection of the ubiquity of excitatory amino acid transmission.

Hayashi (1954) first demonstrated that topical applications of L-Glu to the surface of the cerebral cortex induced convulsions in dogs. Such evidence, at least superficially, implies that excitatory amino acid transmitters might play some role in the genesis of epileptiform discharge of central neurons. This hypothesis was also supported by the report that intravenous injections of excitatory amino acids such as N-methyl-D-aspartic acid (NMDA) evoke convulsions in young mice (Johnston, 1972). Also somewhat suggestive is the description of a fatal convulsive disorder in infants which may be related to excessively high concentrations of L-aspartate (L-Asp) in cerebrospinal fluid (Weitz *et al.*, 1981). Perhaps more convincing evidence is provided by the identification of relatively specific antagonists and blockers of excitatory amino acids which also possess anticonvulsant properties (Croucher *et al.*, 1982; Meldrum *et al.*, 1983; Ryan *et al.*, 1984) provided they can gain access to the CNS. Some of these compounds have only recently been synthesized and likely act as receptor antagonists [e.g., 2-amino-5-phosphonovaleric acid (APV)]. Others, and in particular the divalent cation Mg^{2+} have only recently been identified as physiological blockers of excitatory amino acid channels (see below). In support of the hypothesis that glutamate is involved in epileptiform discharges, hypomagnesemia (usually accompanied by

J. F. MacDonald and Z. Miljkovic • Playfair Neuroscience Unit, University of Toronto, The Toronto Hospital, Toronto, Ontario M5T 2S8, Canada. *J. H. Schneiderman* • Wellesley Hospital, Toronto, Ontario M4Y 1J3, Canada.

hypokalemia and hypocalcemia) is associated with convulsions and magnesium salts are used to treat the seizures associated with acute nephritis and with eclampsia of pregnancy (Mudge, 1985). Of course, some of the effects of magnesium administration are likely to be related to blockade of synaptic transmission (i.e., the neuromuscular junction), but some of its anticonvulsant properties might also be related to central effects.

Attempts to determine the cellular basis of convulsions and epilepsy have often focused upon the hippocampus, the cortical structure with the lowest seizure threshold (Alger, 1984). This structure is also particularly amenable to study *in vitro* as a tissue slice. Usually, inhibitory amino acid antagonists or blockers (e.g., penicillin, bicuculline, picrotoxin) are used to induce synchronous burst discharge in order to provide a model of epilepsy. Focal epileptic discharge is associated with a number of electrophysiological events including the interictal spike which is the recorded EEG counterpart of focal epileptic discharge, synchronous burst discharge which is the recorded synchronous extracellular activity of groups of neurons (see Fig. 6), and the paroxysmal depolarizing shift (PDS) which is the intracellular counterpart of the interictal spike and consists of a slow depolarizing potential upon which ride superimposed regenerative action potentials that make up an actual burst (Alger, 1984).

Several different mechanisms have been proposed to account for the PDS. Currently the PDS is believed to result from a bistable state of the membrane potential (a depolarizing wave of potential) that is a direct consequence of the interaction of a variety of voltage- and time-dependent conductances (e.g., voltage-dependent calcium and potassium) intrinsic to the membrane of the recorded cell (Alger, 1984). However, this is not a sufficient mechanism by itself to account for the synchrony of neurons during the focal discharge. Some mechanism must trigger and maintain the synchrony. This suggests the possibility that the PDS may also contain a component attributable to the activity of synchronized EPSPs (excitatory postsynaptic potentials). Evidence has been provided which suggests that the PDS does contain such a synaptic component (see Johnston and Brown, 1984). Considering the ubiquity of excitatory amino acid transmitters within the hippocampus (Fagg and Foster, 1983), it might be anticipated that they play an important role in synchronous neuronal discharge. Supportive of such a hypothesis is the demonstration that iontophoretic applications of L-Glu to small populations of neocortical neurons can invoke paroxysmal depolarizations (Connors, 1984).

2. Voltage-Sensitive Responses to Excitatory Amino Acids

Some excitatory amino acids, including the most likely transmitter candidates, L-Glu and L-Asp, are capable of activating a receptor and channel which is named for its most specific agonist, the NMDA receptor-channel. The NMDA response is modulated in a voltage-dependent fashion by Mg^{2+} ions (see Fig. 1). Physiological concentrations of this cation block the NMDA channels and the degree of the block is highly voltage dependent (Nowak *et al.*, 1984; Mayer *et al.*, 1984). This voltage dependency is such that the block is most pronounced at hyperpolarized holding potentials suggesting that Mg^{2+} enters and blocks the channel lumen directly. This hypothesis is also supported by the observation that Mg^{2+} ions cause transient channel closures (or "bursting," not to be confused with neuronal bursting) which is consistent with a "fast channel" blocking mechanism (Neher and Steinbach, 1978; Colquhoun and Hawkes, 1983). However, certain aspects of the block are not consistent with this model. For example, the frequency of channel openings was reduced at hyperpolarized potentials when it should have remained unchanged and the duration of each channel burst decreased with increasing Mg^{2+} concentrations rather than increasing as predicted by the model (Nowak *et al.*, 1984).

This voltage-dependent blockade means that some excitatory amino acid transmitters are capable of inducing a bistable state of the membrane potential which is clearly extrinsic in origin to the postsynaptic membrane (MacDonald and Wojtowicz, 1982; MacDonald *et al.*, 1982;

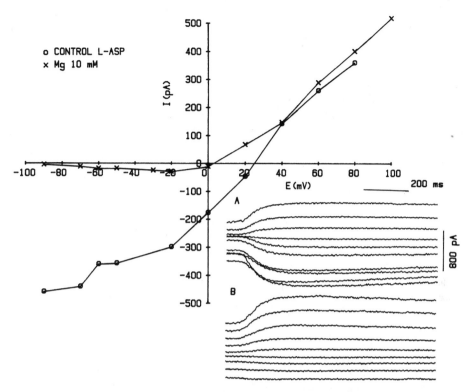

Figure 1. Voltage-dependent block of L-Asp currents by Mg^{2+} in a cultured hippocampal neuron. A single application of L-Asp (100 μM) was given at a series of holding potentials before (○) and following exchange of the bathing solution for one containing 10 mM Mg^{2+} (X). Peak L-Asp currents were plotted against holding potential. Inward currents evoked by L-Asp were strongly depressed but outward currents were unchanged. Inset A shows superimposed L-Asp currents prior to exchanging the bathing solution and inset B shows these currents afterwards. Note that the apparent change in the reversal potential likely was a consequence of our failure to wait for equilibration of the intracellular solution with that of the patch electrode (i.e., shift due to changing concentration of Cs).

Flatman *et al.*, 1983; MacDonald, 1984). In other words, some excitatory amino acids possess the potential to directly generate the PDS.

In earlier electrophysiological experiments this voltage-dependent block was detected as an apparent reduction of input conductance [or no change in input conductance; see MacDonald (1985) for a detailed discussion] during depolarizations evoked by exogenous applications of some excitatory amino acids (e.g., those which activate the NMDA receptor). Under voltage clamp it was possible to demonstrate that the inward currents activated by excitatory amino acids, such as L-Asp, were voltage dependent (in the presence of 0.9 mM extracellular Mg^{2+}) giving N-shaped current–voltage (I–V) curves and providing evidence that excitatory amino acid currents were themselves capable of inducing a bistable membrane state (MacDonald *et al.*, 1982; Flatman *et al.*, 1983). Other excitatory amino acid channels are not subject to this blockade [e.g., kainic acid (Ka)] and, therefore, their I–V curves are relatively linear and their inward currents are not voltage dependent (not able to induce a bistable membrane state).

Even if the PDS is produced purely by intrinsic currents, voltage-sensitive excitatory amino acid currents might sum with them in a variety of complex ways. For example, exposure to the excitatory amino acid might lower the threshold for regenerative potentials (i.e., the PDS) by contributing an extra voltage-dependent inward current at the appropriate membrane potentials.

Supportive of this suggestion is the report that applications of the NMDA antagonist, APV, elevate the threshold for activation of neocortical neurons (Armstrong-James *et al.*, 1985).

Another way in which excitatory amino acids might have a significant action upon the PDS is as a consequence of modulating the influx of an ion such as calcium into the postsynaptic neuron. One possibility is that calcium ions pass directly through the NMDA channels. Evidence now supports this possibility (Dingledine, 1983; MacDonald and Schneiderman, 1984; MacDermott *et al.*, 1986; Morris *et al.*, 1986; Riveros and Orrego, 1986) although sodium and potassium permeability is likely to be more significant (MacDonald, 1984; Nowak *et al.*, 1984; Mayer and Westbrook, 1985).

3. Dissociative Anesthetics

The short-acting anesthetic phencyclidine (PCP), and its congener ketamine, have been shown to selectively block excitatory amino acids which activate the NMDA receptor while sparing those such as Ka (Anis *et al.*, 1983; Duchen *et al.*, 1985; Harrison and Simmonds, 1985; Honey *et al.*, 1985; Martin and Lodge, 1985; Lacey and Henderson, 1986; Thomson, 1986). Whether ketamine and PCP are able to act as receptor antagonists, as channel blockers, or via the lipid phase of the membrane to exert some kind of indirect modulation of the NMDA receptor-channel is unknown. However, evidence does show that the interaction is of the noncompetitive type suggesting that the channel may be the locus of their actions (Harrison and Simmonds, 1985; Martin and Lodge, 1985). The blockade by PCP appears to be at least as potent at blocking NMDA (Lacey and Henderson, 1986) as it is at blocking potassium channels, end-plate channels, and muscarinic receptors (Albuquerque *et al.*, 1983; Bartschat and Blaustein, 1986).

Ketamine, which was developed with the objective of minimizing the hallucinogenic side effects of PCP (White *et al.*, 1982), apparently does not share the ability to block potassium channels although it does block end-plate channels and muscarinic receptors in relatively low concentrations (Maleque *et al.*, 1981; Aronstam *et al.*, 1982; Albuquerque *et al.*, 1983). Ketamine and a series of related compounds, like other specific blockers or antagonists of the NMDA receptor-channel, possess anticonvulsant properties in a number of animal models (Chen *et al.*, 1966; Celesia and Chen, 1974; Callaghan and Schwark, 1980; Hayes and Balster, 1985) and ketamine has been reported to suppress convulsant-like EEG activity in anesthetized patients (Corssen *et al.*, 1974). In addition, ketamine has been employed clinically to suppress seizures in children during febrile convulsions (Davis and Tolstoshev, 1976) and in women with eclampsia (Rucci and Caroli, 1974) when the patients were found resistant to conventional anticonvulsants such as benzodiazepines and pentobarbital. Such evidence suggests that ketamine's anticonvulsant properties might originate in part from its blocking actions upon EPSPs mediated by NMDA receptors (see below). However, ketamine also prolongs inhibitory synaptic currents in hippocampal neurons (Gage and Robertson, 1985) and may potentiate GABA responses (Little and Atkinson, 1984), suggesting an alternate anticonvulsant mechanism.

4. Hippocampal Neurons in Culture

We have attempted to determine the mechanism whereby ketamine and PCP block the NMDA response. The preparation we have employed is hippocampal neurons grown dissociated in tissue culture. Fetal mice were the source of the hippocampal tissue and the only alteration from standard procedures (MacDonald and Wojtowicz, 1982) was that cells were dissociated exclusively by mechanical means and that the dissection and cell separations were performed over ice. Neurons in these cultures cannot be readily identified but almost all respond to excitatory amino acids and the results described subsequently do not appear to be attributable to any particular subpopulation of neurons.

Action potentials and synaptic interactions between the neurons were suppressed by the addition of tetrodotoxin to the extracellular solution which also contained 50 μM bicuculline (see Honey *et al.*, 1985). Ketamine, PCP, Mg^{2+}, and excitatory amino acids were dissolved in this solution. Amino acids were applied by micropressure and blockers by superfusion of the entire culture dish.

Intracellular recordings were made using patch electrodes in a whole-cell voltage-clamp configuration (discontinuous switching single electrode, 20 to 25 kHz). This type of clamp helps to minimize the series resistance, which can be a considerable source of error to measurements of membrane voltage. Furthermore, it was possible to vary membrane potential over a substantial range (-100 to $+100$ mV). The patch electrode solution contained CsCl with calcium buffered to about 10^{-8} M (see Honey *et al.*, 1985).

5. Selectivity and Voltage Dependency

Ketamine and PCP selectively blocked excitatory amino acid currents evoked by L-Asp, NMDA, and L-Glu while sparing those to Ka (Fig. 3), confirming previous reports (see Honey *et al.*, 1985). However, this block was highly voltage dependent, favoring blockade at hyperpolarized potentials, whereas outward excitatory amino acid currents were less influenced by ketamine or PCP (Fig. 2).

This voltage dependency of the block suggests that it results from the movement of positively charged ketamine or PCP molecules, under the influence of a membrane field, into the open NMDA channels. When the field is reversed to a relatively positive potential (inside versus outside), the blocker molecules must overcome this additional barrier. Therefore, the site of

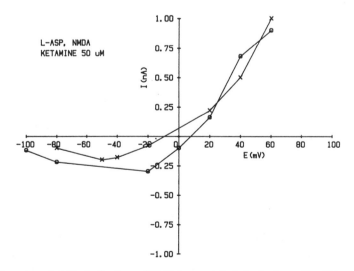

Figure 2. Voltage-dependent block of L-Asp and NMDA currents by ketamine in a cultured hippocampal neuron. I–V curves were constructed as previously described using single applications of L-Asp (50 μM; ○) and NMDA (50 μM; X). Both curves were recorded in the presence of ketamine (50 μM) but absence of Mg^{2+}. The control curves were approximately linear (not shown). Ketamine depressed inward amino acid currents but had less effect upon outward currents.

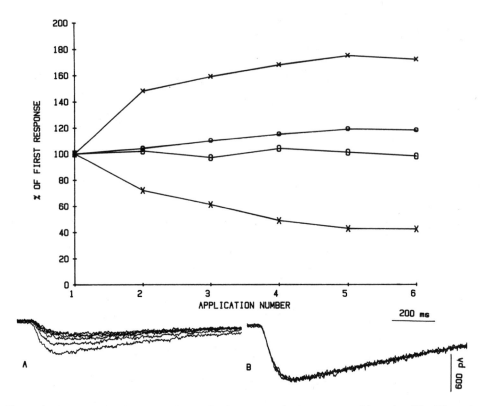

Figure 3. Use-dependent block and unblock of L-Asp currents in the presence of ketamine (20 μM) can be reversed. Results are shown for four series of six applications of L-Asp (100 μM) at a frequency of 0.067 Hz. Peak currents were expressed as a percentage of the first current in each series and plotted against application number. Holding potential was either +60 or −71 mV. The large crosses demonstrate the progressive decrement of peak currents in the presence of ketamine (see inset A for superimposed currents; use-dependent block) whereas the small crosses show an increment (use-dependent unblock). The applications were then repeated following extensive washing of the culture with control solution (small circles, +60 mV holding; large circles, −71 mV holding). Inset B illustrates superimposed currents recorded at −71 mV following this wash.

action of ketamine and PCP would, at least on the basis of circumstantial evidence, seem to be at a binding site associated with the NMDA channel and perhaps located within the channel lumen. Mg^{2+} may also have a binding site within this channel and an interaction between a blocker such as ketamine and this divalent cation might be anticipated. Our experiments have in fact shown that a portion of the ketamine block can be prevented by simultaneous exposure to high concentrations of Mg^{2+} (J. F. MacDonald and Z. Miljkovic, unpublished). In contrast, the antagonist APV selectively reduced responses to these excitatory amino acids (L-Asp, L-Glu, and NMDA but not Ka) equally well at all holding potentials. This result supports other evidence which indicates that APV acts at the NMDA recognition site as a possible competitive antagonist (Foster and Fagg, 1984; Harrison and Simmonds, 1985; Martin and Lodge, 1985).

6. Use Dependency

The repeated presentation of brief pulses (20 to 100 msec) of excitatory amino acids results in a progressive decline of peak inward current provided the frequency of application is greater than about 0.1 Hz. When a short interval free of amino acid is permitted (e.g., 15 sec), peak currents recover spontaneously. This phenomenon resembles desensitization of acetylcholine responses at the end plate and may represent desensitization of the NMDA receptor. However, in the presence of ketamine (or PCP) an additional phenomenon occurs. A decrement of peak inward excitatory amino acid current can be observed which is independent of the frequency at which it is applied (frequency independent) and which does not demonstrate any recovery for periods as long as 5 min. In other words, the blockade by ketamine or PCP requires the repeated presentation of the agonist in order to develop a steady-state block of the inward current (Fig. 3)

This is a true use-dependent block (Strichartz, 1973; Courtney, 1975) because it can only be reversed in the presence of the blocker provided both of the following conditions are met: the membrane field must be reversed, and the membrane must be exposed to the agonist (MacDonald *et al.*, 1987). Depolarization of the membrane without exposure to the agonist will not relieve this block and apparently channels must be activated in order to either relieve (depolarized field: see Fig. 3) or develop (hyperpolarized field) the blockade. Although a number of mechanisms could account for these results, we do not believe that this use dependency is related to occupation of the NMDA recognition site. This is based upon our observations that APV is unable to relieve the ketamine block even though it likely occupies the recognition site but does not activate the channels.

The "Trapping" Phenomenon

Use-dependent and frequency-dependent blockade of voltage-dependent currents by a variety of anesthetics is usually attributed to a cumulative blockade of the underlying channels (see Hille, 1984). Its frequency dependence is thought to be related to the rate of escape of the blocker molecule from the closed state of the channel. This would contrast with fast channel blockers which presumably enter the channel and transiently prevent its closure before they exit. Instead, the blocker molecule may become "trapped" within the closed channel. The more rapidly the blocker escapes from the closed channels, the higher is the frequency of channel activation required to demonstrate the use dependency of the block and the more rapid the recovery once the blocker is washed out. A similar "trapping" phenomenon has also been described for agonist-gated channels in submandibular ganglion neurons (Gurney and Rang, 1984). For example, some methonium compounds, of intermediate chain length (5 to 8 carbons), demonstrate a use-dependent block for which spontaneous recovery occurs at a slow rate unless the membrane is depolarized and agonist reapplied (Gurney and Rang, 1984). This suggests that these blockers escape from the closed channels at a very slow rate.

One of the predictions of this hypothesis would be that the blocker should remain within the closed channel complex even after it has been washed out of the recording bath. We have been able to confirm this prediction for the ketamine block of L-Asp. Once a steady-state block of the inward L-Asp currents was established, the bath was washed for more than 5 min with the control solution. According to our prediction the channels should have remained blocked by ketamine molecules remaining within the closed channels. Consistent with this was our demonstration that the first current evoked by L-Asp was identical in amplitude to the last current (the steady-state current) in the presence of ketamine (Fig. 4). As the L-Asp is repeatedly presented, we would predict that ketamine would begin to leave the open channels (presumably its rate of association with the open channel is concentration dependent) and each subsequent response ought to be larger. This prediction was also confirmed (Fig. 4).

Our experiments have demonstrated that the blockade by ketamine is (1) selective for the NMDA receptor-channel, (2) highly voltage dependent and consistent with a block of this channel, (3) at least partially use dependent and frequency independent (within our experimental constraints) again suggesting a channel block, and (4) consistent with the hypothesis that ketamine is "trapped" within closed NMDA channels. Entry or exit of ketamine from the closed NMDA channels appears to be occurring only at a very slow rate.

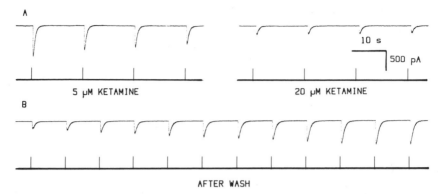

Figure 4. The use-dependent block of L-Asp currents and use-dependent unblock following washout in a cultured hippocampal neuron. The holding potential was set at −70 mV and L-Asp (100 μM) applied at a frequency of 0.067 Hz. Peak inward currents were stable in the control solution (not shown) but when exchanged for 5 μM ketamine a use-dependent block developed (A). In the rightmost panel, four currents are shown with a higher concentration of ketamine (20 μM) after the use-dependent block had reached a steady-state value. Immediately following the fourth of these applications the culture dish was washed with control solution for 5 min. Holding potential was maintained at −70 mV during the wash and no agonist applications were made until those shown in B. This first response in ketamine-free solution was identical to the last in the presence of this blocker. Only repetitive applications of L-Asp were able to relieve the block (use-dependent unblock). Indicators of the pressure applications are given just below evoked currents.

7. Excitatory Transmission Using NMDA Receptors

Recent evidence suggests that some monosynaptic "fast" EPSPs in the spinal cord (Jahr and Jessell, 1985; Jahr and Yoshioka, 1986; Nelson *et al.*, 1986) are probably not mediated by NMDA receptors. For example, these EPSPs are not appropriately voltage dependent in the presence of Mg^{2+} nor are they sensitive to APV. Instead they are blocked by less specific excitatory amino acid antagonists such as kynurenic acid. However, other evidence indicates that repetitive stimulation of some excitatory pathways in hippocampus and cerebral cortex, particularly in the presence of low extracellular Mg^{2+}, is able to reveal "slow" EPSPs which demonstrate the appropriate voltage dependence in the presence of Mg^{2+} and which are sensitive to APV and/or ketamine (Herron *et al.*, 1985; Hablitz and Langmoen, 1986; Thomson, 1986).

A Testable Prediction

The voltage-dependent block of the NMDA channels by Mg^{2+} or by ketamine could have a significant effect on the ability of a neuron to initiate or maintain a bistable membrane potential (i.e., the PDS). This would, however, require that the excitatory amino acid transmitter actually remain in contact with postsynaptic NMDA receptors for a sufficient period. The punctate and rapid delivery of the excitatory amino acid transmitter during a "fast" EPSP, together with its rapid sequestration by uptake systems, would be unlikely to produce sufficient exposure of the postsynaptic neuron to the molecule to permit the induction of a bistable membrane potential. In contrast, the recruitment and summation of "slow" EPSPs would seem more likely to provide a longer exposure to released excitatory amino acid transmitter. Any impairment of excitatory amino acid uptake systems would also favor this circumstance.

However, the concentration of extracellular Mg^{2+} would be critical to the capacity of the excitatory amino acid to directly induce a PDS. In the absence of extracellular Mg^{2+}, depolarizations by excitatory amino acids (NMDA agonists) would not be voltage sensitive and therefore their effects would be indistinguishable from any other source of depolarization (e.g., by other excitatory transmitters). In the presence of concentrations of Mg^{2+} near the physiological range (about 1 mM), the voltage sensitivity of its blockade would potentially induce and/or enhance intrinsic membrane oscillations in the postsynaptic neuron. Still higher concentrations (Fig. 1) would tend to eliminate all inward excitatory amino acid current and block any direct contribution by them to a bistable membrane potential. Therefore, too little Mg^{2+} block would fail to enhance intrinsic oscillations of membrane potential because inward excitatory amino acid currents would not be voltage sensitive, whereas too much block would have a similar action by eliminating these currents altogether.

An alternate scenario might be envisaged if the PDS is purely intrinsic in origin and simply triggered by excitatory synaptic input. The presence of physiological concentrations of Mg^{2+} might actually depress very strongly or hold in check the summation and recruitment of the "slow" EPSPs required to trigger synchronous PDS activity. Synchronization of the PDS would not occur unless summation of "slow" excitatory amino acid EPSPs was permitted perhaps as a consequence of lowered concentrations of extracellular Mg^{2+}. Thus, low extracellular Mg^{2+} would favor the formation and synchronization of the PDS while increasing concentrations would progressively inhibit them.

8. The Hippocampal Slice

We have examined these two possibilities using the hippocampal slice. Extracellular recordings were made from the dendritic region of CA3 as previously described (Schneiderman, 1986). Drugs were dissolved in oxygenated recording solution (Yamamoto's; 2.0 mM Mg^{2+}) and perfused continuously through the entire slice bath. No burst activity is recorded in such slices until a convulsant drug such as penicillin is added. In the presence of penicillin, synchronous burst discharge, representing the population response of the PDS, can be recorded. This provides a model of the mechanism of action of anticonvulsant drugs (Schneiderman and Evans, 1986). A variety of anticonvulsant drugs are effective in suppressing this activity in the presence of relatively high concentrations of Mg^{2+} (2.0 mM). However, this synchronous burst discharge was insensitive to APV at doses as high as 1 mM (Fig. 5). In addition, ketamine had only a weak effect in depressing this synchronous discharge at concentrations as high as 200 μM (Fig. 5). This suggests that the excitatory synaptic activity related to the synchronous discharge is not mediated by the "slow" NMDA EPSPs.

When Mg^{2+} was excluded from the recording solution, we consistently observed synchronous discharge from this region without the addition of a convulsive drug such as penicillin.

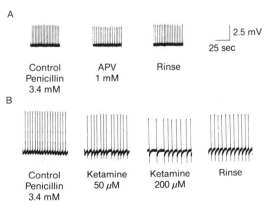

Figure 5. The actions of APV and ketamine on penicillin bursts. (A) APB (1 mM) had little effect on spontaneous field potentials recorded in the CA3 distal dendritic region (approximately 650 μm from the soma) of a guinea pig hippocampal slice perfused with penicillin (3.4 mM). (B) Ketamine reduced the rate and amplitude of population bursts in a penicillin-perfused hippocampal slice but relatively high concentrations (50 to 200 μM) were required. The effect was only partially reversible.

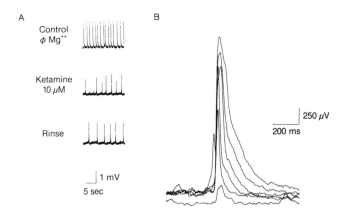

Figure 6. Effects of ketamine on bursts occurring in the absence of Mg^{2+}. (A) Ketamine (10 μM) reduced the rate of spontaneous, synchronous bursts recorded in the CA3 distal dendritic region (approximately 650 μm from the soma) of a guinea pig hippocampal slice perfused with artificial cerebrospinal fluid from which Mg^{2+} was omitted. (B) Ketamine reduced the amplitude and duration of the field potentials. Relatively frequent low-amplitude field potentials (illustrated below the other traces) were also recorded.

Addition of concentrations of Mg^{2+} as low as 250 μM suppressed this spontaneous synchronous discharge. Furthermore, perfusion with 50 μM APV reversibly depressed the amplitude, duration, and frequency of the synchronous discharges and gradually desynchronized them altogether (not shown but see Fig. 6). This effect of APV was readily reversible upon washing it out of the bath. Ketamine (10 μM) and PCP (10 μM) were also highly effective in depressing this spontaneous synchronous discharge (Fig. 6).

Therefore, the latter prediction is supported by these observations. Lowering extracellular levels of Mg^{2+} does not inhibit the PDS and instead favors its spontaneous formation and synchronization. Increasing concentrations of Mg^{2+} progressively inhibit this activity and do not appear to accentuate the PDS. Therefore, at least with regard to this set of experimental conditions, the PDS is unlikely to be a direct consequence of the voltage sensitivity of "slow," NMDA-mediated EPSPs. However, this synaptic activity appears to be significant for the triggering and synchronization of PDS activity. In contrast, if the concentration of Mg^{2+} is relatively high and penicillin is used to induce spontaneous synchronous discharge, it would appear that any

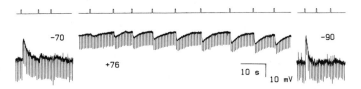

Figure 7. Demonstration of the voltage- and use-dependent block of depolarizing responses to L-Asp in a cultured hippocampal neuron and its unblock at depolarized membrane potential. Three applications of L-Asp (50 μM) were given at a membrane potential of −70 mV (left panel). The depolarization in response to the amino acid declined to zero and did not recover spontaneously (use-dependent block). The cell was then depolarized to +76 mV and the application repeated. The hyperpolarization evoked by L-Asp gradually increases as the ketamine block is relieved (middle panel). When the potential is then set at −90 mV, the depolarizing response to the L-Asp has recovered and with repetition it is reestablished (right panel). Indicators of the pressure applications are given just above evoked currents. A hyperpolarizing 50-msec pulse of constant current was passed across the membrane in order to measure input conductance.

excitatory synaptic activity critical to its triggering and synchronization is mediated by non-NMDA receptors because of its resistance to APV and ketamine.

The spontaneous synchronous discharge of CA3 neurons recorded in the presence of low concentrations of Mg^{2+} provides an alternative model of epileptogenic activity. Furthermore, our results suggest that APV, PCP, and ketamine should be potential anticonvulsant drugs, the effectiveness of which will depend upon the degree of NMDA channel blockade expressed by extracellular Mg^{2+}. It also suggests that some convulsive states, and perhaps some forms of epilepsy, might be associated with an abnormally low concentration of extracellular Mg^{2+} in the brain.

The anticonvulsant properties of ketamine are most likely to be effective under conditions which cause repetitive activation of EPSPs (see Fig. 7). The spontaneous synchronous discharge which occurs in the face of lowered concentrations of Mg^{2+} seems most apt to bring this situation about. The progressive trapping of ketamine within the NMDA channels would also tend to increase its effective potency at these sites of abnormal activity.

References

Albuquerque, E. X., Aguayo, L. G., Warnick, J. E., Ickowicz, R. K., and Blaustein, M. P., 1983, Interactions of phencyclidine with ion channels of nerve and muscle behavioural implications, *Fed. Proc.* **42**:2584–2589.

Alger, B. E., 1984, Hippocampus: Electrophysiological studies of epileptiform activity *in vitro,* in: *Brain Slices* (R. Dingledine, ed.), Plenum Press, New York, pp. 155–193.

Anis, N. A., Berry, S. C., Burton, N. R., and Lodge, D., 1983, The dissociative anaesthetics, ketamine and phencyclidine, selectively reduce excitation of central mammalian neurones by N-methyl-aspartate, *Br. J. Pharmacol.* **79**:565–575.

Armstrong-James, M., Caan, A. W., and Fox, K., 1985, Threshold effects of N-methyl-D-aspartate (NMDA) and 2-amino-5-phosphonovaleric acid (2APV) on the spontaneous activity of neocortical single neurones in the urethane anaesthetised rat, *Exp. Brain Res.* **60**:209–213.

Aronstam, R. S., Narayanan, L., and Wenger, D. A., 1982, Ketamine inhibition of ligand binding to cholinergic receptors and ion channels, *Eur. J. Pharmacol.* **78**:367–370.

Bartschat, D. K., and Blaustein, M. P., 1986, Phencyclidine in low doses selectively blocks a presynaptic voltage-regulated potassium channel in rat brain, *Proc. Natl. Acad. Sci. USA* **83**:189–192.

Callaghan, D. A., and Schwark, W. S., 1980, Pharmacological modifications of amygdaloid-kindled seizures, *Neuropharmacology* **19**:1131–1136.

Celesia, G. G., and Chen, R. C., 1974, Effects of ketamine on EEG activity in cats and monkeys, *Electroencephalogr. Clin. Neurophysiol.* **37**:345–353.

Chen, G., Ensor, C. R., and Bohner, B., 1966, The neuropharmacology of 2-(O-chlorophenyl)-2-methyl-amino-cyclohexanone hydrochloride, *J. Pharmacol. Exp. Ther.* **152**:332–339.

Colquhoun, D., and Hawkes, A. G., 1983, The principles of the stochastic interpretation of ion-channel mechanisms, in: *Single Channel Recording* (B. Sakmann and E. Neher, eds.), Plenum Press, New York, pp. 135–175.

Connors, B. W., 1984, Initiation of synchronized neuronal bursting in neocortex, *Nature* **23**:685–687.

Corssen, G., Little, S. C., and Tavakoli, M., 1974, Ketamine and epilepsy, *Anesth. Analg. (Cleveland)* **53**:319–335.

Courtney, K. R., 1975, Mechanism of frequency-dependent inhibition of sodium currents in frog myelinated nerve by the lidocaine derivative GEA 968, *J. Pharmacol.* **195**:225–236.

Croucher, M. J., Collins, J. F., and Meldrum, B. S., 1982, Anticonvulsant action of excitatory amino acid antagonists, *Science* **216**:889–901.

Curtis, D. R., Phillis, J. W., and Watkins, J. C., 1960, The chemical excitation of spinal neurones by certain acidic amino acids, *J. Physiol. (London)* **158**:296–323.

Davis, R. W., and Tolstoshev, G. C., 1976, Ketamine: Use in severe febrile convulsions, *Med. J. Aust.* **63**:465–466.

Dingledine, R., 1983, N-Methyl aspartate activates voltage-dependent calcium conductance in rat hippocampal pyramidal cells, *J. Physiol. (London)* **343**:385–405.

Duchen, M. R., Burton, N. R., and Biscoe, T. J., 1985, An intracellular study of the interactions of N-methyl-DL-aspartate with ketamine in the mouse hippocampal slice, *Brain Res.* **342**:149–153.

Fagg, G. E., and Foster, A. C., 1983, Amino acid neurotransmitters and their pathways in the mammalian central nervous system, *Neuroscience* **9:**701–719.

Flatman, J. A., Schwindt, P. C., Crill, W. E., and Stafstrom, C. E., 1983, Multiple actions of N-methyl-D-aspartate on cat neocortical neurons *in vitro, Brain Res.* **266:**169–173.

Foster, A. C., and Fagg, G. E., 1984, Acidic amino acid binding sites in mammalian neuronal membranes: Their characteristics and relationship to synaptic receptors, *Brain Res.* **7:**103–164.

Gage, P. W., and Robertson, B., 1985, Prolongation of inhibitory postsynaptic currents by pentobarbitone, halothane and ketamine in CA1 pyramidal cells in rat hippocampus, *Br. J. Pharmacol.* **85:**675–681.

Gurney, A. M., and Rang, H. P., 1984, The channel-blocking action of methonium compounds on rat submandibular ganglion cells. *Br. J. Pharmacol.* **82:**623–642.

Hablitz, J. J., and Langmoen, I. A., 1986, *N*-methyl-D-aspartate receptor antagonists reduce synaptic excitation in the hippocampus, *J. Neurosci.* **6:**102–106.

Harrison, N. L., and Simmonds, M. A., 1985, Quantitative studies on some antagonists of N-methyl-D-aspartate in slices of rat cerebral cortex, *Br. J. Pharmacol.* **84:**318–391.

Hayashi, T., 1954, Effects of sodium glutamate on the nervous system, *Keio J. Med.* **3:**183–192.

Hayes, B. A., and Balster, R. L., 1985, Anticonvulsant properties of phencyclidine-like drugs in mice, *Eur. J. Pharmacol.* **117:**121–125.

Herron, C. E., Lester, R. A. J., Coan, E. J., and Collingridge, G. L., 1985, Intracellular demonstration of an N-methyl-D-aspartate receptor mediated component of synaptic transmission in the rat hippocampus, *Neurosci. Lett.* **60:**19–23.

Hille, B., 1984, *Ionic Channels of Excitable Membranes,* 1st ed., Sinauer Associates, Stanford.

Honey, C. R., Miljkovic, Z., and MacDonald, J. F., 1985, Ketamine and phencyclidine cause a voltage-dependent block of responses to L-aspartic acid, *Neurosci. Lett.* **61:**135–139.

Jahr, C. E., and Jessell, T. M., 1985, Synaptic transmission between dorsal root ganglion and dorsal horn neurons in culture: Antagonism of monosynaptic excitatory postsynaptic potentials and glutamate excitation by kynurenate, *J. Neurosci.* **5:**2281–2289.

Jahr, C. E., and Yoshioka, K., 1986, Ia afferent excitation of motoneurones in the *in vitro* new-born rat spinal cord is selectively antagonized by kynurenate, *J. Physiol. (London)* **370:**515–530.

Johnston, D., and Brown, T. H., 1984, Biophysics and microphysiology of synaptic transmission in hippocampus, in: *Brain Slices* (R. Dingledine, ed.), Plenum Press, New York, pp. 51–86.

Johnston, G. A. R., 1972, Convulsions induced in 10-day-old rats by intraperitoneal injections of monosodium glutamate and related excitant amino acids, *Biochem. Pharmacol.* **22:**137–140.

Lacey, M. G., and Henderson, G., 1986, Actions of phencyclidine on rat locus coeruleus neurons *in vitro, Neuroscience* **17:**485–494.

Little, H. J., and Atkinson, H. D., 1984, Ketamine potentiates the responses of the rat superior cervical ganglion to GABA, *Eur. J. Pharmacol.* **98:**53–59.

MacDermott, A. B., Mayer, M. L., Westbrook, G. L., Smith, S. J., and Barker, J. L., 1986, NMDA-receptor activation increases cytoplasmic calcium concentration in cultured spinal cord neurones, *Nature* **321:**519–522.

MacDonald, J. F., 1984, Substitution of extracellular sodium ions blocks the voltage-dependent decrease of input conductance evoked by L-aspartate, *Can. J. Physiol. Pharmacol.* **62:**109–115.

MacDonald, J. F., 1985, Measurements of transmitter action: The problem of voltage dependence, *Can. J. Physiol. Pharmacol.* **63:**825–830.

MacDonald, J. F., Miljkovic, Z., and Pennefather, P., 1987, Use-dependent block of excitatory amino acid currents in cultured hippocampal neurons by ketamine, *J. Neurophysiol.* **58:**251–266.

MacDonald, J. F., and Schneiderman, J. H., 1984, L-Aspartic acid potentiates "slow" inward current in cultured spinal cord neurones, *Brain Res.* **296:**350–355.

MacDonald, J. F., and Wojtowicz, J. M., 1982, The effects of L-glutamate and its analogues upon the membrane conductance of central murine neurones in culture, *Can. J. Physiol. Pharmacol.* **60:**282–296.

MacDonald, J. F., Porietis, A. V., and Wojtowicz, J. M., 1982, L-Aspartic acid induces a region of negative slope conductance in the current–voltage relationship of cultured spinal cord neurons, *Brain Res.* **237:**248–253.

MacDonald, J. F., Schneiderman, J. H., and Miljkovic, Z., 1986. Excitatory amino acids and regenerative activity in cultured neurones, in: *Excitatory Amino Acids and Epilepsy* (R. Schwarcz and Y. Ben Ari, eds.), Plenum Press, New York, pp. 425–438.

Maleque, M. A., Warnick, J. E., and Albuquerque, E. X., 1981, The mechanism and site of action of ketamine on skeletal muscle, *J. Pharmacol. Exp. Ther.* **219:**638–645.

Martin, D., and Lodge, D., 1985, Ketamine acts as a noncompetitive N-methyl-D-aspartate antagonist on frog spinal cord *in vitro, Neuropharmacology* **24:**999–1003.

Mayer, M. L., and Westbrook, G. L., 1985, The action of N-methyl-D-aspartic acid on mouse spinal neurones in culture, *J. Physiol. (London)* **361**:65–90.

Mayer, M. L., Westbrook, G. L., and Guthrie, P. B., 1984, Voltage-dependent block by Mg^{2+} of NMDA responses in spinal cord neurones, *Nature* **309**:261–263.

Meldrum, B. S., Croucher, M. J., Badman, G., and Collins, J. F., 1983, Antiepileptic actions of excitatory amino acid antagonists in the photosensitive baboon, *Papio papio, Neurosci. Lett.* **39**:101–104.

Morris, M., Friedlich, J., and MacDonald, J. F., 1986, Intracellular calcium in mammalian brain cells: Fluorescence measurements with Quin2, *Exp. Brain Res.* **65**:520–526.

Mudge, G. H., 1985, Agents affecting volume and composition of body fluids, in: *The Pharmacological Basis of Therapeutics,* 7th ed. (A. G. Gilman, L. S. Goodman, T. W. Rall, and F. Murad, eds.), Macmillan Co., New York, pp. 846–878.

Neher, E., and Steinbach, J. H., 1978, Local anaesthetics transiently block currents through single acetylcholine-receptor channels, *J. Physiol. (London)* **277**:153–176.

Nelson, P. G., Pun, R. Y. K., and Westbrook, G. L., 1986, Synaptic excitation in cultures of mouse spinal cord neurones: Receptor pharmacology and behavior of synaptic currents, *J. Physiol. (London)* **372**:169–190.

Nistri, A., and Constanti, A., 1979, Pharmacological characterization of different types of GABA and glutamate receptors in vertebrates and invertebrates, *Prog. Neurobiol.* **13**:117–235.

Nowak, L., Bregestovski, P., Ascher, P., Herbert, A., and Prochiantz, A., 1984, Magnesium gates glutamate-activated channels in mouse central neurones, *Nature* **307**:462–465.

Puil, E., 1981, S-glutamate: Its interactions with spinal neurons, *Brain Res. Rev.* **3**:229–322.

Riveros, N., and Orrego, F., 1986, N-Methylaspartate-activated calcium channels in rat brain cortex slices: Effect of calcium channel blockers and of inhibitory and depressant substances, *Neuroscience* **17**:541–546.

Rucci, F. S., and Caroli, G., 1974, Ketamine and eclampsia, *Br. J. Anaesthesiol.* **46**:546.

Ryan, G. P., Hackman, J. C., and Davidoff, R. A., 1984, Spinal seizures and excitatory amino acid-mediated synaptic transmission, *Neurosci. Lett.* **44**:161–166.

Schneiderman, J. H., 1986, Low concentrations of penicillin rhythmic, synchronous synaptic potentials in hippocampal slice, *Brain Res.* **398**:231–241.

Schneiderman, J. H., and Evans, J. C., 1986, Effects of anticonvulsants on penicillin-induced bursts in guinea pig hippocampal slices, *Epilepsia* **27**:347–353.

Strichartz, G. R., 1973, The inhibition of sodium currents in myelinated nerve by quaternary derivatives of lidocaine, *J. Gen. Physiol.* **62**:37–57.

Thomson, A. M., 1986, A magnesium-sensitive post-synaptic potential in rat cerebral cortex resembles neuronal responses to N-methylapartate, *J. Physiol. (London)* **370**:531–549.

Weitz, M. D., Merlob, P., Amir, J., and Reisner, S. H., 1981, A possible role for aspartic acid in neonatal seizures, *Arch. Neurol.* **38**:258–259.

White, P. F., Way, W. L., and Trevor, A. J., 1982, Ketamine: Its pharmacology and therapeutic uses, *Anesthesiology* **56**:119–136.

9

GABA Neurons and Their Cotransmitters in the Primate Cerebral Cortex

E. G. Jones

1. Introduction

The classical neurotransmitter, γ-aminobutyric acid (GABA), and its synthesizing enzyme, glutamic acid decarboxylase (GAD), have been known to be present in the mammalian cerebral cortex for a relatively long time (Awapara et al., 1950; Roberts and Fenkel, 1950; Albers and Brady, 1959). Along with glutamate, GABA is the compound released in largest amounts when the cortex is subjected to depolarizing stimuli (Jasper and Koyama, 1969; Baughman and Gilbert, 1981). Immunocytochemistry has revealed the existence of a large population of neurons immunoreactive for both GAD and GABA in the cortex of many species of mammal (Ribak, 1978; Emson and Hunt, 1981; Hendrickson et al., 1981; Peters et al., 1982; Hendry et al., 1983a; Houser et al., 1983b, 1985; Bear et al., 1985; Lin et al., 1985). Our quantitative assessments indicate that approximately 25% of the neuronal population in any area of the monkey cortex is GABA- or GAD-immunoreactive (Hendry et al., 1986c). We have also concluded (Jones and Hendry, 1986; Fig. 1) that possibly all the morphological varieties of intrinsic cortical neurons, except the population of small, presumed excitatory, dendritic-spine-bearing neurons of layer IV, are GABA-immunoreactive. Of the several varieties of pyramidal neurons in the cortex, all, from electrophysiological considerations, are undoubtedly also excitatory and it is extremely likely that they use glutamate as a transmitter (Cotman et al., 1981; Streit, 1984; Donoghue et al., 1985).

Apart from GABA and glutamate, a number of brain–gut peptides found in the mammalian cerebral cortex have come to be localized in cortical neurons (Carraway and Leeman, 1976; Hökfelt et al., 1976, 1978; Said and Rosenberg, 1976; Uhl and Snyder, 1976; Dockray, 1976; Muller et al., 1977; Paxinos et al., 1978; Sachs et al., 1978; McDonald et al., 1982a–c, 1983; Peters et al., 1983; Emson and Hunt, 1985; McGinty et al., 1984; Morrison et al., 1983; Hendry et al., 1983b, 1984a). Table I lists the cortical neuropeptides thus far identified and indicates the distribution of cells or fibers immunoreactive for them. Like GABA cells, cells immunoreactive for most peptides appear to be widely distributed to all cortical areas; those immunoreactive for a few are found in more restricted areas. Our studies of cortical cells immunoreactive for the neuropeptides (Hendry et al., 1986b), and a review of reports in the literature, have led us to

E. G. Jones • Department of Anatomy and Neurobiology, University of California, Irvine, California 92717.

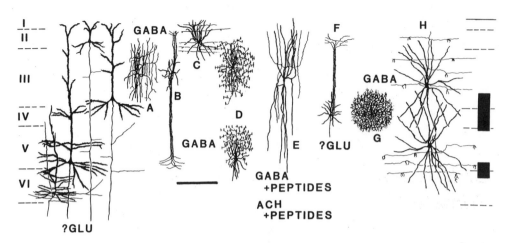

Figure 1. Morphological types of cells identifiable in monkey cerebral cortex, based on studies of Jones (1975) on sensory-motor areas. Cells at left are typical pyramidal cells of layers II–VI which may use glutamate as a transmitter. Cells A–H are intrinsic neurons. All except the small spiny, putatively excitatory cell (F) of layer IV are likely to be GABAergic. Long, bitufted cell (E) is typical type that colocalizes GABA and neuropeptides or (in rat) acetylcholine and neuropeptides. A: cell with axonal arcades; B: double bouquet cell; C, H: basket cells; D: chandelier cells; G: neurogliaform cell. (From Jones, 1986.)

conclude that all the known cortical neuropeptides, rather than defining separate morphological cell varieties, are contained in a cell class that can best be described as having a small rounded soma and a variable number of elongated, "stringy" vertical processes (Figs. 2–4).

Many, perhaps all, of the cortical cells immunoreactive for known neuropeptides show colocalization of immunoreactivity for GABA, GAD, or the biosynthetic enzyme for acetyl-choline (ACh). In 1984, Eckenstein and Baughman identified certain cells in the rat cortex that

Table I. Neocortical Transmitters and Neuropeptides[a]

	Extrinsic (in afferent fibers)		Intrinsic (in cortical neurons)	
	General (to all areas)	Regional (to all areas)	General	Regional
GABA	+	−	++++	−
ACh	++	−	++	−
5HT	+++	−	−	−
NA	+++	−	−	−
DA	−	++	−	−
Glu/Asp	(++)[b]	−	(+++)[b]	−
CCK	−	+	+++	−
NPY	−	−	+++	−
SRIF	−	−	+++	−
VIP	−	−	++	−
SP	−	+	+++	−
DYN	−	−	++	−
CRF	−	−	−	+
NT	−	+	−	−
CGRP	−	−	−	+

[a]From Jones and Hendry (1986).
[b]Likely; not proven conclusively.

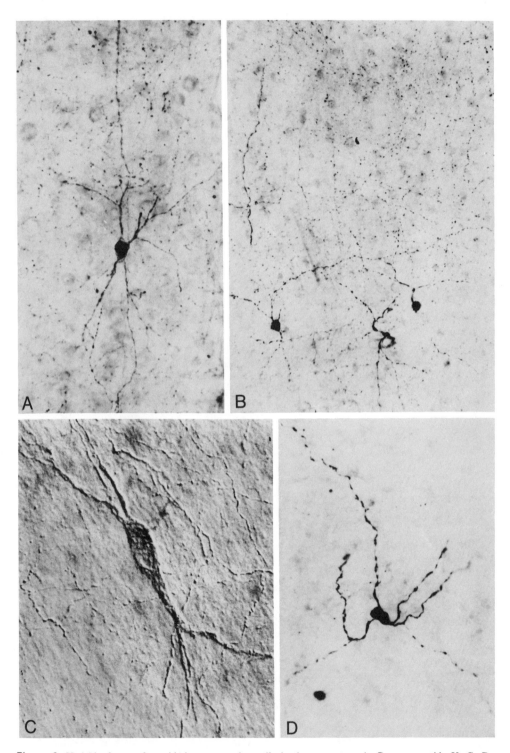

Figure 2. Variable forms of peptide-immunoreactive cells in the neocortex. A, B: neuropeptide Y; C, D: somatostatin. (From Hendry *et al.*, 1984a.)

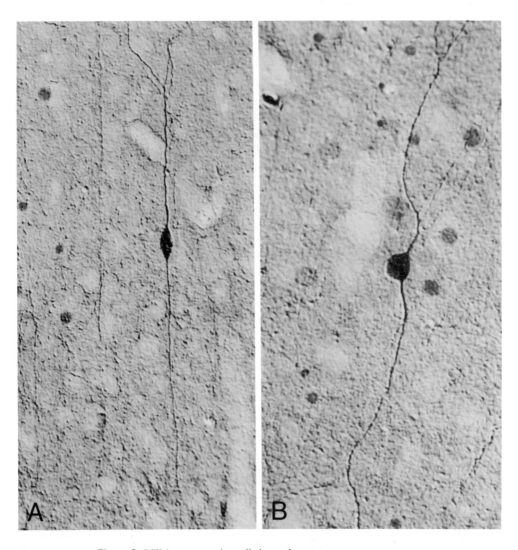

Figure 3. CCK-immunoreactive cells in monkey cortex.

showed colocalization of immunoreactivity for vasoactive intestinal polypeptide (VIP) and choline acetyltransferase (ChAT); in the same year, Schmechel *et al.* reported colocalization of
somatostatin (SRIF) and GAD immunoreactivity in the rat, cat, and monkey cortex; Somogyi *et
al.* identified cells immunoreactive for SRIF and GABA or for cholecystokinin (CCK) and GABA
in the cat cortex and hippocampus; Hendry *et al.* identified cells immunoreactive for SRIF and
GAD, CCK and GAD, or neuropeptide Y (NPY) and GAD in the monkey and cat cortex and
showed quantitatively that at least 95% of cells immunoreactive for any of these peptides were
also immunoreactive for GAD. More recently, we have determined that several other cortical
peptides are almost invariably colocalized with GABA and/or GAD and that more than one
cortical neuropeptide can occur in the same neuron (Jones and Hendry, 1985, 1986; Hendry *et al.*,
1986b). The main purpose of this chapter is to define GABA and peptide-containing cells in terms
of their morphology, synaptic connections, distributions, and proportions relative to other cortical
cells.

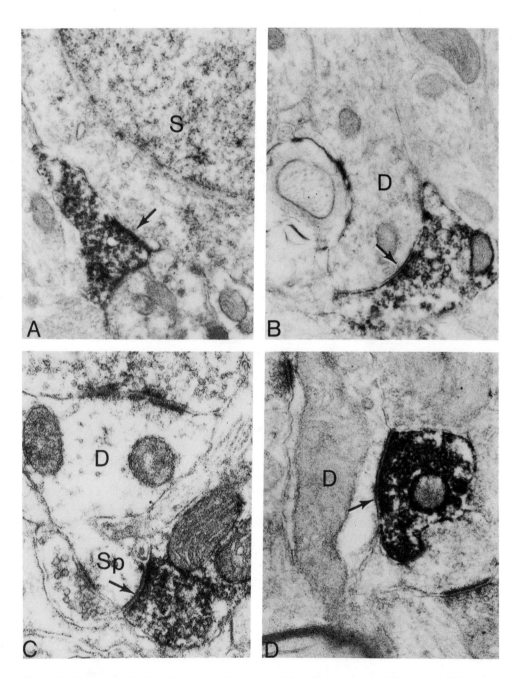

Figure 4. (A) Neuropeptide Y-; (B) vasoactive intestinal peptide-; (C) somatostatin-; (D) cholecystokinin-immunoreactive terminals (arrows) making symmetric synaptic contacts (arrowheads) on somata (S), dendritic spines (Sp), or dendritic shafts (D) in monkey cortex. (From Jones *et al.*, 1986.)

2. Pyramidal Neurons Are Not Immunoreactive for GABA or Known Peptides

Pyramidal neurons (Fig. 1) appear to form between 50 and 60% of the total cell population in any cortical area although these figures are essentially estimates, no extensive quantifications of their numbers yet having been done especially in primates (see Peters, 1986; Winfield et al., 1980). Pyramidal neurons (including those of modified form in layer VI) give rise to the majority of, and in most areas all, the output connections of a cortical area (Jones, 1984a). The output connections go to neighboring and distant cortical areas, to cortical areas in the contralateral hemisphere, and to the large variety of subcortical structures to which the cortex projects. However, pyramidal cells are also major contributors to intracortical circuitry because of their extensive systems of axon collaterals. Stimulation of pyramidal cell axons or their collaterals usually results in the induction of short-latency excitatory postsynaptic potentials in cells on which they synapse, though this may be succeeded at di- and polysynaptic latencies by profound inhibition.

Strong circumstantial evidence suggests that the acidic amino acid glutamate (or possibly aspartate) is the transmitter released from pyramidal cell axon terminals. Specific uptake of these two materials (which share the same high-affinity uptake system) by synaptosomes in cortical projection targets is reduced after decortication; there is specific retrograde axoplasmic transport of D-[^{3}H]aspartate in pyramidal cell axons (Streit, 1984). The demonstration of immunoreactivity for phosphate-dependent glutaminase or aspartate aminotransferase in pyramidal neurons (Donoghue et al., 1985), though supportive of the idea that these cells are glutamatergic or aspartatergic, is unfortunately inconclusive since it could simply reflect the normal involvement of glutamate and aspartate in non-transmitter-related metabolism of the cells.

GABA, GAD, ACh, ChAT, or neuropeptide immunoreactivity has never been convincingly reported in pyramidal neurons. Cell bodies immunoreactive for one or another of these have sometimes been described as "pyramidal" in shape. But this is insufficient, for a true pyramidal neuron can only be defined by the presence of its stereotyped apical and basal dendritic systems covered in dendritic spines and an axon that descends vertically toward the white matter. For most immunoreactive neurons described as pyramidal in the literature, these rigid morphological criteria have not been met. In our own studies we have never stained clear pyramidal cells for the materials mentioned. At the electron microscopic level we have rarely detected dendritic spines immunoreactive for these substances though it has been possible to stain small dendrites of comparable caliber. Finally, virtually all GABA-, GAD-, ChAT-, and peptide-immunoreactive synapses that we have studied in the cortex are of the symmetric variety (Fig. 5), quite unlike the asymmetric synapses of pyramidal cell axon collaterals (Winfield et al., 1981; McGuire et al., 1984).

3. The Proportion of GABA Neurons in Monkey Cerebral Cortex

When stained immunocytochemically for GABA or GAD, any section of the monkey cortex reveals a large proportion of the cortical neuronal population that is immunoreactive for these compounds (Fig. 5). Stained cells appear in all layers of all cytoarchitectonic areas with the largest number apparently in the middle layers, particularly layer IV of the sensory areas. By using relatively thin sections, stained in a manner that maximizes penetration of and staining by the immunoreagents, it is possible to count accurately the GABAergic cell population from area to area (Hendry et al., 1986c). In cynomolgus monkeys, we made counts in 50-µM-wide rectangular, vertical traverses extending from the pia mater to the white matter across the following areas: areas 17 and 18 of the visual cortex, the somatosensory areas 3b and 1–2, the parietal fields areas 5 and 7, the temporal fields 21 and 22, the motor cortex, and the orbitofrontal cortex (Table II). These counts reveal a remarkable constancy of GABA-immunoreactive cell numbers from

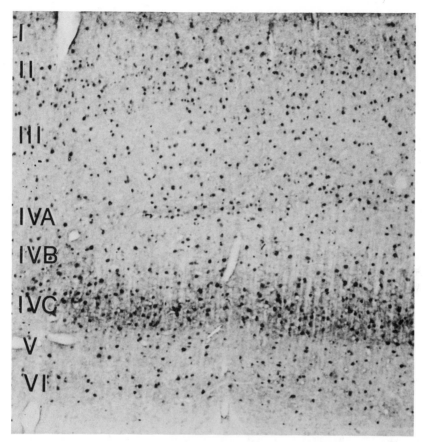

Figure 5. GABA-immunoreactive neurons distributed through all layers of the monkey visual cortex in a 10-μm-thick section. (From Hendry *et al.*, 1986c.) GABA cells account for 25–30% of the cell population in each area.

area to area, except for area 17. In all areas except area 17, there is an average of approximately 30 to 40 GABA- or GAD-immunoreactive cells per 50-μM-wide traverse. In area 17 the number is greater, approximately 54 to 58. When these numbers are compared with our own counts of the total, Nissl-stained neuronal population (Table II) or with the counts made by Rockel *et al.* (1980) in rhesus monkeys, it is clear that GABAergic neurons form approximately 25% of the cell

Table II. Number of GABA-Positive Cells per 50-μm-Wide Traverse (Means of 80–100 Traverses) in Monkey Cortex[a]

	Area 17	Area 18	Area 5	Areas 1–2	Area 3b	Area 4
Animal 1	54.2 ± 2.9	38.4 ± 5.0	38.1 ± 3.2	40.4 ± 3	31.6 ± 3.3	40.0 ± 2.5
Animal 2	54.1 ± 3.1	36.8 ± 5.4	41.7 ± 3.9	39.8 ± 3.1	38.4 ± 2.9	39.7 ± 3.0
Animal 3	57.7 ± 4.5	39.7 ± 4.0	38.6 ± 2.5	39.5 ± 2.8	28.5 ± 4.0	40.4 ± 2.8
Mean	56.2 ± 3.1	38.4 ± 5.1	39.4 ± 3.1	39.8 ± 2.9	32.8 ± 6.1	39.7 ± 2.9

Total number of cells per 50 μm-wide traverse

	Area 17	Area 18	Area 5	Areas 1–2	Area 3b	Area 4
Range	309.0–314.7	152.0–156.1	153.1–154.5	149.7–154.3	152.7–154.9	148.9–151.7
Mean	311.6 ± 19.3	155.1 ± 8.1	153.7 ± 6.4	153.0 ± 7.2	153.66 ± 6.1	150.4 ± 6.1

[a]From Hendry *et al.* (1986c).

population in any area except the visual. In the latter, the consistently higher total cell population results in a GABA population that falls to approximately 20%.

4. Several Varieties of Cortical Intrinsic Neurons Are GABA Neurons

Morphological studies show that there are seven or eight main classes of cortical intrinsic neuron in primates (Jones, 1984); all of them are nonpyramidal in form (Fig. 1). Among the large cortical GABAergic population, there are also a variety of morphological types (Figs. 6, 12). All are nonpyramidal, all lack significant populations of dendritic spines, and all their axons seem to be intrinsic to the cortex and form symmetrical synaptic contacts with flattenable synaptic vesicles (Fig. 15) (Houser *et al.,* 1983b, 1984). These are all features of the six or seven nonspiny types of cortical interneuron. There has been some difficulty in deciding whether all or only some of these morphological forms of nonspiny intrinsic neuron are GABA- or GAD-immunoreactive, because it is rare for the total dendritic tree or complete axonal ramification to be stained immunocytochemically. Two nonspiny forms of cortical interneuron are almost certainly GABAergic, even in the absence of dendritic staining much beyond the primary branches. These are the basket cells, which have an unusually large somal size, and an identifiable proximal dendritic and axon

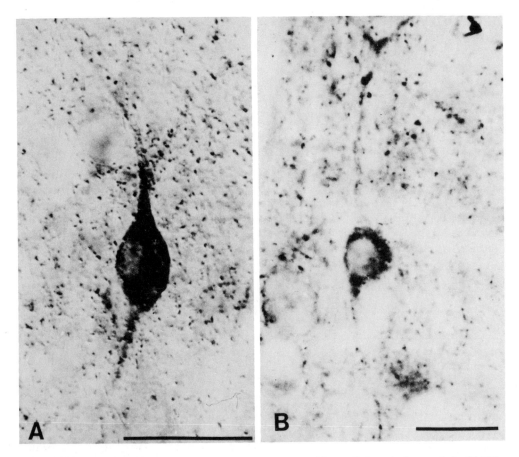

Figure 6. Two neurons immunoreactive for GAD in monkey cortex. These cells have the form typical of GABA neurons that colocalize immunoreactivity for neuropeptides. Bars = 10 μm.

morphology (DeFelipe *et al.*, 1985; Figs. 12, 13) and the chandelier cells whose axons have a unique site of termination on the initial segments of pyramidal cell axons where all synapses are GAD-positive (Peters *et al.*, 1982; Somogyi *et al.*, 1982; DeFelipe *et al.*, 1985; Figs. 1, 17). The proximal dendritic fields and the variety of somal diameters of other GABA-immunoreactive neurons (Hendry *et al.*, 1983a; Houser *et al.*, 1983b, 1984) suggest that possibly all the other types of nonspiny cortical intrinsic neuron are also GABAergic, though it is hard to document this conclusively. Among the types recognizable in studies of GABA and GAD localization are those with small rounded somata from which long thin dendrites arise singly or in tufts and turn vertically, giving the cell a bipolar or bitufted appearance (Fig. 6). The somata of these cells appear to be most common in layer II and the superficial part of layer III, and at the junction of layers V and VI. There is reason to believe (see below and Fig. 1) that this GABAergic cell type is the cortical cell type that contains all or most of the known cortical neuropeptides. Others with very small somata and dendrites recurving toward the soma are likely to be neurogliaform cells (Jones, 1984b) (Fig. 1).

The concentration of the somata of the elongated GABA cells in superficial and deep strata correlates quite well with the two strata of somata that are specifically labeled by transport of [³H]-GABA injected into individual cortical layers in monkeys (Somogyi *et al.*, 1982; DeFelipe and Jones, 1985). When [³H]-GABA is injected into layer II and the superficial part of layer III, small nonpyramidal cell somata are labeled in layers V–VI, immediately deep to the injection focus, but not in intervening layers (Fig. 7A). Conversely, injection of [³H]-GABA into layers V and VI leads to somal labeling in layer II and the superficial part of layer III, again without somal labeling in intervening layers (Fig. 7B). The effect is blocked by intracortical injections of colchicine (DeFelipe and Jones, 1985).

It is the general belief that this form of transmitter-specific, retrograde labeling is a feature of neurons using the transmitter normally (see Streit, 1984). Electron microscopic examination of the autoradiographically labeled, linear profiles that connect injection site and labeled somata, however, reveals labeled dendrites as well as labeled axons (DeFelipe and Jones, 1985). Thus, cells with vertical dendrites as well as axons appear to be involved in the phenomenon and somal labeling may be due to a combination of retrograde axonal and dendritic transport. The elongated GABA neurons of layers II–III and V–VI are obvious candidates to form the basis for this specific translaminar transport of [³H]-GABA.

The extended nature of the axons of basket cells, often as much as 3 mm in the horizontal direction, makes them obvious candidates for mediating horizontal intercolumnar inhibition in the cortex. Neurogliaform cells, by contrast, would act locally, chandelier cells very specifically, and the vertical interlaminar cells could mediate intracolumnar inhibition. Such conjectures, however, need to be confirmed. Apart from proximal dendritic morphology and those special features such as horizontal or vertical axonal distributions, the distribution of GABA synapses on the surfaces of other neurons also leads us to believe that there are many varieties of cortical GABA-containing cells. The selective termination of chandelier cell axons on the initial segments of pyramidal cell axons has already been mentioned. Although no chandelier cell terminals have been reported to end elsewhere, there is considerable variability in the number of such terminals on an individual initial segment (DeFelipe *et al.*, 1985). The significance of this is unknown.

Basket cell terminals are restricted to the somata and proximal portions of the dendrites of pyramidal cells and of other basket cells (Figs. 12, 14) and the multiterminal nature of GAD- and GABA-positive terminals in these positions confirms their basket cell origins.

With basket cells and chandelier cells accounting for most, perhaps all, GABA synapses on pyramidal cell somata, proximal portions of dendrites, and initial axon segments, there remains a very large number of GABA synapses on more distal portions of these dendrites, on secondary and tertiary dendrites, and on dendritic spines (Fig. 16). A logical conclusion, therefore, is that these synapses are formed by other morphological varieties of intrinsic cortical neuron which are also, therefore, GABAergic. Further studies, similar to those that have defined the basket and chandelier cells as GABAergic neurons, will be necessary to establish this.

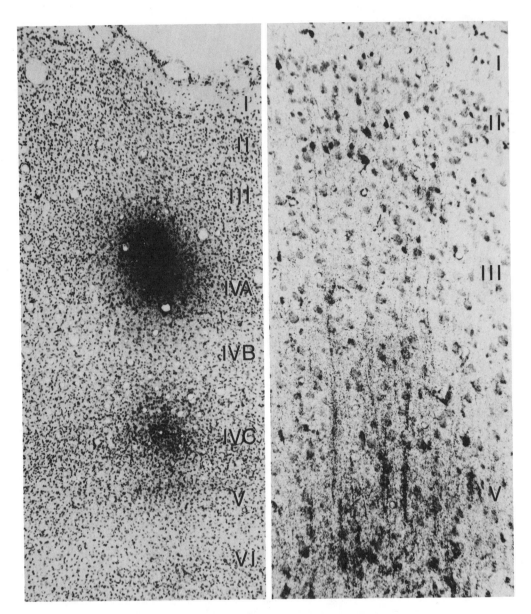

Figure 7. Selective retrograde labeling of neurons by [³H]-GABA. Cells in layers IVc and V of monkey visual cortex (left) are labeled after an injection in layers II–IVa. Cells in layers II–III of monkey motor cortex (right) are labeled after an injection in layer V. (From DeFelipe and Jones, 1985.)

5. Cortical Neuropeptide Neurons Have a Similar Morphology

Our observations in monkeys, cats, rats, and several other mammalian species suggest that all cells immunoreactive for any of the known cortical neuropeptides listed in Table I have an overall similarity in their morphology. Several features distinguish the known cortical neuropeptide cells. All have small, rounded somata, usually less than 10 μm in diameter. The somata are found in all layers but tend to be concentrated in layer II and the superficial part of layer III and in layer VI and the immediately underlying white matter (Figs. 8–10), particularly in monkeys and man. In some areas, additional concentrations of somata can sometimes be found in other layers and a significant concentration of substance P (SP)-immunoreactive somata occurs in the middle layers in most areas (Fig. 10). Most peptide-immunoreactive cells have slender dendrites that can arise in extremely variable numbers from any part of the surface of the soma at any angle. Where, as is common in many immunocytochemical preparations, only the proximal portions of the dendrites are stained, the cells can appear to be bipolar, bitufted, multipolar, stellate, and so on, and even pyramidal. In our own preparations with the staining of secondary and tertiary dendrites enhanced, we have been led to conclude that verticality of dendrites is the *sine qua non* of these cells. Irrespective of how many dendrites arise from a soma and irrespective of their angles of

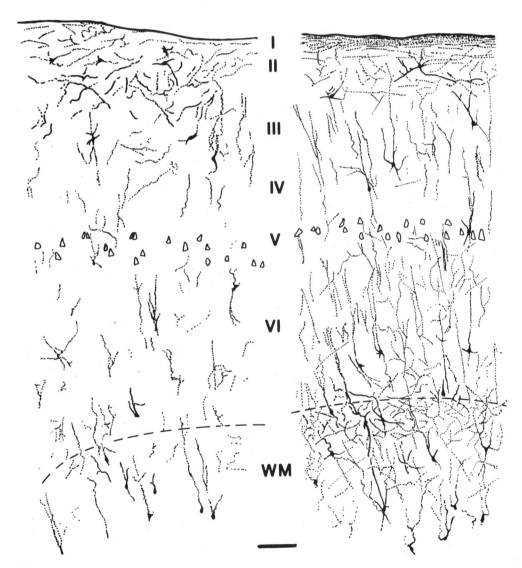

Figure 8. Camera lucida drawing showing distributions of (left) somatostatin- and (right) neuropeptide Y-immunoreactive fibers and cells in monkey motor cortex. Betz cells of layer V are outlined but not labeled. Bar = 250 μm. (From Hendry *et al.*, 1984a.)

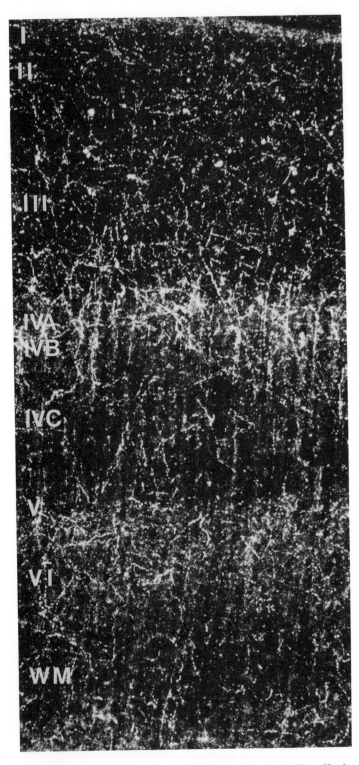

Figure 9. Neuropeptide Y-immunoreactive plexuses in monkey visual cortex. (From Hendry *et al.*, 1984a.)

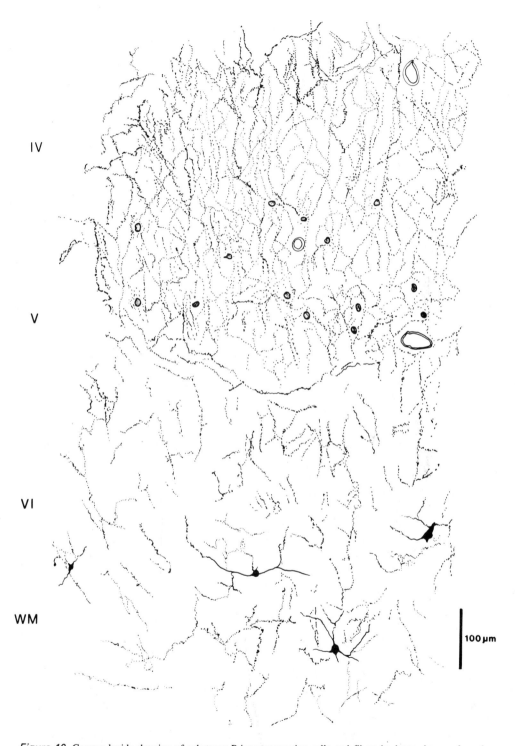

Figure 10. Camera lucida drawing of substance P-immunoreactive cells and fibers in deeper layers of monkey visual cortex. Cells without stained processes in layer IV colocalize GABA immunoreactivity; cells with long stained processes in layer VI and white matter colocalize NPY immunoreactivity. (From Jones, 1986.)

origin, all will branch and/or turn perpendicularly to traverse two or more layers of the cortex. The terminal portions of the processes can branch relatively profusely and so two major plexuses tend to be set up, one in the supragranular layers and one in the infragranular layers and underlying white matter (Fig. 9). Layer IV in some areas is often notably devoid of a peptidergic plexus, except for that formed by SP-immunoreactive processes.

A small number of peptide-immunoreactive neurons have been reported to send axons outside the cerebral cortex in rats. These reports are based upon retrograde labeling of the immunoreactive cell somata by fluorescent dyes injected into certain of the subcortical targets of the cortex. If correct, they imply the existence of either a population of pyramidal neurons immunoreactive for peptides or nonpyramidal projection neurons. We believe it likely that contamination of the plexus of peptidergic processes in the white matter deep to the cortex may account for the reports of extrinsic peptidergic projections from the cortex. This plexus is always evident in white matter overlain by cortex but disappears from deep or exposed white matter such as the internal capsule and corpus callosum (Hendry et al., 1984b). The fact that most cortical peptide cells are also immunoreactive for GABA or GAD (see below) is against their projecting subcortically, since no known subcortical projections are GABAergic.

The axons of peptide neurons in the cortex have not been thoroughly described. The synapses that they form, however, are all very similar. They are small, contain synaptic vesicles that flatten or become pleomorphic in the usual fixatives, and in the vast majority of cases, irrespective of the peptide localized, make symmetric membrane contacts. Contacts have been demonstrated on large and small dendrites of both pyramidal and nonpyramidal neurons and on dendritic spines (Fig. 4). The peptide-immunoreactive cells themselves, including those in the white matter beneath the cortex, receive modest numbers of other, usually nonpeptidergic synapses.

6. Some GABA-Immunoreactive Cortical Neurons Are Also Immunoreactive for Peptides

We have made a systematic effort to quantify the proportions of neurons in the monkey cortex that show colocalization of peptides with classical neurotransmitters, particularly GABA (Figs. 18, 19). Certain neuropeptides such as VIP, which have proven refractory to immunocytochemical staining in the monkey cortex, have been studied in rats only. The population of neurons colocalizing CCK, SRIF, NPY, and GAD or GABA is particularly high. In the monkey (Jones and Hendry, 1986; Hendry et al., 1986b,c) (Fig. 19), virtually all CCK neurons are also GABA- and GAD-immunoreactive. In the rat, some also show VIP immunoreactivity. Approximately 95% of NPY neurons and 95% of SRIF neurons colocalize GABA and GAD. Virtually 100% of SRIF neurons also colocalize NPY and vice versa. Ninety to ninety-five percent of SP neurons (100% of those in the middle layer stratum) colocalize GABA and GAD (Fig. 11). The remaining 5–10% (mainly in layer VI and the white matter) colocalize SRIF and NPY but not GABA or GAD (Figs. 18 and 19).

Hence, most of the neurons immunoreactive for the known cortical peptides are also GABAergic and they also often show immunoreactivity for multiple peptides. It is not known if certain peptides such as dynorphin and corticotrophin releasing factor (CRF), hitherto not stained in the monkey cortex, are also contained in GABA neurons. As mentioned earlier, however, cortical cells immunoreactive for the other peptides in rats have a very similar morphology to those that show colocalization of peptide and GABA immunoreactivity in the monkey. In regard to ACh, its synthetic enzyme, ChAT, is colocalized with VIP in neurons in the rat cortex (Eckenstein and Baughman, 1984). There, the ChAT-immunoreactive cells have the long, stringy morphology typical of peptidergic cells throughout the cortex (Houser et al., 1983a). Whether GAD and ChAT are ever colocalized has not been determined.

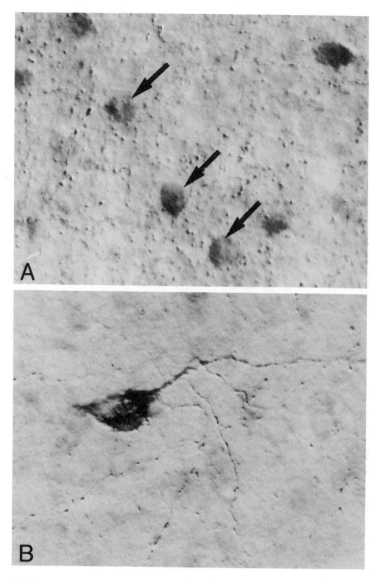

Figure 11. The two types of SP-immunoreactive cells. (A) Cells in layer IV; (B) cells in layer VI.

7. All GABA Neurons Are Not Immunoreactive for Known Peptides

The majority of peptide-positive cortical neurons in the monkey are GAD- and GABA-positive, but our counts show that approximately 70–75% of the GABA-positive neurons do not costain for a known peptide. No somata much larger than 10 μm have ever been stained for a known peptide. Therefore, the larger basket cells cannot be peptide-immunoreactive. Basket cells in monkeys normally have somata 20–50 μm in diameter. The chandelier cells are also unlikely to be included in the costained cells for no chains of peptide-immunoreactive axon terminals have been demonstrated light or electron microscopically on the initial segments of pyramidal cell axons. Although it is possible that several other forms of putatively GABAergic nonpyramidal

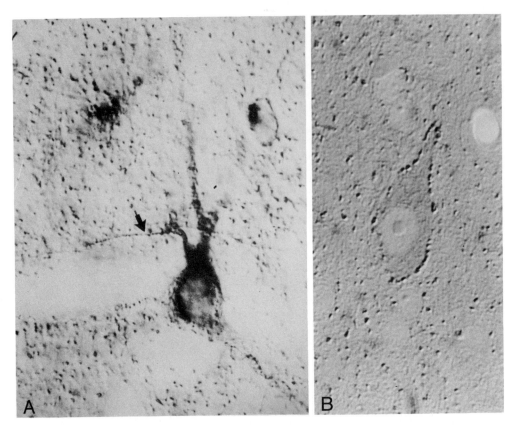

Figure 12. (A) GAD-immunoreactive cell of monkey motor cortex, identified as a basket cell by its large size, multipolar shape, and horizontal axon collaterals (arrow). (From Houser *et al.*, 1984.) (B) Large GAD-immunoreactive cell soma, interpreted as that of a basket cell, showing numerous GAD-positive axon terminals ending on it. (From DeFelipe *et al.*, 1986.)

cells are also immunoreactive for known peptides, the small size and elongated, "stringy" morphology of all the peptide neurons thus far identified tend to place them in a limited, perhaps a single cell class. In Golgi preparations, the type example, in our opinion, is the cell often described as bipolar or bitufted, although obvious bipolar cells are rare in primates and there appear to be gradations in form from one to the other.

Probably many new cortical peptides remain to be discovered and it is likely that some will turn up in basket or chandelier cells or in other types of cortical GABA neurons. It is also conceivable that these cells normally express such small amounts of the known peptides that they simply fail to stain for them. Perhaps, under certain functional states, they might be induced to express these peptides in sufficiently large amounts to be stained immunocytochemically. If the mRNAs for the extended chain precursors of the known peptides are not transcribed at all by certain cells, is it possible that these cells could be induced to transcribe them under novel conditions?

8. Different Classes of GABA–Peptide Cortical Neurons

Morphological classifications of the peptide-immunoreactive neurons of the neocortex are unreliable but there appear to be classes of such cells that can be distinguished either by the constellation of peptides they contain (usually in association with GABA), or in terms of the synaptic targets of their axons. Most cortical SRIF neurons colocalize NPY and vice versa. But neither of these appears to show CCK or VIP immunoreactivity. The majority of SP cells in the middle layers colocalize GABA and not NPY but the layer VI–white matter population colocalizes NPY and not GABA. Other combinations can be seen in Fig. 19. It is possible that these various combinations reflect the presence of a population of GABA neurons in which all the known cortical peptides are potentially present but that differential modulation of their levels occurs. This seems unlikely since certain combinations, e.g., CCK and/or VIP with NPY and/or SRIF, have never been found. This difference may correlate with the tendency for CCK and VIP cells (Fig. 3) to have fewer vertical processes than NPY and SRIF cells (Fig. 2).

Different classes of cortical GABA–peptide neurons might be distinguished by differential distributions of their synaptic terminals. Preliminary evidence suggests that the bulk of SRIF- and NPY-immunoreactive synapses are formed on distal dendritic branches and on dendritic spines of pyramidal neurons. Most CCK- and VIP-immunoreactive synapses, by contrast, appear to terminate on more proximal dendrites of pyramidal neurons (Hendry *et al.*, 1983b, 1984a). SP-immunoreactive synapses appear to be found at all three sites possibly with some differences between the middle layer cell population and the others (Jones *et al.*, 1986). For the present, these qualitative impressions seem to offer a more reliable means of characterizing the GABA–peptide cortical neurons along lines that probably have more functional significance than morphology alone.

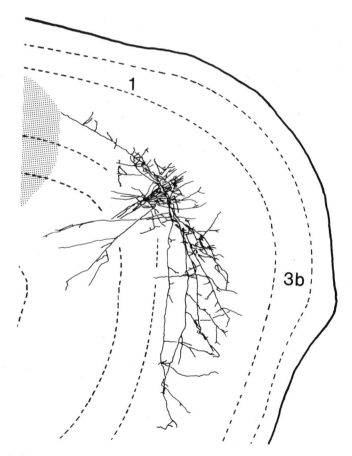

Figure 13. Typical basket cell in monkey somatic sensory cortex (areas 1, 3b) labeled from an injection (stipple) of horseradish peroxidase in area 2. (From DeFelipe *et al.*, 1986.)

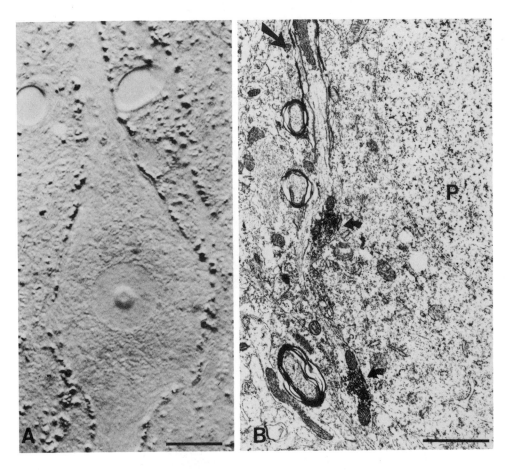

Figure 14. (A) Unstained pyramidal cell in monkey motor cortex, surrounded by GAD-immunoreactive axon terminals. (B) Immunoreactive terminals in the same position on another pyramidal cell soma, and arising from a myelinated axon. Multiterminal endings of this type are those of basket cells. (From Hendry *et al.*, 1983b.)

9. Regulation of GABA and Peptide Levels by Activity

Synaptic activity can regulate levels of transmitters, transmitter-synthesizing enzymes, receptors, and the abundance of related mRNAs in the peripheral nervous system (Ip and Zigmond, 1984; Black *et al.*, 1984, 1985; Roach *et al.*, 1985). Comparable effects can be demonstrated in the central nervous system: In the visual cortex of adult monkeys subjected to monocular visual deprivation for 9–11 weeks, we have found that immunoreactive staining for GABA, GAD, and SP declines markedly in deprived ocular dominance columns (Fig. 20). The reduction in staining is not simply a decline in intensity but an actual reduction in the number of cells that are stained, in comparison with those in adjacent nondeprived columns. NPY-immunoreactive staining is unaffected (Hendry *et al.*, 1985; Hendry and Jones, 1986; Jones and Hendry, 1985). This indicates that GABA levels can be reduced through a reduction in immunoreactive GAD and, moreover, that sensory experience appears to control levels of one peptide expressed by the same cells. In the same animals, levels of immunoreactivity for a calcium/calmodulin-dependent protein kinase, CaM kinase II (Browning *et al.*, 1985; Bennett *et al.*, 1983; DeRiemer *et al.*, 1984), are actually increased in the cells of the deprived columns (Hendry *et al.*, 1985; Hendry and Kennedy, 1986). The GABA–GAD–SP effect may, therefore, be mediated by second messengers associated with changes in intracellular phosphoproteins (Nestler *et al.*, 1984; Nishizuka, 1984; Berridge and Irvine, 1984).

10. Potential Functions of Cortical GABA–Peptide Neurons

Most of the neuropeptides found in the cortex have been studied by iontophoresis onto neocortical or hippocampal neurons. In most studies they have been reported to increase resting levels of discharge and to induce excitatory postsynaptic potentials, with accompanying changes in membrane conductance. The responses can be almost as rapid as those induced by aspartate or glutamate, which are potent excitatory agents. Occasionally, inhibition and complex mixed effects have been reported, especially with SRIF. Any effects that the neuropeptides might have on the receptive fields of sensory cortical neurons have not been reported.

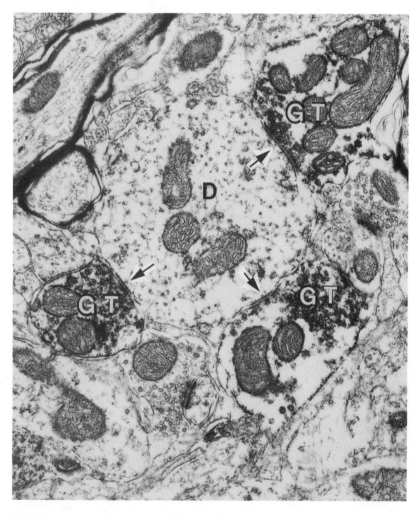

Figure 15. GAD-immunoreactive terminals (GT) ending in symmetrical synapses on a dendrite (D) in monkey motor cortex.

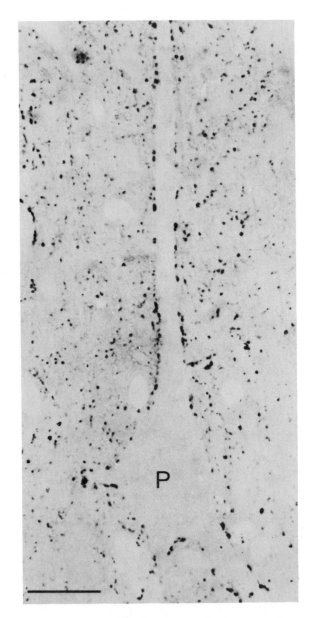

Figure 16. Unstained pyramidal cell soma in monkey motor cortex, showing GAD positive endings on all visible parts of its dendritic tree. (From Houser *et al.*, 1983b.)

It is hard to explain how the release of peptides from a GABAergic terminal might induce excitation in a postsynaptic cell without postulating some special type of mechanism. It should be remembered, however, that there is no evidence to indicate that peptides released from a GABAergic synapse necessarily act directly at that synaptic site. They could, for example, be acting back on receptors located on the terminal from which they are released and through this mechanism might possibly regulate GABA release and therefore lead to disinhibition. For example, NPY acts presynaptically in reducing orthodromically induced population spikes in hippocampal neurons (Colmers *et al.*, 1985).

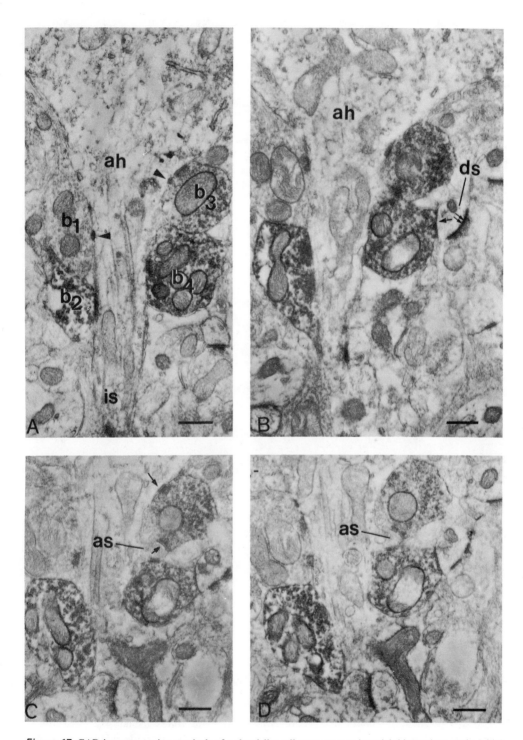

Figure 17. GAD-immunoreactive terminals of a chandelier cell axon, as seen in serial thin sections on the initial segment (is) of the axon of a pyramidal cell in monkey motor cortex. ah, axon hillock; ds, dendritic spine; as, axonal spine. (From DeFelipe *et al.,* 1985.)

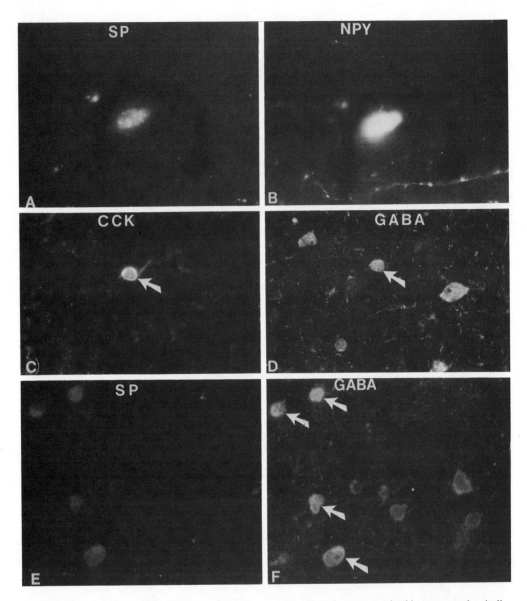

Figure 18. Pairs of fluorescence photomicrographs from sections of monkey cortex stained immunocytochemically for SP and NPY (A, B), for GABA and CCK (C, D), and for GABA and SP (E, F). A small proportion of the GABA-immunoreactive cells are also immunoreactive for the peptides. (From Jones *et al.*, 1986.)

Peptides released from GABA terminals might also exert their effects over wide distances, perhaps affecting populations of neurons removed from the active synapse. Populations of neurons in amphibian sympathetic ganglia appear to be affected in this way by a luteinizing hormone-releasing hormone-like peptide coreleased with ACh (Jan and Jan, 1982).

Other potential actions of neuropeptides in the cerebral cortex include the regulation of vascular perfusion and trophic effects. NPY and VIP are strongly vasoactive (Edvinsson, 1985), and VIP coreleased with ACh from parasympathetic terminals in the submandibular gland leads to vasodilation, increased blood flow, and, thus, to enhancement of the secretomotor effect of ACh (Lundberg *et al.*, 1980). NPY is a vasoconstrictor and the two together might control intracortical vascular perfusion (McCulloch, 1983), perhaps in an activity-mediated manner. However, no experiments relevant to this have been reported.

Some neuropeptides appear to have trophic actions akin to those of the polypeptide growth factors, nerve growth factor, and epidermal growth factor. SP, VIP, and vasopressin induce DNA synthesis and stimulate mitogenesis in mesodermally derived cells and in cultured cell lines (Brenneman *et al.*, 1984; James and Bradshaw, 1984; Nilsson *et al.*, 1985). Some polypeptide growth factors also contain amino acid sequences closely similar to those of known neuropeptides (Gimenez-Gallego *et al.*, 1985). In the peripheral nervous system, certain neuropeptides such as VIP and secretin seem to be capable of inducing tyrosine hydroxylase in sympathetic postganglionic neurons (Ip *et al.*, 1982; Ip and Zigmond, 1984). Hence, modulations of nerve cell chemistry rather than short-term electrical signaling could be one of the more important functions of the peptides.

There are indications that levels of certain peptides in the human neocortex may be altered in demented states. NPY and SRIF levels decline in the cortex in Alzheimer's senile dementia (Davies *et al.*, 1980; Rossor *et al.*, 1982) and SRIF falls in the frontal cortex of parkinsonian patients with dementia. In Alzheimer's disease there is also a large decrease in markers for ACh but no decline in those for GABA with which SRIF and NPY are normally colocalized. The latter suggests a differential regulation of GABA and the peptides in this disease. Perhaps the decline in the two peptides then deprives the cortex of essential trophic agents which in turn causes the destruction of cholinergic neurons and terminals?

11. Conclusions

GABA neurons of the primate cerebral cortex are present in large numbers, consistently forming 20–30% of the neuronal population of any cytoarchitectonic area. They also belong to a variety of morphological types, with selective horizontal, vertical, or local connections and with selective synaptic sites on pyramidal neurons which are non-GABAergic, and sometimes on other GABA neurons. It is possible that GABA neurons account for all the morphological varieties of cortical nonpyramidal neurons, except the small spiny, putatively excitatory neuron typical of layers III and IV.

Approximately 20% of the cortical GABA cell population also shows immunoreactivity for the known cortical neuropeptides. The neuropeptide-containing neurons are a less heterogeneous group than commonly supposed and may belong to a single GABA cell type. One, VIP, may be

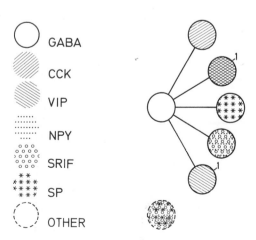

Figure 19. Combinations of GABA and neuropeptide immunoreactivity demonstrated to date in neocortex. "1" indicates combinations demonstrated only in rats. "Other" indicates a small population of neurons showing peptide immunoreactivity only but which may contain another classical neurotransmitter such as ACh. (From Jones and Hendry, 1986.)

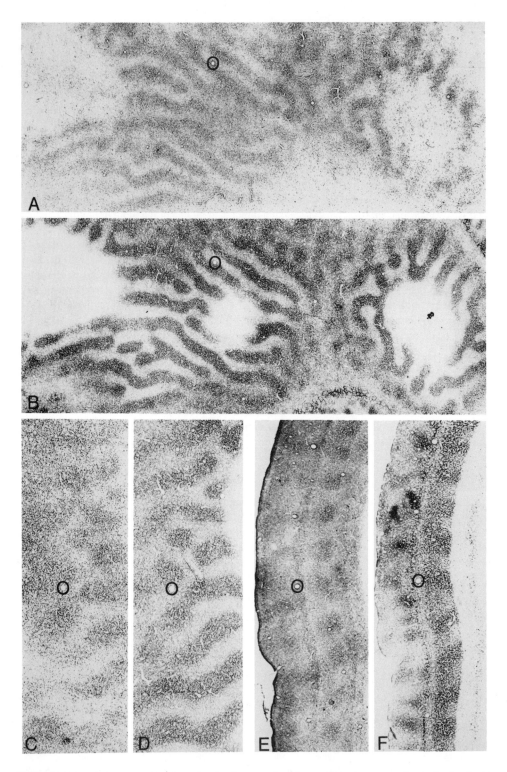

Figure 20. Pairs of alternate sections from the visual cortex of monkeys subjected to monocular deprivation for 11 weeks. The same blood vessels are circled in each pair. (A, B) Tangential sections through layer IV showing GABA immunoreactivity and cytochrome oxidase staining reduced in deprived ocular dominance strips. (C, D) Vertical sections showing reduced GAD immunoreactivity (C) and cytochrome oxidase staining (D) in deprived ocular dominance columns. (E, F) Vertical sections showing reduction in SP immunoreactivity and cytochrome oxidase staining in deprived ocular dominance columns. (From Hendry and Jones, 1986; Jones, 1986.)

more commonly found in a cholinergic neuron that shares the morphological features of the GABA–peptide class. The vast majority of cortical neurons, including all the pyramidal neurons and most varieties of GABAergic intrinsic neurons, are not immunoreactive for known peptides. In the monkey visual cortex, levels of GAD, GABA, and SP are regulated by functional activity.

The roles of the neuropeptides in cortical function are not known and conjectures about them include actions as classical transmitters, actions in the control of levels of activity in populations of neurons, control of regional cortical blood flow, and actions of a trophic nature which, although ill-defined, may yield clues to the role of peptides in cortical disease.

ACKNOWLEDGMENTS. Personal work reported herein was supported by Grant NS-21377 from the National Institutes of Health, United States Public Health Service. I am indebted to Drs. S. H. C. Hendry, C. R. Houser, and J. DeFelipe for their many contributions.

References

Albers, R. W., and Brady, R. O., 1959, The distribution of glutamate decarboxylase in the nervous system of the rhesus monkey, *J. Biol. Chem.* **234:**926–928.

Awapara, J., Landau, A. J., Fuerst, R., and Seale, B., 1950, Free γ-aminobutyric acid in brain, *J. Biol. Chem.* **187:**35–39.

Baughman, R. W., and Gilbert, C. D., 1981, Aspartate and glutamate as possible neurotransmitters in the visual cortex, *J. Neurosci.* **1:**427–439.

Bear, M. F., Schmechel, D. E., and Ebner, F. F., 1985, Glutamic acid decarboxylase in the striate cortex of normal and monocularly deprived kittens, *J. Neurosci.* **5:**1262–1275.

Bennett, M. K., Erondu, N. E., and Kennedy, M. B., 1983, Purification and characterization of a calmodulin-dependent protein kinase that is highly concentrated in brain, *J. Biol. Chem.* **258:**12735–12744.

Berridge, M. J., and Irvine, R. F., 1984, Inositol triphosphate, a novel second messenger in cellular signal-transduction, *Nature* **312:**315–321.

Black, I. B., Adler, J. E., Dreyfus, C. F., Jonakait, G. M., Katz, D. M., LaGamma, E. F., and Markey, K. M., 1984, Neurotransmitter plasticity at the molecular level, *Science* **225:**1266–1270.

Black, I. B., Chkaraishi, D. M., and Lewis, E. J., 1985, Trans-synaptic increase in mRNA coding for tyrosine hydroxylase in a rat sympathetic ganglion, *Brain Res.* **339:**151–153.

Brenneman, D. E., Eider, L. E., and Seigel, R. E., 1984, Vasoactive intestinal peptide increases activity-dependent neuronal survival in developing spinal cord cultures, *Soc. Neurosci. Abstr.* **10:**1050.

Browning, M. D., Huganir, R., and Greengard, P., 1985, Protein phosphorylation and neuronal function, *J. Neurochem.* **45:**11–23.

Carraway, R., and Leeman, S. E., 1976, Characterization of radioimmunoassayable neurotensin in the rat, *J. Biol. Chem.* **251:**1045–1052.

Colmers, W. F., Lukowiak, K., and Pitman, Q. J., 1985, Neuropeptide Y reduces orthodromically evoked population spike in rat hippocampal CAl by a possibly presynaptic mechanism, *Brain Res.* **346:**404–408.

Cotman, C. W., Foster, A., and Lanthorn, T., 1981, An overview of glutamate as a neurotransmitter, *Adv. Biochem. Psychopharmacol.* **27:**1–27.

Davies, P., Katzman, R., and Terry, R., 1980, Reduced somatostatin-like immunoreactivity in cerebral cortex from cases of Alzheimer's disease and Alzheimer senile dementia. *Nature* **288:**279–280.

DeFelipe, J., and Jones, E. G., 1985, Vertical organization of [^{3}H]-aminobutyric acid-accumulating intrinsic neuronal systems in monkey cerebral cortex, *J. Neurosci.* **5:**3246–3260.

DeFelipe, J., Hendry, S. H. C., Jones, E. G., and Schmechel, D., 1985, Variability in the terminations of GABAergic chandelier cell axons on initial segments of pyramidal cell axons in the monkey sensory motor cortex, *J. Comp. Neurol.* **231:**364–384.

DeFelipe, J., Hendry, S. H. C., and Jones, E. G., 1986, A correlative electron microscopic study of basket cells and large GABAergic neurons in the monkey sensory-motor cortex, *Neuroscience* **17:**991–1009.

DeRiemer, S. A., Kaczmarek, L. K., Lai, Y., McGuiness. T. L., and Greengard, P., 1984, Calcium/calmodulin-dependent protein phosphorylation in the nervous system of *Aplysia, J. Neurosci.* **4:**1618–1625.

Dockray, G. J., 1976, Immunochemical evidence of cholecystokinin like peptides in brain, *Nature* **264:**568–570.

Donoghue, J. P., Wenthold, R. J., and Altschuler, R. A., 1985, Localization of glutaminase-like and aspartate aminotransferase-like immunoreactivity in neurons of cerebral neocortex, *J. Neurosci.* **5:**2597–2609.

Eckenstein, F., and Baughman, R. W., 1984, Two types of cholinergic innervation in cortex, one co-localized with vasoactive intestinal polypeptide, *Nature* **314**:153–155.

Edvinsson, L., 1985, Functional role of perivascular peptides in the control of cerebral circulation, *Trends Neurosci.* **8**:126–131.

Emson, P. C., and Hunt, S. P., 1981, Anatomical chemistry of the cerebral cortex, in: *The Organization of the Cerebral Cortex* (F. O. Schmitt, F. C. Worden, G. Adelman, and S. G. Dennis, eds.), MIT Press, Cambridge, Mass., pp. 325–345.

Emson, P. C., and Hunt, S. P., 1985, Peptide-containing neurons of the cerebral cortex, in: *Cerebral Cortex,* Vol. 2 (E. G. Jones and A. Peters, eds.), Plenum Press, New York, pp. 145–172.

Gimenez-Gallego, G., Rodkey, J., Bennett, C., Rios-Candelore, M., DeSalvo, J., and Thomas, K., 1985, Brain-derived acidic fibroblast growth factor: Complete amino acid sequence and homologies, *Science* **230**:1385–1388.

Hendrickson, A. E., Hunt, S. P., and Wu, J.-Y., 1981, Immunocytochemical localization of glutamic acid decarboxylase in monkey striate cortex, *Nature* **292**:605–606.

Hendry, S. H. C., and Jones. E. G., 1986, Reduction in number of immunostained GABA neurons in deprived-eye dominance columns of monkey area 17, *Nature* **320**:750–753.

Hendry, S. H. C., and Kennedy, M. B., 1986, Altered immunoreactivity for a calcium/calmodulin-dependent kinase in neurons of monkey striate cortex deprived of visual input, *Proc. Natl. Acad. Sci. USA* **83**:1536–1540.

Hendry, S. H. C., Houser, C. R., Jones, E. G., and Vaughn, J. E., 1983a, Synaptic organization of immunocytochemically identified GABA neurons in monkey sensory-motor cortex, *J. Neurocytol.* **12**:639–660.

Hendry, S. H. C., Jones, E. G., and Beinfeld, M. C., 1983b, Cholecystokinin-immunoreactive neurons in rat and monkey cerebral cortex make symmetric synapses and have intimate associations with blood vessels, *Proc. Natl. Acad. Sci. U.S.A.* **80**:2400–2404.

Hendry, S. H. C., Jones, E. G., DeFelipe, J., Schmechel, D., Brandon, C., and Emson, P. C., 1984a, Neuropeptide containing neurons of the cerebral cortex are also GABAergic, *Proc. Natl. Acad. Sci. U.S.A.* **81**:6526–6530.

Hendry, S. H. C., Jones, E. G., and Emson, P. C., 1984b, Morphology, distribution and synaptic relations of somatostatin- and neuropeptide Y-immunoreactive neurons in rat and monkey neocortex, *J. Neurosci.* **4**:2497–2517.

Hendry, S. H. C., Jones, E. G., and Kennedy, M. B., 1985, Modulation of GABA, substance P and protein kinase immunoreactivities in monkey striate cortex following eye removal, *Soc. Neurosci. Abstr.* **11**:16.

Hendry, S. H. C., Schwark, H. D., Jones, E. G., and Yan, J., 1986, Proportions of GABA immunoreactive neurons in different areas of monkey cerebral cortex, *J. Neurosci.* **7**:1503–1519.

Hökfelt, T., Meyerson, B., Nilsson, G., Pernow, B., and Sachs, C., 1976, Immunohistochemical evidence for substance P containing nerve endings in the human cortex, *Brain Res.* **104**:181–186.

Hökfelt, T., Elde, R., Johansson, O., Ljungdahl, A., Schultzberg, M., Fuxe, K., Goldstein, M., Nilsson, G., Pernow, B., Terenius, L., Garten, D., Jeffcoate, S. L., Rehfeld, J., and Said, S., 1978, Distribution of peptide-containing neurones, in: *Psychopharmacology: A Generation of Progress* (M. A. Lipton, A. Dimascio, and K. F. Killam, eds.), Raven Press, New York, pp. 39–66.

Houser, C. R., Crawford, C. D., Barber, R. P., Salvaterra, P. M., and Vaughn, J. E., 1983a, Organization and morphological characteristics of cholinergic neurons: An immunocytochemical study with a monoclonal antibody to choline acetyltransferase, *Brain Res.* **266**:97–119.

Houser, C. R., Hendry, S. H. C., Jones, E. G., and Vaughn, J. E., 1983b, Morphological diversity of immunocytochemically identified GABA neurons in monkey sensory motor cortex, *J. Neurocytol.* **12**:617–638.

Houser, C. R., Vaughn, J. E., Hendry, S. H. C., Jones, E. G., and Peters, A., 1984, GABA neurons in the cerebral cortex, in: *Cerebral Cortex,* Vol. 2 (E. G. Jones and A. Peters, eds.), Plenum Press, New York, pp. 63–89.

Houser, C. R., Crawford, G. D., Salvaterra, P. M., and Vaughn, J. E., 1985, Immunocytochemical localization of choline acetyltransferase in rat cerebral cortex: A study of cholinergic neurons and synapses, *J. Comp. Neurol.* **234**:17–33.

Ip, N. Y., and Zigmond, R. E., 1984, Pattern of presynaptic nerve activity can determine the type of neurotransmitter regulating a postsynaptic event, *Nature* **311**:472–474.

Ip, N. Y., Ho, C. K., and Zigmond, R. E., 1982, Secretin and vasoactive intestinal polypeptide acutely increase tyrosine 3-monooxygenase in the rat superior cervical ganglion, *Proc. Natl. Acad. Sci. U.S.A.* **79**:7566–7569.

James, R., and Bradshaw, R. A., 1984, Polypeptide growth factors, *Annu. Rev. Biochem.* **53**:259–292.

Jan, L. Y., and Jan, Y. N., 1982, Peptidergic transmission in sympathetic ganglia of the frog, *J. Physiol. (London)* **327**:219–246.

Jasper, H. H., and Koyama, I., 1969, Rate of release of amino acids from the cerebral cortex of the cat as affected by brainstem and thalamic stimulation, *Can. J. Physiol. Pharmacol.* **47**:889–905.

Jones, E. G., 1984a, Identification and classification of intrinsic circuit elements in the neocortex, in: *Dynamic Aspects of Neocortical Function* (G. M. Edelman, W. E. Gall, and W. M. Cowan, eds.), Wiley, New York, pp. 7–40.

Jones, E. G., 1984b, Neurogliaform or spiderweb cells, in: *Cerebral Cortex,* Vol. 1 (A. Peters and E. G. Jones, eds.), Plenum Press, New York, pp. 409–418.

Jones, E. G., and Hendry, S. H. C., 1985, GABAergic substance P immunoreactive neurons in monkey cerebral cortex, *Soc. Neurosci. Abstr.* **11**:145.

Jones, E. G., and Hendry, S. H. C., 1986, Colocalization of GABA and neuropeptides in neocortical neurons, *Trends Neurosci.* **9**:71–76.

Jones, E. G., Hendry, S. H. C., DeFelipe, J., and Maggio, J. E., 1988, Substance P neurons in monkey cerebral cortex, (submitted).

Lin, C.-S., Lu, S. M., and Schmechel, D. M., 1985, Glutamic acid decarboxylase immunoreactivity in layer IV of barrel cortex of rat and mouse, *J. Neurosci.* **5**:1934–1939.

Lundberg, A., Ånggard, A., Fahrenkrug, J., Hökfelt, T., and Mutt, V., 1980, Vasoactive intestinal polypeptide in cholinergic neurons of exocrine glands: Functional significance of co-existing transmitters for vasodilation and secretion, *Proc. Natl. Acad. Sci. USA* **77**:1651–1655.

McCulloch, J., 1983, Peptides and the microregulation of bloodflow in the brain, *Nature* **304**:129.

McDonald, J. K., Parnavelas, J. G., Karamanlidis, A., Brecha, N., and Koenig, J. I., 1982a, The morphology and distribution of peptide-containing neurons in the adult and developing visual cortex of the rat. I. Somatostatin, *J. Neurocytol.* **11**:809–824.

McDonald, J. K., Parnavelas, J. G., Karamanlidis, A., and Brecha, N., 1982b, The morphology and distribution of peptide-containing neurons in the adult and developing visual cortex of the rat. II. Vasoactive intestinal polypeptide, *J. Neurocytol.* **11**:825–837.

McDonald, J. K., Parnavelas, J. G., Karamanlidis, A., Brecha, N., and Rosenquist, G., 1982c, The morphology and distribution of peptide-containing neurons in the adult and developing visual cortex of the rat. III. Cholecystokinin, *J. Neurocytol.* **11**:881–895.

McDonald, J. K., Parnavelas, J. G., Karamanlidis, A., and Brecha, N., 1983, The morphology and distribution of peptide-containing neurons in the adult and developing visual cortex of the rat. IV. Avian pancreatic polypeptide, *J. Neurocytol.* **11**:985–995.

McGinty, J. F., van der Kooy, D., and Bloom, F. E., 1984, The distribution and morphology of opioid peptide immunoreactive neurons in the cerebral cortex of rats, *J. Neurosci.* **4**:1104–1117.

McGuire, B. A., Hornung, J.-P., Gilbert, C. D., and Wiesel, T. N., 1984, Patterns of synaptic input to layer 4 of cat striate cortex, *J. Neurosci.* **4**:3021–3033.

Morrison, J. H., Benoit, R., Magistretti, P. J., and Bloom, F. E., 1983, Immunohistochemical distribution of pro-somatostatin-related peptides in cerebral cortex, *Brain Res.* **262**:344–351.

Muller, J. E., Starus, E., and Yalow, R. S., 1977, Cholecystokinin and its COOH-terminal octapeptide in the pig brain, *Proc. Natl. Acad. Sci. USA* **74**:3035–3037.

Nestler, E. J., Walaas, S. I., and Greengard, P., 1984, Neuronal phosphoproteins: Physiological and clinical implications, *Science* **225**:1357–1364.

Nilsson, J., von Euler, A. M., and Dalsgaard, C.-J., 1985, Stimulation of connective tissue cell growth by substance P and substance K, *Nature* **315**:61–63.

Nishizuka, Y., 1984, Turnover of inositol phospholipids and signal transduction, *Science* **225**:1365–1370.

Paxinos, G., Emson, P. C., and Cuello, A. C., 1978, The substance P projections to the frontal cortex and the substantia nigra, *Neuroscience* **7**:127–131.

Peters, A., 1987, Number of neurons and synapses in primary visual cortex, in: *Cerebral Cortex,* Vol. 6 (E. G. Jones and A. Peters, eds.), Plenum Press, New York (in press).

Peters, A., Proskauer, C. C., and Ribak, C., 1982, Chandelier cells in rat visual cortex, *J. Comp. Neurol.* **206**:397–416.

Peters, A., Miller, M., and Kimerer, L. M., 1983, Cholecystokinin-like immunoreactive neurons in rat cerebral cortex, *Neuroscience* **8**:431–448.

Ribak, C., 1978, Aspinous and sparsely-spinous stellate neurons contain glutamic acid decarboxylase in the visual cortex of rats, *J. Neurocytol.* **7**:461–476.

Roach, A. H., Adler, J. E., Krause, J., and Black, I. B., 1985, Depolarization regulates the level of pre-protachykinin messenger RNA in the cultured superior cervical ganglion, *Neurosci. Abstr.* **11**:669.

Roberts, E., and Fenkel, S., 1950 γ-Aminobutyric acid in brain: Its formation from glutamic acid, *J. Biol. Chem.* **187**:55–63.

Rockel, A. J., Hiorns, R. W., and Powell, T. P. S., 1980, The basic uniformity in structure of the neocortex, *Brain* **103**:221–244.

Rossor, M. N., Emson, P. C., Mountjoy, C. W., Roth, M., and Iversen, L. L., 1982, Reduced amounts of immunoreactive somatostatin in the temporal cortex in senile dementia of the Alzheimer type, *Neurosci. Lett.* **20**:373–377.

Sachs, C., Hökfelt, T., Meyerson, B., Elde, R., and Rehfeld, J., 1978, Peptide neurons in human cerebral cortex— II, in: *11th World Congress of Neurology* (W. A. den Hartog, G. W. Gruyn, and A. P. J. Heijstee, eds.), Excerpta Medica, Amsterdam.

Said, S. I., and Rosenberg, R. N., 1976, Vasoactive intestinal polypeptide: Abundant immunoreactivity in neural cell lines and normal tissue, *Science* **192**:907–908.

Schmechel, D. E., Vickrey, B. G., Fitzpatrick, D., and Elde, R. P., 1984, GABAergic neurons of mammalian cerebral cortex: Widespread subclass defined by somatostatin content, *Neurosci. Lett.* **47**:227–232.

Somogyi, P., Freund, T. F., and Cowey, A., 1982, The axo-axonic interneuron in the cerebral cortex of the rat, cat and monkey, *Neuroscience* **1**:2577–2608.

Somogyi, P., Hodgson. A. J., Smith, A. D., Nunzi, M. G., Gorio, A., and Wu, J.-Y., 1984, Different populations of GABAergic neurons in the visual cortex and hippocampus of cat contain somatostatin- or cholecystokinin-immunoreactive material, *J. Neurosci.* **4**:2590–2603.

Streit, P., 1984, Glutamate and aspartate as transmitter candidates for systems of the cerebral cortex, in: *Cerebral Cortex*, Vol. 2 (E. G. Jones and A. Peters, eds.), pp. 119–143. New York, Plenum Press.

Uhl, G. R., and Snyder, S. H., 1976, Regional and subcellular distributions of brain neurotensin, *Life Sci.* **19**:1827–1832.

Winfield D. A., Gatter, K. C., and Powell, T. P. S., 1980, An electron microscopic study of the types and proportions of neurons in the cortex of the motor and visual areas of the cat and rat, *Brain* **103**:245–258.

Winfield, D. A., Brooke, R. N. L., Sloper, J. J., and Powell, T. P. S., 1981, A combined Golgi–electron microscopic study of the synapses made by the proximal axon and recurrent collaterals of a pyramidal cell in the somatic sensory cortex of the monkey, *Neuroscience* **6**:1217–1230.

10

Rate-Limiting Steps in the Synthesis of GABA and Glutamate

John C. Szerb

The theme of this symposium, the relationship between the chemical activity of the nervous system and its electrical and behavioral functions, has been Dr. Jasper's major interest during the past 20 years. I would like to contribute to this topic by presenting our recent data on the contrasting mechanisms involved in the control of the synthesis of the transmitters glutamate and GABA. This information can be useful in explaining processes involved in pathological changes in excitability and can suggest measures that are likely to rectify abnormalities in the release of amino acid transmitters. First, however, the rather extensive literature on the metabolic compartments of amino acid synthesis will be briefly reviewed, because the new observations reported here are based on concepts that have evolved during the past 25 years.

1. The Compartmentation of Amino Acid Metabolism

Observations on the rapid labeling of glutamate and GABA following the administration of labeled glucose both *in vitro* (Beloff-Chain *et al.*, 1955) and *in vivo* (Vrba *et al.*, 1962; Waelsch, 1962; Cremer, 1964) were the first indication of a close connection between the tricarboxylic acid cycle and these amino acids. Waelsch (1962) made the significant observation that after the intracerebral administration of [^{14}C]glutamic acid, the specific activity of glutamine exceeded that of glutamate. Since glutamine can be formed only from glutamate, this suggested that not all glutamate present, but only a small compartment, mixes with labeled glutamate. This small glutamate pool, having a higher specific activity, is probably the precursor of glutamine. This was the first evidence for the compartmentalization of amino acid metabolism in the brain, a concept which was to be the subject of numerous investigations during the subsequent 20 years. Early experiments, in which the incorporation of the label into glutamate and GABA was measured, were carried out before the transmitter roles of GABA and glutamate were established. As a consequence, observations were interpreted only in terms of the metabolic roles of these amino acids. However, the realization that GABA and glutamate were transmitters released from nerve

John C. Szerb • Department of Physiology and Biophysics, Dalhousie University, Halifax, Nova Scotia B3H 4H7, Canada.

terminals only served to strengthen the two-compartment model, providing an explanation for the movements of amino acids between the compartments. A brief review of the original observations on compartmentalization will be presented here, followed by a more detailed account of the more recent developments aimed at verifying this concept.

1.1. Original Observations

Both the *in vivo* and *in vitro* observations suggest that there are two groups of labeled precursors of transmitter amino acids, one that preferentially gives rise to labeled GABA and one that produces more labeled glutamine. The members of the first group of precursors are [U-14C]glucose (Vrba *et al.*, 1962; Cremer, 1964) and [2-14C]pyruvate (Albers *et al.*, 1961), while those of the second group, which produces more highly labeled glutamine than glutamate, are [14C]-labeled glutamate (Waelsch, 1962), acetate (Gonda and Quastel, 1966), and GABA (Balazs *et al.*, 1970). The pool of glutamate into which the first group of precursors are preferentially incorporated is large compared to the pool of glutamate to which the second group of precursors contribute.

The interpretation of these results was made easier by the realization that GABA, being a transmitter, is formed exclusively in neurons (Roberts and Kuriyama, 1968). Thus, precursors such as glucose, which preferentially label GABA, must enter a neuronal compartment, while other precursors that label mostly glutamine enter the nonneuronal compartment, presumably glia. The two-compartment model proposed by Van den Berg and Garfinkel (1971) based on these observations consists of a large (neuronal) and a small (glial) compartment, each containing a tricarboxylic acid cycle. According to this model, GABA, formed in the neuronal compartment, is released and then taken up by the glial compartment. In return, glutamine, formed from GABA in the small pool, reenters the large pool. Subsequently, Benjamin and Quastel (1975) concluded that in addition to GABA, synaptically released glutamate is also taken up by glia and turned into glutamine in the small compartment. The identity of this small compartment with astrocytes was confirmed later by Martinez-Hernandez *et al.* (1977) and by Norenberg and Martinez-Hernandez (1979), who showed that only glia contain glutamine synthetase. Simultaneously, van Gelder (1978) described changes in the compartmentalized metabolism of glutamic acid that accompany changes in cortical excitability.

Although assigning two distinct metabolic functions to two different cell types in the brain appeared to be a satisfactory model, subsequently it became evident that the small glutamate pool manifests a heterogeneity which is incompatible with a simple two-compartment model. For instance, Van den Berg *et al.* (1975), in their review, listed eight possible subcompartments of the small glutamate pool which could be distinguished by different yields of labeled glutamine from different precursors, such as acetate or GABA, or in the presence of metabolic inhibitors such as aminooxyacetic acid or fluoroacetate. They suggested that these various subcompartments may reflect the function of different elements within glial cells.

1.2. Verification of the Two-Compartment Hypothesis

The two-compartment hypothesis, formulated from metabolic observations *in vivo* or in preparations, such as slices, which contain both neurons and glia, predicts that neurons and glia should differ clearly in their handling of transmitter amino acids, their precursors and metabolites. Hertz (1979), Schousboe *et al.* (1983), and Hertz *et al.* (1983) examined this prediction by looking at the metabolic fluxes of transmitter amino acids and their precursors in physically isolated neurons and glia and in neurons and glia cultured separately. They assumed that the rates of uptake and metabolism of these compounds in a complete system, consisting of both neurons and glia, are the maximum rates measured separately in astrocytes and neurons. The only exception was the low-affinity glutamine transport, to which a slower rate was assigned. This rate was calculated from the known kinetics of glutamine uptake and the extracellular concentration of glutamine.

They found, as predicted by the two-compartment model, that only neurons had glutamic acid decarboxylase (GAD) activity and only astrocytes contained glutamine synthetase and the complete enzyme system for the metabolism of GABA. Furthermore, glia transported glutamate and aspartate at a much faster rate than did neurons. On the other hand, contrary to the predictions of the two-compartment model, both neurons and glia transported glutamine by a low-affinity system and both contained glutaminase. Since the two-compartment model assumes that the movement of glutamine from glia to neurons compensates for the loss of amino acids that are released and taken up by glia, the approximately equal affinity and capacity of uptake systems for glutamine in neurons and glia and the presence of glutaminase in both were at variance with this model. To account for these observations on isolated neurons and glia, Hertz (1979) proposed a modification of the model, in which nerve terminals and astrocytes are located in the same compartment. The extensive formation of glutamine from injected glutamate was explained by the avid uptake of glutamate by glia, the only constituent containing glutamine synthetase.

While the kinetic parameters of the fluxes and metabolism of amino acid transmitters in neurons and astrocytes observed separately give valuable information about the possible rates of movement of these substances, it is unlikely that these data reflect what actually is happening in the brain *in vivo*. Normally, these processes are not going on in isolation but are linked together, the product of one process being the substrate of the next one. Recent observations on the changing concentration of extracellular glutamine *in vivo* and *in vitro* (Fig. 1) illustrate this point: increased release of glutamate induced by elevated K^+, veratridine, or kainic acid is accompanied by a decrease in extracellular glutamine concentration *in vivo* (Hamberger *et al.*, 1982; Lehmann *et al.*, 1983; Jacobson and Hamberger, 1984) and *in vitro* (Szerb and O'Regan, 1986). Since depolarization, when causing increased glutamate and GABA release, also results in increased glutamate and GABA formation from glutamine (Szerb, 1984), the presynaptic terminals are the likely compartment of increased glutamine utilization responsible for reducing extracellular glutamine levels. Such an intense utilization of glutamine has to be accompanied by an increased transport of glutamine into the compartment which consumes glutamine at a higher rate, while the other compartments, with unchanged glutamine utilization, will transport less or no glutamine with their low-affinity glutamine transport system (Ramaharobandro *et al.*, 1982). Thus, in spite of similar characteristics of glutamine transport in synaptosomes and astrocytes, an increased utilization of glutamine in terminals will result in a net movement of glutamine into terminals, precisely because the glutamine transport systems have a low affinity to glutamine. Would glutamine be transported with a high-affinity system, variations in extracellular glutamine levels in a range actually observed would have no effect on the direction of glutamine flow.

A further method of verifying the two-compartment hypothesis was to follow metabolic changes in brain slices after an increase in the proportion of glia present. This was obtained either by inducing gliosis (Tursky *et al.*, 1979) or by causing the degeneration of terminals through lesions (Nicklas *et al.*, 1979; Molin *et al.*, 1984). As expected from the original two-compartment model, these procedures reduced the incorporation of labeled glucose into glutamate and GABA, which according to the model takes place in terminals, and increased the utilization of labeled acetate for glutamine formation in the glia.

Another possible problem with the originally proposed two-compartment system is the loss of carbon atoms from the tricarboxylic acid cycle of the terminals when α-ketoglutarate is converted to glutamate, which then is released either as such, or after conversion to GABA (Shank and Aprison, 1981). This loss may be compensated for by the excess production of α-ketoglutarate by glia through an anaplerotic process and the subsequent uptake of α-ketoglutarate by the terminals. Indeed, a high-affinity uptake system in synaptosomes for α-ketoglutarate and the formation of glutamate from α-ketoglutarate has been demonstrated (Shank and Campbell, 1984). However, whether α-ketoglutarate is a precursor of releasable glutamate has not yet been shown. In view of the observations that glutamine can cross the blood–brain barrier (Abdul-Ghani *et al.*, 1978; Eriksson *et al.*, 1983), it is not clear why glutamine from plasma, which contains glutamine in just as high concentrations as does the CSF (McGale *et al.*, 1977), cannot also be utilized to replace, through glutamate oxidase or dehydrogenase, the carbon chain lost from the tricarboxylic acid cycle in neurons.

Because of the difficulty in establishing the specific precursor of GABA, Roberts (1981) suggested that ornithine may be the source of GABA. The pathway can go through putrescine, without passing through glutamate, or through glutamate, either directly or through proline. To investigate this possibility, Shank and Campbell (1983a) compared the rate of conversion of labeled ornithine, α-ketoglutarate, and glutamine to glutamate and GABA in fractions of brain homogenates containing predominantly nerve terminals, neuronal or astrocytic cell bodies. They found, however, that the rate of synthesis of glutamate and GABA from glutamine and α-ketoglutarate exceeded by far that from ornithine. The minor role of ornithine as a precursor of transmitter glutamate is also supported by the recent findings of Wroblewski *et al.* (1985), who, after the injection of the ornithine-oxoacid aminotransferase inhibitor, canaline, into the lateral septum, measured the glutamate content of this structure. Canaline caused only a small decrease in glutamate content and this decrease was still present after lesioning the glutamatergic afferents to the septum. Since the lesion itself did not decrease the ornithine-oxoacid aminotransferase activity, the authors concluded that ornithine is the precursor of only a small pool of glutamate, which is likely to be located not only in neurons but also in the glia.

2. Studies on the Sources of GABA and Glutamate

The depolarization-induced release of an amino acid, which depends on the presence of extracellular Ca^{2+}, will, by definition, reflect the function and availability of the transmitter pool and can be used to distinguish it from the metabolic pool. The first study to measure the formation of transmitter GABA in brain slices was that reported by Balazs *et al.* (1970) and Machiyama *et al.* (1970). These authors followed the formation of [^{14}C]-GABA from [U-^{14}C]glucose. Depolarization increased the labeling of glutamate and GABA from [U-^{14}C]glucose four- to fivefold. Later, Szerb (1984) showed that this stimulation was contingent on the presence of Ca^{2+} and therefore due to an increased Ca^{2+}-dependent transmitter release and not to a general stimulation of metabolism. In the studies of Machiyama *et al.* (1970), the specific activity of GABA formed from [^{14}C]glucose was always less than that of glutamate, possibly due to the fact that GABA was also formed from glutamate originating from unlabeled glutamine.

Subsequently, Potashner (1978a,b) used [U-^{14}C]glucose to label transmitter stores of amino acids in guinea pig cortical slices. He estimated the formation of labeled transmitters by measuring their release induced by electrical field stimulation. By carefully choosing the parameters of electrical stimulation, he showed that the stimulation-induced release of aspartate, glutamate, and GABA was greatly reduced by removing Ca^{2+}, and by adding a high concentration of Mg^{2+} to the superfusion medium or by tetrodotoxin. These observations therefore clearly demonstrated that glucose is one of the sources of amino acid transmitters, such as glutamate and GABA, which are released by conducted action potentials through a Ca^{2+}-dependent mechanism.

The two-compartment model predicts that glutamine produced by glia should be taken up by nerve terminals where the accumulated glutamine serves as a precursor for these amino acid transmitters. This prediction was first tested by Shank and Aprison (1977). They found that the hemisected toad spinal cord incubated in 0.2 mM [U-^{14}C]glutamine produced both labeled GABA and glutamate. Some of the labeled glutamate and GABA was released upon incubation with 29 mM K^+ with Na^+ replaced by sucrose. Soon afterwards a number of publications (Tapia and Gonzalez, 1978; Reubi *et al.*, 1978; Kemel *et al.*, 1979; Reubi, 1980) showed that in brain slices, [3,4-^{3}H]glutamine in trace concentrations is readily incorporated into GABA which is released by elevated K^+ in a Ca^{2+}-dependent manner. Similarly, trace amounts of [^{3}H]glutamine were converted into releasable [3H[-GABA *in vivo* (Gauchy *et al.*, 1980). Furthermore, depolarization during incubation with [3H]glutamine increased the specific activity of GABA released by subsequent depolarization (Szerb, 1984). These studies also showed that [3H]glutamate formed from [3H]glutamine is converted directly into GABA. Had [3,4-3H]glutamine employed in these studies been converted first to α-ketoglutarate and then passed around the tricarboxylic acid cycle, it would have lost all its tritium label and no labeled GABA would have been produced.

In summary, observations derived from tracer studies on the formation and metabolism of glutamate and GABA revealed that there are at least two metabolic compartments of transmitter amino acids present: a large one, probably in neurons, in which the formation of these amino acids takes place, and a small one, probably in glia, in which the metabolism of transmitter amino acids occurs. These studies also indicated that both glutamate and GABA can be produced from a variety of sources, including glucose, glutamine, ornithine, or α-ketoglutarate, but no evidence was found that different precursors serve glutamate acting as a transmitter and glutamate acting as the precursor for GABA. However, the central role of glutamine as a precursor of amino acid transmitters moving from glia to terminals has clearly emerged from these studies.

3. The Effect of Different Concentrations of Precursors on the Formation of Transmitter Amino Acids

Once a possible precursor of a substance is established, the determination of the effect of different concentrations of the precursor on the rate of product formation will give an indication whether the availability of a particular precursor determines the rate at which the product is formed. As Shank and Campbell (1983b) state, "The criterion that experimentally induced alterations in the availability and metabolism of potential precursor should significantly affect the content of glutamate and GABA, and more importantly, the amount released by a physiological stimulus, is probably the most valuable of all criteria in that it should give the most definitive information regarding the quantitative relationship between the metabolic precursor and the functional pool of the neurotransmitter." Furthermore, a dependence of transmitter release on precursor concentrations which vary in a range that is normally present, suggests that the observed precursor–product relationship may have functional implications. Technically, the measurement of released transmitter amino acids in the presence of different concentrations of precursors became feasible only with the more recent development of high-performance liquid chromatography, which not only provided a sensitive and easy method for amino acid analysis, but simultaneously allowed the separation of the large amount of precursor from the small amounts of transmitter contained in the medium.

This approach, however, also has its limitations. For the demonstration of the effect of precursor availability on release, the turnover rate of the transmitter pool, hence the rate of synthesis, has to be driven to near its maximum. Therefore, in many of the experiments designed to measure rate-limiting steps, the release of GABA and of the other amino acids had to be stimulated vigorously over a long time (10–40 min).

The validity of such prolonged, intensive stimulation is open to criticism since, under physiological conditions, action potentials produce only a short depolarization of the terminals. Furthermore, some of the voltage-gated Ca^{2+} channels are rapidly inactivated. However, under pathological conditions, such as during seizure activity, prolonged and intense depolarization of terminals does occur. The continuous synthesis of transmitters, or the lack of it, may be of crucial importance in maintaining or terminating such pathological activity. In addition, in all instances when the kinetics of the inactivation of voltage-gated Ca^{2+} has been studied, only about 70% of Ca^{2+} channels were inactivated rapidly, while the rest remained open for an indeterminate time (Nachsen and Blaustein, 1980, 1982; Suszkiw and O'Leary, 1983; Birman and Meunier, 1985). Therefore, Ca^{2+} influx through these noninactivating channels produces the Ca^{2+}-dependent release due to a prolonged depolarization.

In agreement with the central role of extracellular glutamine suggested by the two-compartment model, the CSF contains a high (0.5–0.6 mM) concentration of glutamine (Dickinson and Hamilton, 1966; Perry *et al.*, 1975; McGale *et al.*, 1977). This suggests that not only glucose but also extracellular glutamine may have a quantitatively important role in maintaining transmitter amino acid stores. Indeed, Bradford and Ward (1976) showed that in order to maintain the glutamate and GABA content of a synaptosomal bed, a physiological concentration of glutamine had to be included in the incubation medium in addition to 10 mM glucose. Under these conditions, 0.5 mM [U-^{14}C]glutamine contributed about three times more to the carbon chain of glutamate than to that of GABA. In agreement with the greater contribution of glutamine to glutamate than to GABA, Bradford *et al.* (1978) subsequently found that preincubation of synaptosomal beds with 0.5 mM [^{3}H]- or [U-^{14}C]glutamine in the presence of 2.5 mM glucose increased the veratridine- or high-K$^+$-induced release of glutamate by nearly 100%, but that of GABA only by 10–20%. Although glutamine increased only little the total evoked release of GABA, significant amounts of labeled glutamine were incorporated into both GABA that was released and GABA that remained in the synaptosomes.

Hamberger *et al.* (1978, 1979a,b) carried out detailed studies on the precursor roles of glucose and glutamine in the synthesis of transmitter glutamate in the dentate gyrus of the rabbit hippocampus. Glutamate release in this preparation originates from terminals of the perforant path, because after lesioning the ipsilateral entorhinal cortex, the high-K$^+$-evoked release of glutamate was significantly reduced. In agreement with the findings of Bradford *et al.* (1978), incubation in 0.4 mM glutamine greatly enhanced the high-K$^+$-stimulated, Ca^{2+}-dependent synthesis and release of glutamate. By measuring the formation of [^{14}C]glutamate from [U-^{14}C]glucose or [U-^{14}C]glutamine, they showed that about 70% of released glutamate is derived from glutamine. Furthermore, incubation of the slices with 2 mM glutamate inhibited the conversion of glutamine to glutamate, suggesting that the increased formation of glutamate during release stimulated by high K$^+$ and Ca^{2+} is the result of removal of feedback inhibition of glutaminase by glutamate in the terminals.

More recently, Szerb and O'Regan (1985) reinvestigated the effect of the continuous presence of high extracellular glutamine levels on the depolarization-induced release of glutamate, aspartate, and GABA in rat hippocampal slices. In confirmation of the earlier findings of Bradford *et al.* (1978) and Hamberger *et al.* (1979a), 0.5 mM glutamine increased about fivefold the high-K$^+$-induced release of glutamate, while having no effect on the release of GABA (Fig. 1). The Ca^{2+} dependence of glutamate release, which was enhanced by the presence of 0.5 mM glutamine, was virtually identical with the smaller glutamate release observed without added glutamine, thus confirming the synaptic origin of the large evoked release of glutamate in the

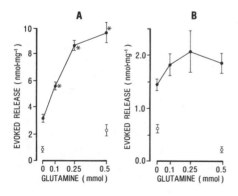

Figure 1. Comparison of the effect of different concentrations of glutamine on the release of glutamate (A) and GABA (B) evoked by 50 mM K$^+$ from rat hippocampal slices. ●, 1.2 mM Ca^{2+} present; ○, 0.1 mM Ca^{2+} present. Values are averages ± S.E.M. of four experiments. Asterisks indicate significant ($p < 0.05$) differences from release observed in the absence of added glutamine. (From Szerb and O'Regan, 1985.)

presence of a physiological concentration of glutamine. The increase in evoked release of glutamate attained a maximum at 0.25 mM glutamine, but 0.1 mM glutamine already had a significant
potentiating action on glutamate release (Fig. 1).

In the light of the ready incorporation of labeled glutamine into releasable GABA, summarized previously, the absence of any effect of the continuous presence of a high concentration of
glutamine on GABA release was puzzling. Recently, a number of experiments were undertaken in
our laboratory (Szerb and O'Regan, 1986, and unpublished observations) to find an explanation
for this discrepancy. One possibility examined was the difference in the method of recycling of
glutamate and GABA: while glutamate taken up by glia is fed back to the terminals via extracellular glutamine, GABA may be taken back straight into the terminals from where it had been
released, causing the synthesis of new GABA to contribute only very little to the total GABA
released. This possibility was tested by measuring the effect of 0.5 mM glutamine on the overflow
of GABA in the presence of 1 mM nipecotic acid, an uptake inhibitor known to increase the
depolarization-induced release of GABA (Szerb, 1982). As shown in Fig. 2, glutamine failed to

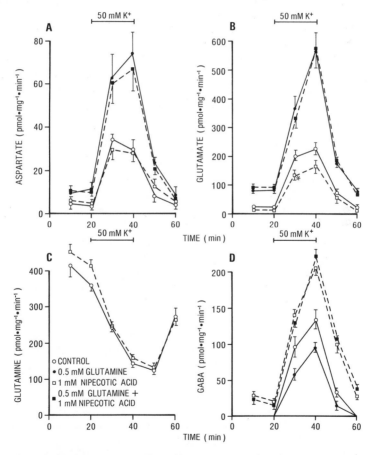

Figure 2. The effect of superfusion with 1 mM nipecotic acid on the release of (A) aspartate, (B) glutamate, (C)
glutamine, and (D) GABA in the absence (open symbols) or presence (filled symbols) of 0.5 mM glutamine.
Circles: release in the absence of nipecotic acid; squares: release in the presence of nipecotic acid. Superfusion with
50 mM K⁺ in third and fourth samples. Values are averages ± SEM of six observations. Asterisk indicates
significant ($p < 0.05$) difference between control and nipecotic acid superfusion. (From Szerb and O'Regan, 1986;
reprinted with permission of Pergamon Press.)

increase the large overflow of GABA due to nipecotic acid, suggesting that the recycling of GABA in the presynaptic terminals is not the reason for the ineffectiveness of glutamine in increasing the release of GABA.

An alternative explanation for the ready labeling of releasable GABA with tracer amounts of glutamine, without large concentrations of glutamine having an effect on GABA release, could be that glutamine is taken up into GABAergic terminals by a high-affinity transport system, which is saturated even by the low concentrations of glutamine that are released spontaneously from the slices. Although low-affinity uptake of glutamine appears to predominate (Hertz *et al.*, 1980; Ramaharobandro *et al.*, 1982; Shank and Campbell, 1984), a minor high-affinity uptake system has also been found by several workers (Balcar and Johnston, 1975; Shank and Campbell, 1984). It seemed possible that this small, high-affinity glutamine uptake system was responsible for glutamine uptake into GABAergic terminals. This was tested by reducing the extracellular concentration of glutamine below what can be expected to be a saturating concentration of a high-affinity transport system and then determining whether added glutamine enhances GABA release. To obtain extremely low glutamine levels, two methods were combined: prolongation of the depolarization by high K^+ and pretreatment of the rats with the glutamine synthetase inhibitor methionine sulfoximine (MSO) (Rothstein and Tabakoff, 1984). While prolonged depolarization by itself greatly reduced glutamine efflux, MSO pretreatment caused an additional 60% drop (Fig. 3C). During this prolonged depolarization the release of GABA declined progressively and the addition of glutamine largely prevented this (Fig. 3D). However, the decline in the release of GABA was the same from hippocampi from MSO-pretreated or control rats, although the release and content of glutamine differed in these two groups by a factor of about two. This suggested that it was not the inadequate supply of glutamine that was responsible for the decline in GABA release with prolonged depolarization but the depletion of another precursor of GABA, whose utilization is also increased by high K^+, namely glucose.

Subsequently, the interaction between glucose and glutamine in the formation of releasable GABA was tested (Szerb and O'Regan, unpublished work). Hippocampal slices were incubated and superfused with Krebs solution containing 5, 1, or 0.2 mM glucose without or with 0.5 mM glutamine and the release of GABA evoked by 50 mM K^+ was measured (Fig. 4). While the release of GABA was not affected by the reduction of the glucose concentration to 1 mM (not shown), it was depressed by more than 50% when glucose was lowered to 0.2 mM. Furthermore, glutamine increased GABA release only when GABA release was depressed in the presence of 0.2 mM glucose (Fig. 4). Thus, in the presence of a low concentration of glucose, either glucose or glutamine was able to augment the release of GABA, although it was unable to restore GABA release fully. This may have been because an additional precursor was also depleted as a result of glucose deprivation.

4. A Model of the Control of GABA and Glutamate Synthesis

A model describing the regulation of GABA synthesis has to take into account the following observations:

1. Releasable labeled GABA can be formed from both labeled glucose (Balazs *et al.*, 1970; Potashner, 1978a; Bradford *et al.*, 1978; Szerb, 1984) and labeled glutamine (Tapia and Gonzalez, 1978; Reubi *et al.*, 1978; Bradford *et al.*, 1978; Szerb, 1984), although the contribution of glucose is greater than that of glutamine (Bradford *et al.*, 1978; Szerb, 1984).

2. In apparent contradiction to the above, in the presence of normal (1–5 mM) glucose, the addition of a physiologically high concentration (0.4–0.5 mM) of glutamine to the medium fails to increase the evoked release of GABA (Bradford *et al.*, 1978; Szerb and O'Regan, 1985). However, when the release of GABA is depressed in the presence of an extremely low (0.2 mM)

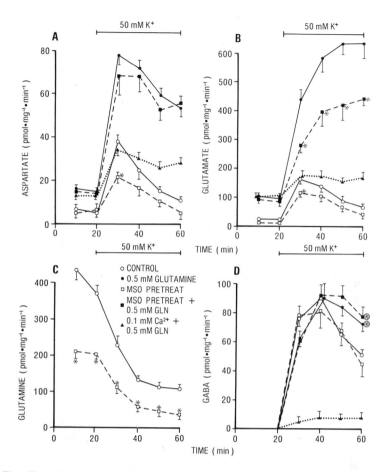

Figure 3. The effect of pretreatment with methionine sulfoximine (MSO) on the release of (A) aspartate, (B) glutamate, (C) glutamine, and (D) GABA in the absence (open symbols) or presence (filled symbols) of 0.5 mM glutamine. Superfusion with 50 mM K$^+$ in third to sixth samples. Values are averages $\pm$ SEM of six experiments. Asterisks indicate significant ($p < 0.05$) differences between slices from control and MSO-pretreated rats; circled asterisks (D) show significant differences between control and glutamine superperfusion. (From Szerb and O'Regan, 1986; reprinted with permission of Pergamon Press.)

concentration of glucose, adding glutamine to the medium about doubles GABA release (Szerb and O'Regan, unpublished observations).

The formation of releasable GABA from either labeled glucose or glutamine indicates that the glutamate pool which is the precursor of GABA can be formed either from α-ketoglutarate or from glutamine, although the former has an approximately 2 : 1 advantage. However, under normal conditions, the rate of GABA formation is not dependent on the size of this glutamate pool, because increasing or decreasing the concentration of either of the glutamate precursors over a wide range does not influence the rate of the evoked release of GABA. For instance, GABA release is essentially unaltered in 1 or 5 mM glucose, or in the presence or absence of 0.5 mM glutamine (Szerb and O'Regan, unpublished observations). However, when both possible precursors are present in very low concentration, such as in a medium containing only 0.2 mM glucose and no added glutamine, the size of the glutamate pool available for GABA synthesis becomes a limiting factor, because increasing the glutamate pool by the addition of either glucose or glu-

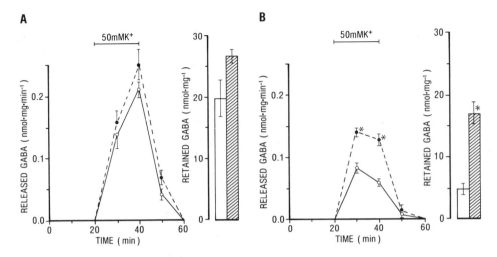

Figure 4. The release and content of GABA in the presence of 5 mM (A) and 0.2 mM (B) glucose. Open symbols: in the absence of glutamine; shaded symbols: in the presence of 0.5 mM glutamine. Values are averages ± SEM of four experiments. Asterisks indicate significant ($p < 0.05$) differences between control and glutamine superfusion. (Szerb and O'Regan, unpublished observations.)

tamine will cause a marked increase in GABA release (Szerb and O'Regan, unpublished observations). All these considerations therefore confirm that under normal conditions the availability of glutamate is not the rate-limiting step in GABA synthesis. Instead, the rate of conversion of glutamate to GABA by the enzyme glutamic acid decarboxylase (GAD) must be the rate-limiting step. This conclusion is in agreement with numerous observations on the susceptibility of GAD to inhibition both by its substrate, glutamate (Seligman 'et al., 1978), and by its product, GABA (Porter and Martin, 1984). Furthermore, depolarization in the presence of Ca^{2+} can increase the activity of GAD (Gold and Roth, 1979).

In contrast to releasable GABA, the rate of formation of releasable glutamate is dependent on the availability of its main precursor, glutamine, in a concentration range found normally in the CSF and brain extracellular fluid. Adding glutamine to the superfusion fluid had two effects on glutamate release: it increased the spontaneous release and the release evoked by depolarization, but only the latter effect was dependent on Ca^{2+} (Fig. 3). The increased spontaneous release of glutamate in the presence of added glutamine probably originates from damaged terminals or glia, both of which contain glutaminase (Hertz, 1979). On the other hand, the depolarization-induced, Ca^{2+}-dependent release, which is also increased by glutamine, is likely to come from intact terminals. The fact that such a depolarization-induced, Ca^{2+}-dependent increase in release can be demonstrated, indicates that the conversion of glutamine to glutamate in terminals is also regulated, contrary to the suggestion of Fonnum (1984) that feedback regulation is missing in slices. Glutamate production by glutaminase is inhibited by glutamate and ammonia, the products of the enzyme (Benjamin, 1981), and Ca^{2+} in the millimolar range increases the enzyme activity (Kvamme et al., 1983). A model which accommodates both product inhibition and marked substrate dependence of glutamate formation in terminals would assign a small compartment of glutamate as the source of synaptically released glutamate. This glutamate pool would be responsible at rest for the inhibition of glutaminase, but as soon as some of this glutamate is released due to the voltage-dependent influx of Ca^{2+}, the inhibition is removed. Since, unlike in the case of GAD, inhibition of glutaminase by its substrate is not known to occur, in the absence of product inhibition, the rate of glutamate formation will largely depend on the concentration of glutamine.

This conclusion is in full agreement with the observations on the enhancing effect of glutamine on glutamate release summarized above.

5. Functional Implications of the Difference in the Control of GABA and Glutamate Synthesis

The observation that the availability of extracellular glutamine has a much greater effect on the release of glutamate than that of GABA, can explain certain pathological shifts in the balance of excitatory and inhibitory transmission. For instance, it can explain why accumulation of ammonium ions in hepatic insufficiency results in CNS depression through a selective decrease in glutamate synthesis and release, without affecting that of GABA (Benjamin, 1981; Hamberger *et al.*, 1982). Ammonium ions, by being its product, potently inhibit glutaminase. Since about 70% of transmitter glutamate is derived from glutamine, its formation is severely depressed by the inhibition of glutaminase. In contrast, the synthesis of GABA, which does not depend on glutamine, is not affected.

In addition, the observation that the availability of glutamine is the major controlling factor in the synthesis of transmitter glutamate but not of GABA, offers an opportunity for a new selective treatment of seizures by restricting the supply of glutamine. This approach looks promising because extracellular glutamine levels are known to decrease only during seizure activity to levels that are submaximal for glutamate production. In contrast, a reduced supply of glutamine should not affect normal asynchronous neuronal activity, when extracellular glutamine levels are sufficient to saturate glutamate formation. Similarly, the supply of GABA, hence inhibition, should also remain normal. For this purpose, however, we will have to learn much more about the transport, sources, and utilization of glutamine in the CNS.

ACKNOWLEDGMENT. The author's work reported herein has been supported by the Medical Research Council of Canada.

References

Abdul-Ghani, A. S., Marton, M., and Dobkin, J., 1978, Studies on the transport of glutamine in vivo between the brain and blood in the resting state and during afferent electrical stimulation, *J. Neurochem.* **31**:541–546.

Albers, R. W., Koval, G., McKhann, G., and Ricks, D., 1961, Quantitative studies of in vivo γ-aminobutyrate metabolism, in: *Regional Neurochemistry* (S. S. Kety and J. Elkes, eds.), Pergamon Press, New York, pp. 340–347.

Balazs, R., Machiyama, Y., Hammond, B. J., Julian, T., and Richter, D., 1970, The operation of the γ-aminobutyrate bypath of the tricarboxylic acid cycle in brain tissue in vitro, *Biochem. J.* **116**:445–467.

Balcar, V. J., and Johnston, G. A. R., 1975, High affinity uptake of glutamine in rat brain slices, *J. Neurochem.* **24**:875–879.

Beloff-Chain, A., Catanzaro, R., Chain, E. B., Massi, I., and Pocchiari, F., 1955, Fate of uniformly labelled ^{14}C glucose in brain slices, *Proc. R. Soc. London Ser. B* **144**:22–28.

Benjamin, A. M., 1981, Control of glutaminase activity in rat brain cortex in vitro: Influence of glutamate, phosphate, ammonium, calcium and hydrogen ions, *Brain Res.* **208**:363–377.

Benjamin, A. M., and Quastel, J. H., 1975, Metabolism of amino acids and ammonia in rat brain cortex slices in vitro: A possible role of ammonia in brain function, *J. Neurochem.* **25**:197–206.

Birman, J., and Meunier, F. M., 1985, Inactivation of acetylcholine release from *Torpedo* synaptosomes in response to prolonged depolarization, *J. Physiol. (London)* **368**:293–307.

Bradford, H. F., and Ward, H. K., 1976, On glutaminase activity in mammalian synaptosomes, *Brain Res.* **110**:115–125.

Bradford, H. F., Ward, H. K., and Thomas, A. J., 1978, Glutamine—A major substrate for nerve endings, *J. Neurochem.* **30**:1453–1459.

Cremer, J. E., 1964, Amino acid metabolism in rat brain studied with ^{14}C-labelled glucose, *J. Neurochem.* **11**:165–185.

Dickinson, J. C., and Hamilton, P. B., 1966, The free amino acids of human spinal fluid determined by ion exchange chromatography, *J. Neurochem.* **13**:1179–1187.

Eriksson, L. S., Law, D. H., Hagenfeldt, L., and Wahren, J., 1983, Nitrogen metabolism of the human brain, *J. Neurochem.* **41**:1324–1328.

Fonnum, F., 1984, Glutamate: A neurotransmitter in the brain, *J. Neurochem.* **42**:1–11.

Gauchy, C., Kemel, M. L., Glowinski, J., and Besson, M. J., 1980, In vivo release of endogenously synthesized [^{3}H]GABA from the cat substantia nigra and the pallido-entopeduncular nuclei, *Brain Res.* **193**:129–141.

Gold, B. I., and Roth, H. R., 1979, Glutamate decarboxylase activity in striatal slices: Characterization of the increase following depolarization, *J. Neurochem.* **32**:883–888.

Gonda, O., and Quastel, J. H., 1966, Transport and metabolism of acetate in rat brain cortex in vitro, *Biochem. J.* **100**:83–94.

Hamberger, A., Chiang, G., Nylen, E. S., Scheff, S. W., and Cotman, C. W., 1978, Stimulus evoked increase in the biosynthesis of putative neurotransmitter glutamate in the hippocampus, *Brain Res.* **143**:549–555.

Hamberger, A. C., Chiang, G. H., Nylen, E. S., Scheff, S. W., and Cotman, C. W., 1979a, Glutamate as a CNS transmitter. I. Evaluation of glucose and glutamine as precursors for the synthesis of preferentially released glutamate, *Brain Res.* **168**:513–530.

Hamberger, A., Chiang, G. H., Sandoval, E., and Cotman, C. W., 1979b, Glutamate as a CNS transmitter. II. Regulation of synthesis in the releasable pool, *Brain Res.* **168**:531–541.

Hamberger, A., Jacobsson, I., Molin, S. O., Nystrom, B., Sandberg, M., and Ungerstedt, U., 1982, Metabolic and transmitter compartments for glutamate, in: *Neurotransmitter Interaction and Compartmentation* (H. F. Bradford, ed.), Plenum Press, New York, pp. 359–378.

Hertz, L., 1979, Functional interaction between neurons and astrocytes. I. Turnover and metabolism of putative amino acid transmitters, *Prog. Neurobiol.* **13**:277–323.

Hertz, L., Yu, A., Svenneby, G., Kvamme, E., Fosmark, H., and Schousboe, A., 1980, Absence of preferential glutamine uptake into neurons—An indication of a net transfer of TCA constituents from nerve endings to astrocytes, *Neurosci. Lett.* **16**:103–109.

Hertz, L., Yu, A. C. H., Potter, R. L., Fisher, T. E., and Schousboe, A., 1983, Metabolic fluxes from glutamate and towards glutamate in neurons and astrocytes in primary cultures, in: *Glutamine, Glutamate and GABA in the Central Nervous System* (L. Hertz, E. Kvamme, E. G. McGeer, and A. Schousboe, eds.), Liss, New York, pp. 327–342.

Jacobson, I., and Hamberger, A., 1984, Veratridine-induced release in vivo and in vitro of amino acids in the rabbit olfactory bulb, *Brain Res.* **299**:103–112.

Kemel, M. L., Gauchy, D., Glowinski, J., and Besson, J. M., 1979, Spontaneous and potassium-evoked release of ^{3}H-GABA newly synthesized from ^{3}H-glutamine in slices of rat substantia nigra, *Life Sci.* **24**:1239–1250.

Kvamme, E., Svenneby, G., and Torgner, I. A., 1983, Calcium stimulation of glutamine hydrolysis in synaptosomes from rat brain, *Neurochem. Res.* **8**:25–38.

Lehmann, A., Isacsson, H., and Hamberger, A., 1983, Effects of in vivo administration of kainic acid on the extracellular amino acid pool in the rabbit hippocampus, *J. Neurochem.* **40**:1314–1320.

McGale, E. H. F., Pye, I. F., Stonier, C., Hutchinson, E. C., and Aber, G. M., 1977, Studies of the interrelationship between cerebrospinal fluid and plasma amino acid concentrations in normal individuals, *J. Neurochem.* **29**:291–297.

Machiyama, Y., Balazs, R., Hammond, B. J., Julian, T., and Richter, D., 1970, The metabolism of γ-aminobutyrate and glucose in potassium ion-stimulated brain tissue in vitro, *Biochem. J.* **116**:469–481.

Martinez-Hernandez, A., Bell, K. P., and Norenberg, M. D., 1977, Glutamine synthetase: Glial localization in brain, *Science* **195**:1356–1358.

Molin, S. O., Nystrom, B., Haglid, K., and Hamberger, A., 1984, Glial contribution to amino acid content and metabolism of deafferented dentate gyrus, *J. Neurosci. Res.* **11**:1–11.

Nachsen, D. A., and Blaustein, M. P., 1980, Some properties of potassium-stimulated calcium influx in presynaptic nerve endings, *J. Gen. Physiol.* **76**:709–728.

Nachsen, D. A., and Blaustein, M. P., 1982, Influx of calcium, strontium, and barium in presynaptic nerve endings, *J. Gen. Physiol.* **79**:1065–1087.

Nicklas, W. J., Nunez, R., Berl, S., and Duvoisin, R., 1979, Neuronal–glial contributions to transmitter amino acid metabolism: Studies with kainic acid-induced lesions of rat striatum, *J. Neurochem.* **33**:839–844.

Norenberg, M. D., and Martinez-Hernandez, A., 1979, Fine structural localization of glutamine synthetase in astrocytes in rat brain, *Brain Res.* **161**:303–310.

Perry, T. L., Hansen, S., and Kennedy, J., 1975, CSF amino acids and plasma-CSF amino acid ratios in adults, *J. Neurochem.* **24**:587–589.

Porter, T. G., and Martin, D. L., 1984, Evidence for feedback regulation of glutamate decarboxylase by γ-aminobutyric acid, *J. Neurochem.* **43**:1464–1467.

Potashner, S. J., 1978a, The spontaneous and electrically evoked release, from slices of guinea-pig cerebral cortex, of endogenous amino acids labelled via metabolism of d-[U-¹⁴C]glucose, *J. Neurochem.* **31**:177–186.

Potashner, S. J., 1978b, Effects of tetrodotoxin, calcium and magnesium on the release of amino acids from slices of guinea-pig cerebral cortex, *J. Neurochem.* **31**:187–195.

Ramaharobandro, N., Borg, J., Mandel, P., and Mark. J., 1982, Glutamine and glutamate transport in cultured neuronal and glial cells, *Brain Res.* **244**:113–121.

Reubi, J. C., 1980, Comparative study of the release of glutamate and GABA, newly synthesized from glutamine, in various regions of the central nervous system, *Neuroscience* **5**:2145–2150.

Reubi, J. C., Van den Berg, C., and Cuenod, M., 1978, Glutamine as precursor for the GABA and glutamate transmitter pools, *Neurosci. Lett.* **10**:171–174.

Roberts, E., 1981, Strategies for identifying sources and sites of formation of GABA-precursor or transmitter glutamate in brain, in: *Glutamate as a Neurotransmitter* (G. Di Chiara and G. L. Gessa, eds.), Raven Press, New York, pp. 91–102.

Roberts, E., and Kuriyama, K., 1968, Biochemical-physiological correlations in studies of the γ-aminobutyric acid system, *Brain Res.* **8**:1–35.

Rothstein, J. D., and Tabakoff, B., 1984, Alteration of striatal glutamate release after glutamine synthetase inhibition, *J. Neurochem.* **42**:1438–1446.

Schousboe, A., Larsson, O. M., Drejer, J., Krogsgaard-Larsen, P., and Hertz, P., 1983, Uptake and release processes for glutamine, glutamate and GABA in cultured neurons and astrocytes, in: *Glutamine, Glutamate and GABA in the Central Nervous System* (L. Hertz, E. Kvamme, E. G. McGeer, and A. Schousboe, eds.), Liss, New York, pp. 297–315.

Seligman, B., Miller, L. P., Brockman, D. E., and Martin, D. L., 1978, Studies on the regulation of GABA synthesis: The interaction of adenine nucleotides and glutamate with brain glutamate decarboxylase, *J. Neurochem.* **30**:371–376.

Shank, R. P., and Aprison, M. H., 1977, Glutamine uptake and metabolism by isolated toad brain: Evidence pertaining to its proposed role as a transmitter precursor, *J. Neurochem.* **28**:1189–1196.

Shank, R. P., and Aprison, M. H., 1981, Present status and significance of the glutamine cycle in neuronal tissue, *Life Sci.* **28**:837–842.

Shank, R. P., and Campbell, G. L., 1983a, Ornithine as a precursor of glutamate and GABA: Uptake and metabolism by neuronal and glial enriched cellular material, *J. Neurosci. Res.* **9**:47–57.

Shank, R. P., and Campbell, G. L., 1983b, Metabolic precursors of glutamate and GABA, in: *Glutamine, Glutamate and GABA in the Central Nervous System* (L. Hertz, E. Kvamme, E. G. McGeer, and A. Schousboe, eds.), Liss, New York, pp. 355–369.

Shank, R. P., and Campbell, G. L., 1984, Amino acid uptake, content and metabolism by neuronal and glial enriched fractions from mouse cerebellum, *J. Neurosci.* **4**:58–69.

Suszkiw, J. B., and O'Leary, M. E., 1983, Temporal characteristics of potassium-stimulated acetylcholine release and inactivation of calcium influx in rat brain synaptosomes, *J. Neurochem.* **41**:868–873.

Szerb, J. C., 1982, Effect of nipecotic acid, a γ-aminobutyric acid transport inhibitor, on the turnover and release of γ-aminobutyric acid in rat cortical slices, *J. Neurochem.* **39**:850–858.

Szerb, J. C., 1984, Storage and release of endogenous and labelled GABA formed from [³H]glutamine and [¹⁴C]glucose in hippocampal slices: Effect of depolarization, *Brain Res.* **293**:293–303.

Szerb, J. C., and O'Regan, P. A., 1985, Effect of glutamine on glutamate release from hippocampal slices induced by high K⁺ or by electrical stimulation: Interaction with different Ca²⁺ concentrations, *J. Neurochem.* **44**:1724–1731.

Szerb, J. C., and O'Regan, P. A., 1986, Possible reasons for the failure of glutamine to influence GABA release in rat hippocampal slices: Effect of nipecotic acid and methionine sulfoximine, *Neurochem. Int.* **8**:389–395.

Tapia, R., and Gonzalez, R. M., 1978, Glutamine and glutamate as precursors of the releasable pool of GABA in brain cortex slices, *Neurosci. Lett.* **10**:165–169.

Tursky, T., Ruscak, M., Lassanova, M., and Ruscakova, D., 1979, [¹⁴C]amino acid formation from labelled glucose and/or acetate with experimentally elicited proliferation of astroglia: Correlation of biochemical and morphological changes, *J. Neurochem.* **33**:1209–1215.

Van den Berg, C. J., and Garfinkel, D., 1971, A simulation study of brain compartments: Metabolism of glutamate and related substances in mouse brain, *Biochem. J.* **123**:211–218.

Van den Berg, C. J., Matheson, D. F., Ronda, G., Reijnierse, G. L. A., Blokhuis, G. G. D., Kroon, M. C., Clarke, D. D., and Garfinkel, D., 1975, A model of glutamate metabolism in brain: Biochemical analysis of a heterogeneous structure, in: *Metabolic Compartmentation and Neurotransmission* (S. Berl, D. D. Clarke, and D. Schneider, eds.), Plenum Press, New York, pp. 515–543.

van Gelder, N. M., 1978, Taurine, the compartmentalized metabolism of glutamic acid, and the epilepsies, *Can. J. Physiol. Pharmacol.* **56:**362–374.

Vrba, R., Gaitonde, M. K., and Richter, D., 1962, The conversion of glucose carbon into protein in the brain and other organs of the rat, *J. Neurochem.* **9:**465–475.

Waelsch, H., 1962, In vivo compartments of glutamic acid metabolism in brain and liver, in: *Amino Acid Pools, Distribution, Formation and Function of Free Amino Acids* (J. T. Holden, ed.), Elsevier, Amsterdam, pp. 722–730.

Wroblewski, J. T., Blaker, W. D., and Meek, J. L., 1985, Ornithine as a precursor of neurotransmitter glutamate: Effect of canaline on ornithine aminotransferase activity and glutamate content in the septum of rat brain, *Brain Res.* **329:**161–168.

11

GABAergic Processes in the Central Visual System

Adam Murdin Sillito and Penelope Clare Murphy

1. Introduction

There is now persuasive evidence that GABA is a primary inhibitory transmitter in the visual cortex and we have a reasonable knowledge of the morphological characteristics of the GABAergic cells (Iversen *et al.*, 1971; Sillito, 1975a, 1984; Ribak, 1978; Peters and Fairén, 1978; Peters and Regidor, 1981; Somogyi *et al.*, 1981, 1984; Freund *et al.*, 1983). My purpose in this account is to provide an overview of the range and types of contributions that GABAergic inhibitory processes make to the functional organization of the primary visual cortex. In so doing it will be necessary to place the comments in the context of our radically changing perspective on many aspects of the synaptic organization of the visual cortex and to consider interactions at the thalamic level. The discussion will be largely based on observations made in the feline visual cortex, which is a primary model for work of this type, and will center around a consideration of those processes involved in the generation of orientation and directional selectivity, ocular dominance, and length preference.

2. Basic Organization of Excitatory and Inhibitory Connections

The cells in the visual cortex can be separated into three broad categories: pyramidal cells (which all bear dendritic spines), spiny stellate cells, and a variety of nonspiny or partially spined cells (LeVay, 1973). The excitatory connections are mediated by the pyramidal and spiny stellate cells and the inhibitory connections by the non- and partially spiny group. The axons of the cells in the dorsal lateral geniculate nucleus (dLGN) make excitatory contacts with cells in all three groups. The most dense input is directed to layer IV of the cortex from the A laminae of the dLGN, bringing input from "X" and "Y" cells, but there is also a projection from the A laminae to the upper part of layer VI. Further input from the C laminae, bringing information from "Y" and "W" cells, is directed to layer I, and the III/IV and IV/V border regions (LeVay and Gilbert,

Adam Murdin Sillito and Penelope Clare Murphy • Department of Physiology, University College, Cardiff CF1 1XL, United Kingdom.

1976; Ferster and LeVay, 1978). The second-order excitatory connections include a projection from layer IV to layers II and III, a projection from layers II and III to layer V, a projection from layer V to layer VI and to layers II and III, and a projection from layer VI to layer IV and the dLGN (Lund *et al.*, 1979; Gilbert and Wiesel, 1979, 1983; Martin and Whitteridge, 1984; McGuire *et al.*, 1984). It is also relevant to note that the apical dendrites of layer VI cells collect excitatory input in layer IV and those of layer V cells collect input from the superficial layers. Some of these excitatory interconnections are summarized in Fig. 1. The excitatory connections made by pyramidal cells also spread extensively in the horizontal domain, and show a clustering pattern in their terminal distribution that may relate to connections specific to orientation columns and ocular dominance columns (Rockland and Lund, 1983; Gilbert and Wiesel, 1983; Matsubara *et al.*, 1985).

While the excitatory connections form an extensive and apparently dominant feature of the neocortical circuit, it is important to emphasize the extent to which this is balanced by a highly organized and varied set of inhibitory connections. It seems in the cat visual cortex that approximately 20% of the cells are GABAergic (Gabbot and Somogyi, 1986) and these make synaptic contacts that are most densely distributed around the cell body, axon initial segment, and proximal dendrites. This differential location of the inhibitory synapses provides the basis for a potent control of a cell's responses in relation to excitatory inputs from dendrites. As a result of their location, inhibitory influences come to dominate many aspects of the response properties of visual cortical cells. The inhibitory inputs reaching any given cortical cell derive from a range of different sources; some of those impinging on pyramidal cells are summarized in highly diagrammatic form in Fig. 2. Thus, a pyramidal cell may be expected to receive specific input to the initial

CORTEX

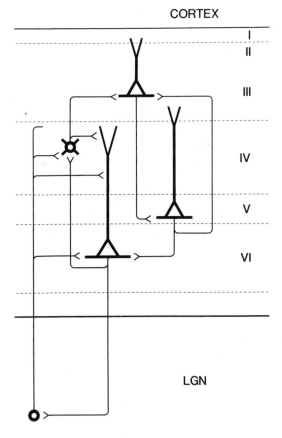

LGN

Figure 1. Diagram summarizing some of the excitatory connections linking different levels in the feline central visual system. The projection from the dorsal lateral geniculate nucleus (LGN) is shown providing input to layer IV and layer VI of the visual cortex (input from the C laminae is not shown). Small cell in layer IV is a spiny stellate one.

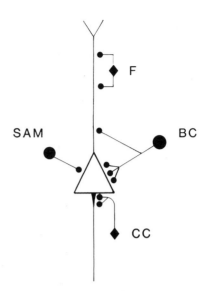

Figure 2. Highly diagrammatic summary of some of the GABAergic inhibitory connections that converge on a pyramidal cell in the visual cortex. Cell receives input to the axon initial segment from chandelier cells (CC), input to the cell body and proximal dendrites from basket cells (BC), further possible input to the cell body from short-axon multipolar cells (SAM), and input to the apical dendrite from bitufted cells (BT) and possibly basket cells (the latter not shown).

segment from chandelier cells (the so-called "axoaxonic" input; Somogyi, 1977), inputs to the cell body from basket cells and short-axon multipolar cells, and inputs to the distal parts of dendrites from several cell types including bitufted cells and basket cells (Peters and Fairén, 1978; Peters and Regidor, 1981; Somogyi and Cowey, 1981; Martin *et al.*, 1983). Not only is there a range of different types of inhibitory interneurons converging on a given cortical cell, but for any one type the input appears to derive from several cells as, for example, in the case of chandelier cells providing the input to the initial segment. There are good grounds for believing that each group of inhibitory inputs may exert effects that are functionally distinct. As the initial segment is considered to be the site for the initiation of the action potential (Spencer and Kandel, 1961), the chandelier cell input to this location may be judged to exert a preemptive control over a cell's activity. Synapses to the cell body, deriving from basket cells, will also evoke a potent control over the cell's responsiveness but one that is likely to be more graded in its interaction with the excitatory input converging on dendrites than that from chandelier cells. A further complexity is introduced by evidence suggesting that GABAergic synapses on dendrites produce a depolarization associated with an increased membrane conductance, as opposed to the hyperpolarization associated with inputs to the cell body (Andersen *et al.*, 1980; Alger and Nicoll, 1982; Kemp, 1984; Scharfman and Sarvey, 1985). It has been suggested that this depolarizing effect could provide the basis for a "discriminative inhibition," because by shunting currents in the vicinity of the inhibitory input, it allows for a selective inhibitory influence on excitatory inputs in that location. Excitatory inputs at other locations may even be facilitated under these conditions. Several additional factors need to be borne in mind, one being that GABA also exerts a slower hyperpolarizing influence on dendrites that appears to be mediated by GABA "B" receptors (Alger and Nicoll, 1982; Nicoll and Newberry, 1984). Another relates to the location of some inhibitory synapses on dendritic spines as opposed to dendritic shafts (Somogyi *et al.*, 1983), since those on spines may be inferred to have the potential for a selective and potent influence on the specific excitatory input to the spines in question.

Even from the present very superficial synopsis of the organization of inhibitory processes within the visual cortex, it is clear that there are sets of distinct mechanisms, each of which may be expected to exert influences on a different aspect of the cell's response profile. Given that there is already evidence to favor the view that different types of inhibitory process may influence direction selectivity, orientation selectivity, length tuning, and binocular interactions (Sillito,

1975b, 1977, 1979; Sillito *et al.,* 1980b; Hammond, 1981; Ganz and Felder, 1984; Bolz and Gilbert, 1986), it does not seem unreasonable to speculate that specific sets of inhibitory mechanisms underlie these functionally discrete influences. Furthermore, it is relevant to question whether, for example, the chandelier cell inputs converging on a specific cortical cell act in synchrony to coordinate one facet of the cell's response profile, or separately to mediate different components. Each chandelier cell may be judged to have the potential for a particularly potent influence on cell activity, although the cell types providing inhibitory input to the cell body must also be considered capable of exerting a very significant control. Effectively such a segregation of control within a given population of inhibitory interneurons would markedly increase the available range of discrete inhibitory mechanisms.

Although one might imagine that a consideration of the role of GABAergic processes in the visual cortex could ignore synaptic operations applying to the dLGN, present knowledge shows that there is a potential for a substantial reciprocal interaction between cortex and dLGN. Consequently, the impact of a cortical mechanism has to be analyzed in the perspective of its potential for modulating the corticofugal feedback to the dLGN, and hence the input to the cortex, as well as the immediate cortical network. In the dLGN, the relay cells receive excitatory input from the retinal afferents on proximal dendrites, and a descending corticofugal excitatory input on distal dendrites of similar magnitude to the retinal input (Wilson *et al.,* 1984). Relay cells are subject to two types of inhibitory input, one from the intrinsic inhibitory interneurons within the dLGN, and the other from cells in the perigeniculate nucleus. In the case of the intrinsic inhibitory interneurons, the dendrites form presynaptic structures in what are referred to as "triadic synapses." These are associated with dendritic spines on the relay cell dendrites and because "X" cells seem to be much more prominently spined than "Y" cells, may be presumed to exert their major influence over "X" cell properties (Rapisardi and Miles, 1984; Wilson *et al.,* 1984). In the triadic synapse, the dendrites of the intrinsic inhibitory interneurons are presynaptic to the relay cell dendrite, but together with the relay cell dendrite they are postsynaptic to the terminals of the retinal afferents (Famiglietti and Peters, 1972). Hence, there is the basis for a very specific control of the transfer of information from the retinal afferent to the relay cell. In addition, it is likely that the axons of the intrinsic inhibitory interneurons make conventional synaptic contacts on the shafts of relay cells. The cells in the perigeniculate nucleus mediate a recurrent collateral inhibitory feedback to the relay cells and intrinsic inhibitory interneurons (Ahlsen *et al.,* 1982). Corticofugal fibers make excitatory contacts on both the intrinsic inhibitory interneurons and the perigeniculate cells. As for the cortex, the inhibitory interactions in the dLGN seem to be mediated by GABA (Sillito and Kemp, 1983; Fitzpatrick *et al.,* 1984; Berardi and Morrone, 1984).

3. Mechanisms Underlying Orientation and Direction Selectivity

As shown in Fig. 3, visual cortical cells display a high degree of selectivity to the orientation and direction of motion of an elongated contour crossing their receptive field. Although there is evidence to support the view that dLGN cells may exhibit some level of orientation and direction bias (Vidyasagar and Urbas, 1982), this is residual in comparison with that seen in the visual cortex and is, moreover, best demonstrated by stimuli of 10° or more in length, while cortical cells can exhibit prominent orientation and direction selectivity to stimuli as short as 2° (Henry *et al.,* 1974). The orientation and direction tuning of a dLGN cell are shown in Fig. 4 and should be compared with records for cortical cells in Figs. 3 and 6. The implication of this is that the orientation and direction selectivity seen in the cortex are strongly dependent on synaptic interactions within the cortex. Hubel and Wiesel (1962) appreciated this point and suggested that orientation selectivity was established in layer IV by the pattern of convergence of geniculate excitatory afferents onto simple cells. The basic tenet here is that simple cells receive input from a

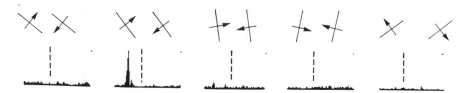

Figure 3. Responses of a simple cell in the striate cortex to a bar of light moving over its receptive field at a range of different orientations. Each peristimulus time histogram (PSTH) shows the response to both directions of motion at one orientation, averaged for 32 trials. The cell only shows a significant response to one direction of motion at one of the test orientations.

number of geniculate afferents with the receptive fields forming a linear array in space, the axis of which then determines the cell's optimal orientation. The subsequent translation of this selectivity into the complex cell population then occurs by the specific organization of second-order excitatory connections. However, this view, as originally expressed, now seems unlikely to be correct. Complex cells retain their visual responsiveness in the absence of an input from simple cells (Hammond and Mackay, 1975), and removal of the input arising in the A laminae of the dLGN, with consequent cessation of visual driving in layers IV and VI, can leave layer II/III complex cells and some layer V complex cells with apparently normal direction and orientation tuning (Malpeli, 1983). Moreover, a significant portion of the complex cell population seems to have direct input from the dLGN (Singer *et al.*, 1975; Toyama *et al.*, 1977; Bullier and Henry, 1979; Martin and Whitteridge, 1984). The implication here is that the process for establishing the orientation and direction tuning of complex cells can occur independently of any operations taking place in layer IV and hence that the synaptic organization underlying these properties is duplicated in several layers.

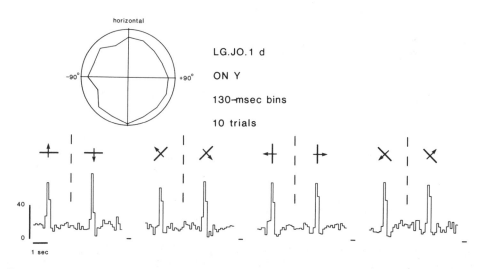

Figure 4. Responses of an ''on'' Y cell in the dorsal lateral geniculate nucleus to a range of orientations similar to those shown in Fig. 3. The PSTHs, averaged for ten trials, show good responses to both directions of motion at each test orientation. The responses of the cell to a wider range of stimulus orientations are plotted on a polar diagram in the top left-hand corner. Here the response magnitude is represented by the distance of each point from the center of the figure. Each point documents the response to a stimulus moving in one direction at a given orientation, with opposite directions of motion for one orientation represented by points 180° apart. This relatively unbiased plot should be compared with the normal responses of visual cortical cells as shown in Fig. 7.

Irrespective of the importance of layer IV to the generation of the properties of cells outside layer IV, there is a general question concerning the nature of the synaptic organization which might be expected to underlie direction and orientation tuning irrespective of the layer in which it is occurring. Taking direction selectivity as an initial example, it is possible to isolate several mechanisms that might underlie the selectivity of a given cell in the visual cortex. In this context, direction selectivity refers to the preference of a cell for one of the two possible directions of motion of an optimally oriented bar of light over the receptive field. The mechanisms are summarized in very simplistic fashion in Fig. 5. The most accessible idea is that of some type of feedforward inhibitory mechanism, whereby a stimulus moving over the receptive field in the nonpreferred direction elicits a wave of inhibition which suppresses the cell's response to its primary excitatory drive. There is considerable evidence for this type of process, from receptive field analysis (Ganz and Felder, 1984), intracellular studies revealing IPSPs in response to the nonpreferred direction of motion (Innocenti and Fiore, 1974; Creutzfeldt et al., 1974), and the effect of a localized blockade of GABAergic inhibitory processes (Sillito, 1975b, 1977, 1984). The latter is demonstrated in Fig. 6. As seen in Fig. 6a, iontophoretic application of the GABA antagonist bicuculline to produce a blockade of the inhibitory processes acting on a layer IV simple cell, eliminates the cell's original directional selectivity. This effect was reversible and commensurate with the fact that the direction selectivity is generated by GABA-mediated inhib-

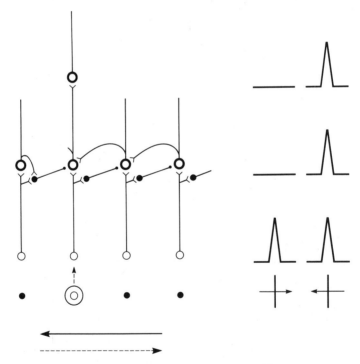

Figure 5. Concept diagram illustrating the broad type of neural connection that might generate direction selectivity in the striate cortex. Records to the right show the hypothetical responses of cells at three levels in the sequence of neurons illustrated to the left. ●, inhibitory interneurons; ○, excitatory cells. The geniculate cell at the first level in the diagram, overlying the ideogram of its concentric receptive field, responds to both directions of motion. The cortical cell at the second level shows a selectivity for motion to the left, following from a combination of two patterns of intrinsic cortical connectivity. First, the feedforward inhibitory connections directed to the right result in a wave of inhibition which suppresses responses to stimuli moving in that direction. In addition, feedforward excitatory connections directed to the left may reinforce the stimulus response in the opposite direction. The cell at the third level in the sequence receives a directionally selective input.

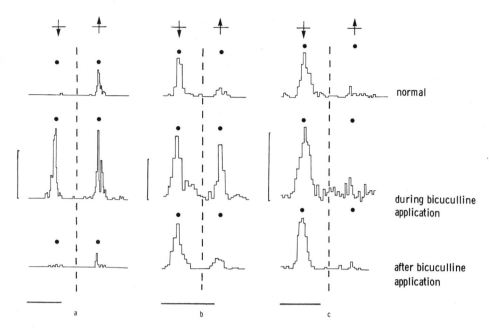

Figure 6. Effect of inhibitory blockade produced by iontophoretically applied bicuculline on the directional selectivity of a simple cell (a), a layer III standard complex cell (b), and a layer V complex cell (c). Records show responses to both directions of motion of an optimally oriented stimulus, averaged over 25 trials. Upper records document normal response, middle records response during inhibitory blockade, and lower records recovery.

itory synapses. Similar results are shown for a layer III complex cell in Fig. 6b, although in this case the direction selectivity is not entirely eliminated. One possibility could be that the bicuculline failed to block all the inhibitory synapses acting on the cell. This cannot be excluded as a contributory factor to this type of data, although the pharmacological effectiveness of bicuculline, as judged by its action on iontophoretically applied GABA, was checked in each case. Another interpretation could be that excitatory mechanisms contribute a component of the direction selectivity. The diagram in Fig. 5 also suggests the presence of an intracortically mediated feedforward excitation in the preferred direction of motion. If the direct excitatory input to a cell studied elicited an effect that was close to threshold, such an intracortically mediated excitation could be very important in generating a level of background facilitation essential to the ability of the main input to elicit an action potential discharge. It is possible that an asymmetry in the excitatory mechanisms generated the residual bias seen in the cell shown in Fig. 6b during inhibitory blockade. On the other hand, the layer V special complex cell, illustrated in Fig. 6c, showed no loss whatsoever of direction selectivity during bicuculline application. This raises the possibility that this cell may have received an excitatory input already tuned for direction selectivity, as suggested for the cell shown at the top of Fig. 5. The difficulty Sillito (1977) experienced in influencing the direction selectivity of layer V cells with bicuculline is interesting in the context of recent evidence suggesting that this layer has the lowest level of GABA-immunoreactive neurons in the striate cortex (Gabbot and Somogyi, 1986). Taken as a whole, the available data from a wide range of studies demonstrate that feedforward inhibitory mechanisms underlie the direction tuning of a significant portion of the population of cortical cells. It is equally clear that some cells appear to receive an excitatory input that is already directionally selective, and laterally directed excitatory connections of the type shown in Fig. 3 must be regarded as exerting a potential influence.

While there is a consensus for the view that inhibitory mechanisms are likely to be one of the major, if not the major, factor generating direction selectivity, the issue of orientation selectivity has provoked some debate. Hubel and Wiesel's original model for orientation selectivity involved purely excitatory connections. Although questioned by some of the early intracellular studies suggesting a role for inhibitory processes (Creutzfeldt and Ito, 1968; Creutzfeldt *et al.*, 1974), this idea was most radically challenged by data obtained from localized application of the GABA antagonist bicuculline. This approach has shown that both simple and complex cells can lose orientation selectivity during inhibitory blockade (Sillito, 1975b, 1979; Tsumoto *et al.*, 1979; Sillito *et al.*, 1980a) as demonstrated by the polar tuning curves in Fig. 7. The effects are reversible and indicate that simple cells and a portion of the complex cell population have access to an excitatory input that does not confer significant orientation bias. The suggestion here is that laterally directed inhibitory interactions driven by orientations outside the range of a cell's preferred orientation are responsible for establishing the orientation tuning (Sillito, 1979, 1984, 1985; Heggelund, 1981a,b). Despite the inability of a recent study to detect this type of inhibition (Ferster, 1986), its presence is supported by studies employing a range of different approaches (Bishop *et al.*, 1971, 1973; Henry *et al.*, 1974; Sillito, 1979; Morrone *et al.*, 1982; Ramoa *et al.*, 1986). Nonetheless, this argument does not apply to all cells. As for direction selectivity there is a population of cells, amounting to approximately half the complex cell population (see Fig. 8), that do not lose orientation tuning during inhibitory blockade (Sillito, 1979) although the tightness of their tuning is reduced. For these cells the excitatory input is certainly orientation biased, either because it derives from cells in which orientation tuning has already been established, or because it involves a particular pattern of convergence of the geniculate input. Certainly some cortical cells appear to receive all their excitatory input via other cortical cells and thus may be presumed to be in a position to receive orientation-biased input.

4. Length Tuning

The views on the mechanisms underlying length tuning have shifted several times since Hubel and Wiesel (1965, 1968) first described "hypercomplex cells" in area 18 of the visual cortex. These cells, subsequently found in the superficial layers of area 17, gave a maximal response to an optimally oriented bar of a certain length, with an increase in stimulus length beyond the optimal provoking a reduction or complete loss of the original response. Hubel and Wiesel postulated that they received an inhibitory input driven by complex cells with receptive fields spatially displaced to either side of that of the cell providing their main excitatory input. These hypercomplex cells were seen as being at the top of the hierarchy processing visual information in area 17, the earlier stages involving interactions at the level of simple and complex cells which were not thought to exhibit length preference. The responses of a hypercomplex cell in the superficial layers of area 17 are illustrated in Fig. 9. The upper records show the normal response pattern, with an optimally oriented bar of light moving through the central region of the receptive field producing a clear excitatory response. Extension of this bar to either side of the central region results in a considerable reduction of the response, and when extended to both sides the response is completely eliminated. These findings are consistent with the presence of powerful inhibitory sidebands. One might therefore anticipate that blockade of inhibition by the iontophoretic application of bicuculline would eliminate the length tuning. As the middle records in Fig. 9 show, it did not. There was some reduction in the power of the two sidebands but a stimulus elongated to both sides of the field still failed to generate a response. Although it was possible that the inhibitory blockade of this cell and other similar cells studied was not complete, the evidence favored the view that they received an excitatory input that was already length tuned (Sillito and Versiani, 1977). The local inhibition appeared to enhance rather than to generate the length tuning. At the time this was a puzzling observation, but seemed to fall into place when simple cells with length-tuned properties were found in layer IV of the striate cortex (Rose, 1977;

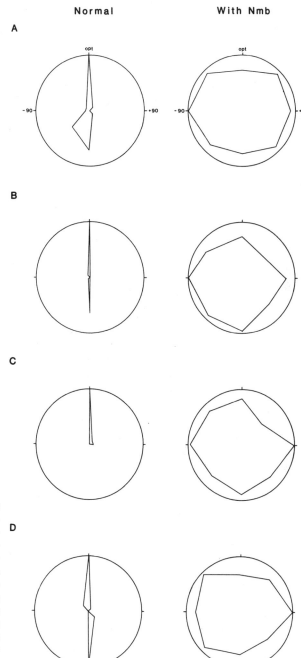

Figure 7. Effect of inhibitory blockade on the orientation tuning of simple (A–C) and complex (D) cells. Polar diagrams show the normal orientation tuning, and orientation tuning during iontophoretic application of bicuculline (Nmb). Polar plots are normalized to the maximum response in each situation; see Fig. 4 for further details. The cells are tightly tuned under normal conditions (cf. geniculate cell in Fig. 4), but this selectivity is lost during inhibitory blockade.

Gilbert, 1977; Kato *et al.*, 1978). Since layer IV provides a major output to layer III (Gilbert and Wiesel, 1979; Martin and Whitteridge, 1984), an obvious interpretation is that layer IV simple cells with length tuning provided the excitatory input to the layer III cells studied by Sillito and Versiani (1977). An important implication here is that cells with length preference are not, as first thought, confined to the top of the cortical hierarchy but occur at the earliest stages.

In a recent paper, Bolz and Gilbert (1986) postulated that the projection from layer VI to

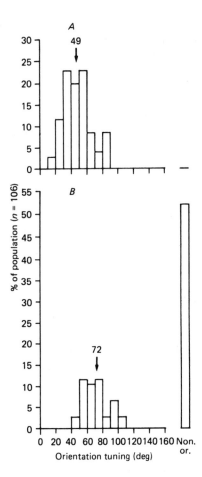

Figure 8. Distribution of the orientation tuning in a population of complex cells (n = 106) before and during bicuculline-induced inhibitory blockade. The orientation tuning was assessed from the width at half-height in the orientation tuning curves; tighter tuning is therefore represented to the left of the distribution. The median tuning for the population of cells under control conditions (A) is 49°. During inhibitory blockade (B), approximately 50% of the population completely loses orientation tuning. The remainder retain an orientation bias, but the median width of tuning for these cells is 72°, indicating a reduction in the absolute selectivity.

layer IV may constitute an important component of the synaptic mechanism establishing length tuning in layer IV. This was based on the observation that some layer VI cells have very long receptive fields (Gilbert, 1977) and the discovery that a component of the layer VI pyramidal cell input to layer IV terminates on smooth dendritic processes thought to be associated with inhibitory interneurons (McGuire *et al.*, 1984). Thus, the layer VI connection might drive inhibitory interneurons in layer IV which in turn could provide an inhibitory input to other layer IV cells. This inhibitory input would increase in magnitude as stimulus length increased and hence might provide the basis for a bias to short stimuli. They tested this hypothesis by reversibly inactivating layer VI and examining the effect of this on length-tuned layer IV cells. Their findings supported the hypothesis; layer IV cells lost their length tuning during the blockade of layer VI. However, the situation is rather more complex than this observation might suggest. As discussed earlier, layer VI cells provide an extensive projection to the dLGN. It is now clear that dLGN cells, when tested with moving bars of the type used to drive cortical cells, exhibit clear length tuning (Cleland *et al.*, 1983; Jones *et al.*, 1987). One possibility is that the length tuning of layer IV simple cells derives from the geniculate input and that it is the length tuning of the geniculate cells that is perturbed by the layer VI blockade. We have examined this issue by checking the length tuning of dLGN cells in the presence and absence of corticofugal feedback. An example of the effect of removing corticofugal feedback on the length tuning of a dLGN cell is given in Fig. 10. There is a clear reduction although not a loss of the original length tuning. Taken across a population of cells, the loss of corticofugal feedback produces a significant shift in length tuning

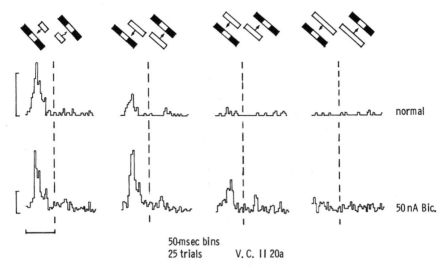

Figure 9. Effect of inhibitory blockade on the length tuning of a superficial layer hypercomplex cell in area 17. Upper records show the normal responses to an optimally oriented bar of varying length moving over the receptive field, averaged for 25 trials. The alignment of the bar with respect to the hypercomplex cell field is shown by the ideograms at the top, in which the inhibitory end zones are shown filled in black to either side of the central excitatory region. As can be seen, extension of the bar length to either or both sides of the central region results in a marked reduction in response magnitude compared to that of the shorter stimulus. During inhibitory blockade produced by iontophoretically applied bicuculline (lower records), there is some reduction in the power of the end zones but the cell still retains a degree of length preference. See text for further discussion.

in the dLGN, as shown in Fig. 11. Basically in the normal situation most dLGN cells tend to show a 50–100% reduction in the optimal response as stimulus length is increased, while they tend to show less than a 50% reduction in the absence of corticofugal feedback. Thus, corticofugal feedback does influence the length tuning of dLGN cells.

Without doubt the situation regarding length tuning is much more complex than it seemed at

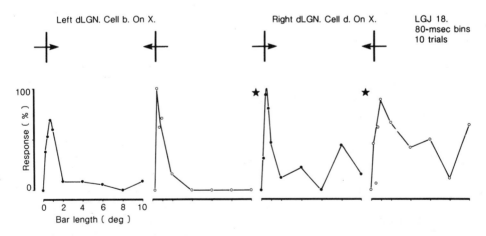

Figure 10. Length tuning curves of dLGN cells with and without corticofugal feedback. Curves show responses as percentage of the maximum, for a bar of light of varying length moving over the receptive field. Data averaged over ten trials, randomly interleaved. The two directions of motion are expressed separately. Curves to the left show responses recorded from a cell in the left dLGN, which retained corticofugal feedback; those on the right for a simultaneously recorded cell in the right dLGN without corticofugal feedback.

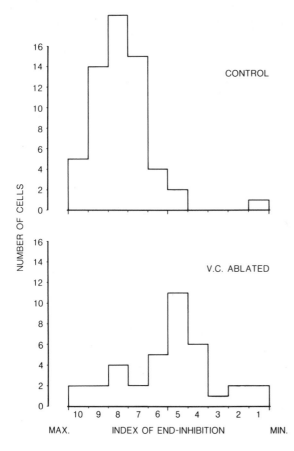

Figure 11. Distribution of end-inhibition in dLGN cells with and without corticofugal feedback. The index of end-inhibition was calculated as the percentage decrease in response magnitude for stimuli 2, 4, and 6° in length as compared to the maximum response, and is divided into ten equal segments incorporating the range of 100% (LHS) to 0% (RHS). In the control situation, the mean reduction in response was 72 ± 2%; following ablation of the visual cortex there was a significant shift to the right, indicating a decrease in end-inhibition, resulting in a mean of 50 ± 4%.

first. Cells in the dLGN exhibit a level of length tuning that is directly comparable to that seen in cortical hypercomplex cells (Cleland *et al.*, 1983; Jones *et al.*, 1987). This, in part, must reflect the operation of GABA-mediated center–surround antagonism in dLGN cells (Cleland *et al.*, 1983; Sillito and Kemp, 1983). However, the full force of the surround antagonism of the center response would not be brought into play by a moving bar stimulus of the type used to drive cortical cells, simply because the bar would only activate a relatively small proportion of the surround relative to the center. This may be reflected in the length tuning of dLGN cells without corticofugal feedback. On the other hand, the corticofugal feedback would be activated by bar stimuli, and certainly some of the cells providing this would be best activated by longer stimuli. The most economical suggestion here is that the corticofugal feedback provides an influence that reinforces the effect of the center–surround antagonism such that responses to bar stimuli show a similar "focus" in the spatial extent of their maximum effectiveness to that seen when the field is tested with contrast spots. It may be part of a general mechanism enhancing the spatial resolution associated with each geniculate input. Moving to the cortex, the most economical explanation for the presence of cells with length preference in layer IV is that this reflects the properties of the geniculate cells providing their primary excitatory drive, as suggested by Cleland *et al.* (1983). This might then be relayed to cells outside layer IV as discussed above. In addition, despite the fact that the geniculate input in the presence of corticofugal feedback displays a level of length tuning that matches that seen in many cortical hypercomplex cells, there is good evidence for an intracortically mediated "end zone" inhibition (Sillito and Versiani, 1977; Orban *et al.*, 1979; Yamane *et al.*, 1985). This might serve two functions: first, it might eliminate the remaining response that many dLGN cells show in the plateau of their tuning curve and, second, it is likely to be responsible for the marked asymmetries that are seen in the strength of end zone inhibition on either side of the receptive field of many hypercomplex cells (e.g., Sillito and Versiani, 1977). This asymmetry may be of some functional significance.

All the above arguments need to be balanced by a range of further considerations. Many cortical cells, including a significant proportion of layer IV cells, do not exhibit length preference. Consequently, the length preference exhibited in the geniculate input must have been eliminated in these cases by the pattern of convergence of the input and the weighting of the various synaptic inputs (for a discussion of this, see Cleland *et al.*, 1983). Given that this occurs in some cases, might it not occur in all, and might not intracortical mechanisms regenerate length preference *de novo?* One argument in favor of this is that the end zone inhibition in cortical cells is itself orientation tuned (Orban *et al.*, 1979). However, it is not clear that Orban *et al.* (1979) could distinguish between the presence of an intracortical inhibitory influence reinforcing length prefer-ence and an underlying geniculate-based mechanism. Further to this, it seems that their best data relate to a single end-stopped complex family cell, and the question of whether end zone inhibi-tion applies throughout the simple cell population is open to some question (Henry, 1985). Bolz and Gilbert (1986) assumed that their data demonstrated a single intracortical mechanism for establishing length preference in layer IV. The fact that loss of the layer VI influence on the dLGN will significantly shift the length tuning of dLGN cells questions this assumption in its most simple form, as does a parallel study showing that length preference in area 17 is strongly influenced by corticoclaustral connections (Sherk and LeVay, 1983). The significance of the claustral input is intriguing, but in the light of present evidence the most logical supposition would be that it influences the properties of the layer VI cells providing the corticofugal feedback and recurrent collateral input to layer IV. Given the degree of length preference established in dLGN relay cells by the concatenation of intrageniculate and corticofugal mechanisms operating on the bias present in the retinal input, it would be slightly surprising if it were not utilized in the

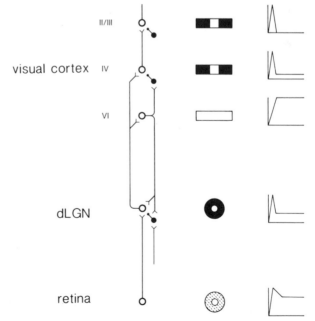

Figure 12. Summary diagram illustrat-ing some of the factors that might con-tribute to the generation of length prefer-ence. Records to the right show hypothetical length tuning curves for cells in retina, dLGN, and cortical layers II/III, IV, and VI. The central figures are ideograms of the related receptive fields, with shaded areas indicating inhibitory zones. To the left are shown some of the connections between these levels which might contribute to their length response characteristics; inhibitory and excitatory neurons are shown as filled and open cir-cles, respectively. Note that the retina shows a small degree of end-inhibition commensurate with its center–surround antagonism, which may be enhanced in the dLGN both by the more powerful an-tagonism and by feedback from layer VI of the visual cortex. Layer IV thus re-ceives a length-tuned input, which may-be further enhanced by intrinsic mechanisms and fed forward to the more superficial layers. The generation of non-endstopped cells in layer VI requires that the tuning of the geniculate input is overcome by the intrinsic circuitry. See text for further discussion.

generation of the length tuning of cortical cells. The orientation bias shown by retinal ganglion and dLGN cells is residual in comparison to their length preference, but a range of arguments indicate that in some way this influences the pattern of orientation selectivity across the cortex (Levick and Thibos, 1982; Vidyasagar and Urbas, 1982; Leventhal, 1983; Schall et al., 1986). A simplified summary of some of the ideas discussed here in relation to length tuning is given in Fig. 12.

5. Ocular Dominance

The subdivision of the visual cortex into ocular dominance columns follows in predictable fashion from the distribution of the geniculate afferents in layer IV of the cortex. The afferents representing the two eyes terminate in alternating bands or stripes in layer IV (Hubel and Wiesel, 1972; Wiesel et al., 1974; Schatz and Stryker, 1978). From this one might predict that the ocular dominance of cortical cells derives entirely from their excitatory connections. This does not seem to be the case since a significant proportion of the population of cortical cells dominated by one eye owe all, or a component of their bias to intracortical inhibitory connections (Sillito et al., 1980b). This is illustrated in Fig. 13, which shows the effect of localized inhibitory blockade on the ocular dominance of a population of cells exclusively dominated by one eye. Some of these cells become equally responsive to both eyes during inhibitory blockade. This is not entirely surprising because ocular dominance is a rather artificial construct; the organization of the input from the two eyes needs to be viewed in the context of the elaboration of binocular vision. Considered in this way it is clear that inhibitory interactions play a role (e.g., Poggio and Fischer, 1977), and that some cells are likely to receive an inhibitory input suppressing their response to a given eye.

In the discussions of the processing of binocular information it is virtually always assumed that all the relevant interactions first occur in the visual cortex. Cells in the dLGN are considered to receive excitatory input that is exclusive to the eye dominating their particular lamina. However, it has been known for some time that dLGN cells often exhibit inhibitory responses to stimulation of the nondominant eye (in this context always the eye that does not provide the main innervation of a given lamina) and very occasionally excitatory responses (Sandersen et al., 1971). We were interested to see whether these binocular inhibitory effects were GABAergic, and

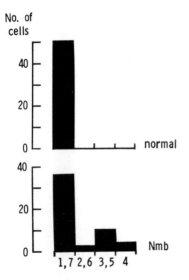

Figure 13. Effect of inhibitory blockade on the ocular dominance of a population of cells in area 17 of the visual cortex, normally dominated exclusively by one eye. The application of bicuculline (Nmb) reveals inputs to many cells from the normally silent eye, in some cases leading to equal dominance (OD 4).

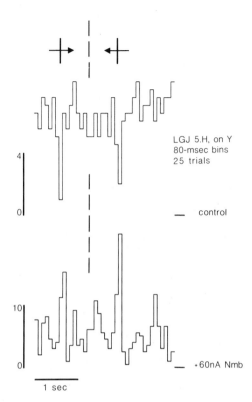

LGJ 5.H, on Y
80-msec bins
25 trials

4

0 ___ control

10

0 ___ +60nA Nmb

1 sec

Figure 14. Effect of inhibitory blockade on the responses of an "on" Y cell in the dLGN to stimulation of the nondominant eye. PSTHs show responses to a bar of light moving back and forth over the receptive field, before and during application of bicuculline (Nmb), averaged for 25 trials. The stimulus normally elicits an inhibition, but this can be seen to mask an underlying excitatory response. See text for further details.

to test visual responses during a blockade of inhibition. As shown in Fig. 14, during such a blockade of the inhibitory input, the inhibitory response to a bar moving over the nondominant eye field is replaced by an excitatory response. This observation applies equally to both "X" and "Y" cells. The excitatory responses were best revealed by a moving bar of light and this led us to suspect that they might be corticofugal in origin. This was not the case, since, surprisingly, removal of the corticofugal projection to the dLGN had no effect on the nondominant eye's excitatory response revealed during inhibitory blockade. Despite the absence of corticofugal effect, it seems that dLGN cells are subject to a relatively complex binocular influence consisting of at least two components of input driven by the nondominant eye. These comprise a GABA-mediated inhibitory input and a subcortically derived excitatory input. It is difficult to imagine that these have no bearing on the processing of binocular information. The absence of any detectable corticofugal binocular excitation is puzzling. As discussed in the preceding sections, the corticofugal projection to the dLGN is very powerful and aside from the fact that the cells providing the projection may exhibit binocular responses (Gilbert, 1977), the fibers of the corticofugal cells cross laminar borders in the dLGN (Robson, 1983). Hence, there is a strong anatomical basis for corticofugal binocular excitatory inputs to dLGN cells. The excitations of the nondominant eye revealed by inhibitory blockade were relatively weak in comparison to the responses of the dominant eye, but these should be viewed in the context of the likely magnitude of the blockade. In contrast to the cortex, the inhibitory synapses in the dLGN are not concentrated around the cell body, but are distributed over the dendrites. Given the spatial extent of the dendrites of dLGN cells it is extremely unlikely that all the inhibitory synapses influencing the cell would be blocked by the iontophoretic application of bicuculline, particularly if some of those involved in binocular interactions occurred on distal dendrites. As corticofugal fibers contact distal dendrites, inhibition controlling their excitation may be particularly difficult to block.

6. Overview

The experiments discussed here outline a range of the components of the influence of GABAergic inhibitory mechanisms in the visual cortex. At the same time, they indicate a series of cases where particular response properties may derive from the excitatory input to cells. This is notable in the case of the input to hypercomplex cells in the superficial laminae of the striate cortex and the apparently orientation-biased input to half the complex cell population. Nevertheless in a range of cases, there are good grounds for believing that the GABAergic inhibitory inputs converging on a cell structure its specificity in the presence of a nonspecific excitatory input. This applies to direction and orientation selectivity in simple cells and some complex cells. However, other aspects of the data suggest that it is wise at this stage to avoid oversimplistic models of the neural organization of particular response properties. In particular, it is clear that the corticofugal input to the dLGN has an important influence over the length tuning of dLGN cells. This means that the information conveyed to cortical cells by the geniculate input is itself subject to the influence of the cortical circuitry and it is no longer valid to consider processes at either level in isolation. Similar comments are likely to apply to the range of interactions between the different cortical laminae, although as yet it is not entirely clear which aspects of receptive field response properties are most influenced by any given set of interconnections.

ACKNOWLEDGMENTS. The support of the Medical Research Council of England and Wellcome Trust is gratefully acknowledged.

References

Ahlsen, G., Lindstrom, S., and Lo, F. S., 1982, Functional distinction of perigeniculate and thalamic reticular neurones in the cat, *Exp. Brain Res.* **45:**118–126.

Alger, B. E., and Nicoll, R. A., 1982, Pharmacological evidence for two kinds of GABA receptor on rat hippocampal pyramidal cells studied in vitro, *J. Physiol. (London)* **328:**125–141.

Andersen, P., Dingledine, R., Gjerstad, L., Langmoen, I. A., and Laursen, A. M., 1980, Two different responses of hippocampal pyramidal cells to application of gamma-aminobutyric acid, *J. Physiol. (London)* **305:**279–296.

Berardi, N., and Morrone, M. C., 1984, The role of γ-aminobutyric acid mediated inhibition on the response properties of cat lateral geniculate nucleus neurones, *J. Physiol. (London)* (in press).

Bishop, P. O., Coombs, J. S., and Henry, G. H., 1971, Responses to visual contours; spatio-temporal aspects of excitation in the receptive fields of striate neurones, *J. Physiol. (London)* **219:**625–657.

Bishop, P. O., Coombs, J. S., and Henry, G. H., 1973, Receptive fields of simple cells in the cat striate cortex, *J. Physiol. (London)* **231:**31–60.

Bolz, J., and Gilbert, C. D., 1986, Generation of end-inhibition in the visual cortex via interlaminar connections, *Nature* **320:**362–365.

Bullier, J., and Henry, G. H., 1979, Ordinal position of first order neurones in cat striate cortex, *J. Neurophysiol.* **42:**1251–1263.

Cleland, B. G., Lee, B. B., and Vidyasagar, T. R., 1983, Response of neurons in the cat's lateral geniculate nucleus to moving bars of different length, *J. Neurosci.* **3:**108–116.

Creutzfeldt, O. D., and Ito, M., 1968, Functional synaptic organization of primary visual cortex neurones in the cat, *Exp. Brain Res.* **6:**324–352.

Creutzfeldt, O. D., Kuhnt, U., and Benevento, L. A., 1974, An intracellular analysis of visual cortical neurones to moving stimuli: Responses in a co-operative neuronal network, *Exp. Brain Res.* **21:**251–274.

Famiglietti, E. W., and Peters, A., 1972, The synaptic glomerulus and the intrinsic neuron in the dorsal lateral geniculate nucleus of the cat, *J. Comp. Neurol.* **144:**285–334.

Ferster, D., 1986, Orientation selectivity of synaptic potentials in neurons of cat primary visual cortex, *J. Neurosci.* **6:**1284–1301.

Ferster, D., and LeVay, S., 1978, The axonal arborization of lateral geniculate neurons in the striate cortex of the cat, *J. Comp. Neurol.* **182:**923–944.

Fitzpatrick, D., Penny, G. R., and Schmechel, D. E., 1984, Glutamic acid decarboxylase-immunoreactive neurons and terminals in the lateral geniculate nucleus of the cat, *J. Neurosci.* **4:**1809–1829.

Freund, T. F., Martin, K. A. C., Smith, A. D., and Somogyi, P., 1983, Glutamate decarboxylase-immunoreactive terminals of Golgi impregnated axo-axonic cells and of presumed basket cells in synaptic contact with pyramidal cells of the cat's visual cortex, *J. Comp. Neurol.* **221:**263–278.

Gabbot, P. L. A., and Somogyi, P., 1986, Quantitative distribution of GABA-immunoreactive neurons in the visual cortex (area 17) of the cat, *Exp. Brain Res.* **61:**323–331.

Ganz, L., and Felder, R., 1984, Mechanism of directional selectivity in simple neurons of the cat's visual cortex analysed with stationary flash sequences, *J. Neurophysiol.* **51:**294–324.

Gilbert, C. D., 1977, Laminar differences in receptive field properties of cells in the cat primary visual cortex, *J. Physiol. (London)* **268:**391–421.

Gilbert, C. D., and Wiesel, T. N., 1979, Morphology and intracortical projections of functionally characterised neurons in cat visual cortex, *Nature* **280:**120–125.

Gilbert, C. D., and Wiesel, T. N., 1983, Clustered intrinsic connections in cat visual cortex, *J. Neurosci.* **3:**1116–1133.

Hammond, P., 1981, Simultaneous determination of directional tuning of complex cells in cat striate cortex for bar and texture motion. *Exp. Brain Res.* **41:**364–369.

Hammond, P., and Mackay, D. M., 1975, Differential responses of cat visual cortex cells to textured stimuli, *Exp. Brain Res.* **22:**427–430.

Heggelund, P., 1981a, Receptive field organization of simple cells in cat striate cortex, *Exp. Brain Res.* **42:**89–98.

Heggelund, P., 1981b, Receptive field organisation of complex cells in cat striate cortex, *Exp. Brain Res.* **42:**99–107.

Henry, G. H., 1985, Physiology of cat striate cortex, in: *The Cerebral Cortex,* Vol. 3 (A. Peters and E. G. Jones, eds.), Plenum Press, New York.

Henry, G. H., Bishop, P. O., and Dreher, B., 1974, Orientation, axis and direction as stimulus parameters for striate cells, *Vision Res.* **14:**766–778.

Hubel, D. H., and Wiesel, T. N., 1962, Receptive fields, binocular interaction and functional architecture in the cat's visual cortex, *J. Physiol. (London)* **160:**106–154.

Hubel, D. H., and Wiesel, T. N., 1965, Receptive fields and functional architecture in two non-striate visual areas (18 and 19) of the cat, *J. Neurophysiol.* **28:**229–289.

Hubel, D. H., and Wiesel, T. N., 1968, Receptive fields and functional architecture of monkey striate cortex, *J. Physiol. (London)* **195:**215–243.

Hubel, D. H., and Wiesel, T. N., 1972, Laminar and columnar distribution of geniculocortical fibres in the macaque monkey, *J. Comp. Neurol.* **146:**421–450.

Innocenti, G. M., and Fiore, I., 1974, Postsynaptic inhibitory components of the response to moving stimuli in area 17, *Brain Res.* **80:**229–289.

Iversen, L. L., Mitchell, J. F., and Srinivasan, 1971, The release of γ-amino butyric acid during inhibition in the cat visual cortex, *J. Physiol. (London)* **212:**519–534.

Jones, H. J., Murphy, P. C., and Sillito, A. M., 1987, Length tuning of cells in the feline dorsal lateral geniculate nucleus when tested with stimulus parameters used for visual cortical studies, (in preparation).

Kato, H., Bishop, P. O., and Orban, G. A., 1978, Hypercomplex and simple/complex cell classifications in cat striate cortex, *J. Neurophysiol.* **41:**1071–1095.

Kemp, J. A., 1984, Intracellular recordings from rat visual cortical cells in vitro and the action of GABA, *J. Physiol. (London)* (in press).

LeVay, S., 1973, Synaptic patterns in the visual cortex of the cat and monkey: Electron microscopy of Golgi preparation, *J. Comp. Neurol.* **150:**53–86.

LeVay, S., and Gilbert, C. D., 1976, Laminar patterns of geniculo-cortical projection in the cat, *Brain Res.* **113:**1–19.

Leventhal, A. G., 1983, Relationship between preferred orientation and receptive field position of neurons in cat striate cortex, *J. Comp. Neurol.* **220:**476–483.

Levick, W. R., and Thibos, L. N., 1982, Analysis of orientation bias in cat retina, *J. Physiol. (London)* **329:**243–261.

Lund, J. S., Henry, G. H., MacQueen, C. L., and Harvey, A. R., 1979, Anatomical organization of the primary visual cortex (area 17) of the macaque monkey, *J. Comp. Neurol.* **184:**559–576.

McGuire, B. A., Hornung, J.-P., Gilbert, C. D., and Wiesel, T. N., 1984, Patterns of synaptic input to layer 4 of cat striate cortex, *J. Neurosci.* **4:**3021–3033.

Malpeli, J. G., 1983, Activity of cells in area 17 of the cat in absence of input from layer A of lateral geniculate nucleus, *J. Neurophysiol.* **49:**595–620.

Martin, K. A. C., and Whitteridge, D., 1984, Form, function and intracortical projections of spiny neurones in the striate visual cortex of the cat, *J. Physiol. (London)* **353**:463–504.

Martin, K. A. C., Somogyi, P., and Whitteridge, D., 1983, Physiological and morphological properties of identified basket cells in the cat's visual cortex, *Exp. Brain Res.* **50**:193–200.

Matsubara, J., Cynader, M., Swindale, N. V., and Stryker, M. P., 1985, Intrinsic projections within visual cortex: Evidence for orientation-specific local connections, *Proc. Natl. Acad. Sci. USA* (in press).

Morrone, M., Durr, D. C., and Maffei, L., 1982, Functional implications of cross-orientation inhibition of cortical visual cells. I. Neurophysiological evidence, *Proc. R. Soc. London Ser. B* **216**:335–354.

Nicoll, R. A., and Newberry, N. R., 1984, A possible synaptic inhibitory action for GABA B receptors on hippocampal pyramidal cells, *Neuropharmacology* **23**:849–850.

Orban, G. A., Kato, H., and Bishop, P. O., 1979, Dimensions and properties of end zone inhibitory areas in receptive fields of hypercomplex cells in cat striate cortex, *J. Neurophysiol.* **42**:833–849.

Peters, A., and Fairén, A., 1978, Smooth and sparsely spined stellate cells in the visual cortex of the rat, a study using combined Golgi electron microscope technique, *J. Comp. Neurol.* **181**:129–172.

Peters, A., and Regidor, J., 1981, A reassessment of the forms of non-pyramidal neurons in area 17 of cat visual cortex, *J. Comp. Neurol.* **203**:685–716.

Poggio, G. F., and Fischer, B., 1977, Binocular interaction and depth sensitivity in striate and prestriate areas of behaving rhesus monkey, *J. Neurophysiol.* **40**:1392–1405.

Ramoa, A. S., Shadlen, M., Skottun, B. C., and Freeman, R. D., 1986, A comparison of inhibition in orientation and spatial frequency selectivity of cat visual cortex, *Nature* **321**:237–239.

Rapisardi, S. C., and Miles, T. P., 1984, Synaptology of retinal terminals in the dorsal lateral geniculate nucleus of the cat, *J. Comp. Neurol.* (in press).

Ribak, C. E., 1978, Aspinous and sparsely-spinous stellate neurons in the visual cortex of rats contain glutamic acid decarboxylase, *J. Neurocytol.* **7**:461–478.

Robson, J. A., 1983, The morphology of corticofugal axons to the dorsal lateral geniculate nucleus of the cat, *J. Comp. Neurol.* **216**:89–103.

Rockland, K. S., and Lund, J. S., 1983, Intrinsic laminar lattice connections in primate visual cortex, *J. Comp. Neurol.* **216**:303–318.

Rose, D., 1977, Responses of single units in cat visual cortex to moving bars of light as a function of bar length, *J. Physiol. (London)* **271**:1–23.

Sandersen, K. J., Bishop, P. O., and Darian-Smith, I., 1971, The properties of the binocular receptive fields of lateral geniculate neurones, *Exp. Brain Res.* **13**:178–207.

Schall, J. D., Vitek, D. J., and Leventhal, A. G., 1986, Retinal constraints on orientation specificity in cat visual cortex, *J. Neurosci.* **6**:823–836.

Scharfman, H. E., and Sarvey, J. M., 1985, Responses to γ-aminobutyric acid applied to cell bodies and dendrites of rat visual cortical neurons, *Brain Res.* **358**:385–389.

Schatz, C. J., and Stryker, M. P., 1978, Ocular dominance in layer IV of the cat's visual cortex and the effects of monocular deprivation, *J. Physiol. (London)* **281**:267–283.

Sherk, H., and LeVay, S., 1983, Contribution of the cortico-claustral loop to receptive field properties in area 17 of the cat, *J. Neurosci.* **3**:2121–2127.

Sillito, A. M., 1975a, The effectiveness of bicuculline as an antagonist of GABA and visually evoked inhibition in the cat's striate cortex, *J. Physiol. (London)* **250**:287–304.

Sillito, A. M., 1975b, The contribution of inhibitory mechanisms to the receptive field properties of neurones in the striate cortex of the cat, *J. Physiol. (London)* **250**:305–322.

Sillito, A. M., 1977, Inhibitory processes underlying the directional specificity of simple complex and hypercomplex cells in the cat's visual cortex, *J. Physiol. (London)* **271**:699–720.

Sillito, A. M., 1979, Inhibitory mechanisms influencing complex cell orientation selectivity and their modification at high resting discharge levels, *J. Physiol. (London)* **289**:33–53.

Sillito, A. M., 1984, Functional considerations of the operation of GABAergic inhibitory processes in the visual cortex, in: *The Cerebral Cortex*, Vol. 2A (A. Peters and E. G. Jones, eds.), Plenum Press, New York.

Sillito, A. M., 1985, Inhibitory circuits and orientation selectivity in the visual cortex, *Models of the Visual Cortex* (D. Rose and V. Dobson, eds.), Wiley, New York.

Sillito, A. M., and Kemp, J. A., 1983, The influence of GABAergic inhibitory processes on the receptive field structure of X and Y cells in cat dorsal lateral geniculate nucleus (dLGN), *Brain Res.* **277**:63–77.

Sillito, A. M., and Versiani, V., 1977, The contribution of excitatory and inhibitory inputs to the length preference of hypercomplex cells in layers II and II of the cat's striate cortex, *J. Physiol. (London)* **273**:775–790.

Sillito, A. M., Kemp, J. A., Milson, J. A., and Berardi, N., 1980a, A reevaluation of the mechanisms underlying simple cell orientation selectivity, *Brain Res.* **194**:517–520.

Sillito, A. M., Kemp, J. A., and Patel, H., 1980b, Inhibitory interactions contributing to the ocular dominance of monocularly dominated cells in the normal cat visual cortex, *Exp. Brain Res.* **41**:1–10.

Singer, W., Tretter, F., and Cynader, M., 1975, Organization of cat striate cortex: A correlation of receptive field properties with afferent and efferent connections, *J. Neurophysiol.* **38**:1080–1098.

Somogyi, P., 1977, A specific "axo-axonal" interneuron in the visual cortex of the rat, *Brain Res.* **136**:345–350.

Somogyi, P., and Cowey, A., 1981, Combined Golgi and electron microscopic study on the synapses formed by double bouquet cells in the visual cortex of the cat and monkey, *J. Comp. Neurol.* **195**:547–566.

Somogyi, P., Cowey, A., Halasz, N., and Freund, T. F., 1981, Vertical organization of neurons accumulating ^{3}H-GABA in the visual cortex of the rhesus monkey, *Nature* **294**:761–763.

Somogyi, P., Kisvarday, Z. F., Martin, K. A. C., and Whitteridge, D., 1983, Synaptic connections of morphologically identified and physiologically characterised large basket cells in the striate cortex of the cat, *Neuroscience* **10**:261–294.

Somogyi, P., Freund, T. F., and Kisvarday, Z. F., 1984, Different types of ^{3}H-GABA accumulating neurons in the visual cortex of the rat: Characterization by combined autoradiography and Golgi impregnation, *Exp. Brain Res.* **54**:45–56.

Spencer, W. A., and Kandel, E. R., 1961, Electrophysiology of hippocampal neurons. III. Firing level and time constant, *J. Neurophysiol.* **24**:260–271.

Toyama, K., Maekawa, K., and Takeda, T., 1977, Convergence of retinal inputs onto visual cortical cells. I. A study of the cells monosynaptically excited from the lateral geniculate body, *Brain Res.* **137**:207–220.

Tsumoto, T., Eckhart, W., and Creutzfeldt, O. D., 1979, Modification of orientation sensitivity of cat visual cortex neurones by removal of GABA mediated inhibition, *Exp. Brain Res.* **34**:351–363.

Vidyasagar, T. R., and Urbas, J. V., 1982, Orientation sensitivity of cat LGN neurones with and without inputs from visual cortical areas 17 and 18, *Exp. Brain Res.* **46**:157–169.

Wiesel, T. N., Hubel, D. H., and Lam, D. M. K., 1974, Autoradiographic demonstration of ocular dominance columns in the monkey striate cortex by means of transneuronal transport, *Brain Res.* **79**:273–279.

Wilson, J. R., Friedlander, M. J., and Sherman, S. M., 1984, Fine structural morphology of identified X- and Y-cells in the cat's lateral geniculate nculeus, *Proc. R. Soc. London Ser. B* **221**:411–436.

Yamane, S., Maske, R., and Bishop, P. O., 1985, Properties of end zone inhibition of hypercomplex cells in cat striate cortex, *Exp. Brain Res.* **60**:200–203.

12

GABAergic Mechanisms and Epileptic Discharges

Massimo Avoli

1. Introduction

Epilepsy is a disorder of brain function characterized by the episodic recurrence of paroxysmal neurological or behavioral manifestations which are caused by abnormal synchronous and excessive discharges of large neuronal populations (Taylor, 1931; Gastaut and Broughton, 1973; Avoli and Gloor, 1987). Based on the fact that normal function in the brain is dependent upon a balance between excitatory and inhibitory processes in neuronal circuits, two types of disturbances of this equilibrium have been considered as possible causes for epileptic discharges: (1) a primary increase of excitatory processes; (2) a decreased efficacy or loss of inhibitory mechanisms which will allow the generation of abnormal paroxysmal neuronal activity.

The aim of this chapter is to review the experimental data related to the second mechanism, namely that of a decreased efficacy of inhibition in the genesis of epileptic discharges. Biochemical, electrophysiological, and pharmacological data suggest that GABA is a ubiquitous inhibitory neurotransmitter in the CNS. Thus, in cortical structures it fully satisfies the criteria required for a substance to be recognized as a transmitter: (1) it is synthesized and accumulates in presynaptic neurons; (2) it is released from their nerve terminals; (3) its action on the postsynaptic neuronal membrane and (4) its inactivation-removal are similar to those of the normally released transmitter; (5) those substances which interfere with the inhibitory postsynaptic potential (IPSP) have similar effects on the neuronal responses to GABA (for review see Krnjević, 1974; Roberts *et al.*, 1976; Johnston, 1978; Nistri and Costanti, 1979).

The first part of this review deals with the physiological actions exerted by both exogenously applied and synaptically released GABA upon cortical neurons. In the second part I shall review different models of epilepsy where a decrease of GABAergic mechanisms has been documented or proposed and discuss the involvement of GABA in the action of several antiepileptic drugs. Finally, the possible role of GABA in human epilepsy will be reviewed.

Massimo Avoli • Montreal Neurological Institute and Department of Neurology and Neurosurgery, McGill University, Montreal, Quebec H3A 2B4, Canada.

2. GABAergic Potentials in Mammalian Cortex

Iontophoretic application of GABA into cortical neurons evokes a quick and reversible depression of the spontaneous firing recorded extracellularly. This powerful inhibitory action, first described by Krnjević and Phillis (1963) and later confirmed in several laboratories (for review see Krnjević, 1974; Nistri and Costanti, 1979), is associated with a membrane hyperpolarization coupled with a marked increase in the membrane conductance to Cl$^-$ ions (Krnjević and Schwartz, 1967). The same ionic mechanism underlies the hyperpolarizing IPSP evoked by the electrical stimulation of a number of pathways in both neocortex and hippocampus (Fig. 1) (Kandel et al., 1961; Andersen et al., 1964a,b; Stefanis and Jasper, 1964; Dreifuss et al., 1969; Renaud et al., 1974; Eccles et al., 1977; Alger and Nicoll, 1982a,b; Avoli, 1986).

Experiments performed in the hippocampus in situ have shown that this hyperpolarizing IPSP is mainly caused by the activation of a recurrent inhibitory system which is mediated by basket cells terminating on or near the soma of pyramidal cells (Andersen et al., 1964a). Accordingly, histochemical studies using either glutamic acid decarboxylase (GAD) activity or GABA histofluorescence as GABA markers have demonstrated this inhibitory transmitter to be largely localized near the stratum pyramidale, where basket cells (i.e., local, presumably inhibitory neurons) are most frequently found (Storm-Mathisen and Fonnum, 1971; Storm-Mathisen, 1975; Barber and Saito, 1976; Ribak et al., 1978). Furthermore, GAD activity is not affected by

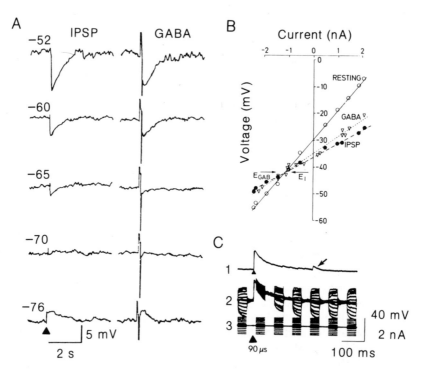

Figure 1. Electrophysiological features of the hyperpolarizing IPSP and of the hyperpolarizing response evoked by GABA iontophoresis in the hippocampus (A) and the neocortex (B, C). In A: intracellular recordings from a pyramidal cell in the CAl subfield of the hippocampal slice reveal a similar behavior for both the IPSP and the GABA-induced response during changes in membrane potential. In B: plot of the voltage–current relationship at resting, at the peak of the IPSP, and during GABA iontophoresis in a cat neocortical neuron recorded in vivo, displays similar membrane potential and conductance change during the IPSP and the action of GABA. In C: synaptic response and associated increase in conductance recorded with a KCl-filled microelectrode in a rat neocortical neuron maintained in vitro. The arrow points to a spontaneously occurring, presumably inverted IPSP. (A from Alger and Nicoll, 1982b; B from Dreifuss et al., 1969; C from Avoli, 1986.)

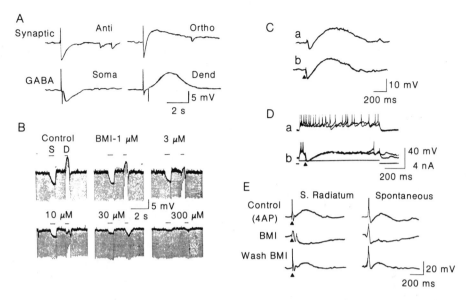

Figure 2. (A) Hyperpolarizing (anti) and depolarizing (ortho) IPSP in the presence of pentobarbital and responses to iontophoresis of GABA into the soma and dendrites of a CAl hippocampal pyramidal cell recorded with a K methyl sulfate-filled electrode. (B) Effects evoked by progressively increasing concentration of bicuculline methiodide (BMI) on the responses to iontophoretic application of GABA into the soma (S) and dendrites (D) of a hippocampal pyramidal cell recorded with a K methyl sulfate-filled electrode (fast deflections in the negative direction in this and the following figure represent intracellularly injected pulses of current to monitor the neuron's input resistance). (C) Similarities between spontaneously occurring (a) and stratum (s.) radiatum-induced (b) long-lasting depolarizing potential in the presence of 4-aminopyridine (4AP) in a hippocampal neuron recorded with K-acetate-filled electrode. (D) Shunting inhibitory effect exerted by the 4AP-induced long-lasting depolarizing potential upon the firing: a shows a repetitive firing evoked by two superimposed depolarizing pulses; b shows the same pulses associated with orthodromic stimulation (▲) in the s. radiatum. (E) Effects evoked by BMI (5μM) upon the s. radiatum-induced and the spontaneously occurring long-lasting depolarizing potential in the presence of 4AP. Action potentials in D and E are truncated. Note in B and E that low concentrations of BMI (i.e., 1–5 μM) blocked the depolarizing component without affecting the hyperpolarizing one. (A and B from Alger and Nicoll, 1982b; C–E from Avoli and Perreault, 1987.)

transection of hippocampal afferents, thus indicating that the GABAergic connections are intrinsic (Storm-Mathisen, 1972). A similar localization has also been suggested for the inhibitory hyperpolarizing inputs which terminate on long-axon cells in the neocortex (Humphrey, 1968; Raabe and Lux, 1972).

The mechanisms underlying the action of GABA and the IPSP have been analyzed further in *in vitro* preparations. In the hippocampal slice, iontophoresis of GABA evokes two distinct effects when applied at two different loci on the same cell: application to the soma causes a hyperpolarization which is reduced by decreasing $[Cl^-]_o$ and has the same equilibrium potential as the hyperpolarization evoked by antidromic or orthodromic stimulation (Fig. 1A) (Andersen *et al.*, 1980; Alger and Nicoll, 1982a,b); application to the dendrites elicits a depolarizing response (Fig. 2A,B) which is most likely produced by a permeability increase to more than one specific ion, including an outward movement of Cl^- (Alger and Nicoll, 1979, 1982b; Andersen *et al.*, 1980; Thalmann *et al.*, 1981). This might imply that in the same hippocampal cell $[Cl^-]_i$ is in fact much higher in the dendrites than in the soma, where GABA induces an inward Cl^- movement (Misgeld *et al.*, 1986). Similar observations have been made in cultured spinal cord cells: in these experiments GABA applications near the soma cause hyperpolarization, whereas applications to dendrite-like processes give di- or multiphasic responses starting with depolarization (Barker and Ransom, 1978a).

The depolarizing potential induced by GABA in the dendrites can also be observed as a postsynaptic phenomenon. Alger and Nicoll (1982a) have recorded, in hippocampal neurons treated with pentobarbital, a slow depolarizing potential which is evoked by orthodromic stimulation (Fig. 2A). Furthermore, in the presence of low doses of 4-aminopyridine, a substance capable of increasing synaptic transmission (Thesleff, 1980; Buckle and Haas, 1982), hippocampal pyramidal cells generate either spontaneously or following orthodromic activation a long-lasting (up to 1.5 sec) depolarizing potential (Fig. 2C) (Avoli and Perreault, 1987). Both the pentobarbital- and the 4-aminopyridine-induced potentials are: (1) associated with an increase in membrane conductance; (2) capable of blocking direct and synaptic activation of the cells (Fig. 2D); and (3) reduced by application of GABA antagonists (Fig. 2E) (Alger and Nicoll, 1982a; Avoli and Perreault, 1987).

A physiological role for the depolarizing response evoked by GABA in the dendrites is in keeping with the presence of interneurons having axonal ramifications in the apical dendritic tree of hippocampal pyramids (Ramón y Cajal, 1893; Lorente de Nó, 1934). In addition, GAD-containing neurons can be found in these dendritic areas (Storm-Mathisen and Fonnum, 1971; Ribak et al., 1978). Thus, the dendritic effect of GABA might represent a new type of inhibitory mechanism capable of shunting selectively some excitatory inputs on the dendrites while facilitating at the same time the effect of other inputs to the same cell (Andersen et al., 1980). This discriminative inhibition stands in contrast to the hyperpolarizing somatic response which has a more global role in stopping any discharge of the cell. It should be noted that in both hippocampus and neocortex a brief depolarizing potential can often be recorded in normal conditions during the hyperpolarization which follows the orthodromically evoked EPSP (Figs. 3Aa, 4).

GABA applications onto the dendrites of hippocampal neurons can also evoke a hyperpolarizing response. As shown by Newberry and Nicoll (1985) this potential is associated with a K^+ conductance and is resistant to bicuculline, a well-known antagonist of the somatic hyperpolarizing and dendritic depolarizing responses to GABA (Fig. 3D,E). Since baclofen is the agonist for this GABA-mediated response (Fig. 3B), the activated receptors have been termed $GABA_B$ in contrast to the $GABA_A$ ones which are linked to the opening of Cl^- channels responsible for the GABA-induced hyperpolarizations at the soma and the depolarizations in the dendrites. A recent report by Andrade et al. (1986) indicates that the opening of the K^+ channels by $GABA_B$ receptors in hippocampal pyramidal cells involves a pertussis toxin-sensitive GTP binding protein.

This $GABA_B$ response is analogous to the late hyperpolarization which follows the EPSP–early IPSP sequence evoked by orthodromic activation of hippocampal or neocortical cells (Figs. 3A, 4) (Fujita, 1979; Connors et al., 1982; Lancaster and Wheal, 1984; Newberry and Nicoll, 1984; Avoli, 1986). This synaptic potential is associated with a K^+ conductance and is enhanced rather than depressed by antagonists of $GABA_A$ receptors (e.g., bicuculline, penicillin, picrotoxin) (Schwartzkroin and Stafstrom, 1980; Thalmann and Ayala, 1982; Newberry and Nicoll, 1984, 1985; Lancaster and Wheal, 1984).

As summarized in Fig. 4, the results reported above suggest that GABA-mediated potentials in cortical neurons are caused by three different mechanisms. These are (1) a hyperpolarizing conductance mediated by Cl^- and caused by the activation of $GABA_A$ receptors located largely in the somatic region; (2) a depolarizing conductance mediated mainly by Cl^- which is due to extrasynaptic or $GABA_A$ receptors in the dendrites; (3) a hyperpolarizing conductance due to a K^+ outward flux which is caused by the activation of $GABA_B$ receptors.

3. GABAergic Mechanisms and Experimental Epileptic Discharges

3.1. Acute Models of Epilepsy

Decrease or loss of efficacy of GABAergic mechanisms has been demonstrated to underlie epileptiform discharges in several preparations. Thus, substances capable of interfering with

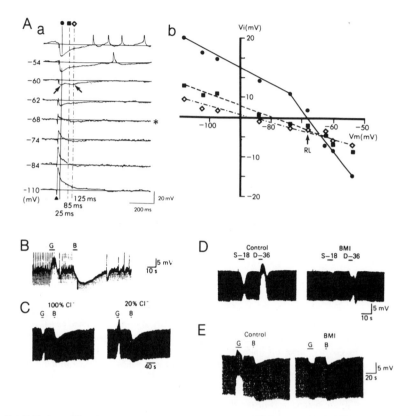

Figure 3. (A) Early and late hyperpolarizing potentials in a rat neocortical neuron maintained *in vitro* following stimulation of the white matter. In b, plot of the amplitudes (Vi) of the synaptic responses shown in a over the membrane potential (Vm) at three different latencies displays two different slopes and two different reversal levels for the early and late hyperpolarizing potentials. This neuron was recorded intracellularly with a K-acetate-filled electrode. Action potentials in a are truncated. (B) Responses evoked by GABA (G) and baclofen (B) in a hippocampal neuron recorded with KCl-filled microelectrode: the GABA response is depolarizing while the baclofen one is still hyperpolarizing, suggesting a Cl⁻ independence of the baclofen response. (C) Same conclusions can be made from this experiment where the external Cl⁻ concentration was reduced while recording with K methyl sulfate-filled electrode; superfusion with a medium containing only 20% Cl⁻ (thionate substitution) for 12 min reverses the GABA- but not the baclofen-induced response. (D) Effects induced by BMI on the responses evoked by GABA application onto the somatic (S) and dendritic (D) regions. Note that BMI blocks the somatic hyperpolarization and the dendritic depolarizing responses, disclosing in the latter cases a hyperpolarization. (E) Dendritic application of both GABA (G) and baclofen (B) in control and during superinfusion of BMI. Note that BMI blocks the dendritic depolarizing response and discloses a hyperpolarizing one while not affecting the baclofen-induced potential (A from Avoli, 1986; B–E from Newberry and Nicoll, 1985.)

GABA synthesis, release, or postsynaptic effects have all displayed potent convulsive effects (see Krnjević, 1983).

Thiosemicarbazide (Killam and Bain, 1957) or methoxypyridoxine (Ozawa and Okada, 1976) induce epileptiform discharges while decreasing the GABA content in the brain through a reduction of GAD activity. Furthermore, a similar mechanism has been shown to account for the genesis of seizures in mice exposed to hyperbaric oxygen (Wood *et al.*, 1966). A relation between the appearance of epileptiform activity and interference with GABA release can be found in experiments where 3-mercaptopropionic acid has been employed (Fan *et al.*, 1981). Also, since tetanus toxin can prevent GABA release in the basal ganglia (Davies and Tongroach, 1979), epileptic activity induced by this toxin might represent a model based on a selective block of GABA release (Krnjević, 1983).

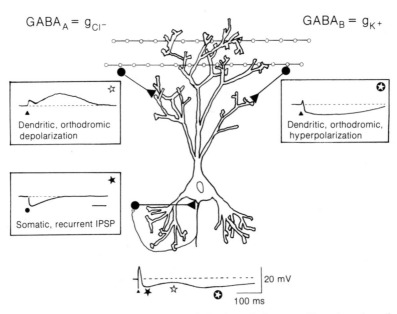

Figure 4. Summary of the different actions exerted by GABA in cortical neurons. Framed panels on the left show drawings of a dendritic, orthodromic depolarizing potential and somatic hyperpolarizing recurrent IPSP. Both responses are caused by GABA$_A$ receptors linked with the opening of Cl$^-$ channels. In the right panel, dendritic orthodromic hyperpolarization caused by activation of GABA$_B$ receptors which are linked with the opening of K$^+$ channels. Note that the latter mechanism might occur at the soma as well. The cell drawn is a pyramidal hippocampal cell, though this basic mechanism should also apply to long-axon pyramidal neurons in the neocortex. Orthodromic response in the bottom part of the figure is an actual intracellular recording from a hippocampal pyramidal neuron in control medium displaying the three different GABAergic mechanisms as indicated by the filled star, open star, and circled star. (P. Perreault and M. Avoli, unpublished data.)

The most detailed studies on the relation between a decrease of GABAergic mechanisms and epileptogenesis have. however, been carried out on the action of chemical convulsants such as penicillin, bicuculline, or picrotoxin. These drugs, when applied topically on a restricted region of the cortex *in situ* or in the artificial cerebrospinal fluid bathing cortical slices maintained *in vitro,* are capable of inducing recurrent epileptiform discharges. This type of activity, when recorded in the EEG, resembles the interictal focal "spikes" or "sharp waves" observed in epileptic patients and is characterized at the intracellular level by the occurrence of large-amplitude depolarizations associated with bursts of action potentials (so-called paroxysmal depolarizing shift) (Ayala *et al.,* 1973; Prince and Connors, 1986) (Fig. 5A). Several investigators have reported that the appearance of epileptiform bursts is accompanied by a decrease or blockade of the recurrent, somatic IPSP (Fig. 5B) and by a striking reduction of the membrane conductance increase invoked by iontophoretic applications of GABA (Wong and Prince, 1979; Dingledine and Gjerstad, 1980; Schwartzkroin and Prince, 1980; Lebeda *et al.,* 1982).

However, low concentrations of these convulsants are capable of increasing the excitability of cortical neurons without changing the efficacy of recurrent inhibitory systems (Fig. 6) (Avoli, 1984). This effect may be related to an alteration of the inhibitory mechanisms located in the dendrites, a notion supported by experiments in the *in vitro* hippocampal slice where: (1) the inhibitory depolarizing responses to iontophoretic GABA applications onto the dendrites of pyramidal cells are reduced by concentrations of convulsants (e.g., 0.1 mM penicillin or 1–3 μM bicuculline) which are lower than those required to affect GABA-induced hyperpolarization at the soma (Fig. 2B) (Alger and Nicoll, 1982b); (2) the dendritic depolarizing GABAergic potential

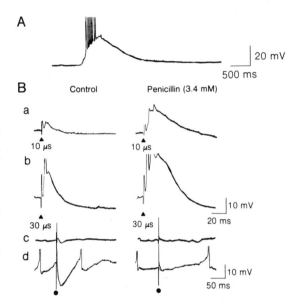

Figure 5. (A) Paroxysmal depolarizing shift recorded intracellularly in a CA1 pyramidal neuron of a hippocampal slice bathed in 20 µM BMI. (B) Effects induced by penicillin upon orthodromic (a, b) and antidromic (c, d) responses of a hippocampal pyramidal neuron in the CA1 subfield. a and b represent two stimuli in s. radiatum at different strengths as obtained by varying the width of the stimulus. c and d are antidromic responses evoked at resting level (c) and at a depolarized level (d). (V. Tancredi and M. Avoli, unpublished data.)

disclosed by 4-aminopyridine is blocked by concentrations of bicuculline (2–5 µM) which do not reduce the recurrent IPSP (Fig. 2E) (Avoli and Perreault, 1987).

Generalized spike and wave discharges induced by intramuscular injections of penicillin in the cat, an experimental model for human absence attacks (Gloor, 1984), may represent a type of epileptic activity caused by such a selective decrease of GABAergic dendritic mechanisms. Both extracellular and intracellular recordings from cat neocortical neurons have shown that well-known GABAergic mechanisms such as those evoked by antidromic stimulation of the pyramidal tract (Stefanis and Jasper, 1964; Renaud et al., 1974) or cortical shock (Krnjević et al., 1966; Dreifuss et al., 1969) as well as neuronal responses to GABA iontophoresis remain essentially unchanged after intramuscular injections of doses of penicillin sufficient to produce spike and wave discharges (Fig. 7) (Kostopoulos et al., 1983; Giaretta et al., 1985, 1987; Kostopoulos, 1986). Furthermore, the rhythmic hyperpolarizations observed during each spike and wave burst are associated with a Cl$^-$ conductance increase as suggested by the reduction and inversion of the early phase during and following Cl$^-$ injections (Fig. 8) (Fisher and Prince, 1977; Giaretta et al.,

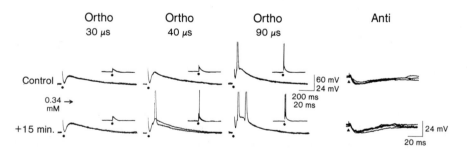

Figure 6. Effects induced by penicillin upon the EPSP (ortho) and the recurrent IPSP (anti). Penicillin at low concentration (0.34 mM) induces an increase of the amplitude and half-width of the EPSP (30 µsec) while at higher intensities of stimulation one (40 µsec) or two (90 µsec) action potentials are evoked. In spite of these changes, the recurrent IPSP is not modified. Small frames show the same responses at lower amplification and speed. (From Avoli, 1984.)

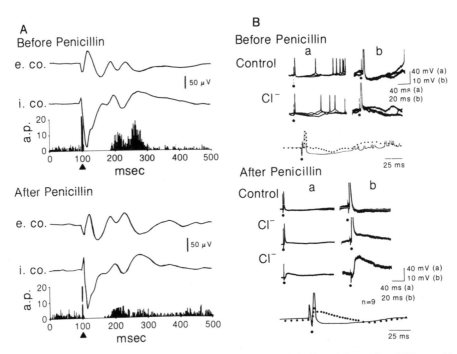

Figure 7. Preservation of the current inhibition after intramuscular injection of doses of penicillin capable of inducing the pattern of generalized spike and wave discharges. (A) Focal potential (e.co. and i.co.) and peristimulus time histogram of a neuron before and after penicillin at a stage of spike and wave discharges. (B) Intracellular responses of two different pericruciate neurons to stimulation of cerebral peduncles and effects induced by intracellular Cl$^-$ injection (records in column b are the same as those in column a, but recorded with a higher amplification and a faster sweep). Lowest traces in upper and lower panels show averages triggered by the stimulus in the cerebral peduncle. Solid line, before Cl$^-$ injection; dotted line, after Cl$^-$ injection. The first neuron (upper panel) was recorded before penicillin administration; the second (lower panel) after penicillin at the time of fully developed SW discharge (Cl$^-$ injected current strength: upper record, 1 nA; lower, 2 nA). (A from Kostopoulos *et al.*, 1983; B from Giaretta *et al.*, 1987.)

1987). As reported by Quesney and Gloor (1978) and Davenport *et al.* (1979), the concentrations of penicillin found in the brain during spike and wave discharges are by one or two orders of magnitude lower than those required to block somatic hyperpolarizing GABAergic potentials, but they are well within the range sufficient to affect, at least in the hippocampus, dendritic responses to GABA (Alger and Nicoll, 1982b).

However, in this model of generalized epilepsy the depression of firing associated with recurrent inhibition or following thalamic or cortical stimulation disappears shortly before the onset as well as during tonic–clonic EEG seizure. This suggests that the transition from spike and wave discharges to generalized tonic–clonic seizures is caused by a breakdown of postsynaptic inhibition (Fig. 9). Such a breakdown of inhibition is also seen to develop during paroxysmal hippocampal discharges evoked in the rat by repetitive electrical stimulation (i.e., in the absence of any GABA$_A$ antagonist) as shown by the blockage of the IPSP and the disappearance of responses to GABA iontophoresis (Ben Ari *et al.*, 1981). Furthermore, in slices of the guinea pig olfactory cortex treated with 4-aminopyridine, a convulsant capable of increasing both excitatory and inhibitory postsynaptic potentials (Thesleff, 1980; Buckle and Haas, 1982), a late, orthodromically induced hyperpolarizing potential is reduced in amplitude and abolished a few seconds before the appearance of seizure-like discharges (Galvan *et al.*, 1982). Thus, findings

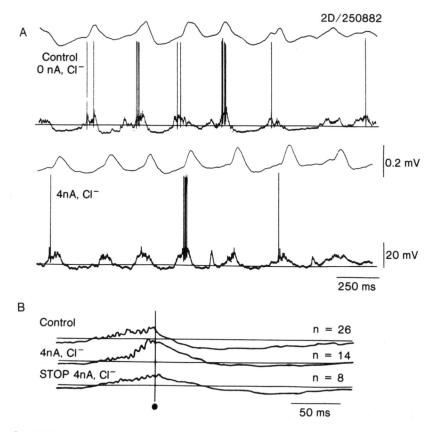

Figure 8. (A) EEG (upper) and intracellular (lower) recordings of a pericruciate neuron during spike and wave discharge before (control: 0 nA, Cl⁻) and during injection of negative current (4 nA, Cl⁻); (B) averages of intracellular recordings triggered by the last action potential in each burst associated with the spike component of the spike and wave discharge (black dot and vertical line) before (control), during (4 nA, Cl⁻), and after cessation of steady negative current (stop 4 nA, Cl⁻). (From Giaretta *et al.*, 1987.)

from both *in vitro* and *in vivo* models point to a loss of synaptic inhibitory mechanisms, presumably hyperpolarizing potentials of both $GABA_A$ and $GABA_B$ type, as causal factor for the onset and maintenance of ictal, seizure-like activity (except for that characterized by spike and wave discharges).

Several interrelated mechanisms may explain the decrease and/or disappearance of synaptic inhibitory potentials immediately before and during sustained seizure discharges. First, hyperpolarizing Cl⁻ IPSPs display a use-dependent depression caused by a decrease in the associated conductance (presumably through a presynaptic mechanism) as well as by a shift in its equilibrium potential (McCarren and Alger, 1985). Second, GABA-induced effects display a rapid decline during maintained application (i.e., desensitization occurs), a phenomenon which might also occur during repetitive inhibitory synaptic activation (Krnjević, 1983). Third, seizure activity is accompanied and in some case shortly preceded by an increase in $[K^+]_o$ (Heinemann *et al.*, 1986; Lux *et al.*, 1986): this will cause a shift of the Cl⁻ equilibrium through a Donnan-like phenomenon as well as a shift in K^+ equilibrium potential for the late $GABA_B$ potential. Four $[Ca^{2+}]_o$ decreases immediately before and during ictal paroxysmal activity (Pumain *et al.*, 1983; Heinemann *et al.*, 1986), thus depressing inhibitory synaptic transmission. It should be noted that

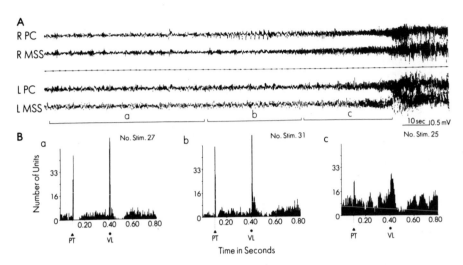

Figure 9. (B) Peristimulus time histograms of an identified pyramidal tract neuron recorded at a stage when spike and wave discharges were cyclically turning into EEG tonic–clonic activity. Computation of each histogram was limited at the period associated with one of three different types of EEG activity as shown in A (i.e., SW discharges in a; initial focal seizure in b; tonic–clonic EEG seizure in c). MSS, middle suprasylvian gyrus; PC, pericruciate gyrus; R, right; L, left. Single cell stimuli were delivered into cerebral peduncles (▲) and nucleus ventralis lateralis (●) of the thalamus.

in the hippocampus $[Ca^{2+}]_o$ falls sharply in the cell body layer where Cl^- hyperpolarizing IPSPs are generated (Krnjević *et al.*, 1982). Thus, in this case, the deficiency of Ca^{2+} would depress particularly the release of GABA and therefore the efficacy of the IPSPs.

3.2. Chronic Models of Epilepsy

A decreased effectiveness of GABAergic mechanisms might also be a feature of several models of chronic epileptic discharge. Ribak *et al.* (1979) have observed a selective loss of GAD-containing cells in epileptic lesions evoked by the application of alumina gel. Findings which are in line with those of Ribak *et al.* have been reported by Bakey and Harris (1981), who demonstrated in monkey cortical epileptic foci a diminution of both GAD activity and GABA receptors without any comparable depletion of other transmitter-related enzymes or receptors. Evidence for a decrease of GABAergic mechanisms has also been shown in epileptogenic lesions induced by the topical application of Co^{2+} to the cortex. Here, however, the fall in GAD activity and GABA content is accompanied by an elevation of GABA binding indicating a possible compensatory increase of receptors to GABA perhaps as the result of denervation supersensitivity (Ross and Craig, 1981).

Histological studies of isolated cortical slabs (Ribak and Reiffenstein, 1982) generating epileptiform activity or motor cortex exposed to severe hypoxia (Sloper *et al.*, 1980) have shown a decrease of symmetrical, type II synapses which are characteristic of inhibitory terminals (Gray, 1959; Eccles, 1969; Peters *et al.*, 1970). Since some human epilepsies may be caused by a hypoxic episode occurring at birth, the evidence of degenerating symmetrical synapses in the motor cortex of young monkeys exposed to severe hypoxia might reveal a fundamental mechanism relevant to human epileptogenesis.

A less clear pattern of changes in inhibitory mechanisms occurs in the kindling model where periodic administration of initially subconvulsive electrical stimuli to a brain structure leads to limbic and clonic motor seizures (Goddard *et al.*, 1969). Several biochemical studies have failed to prove an impairment of GABAergic function in this model of epilepsy (Fabisiek and Schwark, 1982; Lerner-Natoli *et al.*, 1985). However, by using synaptosomal fractions of different regions of amygdaloid-kindled rats a decrease of GAD activity has been shown to occur in the substantia nigra (Löscher and Schwark, 1985). On the other hand, it has been shown that prevention of amygdala kindling can be achieved by inhibiting GABA uptake (Schwark and Halusa, 1986) while an increase of GABA release has been documented in hippocampal slices from kindled rats (Liebowitz *et al.*, 1978). When assessed with electrophysiological techniques, inhibitory mechanisms appear to increase or decrease depending upon the hippocampal regions analyzed or the stage of kindling (Oliver and Miller, 1985; King *et al.*, 1985).

Changes in GABAergic mechanisms appear to occur in some genetic models of epilepsy. In a mouse strain (DBA/2) susceptible to audiogenic seizures, GABA receptor binding is lower than in nonsusceptible strains (Ticku, 1979; Horton *et al.*, 1982). Also, an interesting set of biochemical and morphological data suggestive for changes in GABA function has been reported in the seizure susceptible Mongolian gerbil, a genetic model for generalized epilepsy (Olsen *et al.*, 1986; Ribak, 1986).

4. GABAergic Potentials and Antiepileptic Drugs

The possible relation between epileptic discharge and decreased efficacy of inhibitory mechanisms is supported by the fact that several antiepileptic drugs enhance GABA-mediated inhibition in a variety of preparations.

Barbiturates increase GABAergic potentials through an interaction with the picrotoxin binding site on the GABA–receptor complex (see also Lambert *et al.*, this volume). The end result of this type of interaction is an increase in GABA binding and consequently a modification of the kinetics of the Cl^- channel function (Fig. 10). In line with such a mechanism, pentobarbital prolongs GABAergic IPSPs, presynaptic inhibition, and postsynaptic GABA responses suggesting that it might increase the time of opening of the Cl^- channel (Nicoll, 1975a,b; Nicoll *et al.*, 1975; Barker and Ransom, 1978b; MacDonald and Barker, 1979a,b). Barker and McBurney (1979) have indeed shown that in mouse spinal cord neurons, mean channel opening duration increases severalfold during iontophoresis of phenobarbital while mean channel conductance is not altered significantly.

It should be emphasized that the enhancement of GABA responses is selective since barbiturates do not increase the responses of mouse spinal cord neurons in cell culture to β-alanine, glycine, or taurine (MacDonald and Barker, 1979a,b) (Fig. 10A). Furthermore, although barbiturates can display multiple actions on central neurons (e.g., antagonism of glutamate-induced responses, reduction of Ca^{2+}-dependent action potentials, block of Ca^{2+} uptake by synaptosomes, reduction of neurotransmitter release), the enhancement of GABA responses occurs at concentrations lower than those required for reducing Ca^{2+}-dependent action potential duration but well within the range of anticonvulsant therapeutic free-serum concentrations (for review see MacDonald, 1984).

Benzodiazepines are another group of drugs with anticonvulsant effects which are capable of enhancing GABA-mediated inhibition. Furthermore, as suggested by both *in vivo* and *in vitro* studies (MacDonald and Barker, 1979b; Choi *et al.*, 1977; Tancredi *et al.*, 1983), this effect is highly selective since neuronal responses to glycine, taurine, β-alanine, and glutamic acid are not affected (Fig. 11). Further information on the relation between benzodiazepines and GABA receptors can be found elsewhere in this book (Chapter 13).

Although less compelling than for barbiturates and benzodiazepines, experimental evidence supports a potentiation of GABA-mediated inhibition as mechanisms of action of two other antiepileptic drugs, namely phenytoin and valproic acid. Electrophysiological studies have shown that phenytoin is capable of increasing GABA-mediated presynaptic inhibition and IPSPs in the

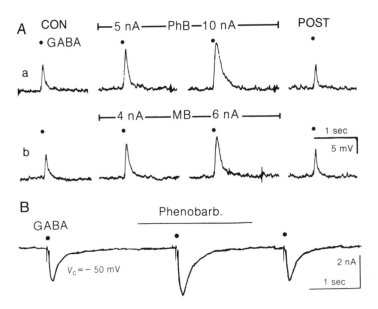

Figure 10. Enhancement of GABA-mediated postsynaptic inhibition by barbiturates in mouse spinal cells in dissociated culture. (A) Responses to GABA iontophoresis increase in amplitude and duration during iontophoresis of phenobarbital (PhB) in a or methobarbital (MB) in b. (B) Potentiation of GABA-induced responses by phenobarbital in a spinal neuron grown in cell culture and recorded in voltage-clamp mode. In these experiments, recordings were done with 3 M KCl-filled electrodes. (A from MacDonald and Barker, 1979a; B from Barker and McBurney, 1979.)

spinal cord, cuneate nucleus, cortex, and crayfish stretch receptors (Davidoff, 1972; Raabe and Ayala, 1976; Deisz and Lux, 1977; Ayala *et al.*, 1977). Valproic acid has been shown to increase selectively the levels of GABA in the brain via an interaction with some of the enzymes involved in the synthesis and degradation of GABA (Godin *et al.*, 1969; Iadarola and Gale, 1979; Löscher, 1981). Furthermore GABA-induced responses are enhanced by application of valproic acid both *in vivo* and *in vitro* (MacDonald and Bergey, 1979; Gent and Phillips, 1980; Baldino and Geller, 1981; Hackman *et al.*, 1981).

5. GABAergic Mechanisms and Human Epilepsies

The clearest demonstration of a relation between GABA and seizures in humans rests on the occurrence of convulsions in infants caused by pyridoxine deficiency (Malony and Parmalee, 1954; Hunt *et al.*, 1954; Coursin, 1954; for a historical review, see Jasper, 1984). Pyridoxine, known also as vitamin B_6, is the coenzyme for the formation of GABA from glutamic acid by means of the enzyme GAD. Thus, following a diet with milk accidentally made deficient in pyridoxine during processing, seizures developed in infants fed on this formula and could be arrested within minutes by administration of pyridoxine (Coursin, 1954).

However, in spite of several attempts to show a change in the content of GABA and related enzymatic activities in human chronic epileptogenic brain tissue, there was no significant difference between cortical areas found to be spiking and nonspiking at the electrocorticography (for review see Sherwin and van Gelder, 1986). Tursky *et al.* (1976) found no difference in the GAD activity of stereotaxic biopsy samples of human hippocampus as compared to nonepileptic tissue removed for other types of pathology. A similar negative finding has been reported by Babb and Brown (1986). Furthermore, Sherwin *et al.* (1984) failed to find a significant change in the mean

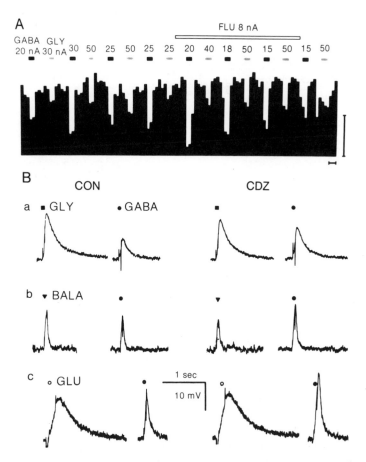

Figure 11. Selective increase by benzodiazepine of GABA-induced responses. (A) Flurazepine (FLU) enhances the decreases of spontaneous firing evoked by iontophoresis of GABA without changing those evoked by glycine (GLY) in a rat cortical neuron recorded *in situ.* (B) Changes induced by chlordiazepoxide (CDZ) upon GABA-induced but not glycine-, β-alanine (BALA)-, or glutamic acid (GLU)-induced responses in a mouse spinal neuron in dissociated culture. (A from Tancredi *et al.,* 1983; B from MacDonald and Barker 1979a.)

activity of GAD in actively spiking neocortical foci. It should be noted that the only report indicating a diminution of GAD activity in nearly half of the samples from human epileptic foci (Lloyd *et al.,* 1983) might have been biased by the presence of reactive astroglia formation which should dilute neuronal elements and consequently lower the GAD activity.

More recently, by using the *in vitro* slice preparation, inhibitory mechanisms have been studied directly in human neurons located in epileptogenic cortical areas. Schwartzkroin *et al.* (1983) had reported that in slices obtained from active epileptogenic areas (as determined with intra-operative electrocorticography), neurons have less effective IPSPs as compared with cells in slices taken from nearby tissue. However, in a more recent paper from the same laboratory, it has been shown that the spontaneous and rhythmic synaptic events recorded in human neurons in epileptic mesial temporal (i.e., probably hippocampal) tissue are GABAergic in nature (Schwartzkroin and Haglund, 1986). Furthermore, a similar type of activity could also be recorded in neurons of normal monkey hippocampus, which was used as normal control.

The ability of human neurons from the epileptic hippocampus to produce spontaneous presumably GABAergic postsynaptic potentials has also been confirmed in our laboratory (Fig.

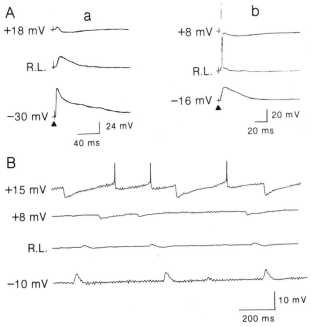

Figure 12. Intracellular recordings in human neocortical (A) and hippocampal (B) neurons with K-acetate-filled electrode. (A) Stimulus-induced synaptic potentials in two different neurons located in epileptic (a) and nonepileptic neocortex (b) display a short-latency hyperpolarizing potential, presumably an IPSP. (B) Spontaneously occurring postsynaptic potential in a hippocampal neuron from an epileptic patient. Note that the spontaneous synaptic potentials were mainly depolarizing at resting levels (R.L.) while they became clearly hyperpolarizing at depolarized membrane levels. (From M. Avoli, unpublished data.)

12B). In addition, we have been able to record stimulus-induced IPSPs which appear to be hyperpolarizing at a depolarizing membrane potential and are associated with an increase in conductance to Cl^- ions. These IPSPs could be recorded in neocortical neurons from brain tissue obtained from patients operated for epileptic as well as nonepileptic pathologies. Although preliminary, these data suggest that inhibitory potentials are not qualitatively different in human epileptogenic neocortex as compared to nonepileptogenic neocortex. However, we still lack information on possible quantitative measures of inhibitory mechanisms in human epileptogenic cortex. At the same time the question whether epileptic human tissue may display abnormalities in inhibitory mechanisms other than those located near the soma (i.e., hyperpolarizing ones), remains unexamined.

ACKNOWLEDGMENTS. This work was supported by the Medical Research Council of Canada (MA 8109) and the Fond de la Recherche en Santé du Québec. I am grateful to Ms. G. Robillard for secretarial assistance.

References

Alger, B. E., and Nicoll, R. A., 1979, GABA-mediated biphasic inhibitory responses in hippocampus, *Nature* **281:**315–317.

Alger, B. E., and Nicoll, R. A., 1982a, Feed-forward dendritic inhibition in rat hippocampal pyramidal cells studied in vitro, *J. Physiol. (London)* **328:**105–123.

Alger, B. E., and Nicoll, R. A., 1982b, Pharmacological evidence for two kinds of GABA receptors on rat hippocampal pyramidal cells studied in vitro, *J. Physiol. (London)* **328:**125–141.

Andersen, P., Eccles, J. C., and Loyning, Y., 1964a, Location of postsynaptic inhibitory synapses on hippocampal pyramids, *J. Neurophysiol.* **27:**592–607.

Andersen, P., Eccles, J. C., and Loyning, Y., 1964b, Pathway of postsynaptic inhibition in the hippocampus, *J. Neurophysiol.* **27:**608–619.

Andersen, P., Dingledine, R., Gjerstad, L., Langmoen, I. A., and Mosfeldt-Laursen, A., 1980, Two different responses of hippocampal pyramidal cells to application of gamma-aminobutyric acid, *J. Physiol. (London)* **305**:279–296.

Andrade, R., Malenka, R. C., and Nicoll, R. A., 1986, A G-protein couples serotonin and GABA_B receptors to the same channels in hippocampus, *Science* **234**:1261–1265.

Avoli, M., 1984, Penicillin-induced hyperexcitability in the "in vitro" hippocampal slice can be unrelated to impairment of somatic inhibition, *Brain Res.* **370**:154–158.

Avoli, M., 1986, Inhibitory potentials in neurons of the deep layers of the "in vitro" neocortical slice, *Brain Res.* **370**:165–170.

Avoli, M., and Gloor, P., 1987, Epilepsy, in: *Encyclopedia of Neuroscience,* Vol. I (G. Adelman, ed.), Birkhäuser, Basel, Stuügard, pp. 400–403.

Avoli, M., and Perreault, P. A., 1987, GABAergic depolarizing potential in the hippocampus disclosed by the convulsant 4-aminopyridine, *Brain Res.* **400**:191–195.

Ayala, G. F., Dichter, M., Gumnit, R. J., Matsumoto, H., and Spencer, W. A., 1973, Genesis of epileptic interictal spikes: New knowledge of cortical feedback systems suggests a neurophysiological explanation of brief paroxysms, *Brain Res.* **52**:1–17.

Ayala, G. F., Lin, S., and Johnston, D., 1977, The mechanism of action of diphenylhydantoin on invertebrate neurons. II. Effects on synaptic mechanisms, *Brain Res.* **121**:259–270.

Babb, T. L., and Brown, W. J., 1986, Neuronal, dendritic and vascular profiles of human temporal lobe epilepsy correlated with cellular physiology "in vivo," *Adv. Neurol.* **44**:949–966.

Bakey, R. A. E., and Harris, A. B., 1981, Neurotransmitter, receptor and biochemical changes in monkey cortical epileptic foci, *Brain Res.* **206**:387–404.

Baldino, F., and Geller, H. M., 1981, Sodium valproate enhancement of gamma-aminobutyric acid (GABA) inhibition—Electrophysiological evidence for anticonvulsant activity, *J. Pharmacol. Exp. Ther.* **217**:445–450.

Barber, R., and Saito, K., 1976, Light microscopic visualization of GAD and GABA-T in immunocytochemical preparations of rodent CNS, in: *GABA in Nervous System Function* (E. Roberts, T. N. Chase, and D. B. Tower, eds.), Raven Press, New York, pp. 113–132.

Barker, J. L., and McBurney, R. N., 1979, Phenobarbitone modulation of postsynaptic GABA receptor function on cultured mammalian neurons, *Proc. R. Soc. London Ser. B* **206**:319–327.

Barker, J. L., and Ransom, B. R., 1978a, Amino acid pharmacology of mammalian central neurones grown in tissue culture, *J. Physiol. (London)* **280**:331–354.

Barker, J. L., and Ransom, B. R., 1978b, Pentobarbitone pharmacology of mammalian central neurones grown in tissue culture, *J. Physiol. (London)* **280**:355–372.

Ben Ari, Y., Krnjević, K., Reiffenstein, R. J., and Reinhardt, W., 1981, Inhibitory conductance changes and action of GABA in rat hippocampus, *Neuroscience* **6**:2445–2463.

Buckle, P. J., and Haas, H. L., 1982, Enhancement of synaptic transmission by 4-aminopyridine in hippocampal slices of the rat, *J. Physiol. (London)* **326**:109–122.

Choi, D. W., Farb, D. H., and Fischbach, G. D., 1977, Chlordiazepoxide selectively augments GABA action in spinal cord cultures, *Nature* **269**:342–344.

Connors, B. W., Gutnick, M. J., and Prince, D. A., 1982, Electrophysiological properties of neocortical neurons in vitro, *J. Neurophysiol.* **48**:1302–1320.

Coursin, D. B., 1954, Convulsive seizures in infants with pyridoxine-deficient diet, *J. Am. Med. Assoc.* **154**:406.

Davenport, J., Schwindt, P. C., and Crill, W. E., 1979, Epileptic doses of penicillin do not reduce a monosynaptic GABA-mediated post-synaptic inhibition in the intact anesthetized cat, *Exp. Neurol.* **65**:552–572.

Davidoff, R. A., 1972, Diphenylhydantoin increases spinal presynaptic inhibition, *Trans. Am. Neurol. Assoc.* **97**:193–196.

Davies, J., and Tongroach, P., 1979, Tetanus toxin and synaptic inhibition in the substantia nigra and striatum of the rat, *J. Physiol. (London)* **290**:23–36.

Deisz, R. A., and Lux, H. D., 1977, Diphenylhydantoin prolongs postsynaptic inhibition and iontophoretic GABA action in the crayfish stretch receptor, *Neurosci. Lett.* **51**:199–203.

Dingledine, R., and Gjerstad, L., 1980, Reduced inhibition during epileptiform activity in the *in vitro* hippocampal slice, *J. Physiol. (London)* **305**:297–313.

Dreifuss, J. D., Kelly, J. S., and Krnjević, K., 1969, Cortical inhibition and gamma-aminobutyric acid, *Exp. Brain Res.* **9**:137–154.

Eccles, J. C., 1969, *The Inhibitory Pathways of the Central Nervous System,* Thomas, Springfield, Ill.

Eccles, J. C., Nicoll, R. A., Oshima, T., and Rubia, F. J., 1977, The anionic permeability of the inhibitory postsynaptic membrane of hippocampal pyramidal cells, *Proc. R. Soc. London Ser. B* **198**:345–361.

Fabisiek, J. P., and Schwark, W. S., 1982, Cerebral amino acids in the amygdala kindling model of epilepsy, *Neuropharmacology* **21:**179–182.

Fan, S. G., Wusteman, M., and Iversen, L. L., 1981, 3-Mercaptopropionic acid inhibits GABA release from rat brain slices in vitro, *Brain Res.* **228:**379–387.

Fisher, R. S., and Prince, D. A., 1977, Spike–wave rhythms in cat cortex induced by parenteral penicillin. II. Cellular features, *Electroencephalogr. Clin. Neurophysiol.* **42:**625–639.

Fujita, Y., 1979, Evidence for the existence of inhibitory postsynaptic potentials in dendrites and their functional significance in hippocampal pyramidal cells of adult rabbits, *Brain Res.* **175:**59–69.

Galvan, M., Grafe, P., and ten Bruggengate, G., 1982, Convulsant actions of 4-aminopyridine on the guinea pig olfactory cortex slice, *Brain Res.* **241:**75–86.

Gastaut, H., and Broughton, R., 1973, Epileptic seizures: Their clinical nature, pathophysiologic and differential diagnosis, in: *Anticonvulsant Drugs*, Vol. I (J. Mercier, ed.), Pergamon Press, New York, pp. 3–44.

Gent, J. P., and Phillips, N. I., 1980, Sodium di-n-propylacetate (valproate) potentiates responses to GABA and muscimol on single central neurons, *Brain Res.* **197:**275–278.

Giaretta, D., Kostopoulos, G., Gloor, P., and Avoli, M., 1985, Intracortical inhibitory mechanisms are preserved in feline generalized penicillin epilepsy, *Neurosci. Lett.* **59:**203–208.

Giaretta, D., Avoli, M., and Gloor, P., 1987, Intracellular recordings in pericruciate neurons during spike and wave discharges of feline generalized penicillin epilepsy, *Brain Res.* **405:**68–79.

Gloor, P., 1984, Electrophysiology of generalized epilepsy, in: *Electrophysiology of Epilepsy* (P. A. Schwartzkroin and H. Wheal, eds.), Academic Press, New York, pp. 109–136.

Goddard, G. V., McIntyre, D. C., and Leech, C. K., 1969, A permanent change in brain function resulting from daily electrical stimulation, *Exp. Neurol.* **25:**295–330.

Godin, Y., Heiner, L., Mark, J., and Mandel, P., 1969, Effects of di-n-propyl-acetate, an anticonvulsant compound on GABA metabolism, *J. Neurochem.* **16:**869–873.

Gray, E. G., 1959, Axo-somatic and axo-dendritic synapses of the cerebral cortex: An electron microscope study, *J. Anat.* **93:**420–433.

Hackman, J. C., Grayson, V., and Davidoff, R. O., 1981, The presynaptic effects of valproic acid in the isolated frog spinal cord, *Brain Res.* **220:**269–285.

Heinemann, U., Konnerth, A., Pumain, R., and Wadman, W., 1986, Extracellular calcium and potassium concentration changes in chronic epileptic brain tissue, *Adv. Neurol.* **44:**641–661.

Horton, R. W., Prestwick, S. A., and Meldrum, B. S., 1982, Gaba and benzodiazepine binding sites in audiogenic seizure susceptible mice, *J. Neurochem.* **39:**864–770.

Humphrey, D. E., 1968, Reanalysis of the antidromic cortical response. II. On the contribution of cell discharge and PSPs to the evoked potentials, *Electroencephalogr. Clin. Neurophysiol.* **25:**421–442.

Hunt, A. D., Stokes, J., McCrory, W. W., and Stroud, H. H., 1954, Pyridoxine dependency: Report of a case of intractable convulsions in an infant controlled by pyridoxine, *Pediatrics* **13:**140.

Iadarola, M. J., and Gale, K., 1979, Dissociation between drug-induced increase in nerve terminal and non-nerve terminal pools of GABA in vivo, *Eur. J. Pharmacol.* **59:**125–129.

Jasper, H. H., 1984, The saga of K. A. C. Elliott and GABA, *Neurochem. Res.* **9:**449–460.

Johnston, G. A. R., 1978, Neuropharmacology of amino acid inhibitory transmitters, *Annu. Rev. Pharmacol. Toxicol.* **18:**269–289.

Kandel, E. R., Spencer, W. A., and Brinley, F. J., 1961, Electrophysiology of hippocampal neurons. I. Sequential invasion and synaptic organization, *J. Neurophysiol.* **24:**225–242.

Killam, K. F., and Bain, J. A., 1957, Convulsant hydrozides. I. In vitro and in vivo inhibition of vitamin B6 enzymes by convulsant hydrazides, *J. Pharmacol. Exp. Ther.* **119:**255–262.

King, G. L., Dingledine, R., Giacchino, J. L., and McNamara, J. A., 1985, Abnormal neuronal excitability in hippocampal slices from kindled rats, *J. Neurophysiol.* **54:**1295–1304.

Kostopoulos, G., 1986, Neuronal sensitivity to GABA and glutamate in generalized epilepsy with spike and wave discharges, *Exp. Neurol.* **92:**20–36.

Kostopoulos, G., Avoli, M., and Gloor, P., 1983, Participation of cortical recurrent inhibition in the genesis of the spike and wave discharges in feline generalized penicillin epilepsy, *Brain Res.* **267:**101–112.

Krnjević, K., 1974, Chemical nature of synaptic transmission in vertebrates, *Physiol. Rev.* **54:**419–450.

Krnjević, K., 1983, GABA mediated inhibitory mechanisms in relation to epileptic discharge, in: *Basic Mechanisms of Neuronal Hyperexcitability* (H. H. Jasper and N. M. van Gelder, eds.), Liss, New York, pp. 249–280.

Krnjević, K., and Phillis, J. W., 1963, Iontophoretic studies of neurons in the mammalian cerebral cortex, *J. Physiol. (London)* **165:**274–304.

Krnjević, K., and Schwartz, S., 1967, The action of γ-aminobutyric acid on cortical neurons, *Exp. Brain Res.* **3:**320–336.

Krnjević, K., Randic, M., and Straughan, D. W., 1966, Nature of a cortical inhibitory process, *J. Physiol. (London)* **184**:49–77.

Krnjević, K., Morris, M. E., and Reiffenstein, R. J., 1982, Stimulation evoked changes in extracellular K^+ and Ca^{++} concentrations in pyramidal layer of the rat hippocampus, *Can. J. Physiol. Pharmacol.* **60**:1643–1657.

Lancaster, B., and Wheal, H. V., 1984, The synaptically evoked hyperpolarization in hippocampal CA1 pyramidal cells is resistant to intracellular EGTA, *Neuroscience* **12**:267–275.

Lebeda, F. J., Hablitz, J. J., and Johnston, D., 1982, Antagonism of GABA-mediated responses by d-tubocurarine in hippocampal neurons, *J. Neurophysiol.* **48**:622–632.

Lerner-Natoli, M., Heaulme, M., Leyris, R., Biziere, K., and Londouin, G., 1985, Absence of modifications in GABA metabolism after repeated generalized seizures in amygdala-kindled rats, *Neurosci. Lett.* **62**:271–276.

Liebowitz, N., Pedley, T., and Cutler, W., 1978, Release of GABA from hippocampal slices of the rat following generalized seizures induced by daily electrical stimulation of entorhinal cortex, *Brain Res.* **138**:369–373.

Lloyd, K. G., Munari, C., Worms, P., Bossi, L., and Morselli, P. L., 1983, Indications for the use of gamma-aminobutyric acid (GABA)-agonists in convulsant disorders, in: *Progress in Clinical and Biological Research,* Vol. 124 (G. Nistico, R. Di Perri, and H. Meinardi, eds.), Liss, New York, pp. 285–297.

Lorente de Nó, R., 1934, Studies on the structure of the cerebral cortex. II. Continuation of the study of the ammonic system, *J. Psychol. Neurol.* **46**:113–177.

Löscher, W., 1981, Valproate induced changes in GABA metabolism at the subcellular level, *Biochem. Pharmacol.* **30**:1364–1366.

Löscher, W., and Schwark, W. S., 1985, Evidence for impaired GABAergic activity in the substantia nigra of amygdaloid kindled rats, *Brain Res.* **339**:146–150.

Lux, H. D., Heinemann, U., and Dietzel, I., 1986, Ionic changes and alterations in the site of the extracellular space during epileptic activity, *Adv. Neurol.* **44**:619–638.

McCarren, M., and Alger, B. E., 1985, Use-dependent depression of IPSPs in rat hippocampal pyramidal cells in vitro, *J. Neurophysiol.* **53**:557–571.

MacDonald, R. L., 1984, Anticonvulsant and convulsant drug actions on vertebrate neurones in primary dissociated cell culture, in: *Electrophysiology of Epilepsy* (P. A. Schwartzkroin and H. Wheal, eds.), Academic Press, New York, pp. 353–387.

MacDonald, R. L., and Barker, J. L., 1979a, Enhancement of GABA-mediated postsynaptic inhibition in cultured mammalian spinal cord neurons: A common mode of anticonvulsant action, *Brain Res.* **167**:323–336.

MacDonald, R. L., and Barker, J. L., 1979b, Anticonvulsant and anesthetic barbiturates: Different postsynaptic actions on cultured mammalian neurons, *Neurology* **29**:432–447.

MacDonald, R. L., and Bergey, G. K., 1979, Valproic acid augments GABA-mediated postsynaptic inhibition in cultured mammalian neurones, *Brain Res.* **170**:558–562.

Malony, C. J., and Parmalee, A. H., 1954, Convulsions in young infants as a result of pyridoxine (vitamin B6) deficiency, *J. Am. Med. Assoc.* **154**:405.

Misgeld, U., Deisz, R. A., Dodt, H. V., and Lux, H. D., 1986, The role of chloride transport in post-synaptic inhibition of hippocampal neurons, *Science* **232**:1413–1415.

Newberry, N. R., and Nicoll, R. A., 1984, A bicuculline-resistant inhibitory post-synaptic potential in rat hippocampal pyramidal cells in vitro, *J. Physiol. (London)* **348**:239–254.

Newberry, N. R., and Nicoll, R. A., 1985, Comparison of the action of baclofen with γ-aminobutyric acid on rat hippocampal pyramidal cells in vitro, *J. Physiol. (London)* **360**:161–185.

Nicoll, R. A., 1975a, Pentobarbital: Action on frog motoneurons, *Brain Res.* **96**:119–123.

Nicoll, R. A., 1975b, Presynaptic action of barbiturates on the frog spinal cord, *Proc. Natl. Acad. Sci. USA* **72**:1460–1463.

Nicoll, R. A., Eccles, J. C., Oshima, T., and Rubia, F., 1975, Prolongation of hippocampal inhibitory post-synaptic potentials by barbiturates, *Nature* **258**:625–627.

Nistri, A., and Costanti, A., 1979, Pharmacological characterization of different types of GABA and glutamate receptors in vertebrate and invertebrates, *Prog. Neurobiol.* **13**:117–235.

Oliver, M. W., and Miller, J. J., 1985, Alterations of inhibitory processes in the dentate gyrus following kindling-induced epilepsy, *Exp. Brain Res.* **57**:443–447.

Olsen, R. W., Wamsley, J. K., Lee, R. J., and Lomax, P., 1986, Benzodiazepine barbiturate–GABA receptor chloride ionophore complex in a genetic model for generalized epilepsy, *Adv. Neurol.* **44**:365–378.

Ozawa, S., and Okada, Y., 1976, Decrease of GABA and appearance of depolarization shift in thin hippocampal slices "in vitro," in: *GABA in Nervous System Function* (E. Roberts, T. N. Chase, and D. B. Tower, eds.), Raven Press, New York, pp. 449–454.

Peters, A., Palay, S. L., and Webster, H. de F., 1970, *The Fine Structure of the Nervous System: The Cells and Their Processes,* Harper & Row, New York.

Prince, D. A., and Connors, B. W., 1986, Mechanisms of interictal epileptogenesis, *Adv. Neurol.* **44**:275–299.

Pumain, R., Kurcewicz, I., and Louvel, J., 1983, Fast extracellular calcium transients: Involvement in epileptic processes, *Science* **222**:177–179.

Quesney, L. F., and Gloor, P, 1978, Generalized penicillin epilepsy in the cat: Correlation between electrophysiological data and distribution of ^{14}C-penicillin in the brain, *Epilepsia* **19**:34–45.

Raabe, W., and Ayala, G. F., 1976, Diphenylhydantoin increases cortical postsynaptic inhibition, *Brain Res.* **105**:597–601.

Raabe, W., and Lux, H. D., 1972, Studies on extracellular potentials generated by synaptic activity on single cat motor cortex neurons, in: *Synchronization of EEG Activity in Epilepsy* (H. Petsche and M. A. B. Brazier, eds.), Springer-Verlag, Berlin, pp. 46–58.

Ramón y Cajal, S., 1893, Beiträge zur feineren Anatomie des grossen Hirns. I. Über die feinere Struktur des Ammonhornes, *Z. Wiss. Zool.* **56**:615–663.

Renaud, L. P., Kelly, J. S., and Provini, L., 1974, Synaptic inhibition in pyramidal tract neurons: Membrane potential and conductance changes evoked by pyramidal tract and cortical stimulation, *J. Neurophysiol.* **37**:1144–1155.

Ribak, C. E., 1986, Contemporary methods in neurocytology and their application to the study of epilepsy, *Adv. Neurol.* **44**:739–765.

Ribak, C. E., and Reiffenstein, R. J., 1982, Selective inhibitory synapse loss in chronic cortical slabs: A morphological basis for epileptic susceptibility, *Can. J. Physiol. Pharmacol.* **60**:864–870.

Ribak, C. E., Vaughn, J. E., and Saito, K., 1978, Immunocytochemical localization of glutamic acid decarboxylase in neuronal somata following colchicine inhibition of axonal transport, *Brain Res.* **140**:315–322.

Ribak, C. E., Harris, A. B., Vaughn, J. E., and Roberts, E., 1979, Inhibitory GABAergic nerve terminals decrease at sites of focal epilepsy, *Science* **205**:211–214.

Roberts, E., Chase, T. N., and Tower, D. B. (eds.), 1976, *GABA in Nervous System Function*, Raven Press, New York.

Ross, S. M. E., and Craig, C. R., 1981, GABA concentration, L-glutamate-1-decarboxylase activity and properties of the GABA postsynaptic receptor in cobalt epilepsy in the rat, *J. Neurosci.* **1**:1338–1396.

Schwark, W. S., and Halusa, M., 1986, Prevention of amygdala kindling with an inhibitor of γ-aminobutyric acid uptake, *Neurosci. Lett.* **69**:65–69.

Schwartzkroin, P. A., and Haglund, M. M., 1986, Spontaneous rhythmic synchronous activity in epileptic human and normal monkey temporal lobe, *Epilepsia* **27**:523–533.

Schwartzkroin, P. A., and Prince, D. A., 1980, Changes in excitatory and inhibitory synaptic potentials leading to epileptogenic activity, *Brain Res.* **183**:61–76.

Schwartzkroin, P. A., and Stafstrom, C. E., 1980, Effects of EGTA on the calcium activated afterhyperpolarization in hippocampal CA3 pyramidal cells, *Science* **210**:1125–1126.

Schwartzkroin, P. A., Turner, D. A., Knowles, W. D., and Wyler, A. R., 1983, Study on human and monkey "epileptic" neocortex in the in vitro slice preparation, *Ann. Neurol.* **13**:249–257.

Sherwin, A. L., and van Gelder, N., 1986, Amino acid and catecholamine markers of metabolic abnormalities in human focal epilepsy, *Adv. Neurol.* **44**:1011–1032.

Sherwin, A. L., Quesney, L. F., Gauthier, S., Olivier, A., Robitaille, Y., McQuaid, P., Harvey, C., and van Gelder, N., 1984, Enzyme changes in actively spiking areas of human epileptic cerebral cortex, *Neurology* **34**:927–933.

Sloper, J. J., Johnson, P., and Powell, T. P. S., 1980, Selective degeneration of interneurons in the motor cortex of infant monkeys following controlled hypoxia: A possible cause of epilepsy, *Brain Res.* **198**:204–209.

Stefanis, C., and Jasper, H. H., 1964, Recurrent collateral inhibition in pyramidal tract neurons, *J. Neurophysiol.* **27**:855–877.

Storm-Mathisen, J., 1972, Glutamate decarboxylase in the rat hippocampal region after lesions of the afferent fibre systems: Evidence that the enzyme is localized in intrinsic neurons, *Brain Res.* **40**:215–235.

Storm-Mathisen, J., 1975, High activity uptake of GABA in presumed GABAergic nerve endings in the rat brain, *Brain Res.* **84**:409–427.

Storm-Mathisen, J., and Fonnum, F., 1971, Quantitative histochemistry of glutamate decarboxylase in the rat hippocampal region, *J. Neurochem.* **18**:1105–1111.

Tancredi, V., Frank, C., Brancati, A., Avoli, M., and White, P., 1983, Interactions between amino acid and neurotransmitters and flurazepam in the neocortex of unanesthetized rats. *J. Neurosci. Res.* **9**:159–164.

Taylor, J., 1931, *Selected Writing of John Hughlings Jackson, on Epilepsy and Epileptiform Convulsion*, Vol. I, Hodder & Stoughton, London.

Thalmann, R. H., and Ayala, G. F., 1982, A late increase in K conductance follows synaptic stimulation of granule neurons of the dentate gyrus, *Neurosci. Lett.* **23**:243–248.

Thalmann, R. H., Peck, E. J., and Ayala, G. F., 1981, Biphasic response of hippocampal pyramidal neurons to GABA, *Neurosci. Lett.* **21**:319–324.

Thesleff, S., 1980, Aminopyridines and synaptic transmission, *Neuroscience* **5**:1413–1419.

Ticku, M. K., 1979, Differences in GABA receptor sensitivity in inbred strains of mice, *J. Neurochem.* **33**:1136–1138.

Tursky, T., Lassanova, M., Sramka, M., and Nadvornik, P., 1976, Formation of glutamate and GABA in epileptogenic tissue from human hippocampus in vitro, *Acta Neurochir. Suppl.* **23**:111–118.

Wong, R. K. S., and Prince, D. A., 1979, Dendritic mechanisms underlying penicillin-induced epileptiform activity, *Science* **204**: 1228–1231.

Wood, J. D., Watson, W. J., and Stacey, N. E., 1966, A comparative study of hyperbaric oxygen-induced and drug-induced convulsions with particular reference to γ-aminobutyric acid metabolism, *J. Neurochem.* **13**:361–370.

13

Modulatory Sites Associated with the GABA Receptor–Ionophore Complex and the Development of New, Potentially Specific Therapeutic Agents

J. D. C. Lambert, E. N. Petersen, M. S. Jensen, and L. H. Jensen

1. General Introduction

Most drugs which act on the central nervous system (CNS) do so by interfering with chemical transmission between nerve cells. This may be achieved in many ways, e.g., receptor blockade, stimulation or depression of presynaptic transmitter synthesis, blockade of transmitter uptake or inactivation, and so on. Most of the centrally active drugs which have been in use for a long time were originally discovered on an empirical basis. Examples are naturally occurring alkaloids (many of which had been known for generations to be psychoactive, analgesic, and so on) and more or less randomly synthesized molecules (e.g., barbiturates, neuroleptics). Many of these agents have proved to be very useful tools to the basic scientist in his efforts to investigate and understand the workings of the nervous system. With this understanding of transmitters, receptors, and synaptic mechanisms, it has in turn been possible to transform the art of drug molecule design into more of a science. Ultimately, it becomes possible to predict the pharmacological profile of a new molecule before it is synthesized. In this way, drugs can be designed which have a sharper profile of action, so increasing specificity and eliminating unwanted side effects. There are, however, other considerations to be made before a substance which performs well in experimental models can be considered to have a future in the clinic. It must be able to cross the blood–brain barrier, either directly or as a precursor; its biological half-time should not be inappropriately short or long; it should not have side effects (e.g., on visceral organs) which are unrelated to its central action.

A case in point is provided by agents which are active at the benzodiazepine (BZ) receptor. BZs (e.g., chlordiazepoxide, valium) were first introduced into the clinic in the 1960s as minor tranquilizers. The pharmacological profile of BZ action is (in order of increasing dose) anxiolytic,

J. D. C. Lambert and M. S. Jensen • Institute of Physiology, Århus University, 8000 Århus C, Denmark.   E. N. Petersen and L. H. Jensen • A/S Ferrosan Research Division, Sydmarken 5, 2860 Søborg, Denmark.   Present address for E. N. P.: Als Dumex, DK-2300, Copenhagen, Denmark.

antiepileptic, hypnotic, amnesic, and muscle relaxant. In view of their low toxicity, BZs quickly became the drug of choice for many conditions where barbiturates had previously been indicated. BZs are now a panacea of the Western world. In a given year about 20% of the population will consume a BZ preparation. It was not until about 20 years after their discovery that significant progress was made in determining the site and mechanism of action of BZs. Specific receptors for BZs were then demonstrated in the CNS, and BZs were found to prolong inhibition at synapses where GABA is the transmitter. With the precedent provided by the morphine-opiate system, a search was made for an endogenous ligand. This unearthed a totally different class of molecules—the β-carboline esters—which were active at the same receptor as BZs. Surprisingly, the behavioral profile of these first β-carbolines was opposite that of the BZs. They were anxiogenic and either frank convulsants or proconvulsants. They could also be shown to reduce GABA responses. Two important pharmacological principles were demonstrated by this system. (1) The BZ receptor is connected to the GABA receptor–ionophore complex in such a way that occupation of the former by an appropriate ligand modulates the efficacy of GABA as an inhibitory transmitter. (2) The structure of the ligand determines whether the modulation is positive (GABA action enhanced) or negative (GABA action depressed).

Although it now seems unlikely that an endogenous BZ ligand will be found among the ranks of the β-carbolines, these substances have proved to be valuable in determining the molecular configuration and operation of the BZ receptor. It also seems likely that β-carbolines will provide some clinically useful drugs for the future. A range of β-carbolines has now been synthesized which have actions ranging from BZ-like to BZ-opposite. Within this range it is possible to select for a sharper profile of activity (i.e., fewer side effects), e.g., antiepileptic, anxiolytic, memory and awareness enhancement.

This chapter will deal with GABAergic inhibitory mechanisms and the associated modulatory sites which alter the efficacy whereby interaction of GABA with its receptor is translated into an increase in ionic permeability and neuronal inhibition. The greatest emphasis will be placed on the BZ receptor. The system will be considered at three levels of organization: (1) the molecular level, where the structure and function of the receptors will be briefly reviewed; (2) the cellular level, where electrophysiological techniques have been used to determine how the response of the neuron as a whole is modulated by interaction at the receptors; (3) the whole animal level, where the behavioral profile (and preliminary clinical tests) of β-carboline derivatives will be presented. This division has not been applied dogmatically, but relaxed where the nature of the material demands extensive cross-referencing between the categories.

2. Molecular Structure and Function of the GABA Receptor–Ionophore Complex

GABA has been established as a major transmitter of inhibition in the CNS (Nistri and Constanti, 1979). On a pharmacological and mechanistic basis, at least two receptors for GABA have been identified. These have been termed $GABA_A$ and $GABA_B$, respectively. The latter are activated specifically by baclofen and probably mediate an inhibition of adenylate cyclase (Dolphin, 1984). This chapter will concentrate on $GABA_A$ receptors, which are coupled to an anion-selective ionophore, Cl^- being the major charge carrier *in vivo*. Operation of the ionophore is rapid and the synaptic current flows for a few milliseconds (Nistri *et al.*, 1980). This usually causes a transient hyperpolarization of the postsynaptic membrane—the inhibitory postsynaptic potential (IPSP). The $GABA_A$ receptor is blocked by bicuculline in a competitive manner.

The GABA receptor–ionophore complex is also coupled to a number of modulatory receptors (Olsen, 1982; Bræstrup and Nielsen, 1983). The presence of an appropriate ligand at these sites causes either enhancement or depression of GABAergic transmission. Many centrally acting drugs exert their action through this system. Two major groups of drugs which potentiate GABAergic transmission are the BZs and the barbiturates. That barbiturates are generally stronger depressants than BZs probably results from the fact that they also depress synaptic excitation mediated by excitatory amino acids (Barker and Ransom, 1978b; Lambert and Flatman, 1981). Convulsants such as picrotoxin and the bicyclic cage convulsants (e.g., *t*-butylbicyclo-phos-phorothionate, TBPS) depress GABAergic transmission by acting at a site associated with the Cl^- ionophore (Tallman and Gallagher, 1985).

2.1. The GABA$_A$ Receptor

Binding studies on GABA$_A$ receptors (as distinct from uptake sites) in membrane fragments show receptor heterogeneity with affinities (K_a) ranging from $\sim 10^{-8}$ M to 10^{-7} M (see Olsen, 1982). This contrasts with an ED$_{50}$ value for enhancement of BZ binding by GABA of around 10^{-6} M (Bræstrup *et al.*, 1979b), while from electrophysiological experiments, the dose of GABA necessary to evoke a detectable response is around 10^{-5} M (Farb *et al.*, 1984). In the intact neuron it is probably the low-affinity receptor which mediates the increase in Cl^- permeability. The high-affinity receptors may represent a conformational state which is a function of the membrane fragment preparation (Tallman and Gallagher, 1985), and assay conditions may also explain discrepancies between affinity constants (Olsen, 1982). The nature of the GABA receptor which is coupled to the BZ receptor is dealt with in greater detail in Section 3.

2.2. BZ Receptors

High-affinity (K_D around 10^{-9} M), specific binding sites for BZs have been demonstrated in the CNS of vertebrates which are phylogenetically younger than the bony fishes (Möhler and Okada, 1977; Squires and Bræstrup, 1977). There is a strong (though not absolute) correlation between the ability of a range of BZ analogues to displace ^{3}[H]diazepam from its binding sites and their potency in animal models designed to test behavioral actions (Bræstrup and Squires, 1978; Möhler and Okada, 1978). This strongly suggests that the BZ binding sites are indeed the receptors through which BZs exert their behavioral actions. These BZ receptors are located on neurons (Bræstrup *et al.*, 1979a) and at GABAergic synapses (Möhler *et al.*, 1981).

Although biochemical evidence suggests a linkage of GABA and BZ receptors at the molecular level, the correlation between anatomical localization of GABA and BZ binding sites is not very good when studied in the whole CNS. For example, BZ binding sites can be shown autoradiographically in areas of the CNS with poor expression of binding sites for the GABA-mimetic, muscimol (Unnerstall *et al.*, 1981). The colocalization of the receptors has also been studied extensively in the cerebellum. GABA$_A$ binding sites are preferentially located in the granule and Purkinje cell layers (Chan-Palay, 1978), which is also the location of GABAergic synapses. On the other hand, BZ binding sites are mainly concentrated in the molecular layer. Fry *et al.* (1985) have studied binding site distribution in a mouse mutant ("Lurcher"), which has lost all Purkinje cells and 90% of granule cells. While they have shown the expected large decrease in GABA$_A$ receptors when compared to the control, no difference in BZ binding was seen, either with ^{3}[H]flunitrazepam or quantitative autoradiography. The majority of GABA receptors do not, therefore, appear to be linked with BZ receptors. These apparent contradictions may be resolved with a better understanding of the subtypes of BZ receptors (see below) and their coupling to the GABA receptor.

Another type of BZ receptor, characterized by its high affinity for the BZ analogue Ro 5-4864, exists on glial cells (Gallagher *et al.*, 1981) and on peripheral, nonneuronal structures (Wang *et al.*, 1980), but is probably not involved in the behavioral manifestations of BZs.

2.2.1. Ligands that Bind at the BZ Receptor—The Concept of Agonist and Inverse Agonist

In their search for an endogenous BZ ligand, Bræstrup and colleagues screened human urine for compounds which were able to inhibit competitively diazepam binding. This led to the discovery of the β-carbolines (Nielsen *et al.*, 1979; Bræstrup *et al.*, 1980). The first β-carboline derivative tested was the ester, ethyl-β-carboline-3-carboxylate (β-CCE), which was probably formed during alcoholic extraction. Its affinity for BZ binding sites (K_D around 10^{-9} M) proved to be comparable with, or even greater than, diazepam and other potent BZ ligands (Bræstrup and Nielsen, 1983; Bræstrup *et al.*, 1983b).

The behavioral profile of the original β-carbolines, however, proved to be opposite to that of BZs (see Section 4). Not only did they antagonize the action of BZs, but they were shown to be convulsant or proconvulsant and anxiogenic in their own right (Oakley and Jones, 1980; Bræstrup *et al.*, 1982; Nutt *et al.*, 1982). This was the first time that agents which act at the same receptor were shown to have opposite effects and this new concept required a new nomenclature for ligands acting at the BZ receptor. Strictly speaking, a receptor should be named according to the endogenous ligand. This was not available for the present system. Thus, on the historical basis that BZs were the first substances studied, Polc *et al.* (1982) suggested that ligands producing classical BZ-like effects (including more recently synthesized β-carbolines) be termed *agonists* at the receptor while ligands whose behavioral profile was opposite to BZs be termed *inverse*

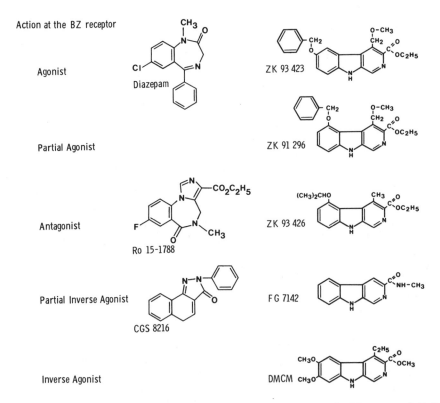

Figure 1. Examples of the structural diversity of molecules which are active at the BZ receptor. β-Carboline derivatives (right) represent the complete spectrum of action at the receptor of full agonist to full inverse agonist. The other molecules represent examples of a benzodiazepine (diazepam); imidazodiazepine (Ro 15-1788); pyrazolo-quinoline (CGS 8216).

agonists. Active agents which are not able to evoke the maximum response available are termed *partial agonists* and *partial inverse agonists,* respectively. Compounds which are able to block the activity of the aforementioned agents and are without (or with only slight) intrinsic activity are termed receptor *antagonists.* Figure 1 shows the molecular diversity of ligands which are active at the BZ receptor. β-Carboline derivatives span the complete spectrum from full agonist to full inverse agonist. BZs (e.g., diazepam) are mainly agonists, the imidazodiazepine Ro 15-1788 is an antagonist, while the pyrazoloquinoline CGS 8216 is a partial inverse agonist.

2.2.2. Multiplicity of BZ Receptors

Many lines of evidence suggest that BZ agonists and β-carboline inverse agonists are competing for exactly the same site (see Bræstrup *et al.,* 1983b). Evidence includes: the effects of both groups are inhibited by receptor antagonists; β-CCM and DMCM (methyl 6,7-dimethoxy-4-ethyl-β-carboline-3-carboxylate) completely inhibit ^{3}[H]flunitrazepam (FNM) binding in several brain regions, the K_D values for β-CCM and DMCM agreeing with the IC_{50} values for inhibition of ^{3}[H]-FNM binding; the anatomical distribution of binding sites for β-CCM, DMCM, and FNM and the total number of binding sites for the three ligands are similar; the molecular sizes of the binding sites are identical. There are, nevertheless, several lines of evidence which suggest receptor heterogeneity, or different conformational states of the same receptor.

a. Photoshift. When irradiated with UV light in the presence of FNM, 25% of the BZ sites are labeled irreversibly (perhaps one site of the functional tetramer; see Section 2.5), while the affinity of the remaining sites for BZ ligands is markedly decreased (Möhler, 1982; Bræstrup *et al.,* 1983a). On the other hand, the affinity for inverse agonists—especially DMCM—is increased (Bræstrup *et al.,* 1983a). In the electrophysiological situation, the ability of BZ agonists to increase the response to GABA was reduced 75% by photoinactivation, while the effect of β-CCM and DMCM on the response to GABA was unaltered. BZs and β-CCM were, however, still able to compete for the remaining sites (Farb *et al.,* 1984).

b. Binding Studies. The first indications of BZ receptor heterogeneity or negative cooperativity were obtained with CL 218,872—a triazolopyridazine (Squires *et al.,* 1979). A Hill coefficient of significantly less than one was obtained in all brain regions tested except the cerebellum (where a coefficient of one is indicative of a single receptor). The binding of β-carboline derivatives has also been used to demonstrate at least two different binding sites (BZ$_1$ and BZ$_2$) in the rat brain (Bræstrup and Nielsen, 1983; Sieghart *et al.,* 1983). PrCC binds preferentially to BZ$_1$ receptors and DMCM to BZ$_2$ receptors, the differences in affinities being about tenfold. Based on ratios of binding between these two β-carbolines and ^{3}[H]-FNM, it has been shown that BZ$_1$ receptors predominate in the cerebellum, while the highest concentration of BZ$_2$ receptors was found in the hippocampus.

2.3. The Anion-Selective Channel and Associated Binding Sites

The ionophore is permeable to a number of small anions including the halides, nitrate, and thiocyanate (Costa *et al.,* 1979). Cl^- is the charge carrier *in vivo.* The channel may be envisaged as a water-filled pore, ionic selectivity being conferred by the presence of appropriately charged amino acids. Picrotoxin binds to a site which is close to the anion channel and acts to prevent ion movement through the ionophore. Picrotoxin is thus a noncompetitive inhibitor of GABA action (Simmonds, 1980). The picrotoxin binding site and its vicinity is also the locus for the binding of a large number of structurally different, centrally active drugs (Olsen, 1982). The so-called cage convulsants (e.g., TBPS) also interact at this site to depress GABAergic transmission in a manner similar to that of picrotoxin (Bowery *et al.,* 1977).

All barbiturates (ranging from convulsant to anticonvulsant) compete with dihydropicrotoxinin for binding to the picrotoxin (PTX) site (Ticku and Olsen, 1978). The action of sedative/hypnotic barbiturates is to potentiate GABA responses, which is consonant with their clinical picture. In the presence of these barbiturates, the duration of individual channel openings is increased (Study and Barker, 1981).

2.4. Interactions between the Components of the GABA Receptor–Ionophore Complex

The GABA receptor–ionophore is comprised of essentially three receptive sites (see Fig. 2)—those for GABA, BZs, and PTX. The intimate linkage between these sites is amply illustrated by their interactions, which have been reviewed extensively by Olsen (1982). Ligands which act at one of these sites will mutually displace (antagonize) each other to a greater or lesser extent. However, there are also allosteric interactions. In general terms, when a ligand acts at one of the sites to alter the efficiency of GABAergic transmission, concomitant changes will occur at the other sites, which will strengthen the effect of the primary ligand. This effect could be termed "provoked synergism." Thus, in the presence of a sedative barbiturate, the affinities of both the BZ and the GABA receptors are increased (Willow and Johnston, 1980; Skolnick et al., 1981) in an additive fashion. Convulsant barbiturates, on the other hand, have no effect on BZ binding (Olsen and Leeb-Lundberg, 1981). Stimulatory action at the receptors usually requires the presence of anions which can penetrate the ionophore (Olsen, 1982).

There is an allosteric interaction between GABA and BZ receptors such that the occupation of one receptor by the appropriate ligand influences the affinity of the other. In the presence of GABA, the affinity of the BZ receptor is more than doubled, depending on the BZ ligand (Bræstrup et al., 1983a). This action is blocked by (+)bicuculline (Tallman et al., 1978), which is a competitive antagonist at the $GABA_A$ receptor. GABA has little or no effect on the binding of BZ receptor antagonists (Möhler and Richards, 1981), but causes a decrease in affinity for inverse agonists, by up to 50% for DMCM (Bræstrup et al., 1983a). This change in affinity of the BZ receptor has been called the "GABA shift" and is a useful test to predict the pharmacological and behavioral action of analogues (Bræstrup et al., 1983a). The converse, i.e., that occupation of the BZ receptor can modulate the affinity of the GABA receptor, probably occurs (Skerritt et al., 1982; Bræstrup and Nielsen, 1983; Skerritt and Johnston, 1983), but is still a matter of dispute (see Olsen, 1982). On the other hand, inverse agonists such as β-CCE and β-CCM have no effect on GABA binding (Skerritt et al., 1983).

With respect to interactions between the BZ receptor and sites associated with the ionophore, BZ agonists decrease the binding of DHP (Leeb-Lundberg et al., 1981). On the other hand, the binding of the convulsant TBPS is enhanced by BZ agonists and depressed by inverse agonists (Nielsen et al., 1985). As expected, TBPS binding is reduced (strongly) by the GABA-mimetic muscimol (Nielsen et al., 1985).

2.5. Molecular Structure of the GABA Receptor and Modulatory Sites

There have been numerous attempts to isolate and purify the GABA receptor with its attendant modulatory sites and ionophore. A number of proteins with molecular weights of 50,000–60,000 have been reported to bind FNM covalently (Sieghart et al., 1983) and may therefore represent the BZ receptor protein of the complex. Since at least four BZ-binding proteins were identified, it is possible that these represent different BZ receptors. This is supported by the fact that triazolopyridazines inhibited labeling of the three heavier proteins.

Based on results from radiation experiments, Nielsen et al. (1985) have proposed a model of the GABA/BZ receptor/Cl⁻ ionophore complex, which is reproduced in Fig. 2. The results show that the GABA receptor is intimately associated with the TBPS binding site (i.e., the anion gating

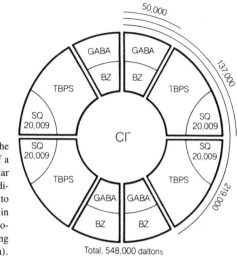

Figure 2. A diagrammatic representation of the GABA/BZ/ionophore complex. The complex consists of a tetramer made up of four identical subunits. The molecular weight of the component parts has been determined by radiation inactivation. Binding sites for some agents known to be active on the complex are illustrated. All are discussed in the text except for SQ 20,009 (a pyrazolopyridazine etazolate, an anxiolytic) which interacts with the Cl^- gating mechanism. (From Nielsen *et al.*, 1985, with permission).

mechanism) and that this interacts allosterically with the BZ receptor. Overall, the results led the authors to conclude that the GABA/BZ receptor/Cl^- ionophore probably exists as a tetramer (Fig. 2) with a total molecular weight of 548,000.

3. Electrophysiology

Electrophysiological recordings from a number of tissues have shown that BZs potentiate the action of exogenously applied GABA and IPSPs at presumed GABAergic synapses (Polc and Haefely, 1976; MacDonald and Barker, 1978; Choi *et al.*, 1981). The action of BZs is accompanied by an increase in frequency of opening of GABA-operated ionophores (Study and Barker, 1981), which contrasts with the fact that convulsants generally reduce the frequency of opening of ion channels operated by neutral amino acids (Barker *et al.*, 1983).

We have used intracellular recordings from mouse neurons grown in tissue culture to investigate how agents which act at the modulatory sites modify postsynaptic responses to GABA. The manner in which these agents change natural GABAergic inhibition and the consequence of this for neuronal output may therefore be inferred. It is known that the BZ receptors in cultures closely resemble those isolated from the intact nervous system (Huang *et al.*, 1980; White *et al.*, 1981) and that (for cortex cultures) low-affinity BZ-binding sites (K_d 2.4 × 10^{-7} M) may be located preferentially on neurons (Sher and Machen, 1984). In cultured chick neurons, the high-affinity "functional" BZ receptor is fully expressed at 3 weeks (Farb *et al.*, 1984).

Our neurons were usually impaled with KCl recording electrodes (Jensen and Lambert, 1984, 1986), and responses to GABA were depolarizing in accordance with the positive shift in E_{Cl} (to around −25 mV).

3.1. Agents That Act at the BZ Receptor

As would be expected from the binding studies outlined in Section 2, GABA responses were found to be depressed by DMCM. An example of this interaction for a single dose of GABA is shown in Fig. 7. Examination of the dose–response curve for GABA in the absence and presence of DMCM revealed a relationship which is characteristic of noncompetitive inhibition (Fig. 3). The response to each dose of GABA was reduced by the same amount while the ED_{50} for GABA

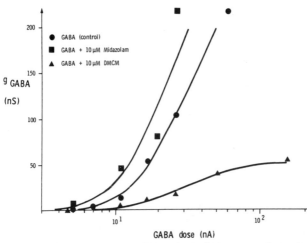

Figure 3. Effect of midazolam and DMCM on dose–response curve to GABA. A cultured neuron was impaled with a 3 M KCl electrode through which constant-current pulses were injected to measure the membrane conductance (G_M). The response to GABA (g_{GABA} in siemens $\times 10^{-9}$) was calculated by subtracting the resting G_M from the G_M value recorded during an iontophoretic application of GABA (dose in A $\times 10^{-9}$ on abscissa). Values of g_{GABA} for large responses in the control situation and in the presence of midazolam were too large to measure because the neuron was effectively short-circuited. Supramaximal doses of midazolam and DMCM (both 10^{-5} M) were applied to the neuron by pressure from a blunt pipette. Midazolam caused a shift to the left of the dose–response curve. DMCM behaved as a noncompetitive inhibitor (i.e., the maximum response to GABA is reduced with no change in the ED_{50}). This has also been established for other neurons where it was possible to determine a value for a close-to-maximum response to GABA in the control situation (e.g., Fig. 6; Jensen and Lambert, 1986). (From Jensen and Lambert, 1984.)

was unaltered. The maximum depression of the GABA response attained in the presence of DMCM was usually about 70% (although it is around 80% in Fig. 3). Since DMCM is a full inverse agonist, this would represent the maximum compliance of the GABA/BZ complex in the negative direction. These results indicate that DMCM and GABA are not competing for a common site, i.e., the depression caused by DMCM cannot be overcome by increasing the dose of GABA. In this respect DMCM behaves in a manner similar to PTX, which interferes with the operation of the ionophore (see below).

In 74 neurons tested, the dose of DMCM necessary to cause a just-detectable decrease in the GABA response varied between 10^{-8} and 10^{-6} M (Jensen and Lambert, 1986). An explanation for this hundredfold range of threshold doses for DMCM may be that the BZ receptor can exist in more than one conformational state (Bræstrup *et al.*, 1983a). One conformation has a higher affinity for a BZ agonist, while the other favors an inverse agonist. It is also possible that two distinct BZ receptors (Petersen *et al.*, 1983; Sieghart *et al.*, 1983) are present in our cultured neurons, but their occurrence and distribution are unknown. It is noteworthy that, using cultured chick neurons, Farb *et al.* (1984) obtained an ED_{50} of 10^{-8} M for the action of DMCM on GABA responses.

The water-soluble BZ agonist, midazolam, potentiated GABA responses with a parallel shift to the left of the dose–response curve (Fig. 3; see also MacDonald and Barker, 1978; Choi *et al.*, 1981; Jensen and Lambert, 1984).

In accordance with biochemical and behavioral studies, the β-carboline-type agonist ZK 93423 (Fig. 1) can be shown to enhance specifically GABA responses on cultured neurons (Fig. 4). It should be noted that electrophysiological experiments with this substance are complicated by the fact that it binds strongly to glass and plastics and to cortex membranes with a very slow dissociation rate (Tage Honoré and Jørgen Drejer, personal communication).

Following pressure pulse application of either midazolam or DMCM to a given neuron, the time course of recovery from the action of both agents was very similar: $t_{1/2}$ was usually 20–30 sec (e.g., see Fig. 7).

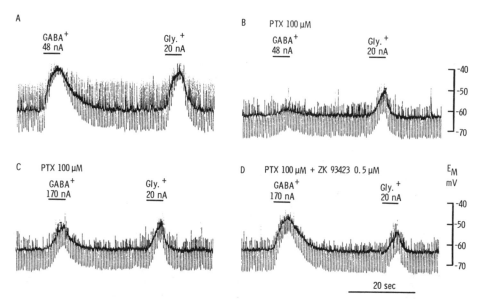

Figure 4. Response to GABA is depressed by picrotoxin and enhanced by the β-carboline agonist, ZK 93423. A cultured neuron was impaled with a 3 M KCl electrode so that the responses to GABA and glycine (Gly.) caused a depolarization of the membrane potential (E_M). Constant-current pulses injected through the recording electrode evoke the negative-going voltage transients on the records. The size of these transients is inversely proportional to G_M. (A) Iontophoretic applications of GABA and glycine have been chosen to evoke similarly sized responses (depolarization with increase in G_M). Note the marked spontaneous activity in the neuron, which is represented by the positive-going deflections from the baseline. (B) In the presence of picrotoxin (PTX, 10^{-4} M), the GABA response was nearly obliterated, while the response to glycine and the spontaneous activity were also reduced. (C) The dose of GABA was increased three-to fivefold so that the response was again comparable to that of glycine. (D) ZK 93423 (5×10^{-7} M) was added to the perfusion medium. The GABA response increased (by about 200% as measured from the change in g_{GABA}), while the response to glycine was slightly reduced.

Interaction of an Agonist and Inverse Agonist at the BZ Receptor

Since DMCM and midazolam have opposite actions on GABA responses, a mutual antagonism between these agents would be predicted. This would be irrespective of whether the same receptor was involved or not (e.g., the degree of enhancement of GABA responses by BZ agonists is quantitatively the same following the addition of picrotoxin). On occasions, however, doses of DMCM which had little or no effect on GABA responses in themselves could attenuate markedly the potentiating action of midazolam. Such an experiment is shown in Fig. 5 (see also Jensen and Lambert, 1986). For this individual neuron and the chosen doses of modulators, DMCM appears to act as an antagonist with weak inverse agonist activity. DMCM (10^{-8} M) caused only a small reduction in the response to GABA. This same dose of DMCM markedly reduced the potentiation of the GABA response caused by a hundredfold larger dose of midazolam (10^{-6} M). This result suggests either that the two agents are competing for the same binding site or that the sites are distinct, but there is a strong allosteric interaction. As outlined in Section 2, there is an overlapping of the recognition sites for BZ and β-carboline ligands, but discrete differences within the site itself can be demonstrated.

Current evidence suggests that a single ionic channel is associated with a tetramer consisting of identical subunits (Fig. 2). There is no cooperativity between the subunits. Simultaneous binding of two GABA molecules is obligatory for operation of the ionophore (Barker and

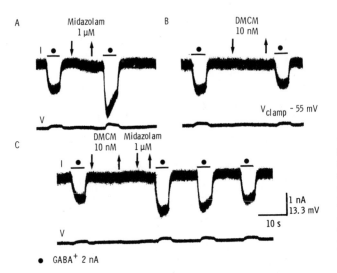

Figure 5. DMCM antagonizes the midazolam-induced potentiation of a response to GABA. A voltage-clamp experiment with the same experimental protocol as shown in Fig. 7. (A) Midazolam (10^{-6} M) caused a marked potentiation (by 125%) of the response to GABA. (B) A hundredfold lower concentration of DMCM (10^{-8} M) caused only a small reduction (by 14%) of the GABA-evoked current. (C) When DMCM was applied before midazolam, the potentiation of the GABA response (by 55%) was much less than that seen when midazolam was applied alone, in spite of the fact that the midazolam-containing solution quickly displaced the DMCM-containing solution from the vicinity of the neuron (A).

Ransom, 1978a). Presumably there is no priority as to which two of the four GABA receptors are occupied. However, the presence of a BZ ligand at one of the sites will increase the affinity of the associated GABA receptor, thus conferring a higher priority on this subunit. Presumably, therefore, at least two BZ ligands must bind to each tetramer in order that GABAergic transmission can be modified. Low concentrations of a BZ receptor ligand, which are insufficient to cause significant alteration in the operation of the ionophore, would nevertheless interfere with the access to the receptors of another ligand. This would explain why DMCM at low doses has predominantly antagonistic activity (Fig. 5), while larger doses are required to reveal inverse agonist activity (e.g., Figs. 3 and 7).

3.2. Agents That Act at Sites Associated with the Ionophore

PTX inhibits GABA in a noncompetitive manner. An example of an interaction is shown in Fig. 4, where PTX (10^{-4} M) nearly abolished the response to GABA. This inhibition could not be overcome by increasing the dose of GABA. This dose of PTX also reduced the response to glycine, which acts at a pharmacologically distinct receptor. Figure 4C,D, shows that PTX had not affected the ability of the β-carboline agonist, ZK 93423, to potentiate specifically the response to GABA.

The barbiturate anesthetic, pentobarbitone (PB), has dual actions on cultured neurons (Barker and Ransom, 1978b). At low doses it enhances GABA responses, while at higher doses it has a direct GABA-mimetic action. Both these effects are shown in Fig. 6, where the dose of PB is changed according to the dilution of a 5×10^{-4} M solution applied from a blunt pipette. Responses to both GABA and PB were reduced by PTX (5×10^{-4} M). The blockade of the GABA response by PTX was greatly reduced by PB (Fig. 6B), an observation consistent with the fact that PB and PTX are competing for the same site.

3.3. Identity of the GABA Receptor That is Coupled to the BZ Receptor

Enhancement of BZ agonist binding by GABA probably occurs following interaction of GABA with a low-affinity domain of its receptor (K_a ca. 10^{-6} M; Browner *et al.*, 1981; Skerritt

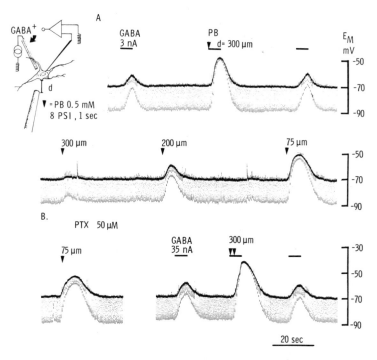

Figure 6. Pentobarbitone (PB) at low doses enhances response to GABA and has a direct, GABA-mimetic action at higher doses. The insert at the top left shows the experimental setup where a cultured neuron is impaled with a 3 M KCl electrode. G_M is measured by injection of constant-current pulses (negative voltage deflections on E_M trace). GABA was applied by iontophoresis to the soma, while PB (5×10^{-4} M) was applied from a blunt, pressure electrode at various distances (d) from the neuron (1-sec-duration applications at the points indicated by the downward-pointing arrowheads above the traces). (A) Response to GABA was markedly potentiated (g_{GABA} increased about 12-fold with respect to the control response) when PB was applied from a distance of 300 μm just at the start of the iontophoretic pulse of GABA. The recordings on the middle line show the direct effect of PB when applied at different distances (hence doses, although the exact concentration of PB at the membrane is not known). At 300 μm the response to PB is just-threshold, while at 200 μm it is about the same size as the response to GABA. At 75 μm there is a marked depolarization and increase in G_M. (B) Four minutes after the start of picrotoxin (PTX, 5 $\times$ 10^{-5} M) perfusion. The response to PB was markedly reduced (g_{PB} had decreased to about 40% of that of the last response shown in A). The response to GABA was also nearly abolished (not shown) and the GABA-ejecting current had to be increased by about 12 times to obtain the same response as seen in A. PB applied from 300 μm potentiated this response to a much greater extent than was seen before PTX. The membrane was effectively short-circuited (no voltage transient could be seen in response to current injection).

et al., 1982; Krogsgaard-Larsen *et al.*, 1984). A low-affinity GABA receptor is probably also responsible for the neuronal inhibitory response as measured with electrophysiological techniques. To investigate whether these receptors were identical, compounds which were known to be potent GABA-mimetics from electrophysiological studies were studied for their ability to stimulate BZ binding. To increase the sensitivity of the assay, the experiments were performed at 0°C and in the absence of Cl⁻ ions. There appeared to be a poor correlation between the performance of the agonists in the two situations. On the one hand, some potent GABA-mimetics (typified by muscimol) stimulated diazepam binding while, for example, 4,5,6,7-tetrahydroisoxazolo[5,4-*c*]pyridin-3-ol (THIP) had little effect on the binding of BZs, and piperidine-4-sulfonic acid (P4S) actually decreased BZ binding (Bræstrup *et al.*, 1979b). Not suspecting that the assay conditions had influenced the results, Bræstrup *et al.* (1979b) proposed that THIP behaved as a partial agonist and P4S a competitive antagonist at the GABA receptor which was coupled to the BZ receptor. Karobath *et al.* (1979) suggested that the GABA receptor was of a novel type.

We have investigated the action of agents which are active at the BZ receptor on responses to these GABA-mimetics in electrophysiological experiments (Jensen and Lambert, 1984). These recordings were performed under "physiological conditions," i.e., in Hanks balanced salt solution at 34–36°C. From the results shown in Fig. 7, it can be seen that the responses to GABA and its two mimetics. THIP and P4S, are modulated by both the agonist, midazolam, and the inverse agonist, DMCM. The enhancement by midazolam and depression by DMCM are similar in extent for all three GABA-mimetics, and the time courses of recovery following modulator application are also similar. This test has therefore not exposed differences between the GABA receptors. Later binding studies have shown that, when assayed in warm, Cl^--containing media, both THIP and P4S stimulated BZ binding (Krogsgaard-Larsen et al., 1984). There may, nevertheless, be more subtle differences between the GABA receptors, or domains of the GABA receptor. This is exemplified by the work of Skerritt and Johnston (1983), who have shown that, while binding of [3H]diazepam is stimulated by GABA, muscimol, and THIP, in the complementary situation diazepam stimulated the binding of GABA and muscimol, but was without effect on THIP binding.

4. Behavioral Actions

The discovery of the first potent β-carboline acting at the BZ receptor (β-CCE) by Bræstrup et al. (1980) initiated an intensive investigation of its expected BZ-like pharmacological properties. However, it soon became apparent that β-CCE antagonized the effects of BZs (Tenen and Hirsch, 1980) and even evoked effects opposite to the BZs when the threshold of seizure caused by electrical stimulation or convulsants like pentylenetetrazol and bicuculline were studied (Cowen et al., 1981; Nutt et al., 1982). β-CCM and, in particular, DMCM (a more stable derivative of β-CCM) produced frank convulsions in rodents as well as in baboons (Croucher and Meldrum, 1983; Petersen, 1983). These seizures as well as the proconvulsant effect of β-CCE were antagonized by the BZ antagonist Ro 15-1788 (Nutt et al., 1982; Bræstrup et al., 1982; Petersen, 1983).

Bræstrup et al. (1982, 1983) have described the BZ receptor ligands as a continuum possessing efficacies ranging from full agonists over partial agonists to receptor antagonist and further over partial inverse agonists to full inverse agonists. Examples of these and their behavioral actions are given in Table I. Very weak efficacies in this continuum can only be detected in very sensitive tests such as the sound-induced seizure paradigm using DBA/2 mice (Jensen et al., 1983). Petersen et al. (1983, 1986) have suggested that differential efficacy observed in various pharmacological paradigms may be caused by differential interaction of various BZ ligands on the BZ receptors or domains within these. Consequently, a single continuum of ligands cannot be defined since it is dependent on the paradigm in question.

4.1. Anticonvulsant–Convulsant Effects

Several tests of seizure threshold have been utilized to demonstrate a continuum of BZ ligands. Seizures induced by electrical stimulation of the cornea showed a full span of effects measured as dose-dependent changes in the threshold for seizures. The BZs produced marked elevation of the threshold whereas DMCM in nonconvulsant doses lowered the threshold to about 60% of the control (Fig. 8). Similar effects have been obtained using bicuculline- (Cowan et al., 1981), pentylenetetrazol- (Tenen and Hirsch, 1980), and PTX-induced seizures (Jensen and Petersen, 1983).

Three paradigms utilizing animals which are genetically prone to epilepsy showed the same bidirectional effects. Sound-induced seizures in DBA/2 mice are highly sensitive to the proconvulsant and anticonvulsant effect of BZ receptor ligands. In this paradigm the BZ receptor

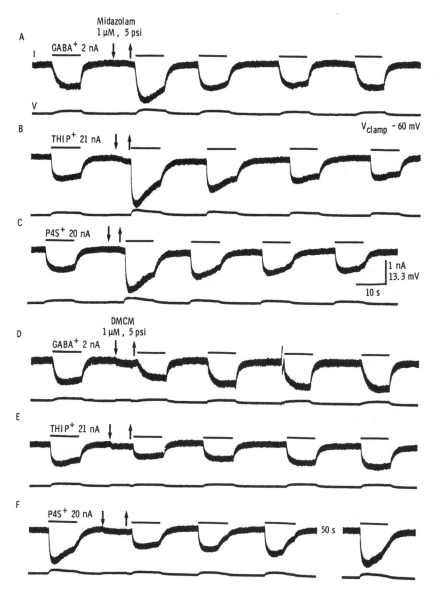

Figure 7. Neuronal responses to GABA, THIP, and P4S are potentiated by midazolam and depressed by DMCM. Single-electrode voltage-clamp experiment on a neuron impaled in the soma with a 3 M KCl electrode. Upper trace of each pair shows the current (inward downwards) necessary to clamp the membrane at −60 mV during application of the GABA-mimetics to the soma, while the voltage is monitored on the lower trace. (A–C) Iontophoretic doses of GABA (A), THIP (B), and P4S (C) were chosen to evoke similarly sized responses before a solution containing midazolam (10^{-6} M) was applied from a blunt, pressure pipette. Midazolam caused a marked potentiation of the responses to all three agents. The extent of the potentiation, and the time course of return to the control response were similar in each case. (D–F) Similar experiment; except that DMCM (10^{-6} M) was applied from the pressure electrode. This depressed the response to each agonist to a similar extent.

In quantitative terms, the response to GABA was, in fact, altered to a slightly lesser extent by midazolam and DMCM than those to THIP and P4S. (From Jensen and Lambert, 1984.)

Table I. Classification of Ligands That Bind with the BZ Receptor According to Their Efficacy and Actions

	Examples	Efficacy	Actions
Agonist	Diazepam ZK 93423	High positive efficacy	Anticonvulsant, anticonflict, ataxic, sedative, amnesic
Partial agonist	ZK 91296 CGS 9896	Low positive efficacy	Anticonvulsant, anticonflict, amnesic
Antagonist	Ro 15-1788 ZK 93426	No efficacy	Antagonize effects of agonists and inverse agonists
Partial inverse agonist	β-CCE FG 7142 CGS 8216 Ro 15-3505	Low negative efficacy	Proconvulsant, proconflict, nootropic
Inverse agonist	β-CCM DMCM	High negative efficacy	Convulsant, proconflict, nootropic

occupancies of effective doses of the compounds have been calculated and a proper efficacy spectrum of the ligands has therefore been given (Jensen *et al.*, 1983). Photoepileptic baboons are very sensitive to the action of BZ receptor inverse agonists. β-CCE and β-CCM produce frank convulsions in these baboons and non-light flash-sensitive baboons become light sensitive (Cepeda *et al.*, 1981; Croucher and Meldrum, 1983). Even the partial agonist ZK 91296 proved to be very potent in protecting against the myoclonic seizures in baboons (Meldrum *et al.*, 1983).

Inbred rats with spontaneous petit mal epilepsy are very sensitive to the effect of BZ receptor ligands. The frequency of spikes and waves on the EEG is markedly increased by the inverse agonists FG 7142 and DMCM, whereas agonists such as ZK 93423 and diazepam eliminated these discharges. It is noteworthy that the partial agonist ZK 91296 was effective without inducing sedation or changes in the background EEG, whereas ZK 93423 and diazepam evoked both these effects (Marescaux *et al.*, 1987). All these actions are antagonized by Ro 15-1788.

4.2. Muscle Relaxant–Muscle Stimulant Effects

In high doses, BZs produce muscle relaxation associated with marked sedative effects. In genetically spastic rats, the EMG from the gastrocnemius–soleus muscles shows a high tonic activity. This hyperactivity is further enhanced by bicuculline and by inverse agonists at the BZ

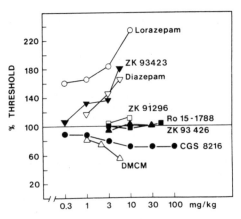

Figure 8. Effects of a full spectrum of BZ receptor ligands on the threshold for electroshock-induced tonic seizures in mice. Drugs were injected intraperitoneally, and the test was carried out 30 min later. The current was applied by corneal electrodes (50 Hz, 0.2 sec) and titrated by the up-and-down method to a level where tonic seizures were evoked in 50% of the mice (control 10–12 mA). DMCM became convulsant in doses above 3 mg/kg.

receptors, β-CCM, FG 7142, and CGS 216 (a pyrazoloquinoline; Ikonomidou *et al.*, 1985). On the other hand, sedative doses of the potent agonists, diazepam and ZK 93423, completely abolished this hyperactivity. Surprisingly, the partial agonist ZK 91296 did not influence hyperactivity (Klockgether *et al.*, 1985a). Ro 15-1788 effectively antagonized the effect of both inverse agonists and agonists (Ikonomidou *et al.*, 1985; Klockgether *et al.*, 1985b).

4.3. Hypnotic/Amnesic–Stimulant Effects

The hypnotic and amnesic effects of BZs are easily demonstrated in the clinic as well as in experimental animals. The hypnotic effect can be observed directly or as an increased sleeping time in barbiturate-treated rats. The full continuum of ligands can also be demonstrated in this paradigm and DMCM very significantly reduces the sleeping time (Jensen *et al.*, 1986; Fig. 9).

Amnesia can be demonstrated using the passive avoidance paradigm where mice are trained to avoid entering a compartment of the test box where foot shocks are given. This task is easily learned and recalled 4 days later. Mice treated with a BZ agonist also learn the task although more shocks are taken before criterion is reached. The mice are, however, unable to consolidate this information, and when exposed to the test situation 4 days later they are unable to recall the previous experience. Since mice are very good in learning the task, no improvement can be demonstrated with inverse agonists. However, when the mice are impaired in performing the task by (e.g.) scopolamine injection, inverse agonists are capable of reversing this impairment in performance (Jensen *et al.*, 1987; Venault *et al.*, 1987). This antiamnesic effect of inverse agonists may hold promises for the development of agents for the treatment of patients with diseases due to hyperactivity in the GABA system. One condition that might be treatable with weak partial inverse agonists is memory disturbances in senile dementia.

4.4. Anxiolytic–Anxiogenic Effects

Anxiety is a state of the individual which is very difficult to quantify, particularly in animals. Tests for anxiolytic effects in animals are therefore performed utilizing approach–withdrawal paradigms, the so-called conflict paradigms where animals are punished for trying to obtain a reward. Anxiolytics disinhibit the animals, which means that they become oblivious to punishment (Fig. 10). BZ receptor agonists generally possess anxiolytic effects when the intrinsic

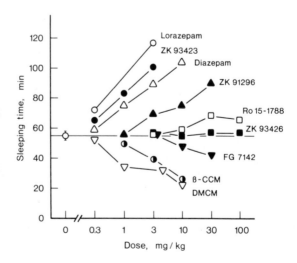

Figure 9. Effects of a full spectrum of BZ receptor ligands on the duration of pentobarbital-induced loss of righting reflex in rats. The compounds were injected intraperitoneally 15 min after pentobarbital sodium 30 mg/kg i.v. and the time with loss of righting reflex was recorded. The righting reflex was defined to be present when the rat succeeded in turning over from lying on its back in response to a pinch to one hind paw. The test was carried out every 2 min.

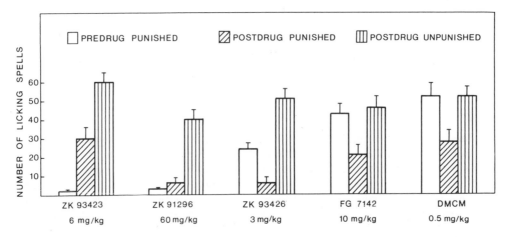

Figure 10. Effects of a full spectrum of β-carbolines in the water lick conflict test. The rats were water deprived for 48 hr and then allowed access to a water bottle with a 0.4-A current on the spout for 6 min (predrug punished session). Rats with high licking activity were administered ZK 93426, FG 7142, or DMCM i.p. and retested 30 min later (DMCM 10 min) for another 6-min period. The rats were then transferred from the test box to a familiar cage where nonpunished licking activity was measured for 6 min. Rats with low control predrug punished licking activity were administered ZK 93423 or ZK 91296 and subjected to the same schedule as above. Saline administration had no effect on the licking activity in either the high-conflict or the low-conflict rats.

efficacy of the ligand in this respect is sufficiently high. Some partial agonists therefore possess only weak or inconsistent effects in these paradigms (Petersen *et al.*, 1984).

Inverse agonists make the animals more reluctant to accept punishment for obtaining the reward. In other words, they increase the level of conflict in the animals. Such proconflict effects have been observed in mice (Prado de Carvalho *et al.*, 1983) and in rats (Corda *et al.*, 1983; Petersen and Jensen, 1984). Figure 10 shows results from a water lick conflict paradigm utilizing rats which had been deprived of water for 48 hr. The effects are very consistent and other compounds such as PTZ, bicuculline, and PTX, which reduce the GABA-mediated increase in chloride conductance, appear to produce similar effects. These findings indicate that the functional state of the GABA-operated chloride channel may be very crucial for the level of anxiety within the animals. This does not, however, exclude that other neuronal mechanisms are also important in this respect. Great care should be exercised in the interpretation of this kind of information since proconflict effects do not necessarily predict anxiogenic effects. In the case of inverse agonists, however, there seems to be a good correlation (see Section 4.5).

Several other tests, e.g., the four-plate paradigm (Stephens and Kehr, 1985), the social interaction test between rats (File and Lister, 1983), and the elevated plus maze (Pellow *et al.*, 1985), have also been able to detect the anxiolytic effect of BZ receptor agonists. Inverse agonists have been shown to produce effects opposite those of the BZ agonists in the four-plate paradigm (Stephens and Kehr, 1985) and in the social interaction test (File and Lister, 1983).

An anxiety-like state can be induced in rhesus monkeys by the injection of β-CCE (Ninan *et al.*, 1982). This effect is blocked by Ro 15-1788.

4.5. Clinical Effects of BZ Agonists and Inverse Agonists

The sedative–hypnotic effects of the BZs have been shown to be rapidly and fully reversible by the BZ receptor antagonists Ro 15-1788 in animals as well as man (Hunkeler *et al.*, 1981; Darragh *et al.*, 1981). Ro 15-1788 by itself had no effect (Darragh *et al.*, 1981). The prediction that the partial agonist ZK 91296 would not possess sedative–hypnotic effects has been confirmed by intravenous application in man (Dorow, personal communication). The partial inverse agonist FG 7142 has been shown to possess marked anxiogenic effects in two volunteers where plasma concentrations of FG 7142 exceeded 200 ng/ml. Peripheral symptoms such as flushing of the trunk and face were observed in several other volunteers with lower plasma concentrations of FG 7142 (Dorow *et al.*, 1983). This latter study is extremely important since it substantiates in a clinical sense the findings from animal experiments. Inverse agonists will therefore most probably induce the opposite effects of BZs in man. With the advent of the β-carbolines we have a chemical series which covers the spectrum from full inverse agonists to full agonists at the BZ receptor.

ACKNOWLEDGMENTS. We thank Finn Marquard and Kirsten Kandborg for technical assistance and Karen Damgaard Ottesen, Bodil Ussing Nielsen, and Lis Skjøt for typing the manuscript. This work was supported by the Danish Medical Research Council.

References

Barker, J. L., and Ransom, B. R., 1978a, Amino acid pharmacology of mammalian central neurones grown in tissue culture, *J. Physiol. (London)* **280:**331–354.

Barker, J. L., and Ransom, B. R., 1978b, Pentobarbitone pharmacology of mammalian central neurones grown in tissue culture, *J. Physiol. (London)* **280:**355–372.

Barker, J. L., McBurney, R. N., and Mathers, D. A., 1983, Convulsant-induced depression of amino acid responses in cultured mouse spinal neurones studied under voltage clamp, *Br. J. Pharmacol.* **80:**619–629.

Bowery, N. G., Collins, J. F., Hill, R. G., and Pearson, S., 1977, t-Butylbicyclo phosphate: A convulsant and GABA antagonist more potent than bicuculline, *Br. J. Pharmacol.* **60:**175–176.

Bræstrup, C., and Nielsen, M., 1983, Benzodiazepine receptors, in: *Handbook of Psychopharmacology,* Vol. 17 (L. L. Iversen, S. D. Iversen, and S. H. Snyder, eds.), Plenum Press, New York, pp. 258–384.

Bræstrup, C., and Squires, R. F., 1978, Brain specific benzodiazepine receptors, *Br. J. Psychiatry* **133:**249–260.

Bræstrup, C., Nielsen, M., Biggio, G., and Squires, R. F., 1979a, Neuronal localization of benzodiazepine receptors in cerebellum, *Neurosci. Lett.* **13:**219–224.

Bræstrup, C., Nielsen, M., Krogsgaard-Larsen, P., and Falch, E., 1979b, Partial agonists for brain GABA/benzodiazepine receptor complex, *Nature* **280:**331–333.

Bræstrup, C., Nielsen, M., and Olsen, C. E., 1980, Urinary and brain beta-carboline-3-carboxylates as potent inhibitors of brain benzodiazepine receptors, *Proc. Natl. Acad. Sci. USA* **77:**2288–2292.

Bræstrup, C., Schmiechen, R., Neef, G., Nielsen, M., and Petersen, E. N., 1982, Interaction of convulsive ligands with benzodiazepine receptors, *Science* **216:**1241–1243.

Bræstrup, C., Nielsen, M., Honoré, T., Jensen, L. H., and Petersen, E. N., 1983a, Benzodiazepine receptor ligands with positive and negative efficacy, *Neuropharmacology* **22:**1451–1457.

Bræstrup, C., Nielsen, M., and Honoré, T., 1983b, Binding of [³H]-DMCM, a convulsive benzodiazepine ligand, to rat brain membranes: Preliminary studies, *J. Neurochem.* **41:**454–460.

Browner, M., Ferkany, J. W., and Enna, S. J., 1981, Biochemical identification of pharmacologically and functionally distinct GABA receptors in rat brain, *J. Neurosci.* **1:**514–518.

Cepeda, C., Tanaka, T., Besselievre, R., Potier, P., Naquet, R., and Rossier, J., 1981, Proconvulsant effects in baboons of β-carboline, a putative endogenous ligand for benzodiazepine receptors, *Neurosci. Lett.* **24:**53–57.

Chan-Palay, V., 1978, Autoradiographic localization of γ-aminobutyric acid receptors in rat central nervous system using ³H-muscimol, *Proc. Natl. Acad. Sci. USA* **75:**1024–1028.

Choi, D. W., Farb, D. H., and Fischbach, G. D., 1981, Chlordiazepoxide selectively potentiates GABA conductance of spinal cord and sensory neurons in cell culture, *J. Neurophysiol.* **45:**621–631.

Corda, M. G., Blaker, W. D., Mendelson, W. B., Guidotti, A., and Costa, E., 1983, β-Carbolines enhance shock-induced suppression of drinking in rats, *Proc. Natl. Acad. Sci. USA* **80:**2072–2076.

Costa, T., Rodbard, D., and Pert, C. B., 1979, Is the benzodiazepine receptor coupled to a chloride anion channel? *Nature* **177:**315–317.

Cowen, P. J., Green, A. R., Nutt, D. J., and Martin, I. L., 1981, Ethyl β-carboline carboxylate lowers seizure threshold and antagonizes flurazepam-induced sedation in rats, *Nature* **290:**54–55.

Croucher, M. J., and Meldrum, B. S., 1983, Actions of the benzodiazepine receptor "inverse agonist", DMCM, in the primate, *Papio papio, Br. J. Pharmacol.* **79:**433P.

Darragh, A., Scully, M., Lambe, R., Brick, I., O'Boyle, C., and Downie, W. W., 1981, Investigation in man of the efficacy of a benzodiazepine antagonist, Ro 15-1788, *Lancet* **2:**8–10.

Dolphin, A. C., 1984, GABA$_B$ receptors: Has adenylate cyclase inhibition any functional relevance? *Trends Neurosci.* **7:**363–364.

Dorow, R., Horowski, R., Paschelke, G., Amin, M., and Bræstrup, C., 1983, Severe anxiety induced by FG 7142, a β-carboline ligand for benzodiazepine receptors, *Lancet* **2:**98–99.

Farb, D. H., Borden, L. A., Chan, C. Y., Czajkowski, C. M., Gibbs, T. T., and Schiller, G. D., 1984, Modulation of neuronal function through benzodiazepine receptors: Biochemical and electrophysiological studies on neurons in primary monolayer cell culture, *Ann. N.Y. Acad. Sci.* **435:**1–31.

File, S. E., and Lister, R. G., 1983, Interactions of ethyl-β-carboline-3-carboxylate and Ro 15-1788 with CGS 8216 in an animal model of anxiety, *Neurosci. Lett.* **39:**91–94.

Fry, J. P., Rickets, C., and Biscoe, T. J., 1985, On the location of γ-aminobutyrate and benzodiazepine receptors in the cerebellum of the normal C3H and lurcher mutant mouse, *Neuroscience* **14:**1091–1101.

Gallagher, D. W., Mallorga, P., Oertel, W., Henneberry, R., and Tallman, J. F., 1981, ^{3}H diazepam binding in a mammalian central nervous system: A pharmacological characterization, *J. Neurosci.* **1:**218–225.

Huang, A., Barker, J. L., Paul, S. M., Moncada, V., and Skolnick, P., 1980, Characterization of benzodiazepine receptors in primary cultures of fetal mouse brain and spinal cord neurons, *Brain Res.* **190:**485–491.

Hunkeler, W., Möhler, H., Pieri, L., Polc, P., Bonetti, E. P., Cumin, R., Schaffner, R., and Haefely, W., 1981, Selective antagonists of benzodiazepines, *Nature* **290:**514–516.

Ikonomidou, C., Turski, L., Klockgether, T., Schwarz, M., and Sontag, K., 1985, Effects of methyl β-carboline-3-carboxylate, Ro 15-1788 and CGS 8216 on muscle tone in genetically spastic rats, *Eur. J. Pharmacol.* **113:**205–213.

Jensen, L. H., and Petersen, E. N., 1983, Bidirectional effects of benzodiazepine receptor ligands against picrotoxin- and pentylenetetrazol-induced seizures, *J. Neural Transm.* **58:**183–191.

Jensen, L. H., Petersen, E. N., and Bræstrup, C., 1983, Audiogenic seizures in DBA/2 mice discriminate sensitively between low efficacy benzodiazepine receptor agonists and inverse agonists, *Life Sci.* **33:**393–399.

Jensen, L. H., Petersen, E. N., Honoré, T., and Drejer, J., 1986, Bidirectional modulation of GABA function by β-carbolines, *Adv. Biochem. Psychopharmacol.* **41:**79–90.

Jensen, L. H., Stephens, D. N., Sarter, M., and Petersen, E. N., 1987, Bidirectional effects of β-carbolines and benzodiazepines on memory processes, *Brain Res. Bull.* **19**(4):(in press).

Jensen, M. S., and Lambert, J. D. C., 1984, Modulation of the responses to the GABA-mimetics, THIP and piperidine-4-sulphonic acid, by agents which interact with benzodiazepine receptors, *Neuropharmacology* **23:**1441–1450.

Jensen, M. S., and Lambert, J. D. C., 1986, Electrophysiological studies in cultured mouse CNS neurones of the actions of an agonist and an inverse agonist at the benzodiazepine receptor, *Br. J. Pharmacol.* **88:**717–731.

Karobath, M., Placheta, P., Lippitsch, M., and Krogsgaard-Larsen, P., 1979, Is stimulation of benzodiazepine receptor binding mediated by a novel GABA receptor? *Nature* **278:**748–749.

Klockgether, T., Schwarz, M., Turski, L., and Sontag, K.-H., 1985a, ZK 91296, an anticonvulsant β-carboline which lacks muscle relaxant properties, *Eur. J. Pharmacol.* **110:**309–315.

Kockgether, T., Pardowitz, I., Schwarz, M., Sontag, K.-H., and Turski, L., 1985b, Evaluation of the muscle relaxant properties of a novel β-carboline, ZK 93423 in rats and cats, *Br. J. Pharmacol.* **86:**357–366.

Krogsgaard-Larsen, P., Falch, E., and Jacobsen, P., 1984, GABA agonists: Structural requirements for interaction with the GABA–benzodiazepine receptor complex, in: *Actions and Interactions of GABA and Benzodiazepines* (N. G. Bowery, ed.), Raven Press, New York, pp. 109–132.

Lambert, J. D. C., and Flatman, J. A., 1981, The interaction between barbiturate anaesthetics and excitatory amino acid responses on cat spinal neurones, *Neuropharmacology* **20:**227–240.

Leeb-Lundberg, F., Napias, C., and Olsen, R. W., 1981, Dihydropicrotoxinin binding sites in mammalian brain: Interactions with convulsant and depressant benzodiazepines, *Brain Res.* **216:**399–408.

MacDonald, R., and Barker, J. L., 1978, Benzodiazepines specifically modulate GABA-mediated postsynaptic inhibition in cultured mammalian neurons, *Nature* **271:**563–564.

Marescaux, C., Vergnes, M., Jensen, L., Petersen, E. N., Depaulis, A., Micheletti, G., and Warter, J. M., 1987, Bidirectional effects of beta-carbolines in rats with spontaneous petit mal-like seizures, *Brain Res. Bull.* **19**(4):(in press).

Meldrum, B. S., Evans, M. C., and Bræstrup, C., 1983, Anticonvulsant action in the photosensitive baboon, *Papio papio*, of a novel β-carboline derivative, ZK 91296, *Eur. J. Pharmacol.* **91:**255–259.

Möhler, H., 1982, Benzodiazepine receptors: Differential interaction of benzodiazepine agonists and antagonists after photo-affinity labelling with flunitrazepam, *Eur. J. Pharmacol.* **80:**435–436.

Möhler, H., and Okada, T., 1977, Gamma-amino-butyric acid receptor binding with (+) bicuculline methiodide in rat CNS, *Nature* 267:65–67.

Möhler, H., and Okada, T., 1978, The benzodiazepine receptor in normal and pathological human brain, *Br. J. Psychiatry* 133:261–268.

Möhler, H., and Richards, J. G., 1981, Agonist and antagonist benzodiazepine receptor interaction in vitro, *Nature* 294:763–765.

Möhler, H., Richards, J. G., and Wu, J. Y., 1981, Autoradiographic localization of benzodiazepine receptors in immunocytochemically identified gamma-aminobutyrergic synapses, *Proc. Natl. Acad. Sci. USA* 78:1935–1938.

Nielsen, M., Gredal, O., and Bræstrup, C., 1979, Some properties of ^{3}H-diazepam displacing activity from human urine, *Life Sci.* 25:679–686.

Nielsen, M., Honoré, T., and Bræstrup, C., 1985, Radiation inactivation of brain [^{35}S]*t*-butylbicyclophosphorothionate binding sites reveals complicated molecular arrangements of the GABA/benzodiazepine receptor chloride channel complex, *Biochem. Pharmacol.* 34:3633–3642.

Ninan, P. T., Insel, T. M., Cohen, R. M., Cook, J. M., Skolnick, P., and Paul, S. M., 1982, Benzodiazepine receptor-mediated experimental "anxiety" in primates, *Science* 218:1332–1334.

Nistri, A., and Constanti, A., 1979, Pharmacological characterization of different types of GABA and glutamate receptors in vertebrates and invertebrates, *Prog. Neurobiol.* 13:117–235.

Nistri, A., Constanti, A., and Krnjević, K., 1980, Electrophysiological studies of the mode of action of GABA on vertebrate central neurons, *Adv. Biochem. Psychopharmacol.* 21:81–90.

Nutt, D. J., Cowen, P. J., and Little, H. J., 1982, Unusual interactions of benzodiazepine receptor antagonists, *Nature* 295:436–438.

Oakley, N. R., and Jones. B. J., 1980, The proconvulsant and diazepam-reversing effects of ethyl-beta-carboline-3-carboxylate, *Eur. J. Pharmacol.* 68:381–382.

Olsen, R. W., 1982, Drug interactions at the GABA receptor–ionophore complex, *Annu. Rev. Pharmacol. Toxicol.* 22:245–277.

Olsen, R. W., and Leeb-Lundberg, F., 1981, Convulsant and anticonvulsant drug binding sites related to the GABA receptor/ionophore system, in: *Neurotransmitters, Seizures and Epilepsy* (P. L. Morselli, K. G. Lloyd, W. Löscher, B. S. Meldrum, and E. H. Reynolds, eds.), Raven Press, New York, pp. 151–163.

Pellow, S., Chopin, P., File, S. E., and Briley, M., 1985, Validation of open:closed arm entries in an elevated plus-maze as a measure of anxiety in the rat, *J. Neurosci. Methods* 14:149–167.

Petersen, E. N., 1983, DMCM: A potent convulsive benzodiazepine receptor ligand, *Eur. J. Pharmacol.* 94:117–124.

Petersen, E. N., and Jensen, L. H., 1984, Proconflict effect of benzodiazepine receptor inverse agonists and other inhibitors of GABA function, *Eur. J. Pharmacol.* 103:91–97.

Petersen, E. N., Jensen, L. H., Honoré, T., and Bræstrup, C., 1983, Differential pharmacological effects of benzodiazepine receptor inverse agonists, in: *Benzodiazepine Recognition Site Ligands: Biochemistry and Pharmacology* (G. Biggio and E. Costa, eds.) Raven Press, New York, pp. 57–64.

Petersen, E. N., Jensen, L. H., Honoré, T., Bræstrup, C., Kehr, W., Stephens, D. N., Wachtel, H., Seidelman, D., and Schmiechen, R., 1984, ZK 91296, a partial agonist at benzodiazepine receptors, *Psychopharmacology* 83:240–248.

Petersen, E. N., Jensen, L. H., Drejer, J., and Honoré, T., 1986, New perspectives in benzodiazepine receptor pharmacology, *Pharmacopsychiatry* 19:4–6.

Polc, P., and Haefely, W., 1976, Effects of two benzodiazepines, phenobarbitone, and baclofen on synaptic transmission in the cat cuneate nucleus, *Naunyn-Schmiedebergs Arch. Pharmacol.* 292:121–131.

Polc, P., Bonetti, E. P., Schaffner, R., and Haefely, W., 1982, A three-state model of the benzodiazepine receptor explains the interactions between the benzodiazepine antagonist Ro 15-1788, benzodiazepine tranquilizers, β-carbolines, and phenobarbitone, *Naunyn-Schmiedebergs Arch. Pharmacol.* 321:260–264.

Prado de Carvalho, L., Grecksch, G., Chapouthier, G., and Rossier, J., 1983, Anxiogenic and non-anxiogenic benzodiazepine antagonists, *Nature* 301:64–66.

Sher, P. K., and Machen, V. L., 1984, Properties of [^{3}H]diazepam binding sites on cultured murine glia and neurons, *Dev. Brain Res.* 14:1–6.

Sieghart, W., Mayer, A., and Drexler, G., 1983, Properties of [^{3}H]flunitrazepam binding to different benzodiazepine binding proteins, *Eur. J. Pharmacol.* 88:291–299.

Simmonds, M. A., 1980, Evidence that bicuculline and picrotoxin act at separate sites to antagonize γ-amino butyric acid in rat cuneate nucleus, *Neuropharmacology* 19:39–45.

Skerritt, J. H., and Johnston, G. A. R., 1983, Diazepam stimulates the binding of GABA and muscimol but not THIP to rat brain membranes, *Neurosci. Lett.* 38:315–320.

Skerritt, J. H., Willow, M., and Johnston, G. A. R., 1982, Diazepam enhancement of low affinity GABA binding to rat brain membranes, *Neurosci. Lett.* **29:**63–66.

Skerritt, J. H., Johnston, G. A. R., and Bræstrup, C., 1983, Modulation of GABA binding to rat brain membranes by alkyl β-carboline-3-carboxylate esters, *Eur. J. Pharmacol.* **86:**299–301.

Skolnick, P., Moncada, V., Barker, J. L., and Paul, S. M., 1981, Pentobarbital: Dual actions to increase brain benzodiazepine receptor affinity, *Science* **211:**1448–1450.

Squires, R. F., and Bræstrup, C., 1977, Benzodiazepine receptors in rat brain, *Nature* **166:**732–734.

Squires, R. F., Benson, D. I., Bræstrup, C., Coupet, J., Klepner, C. A., Myers, V., and Beer, B., 1979, Some properties of brain specific benzodiazepine receptor: New evidence for multiple receptors, *Pharmacol. Biochem. Behav.* **10:**825–830.

Stephens, D. N., and Kehr, W., 1985, β-Carbolines can enhance or antagonize the effects of punishment in mice, *Psychopharmacology* **85:**143–147.

Study, R. E., and Barker, J. L., 1981, Diazepam and (−) pentobarbital: Fluctuation analysis reveals different mechanisms for potentiation of GABA responses in cultured central neurons, *Proc. Natl. Acad. Sci. USA* **78:**7180–7184.

Tallman, J. F., and Gallagher, D. W., 1985, The GABA-ergic system: A locus of benzodiazepine action, *Annu. Rev. Neurosci.* **8:**21–44.

Tallman, J. F., Thomas, J. W., and Gallager, D. W., 1978, GABAergic modulation of benzodiazepine binding site sensitivity, *Nature* **274:**383–385.

Tenen, S. S., and Hirsch, J. D., 1980, β-Carboline-3-carboxylic acid ethyl ester antagonizes diazepam activity, *Nature* **288:**609–610.

Ticku, M. K., and Olsen, R. W., 1978, Interaction of barbiturates with dihydropicrotoxinin binding sites related to the GABA receptor–ionophore system, *Life Sci.* **22:**1643–1651.

Unnerstall, J. R., Kuhar, M. J., Niehoff, D. L., and Palacios, J. M., 1981, Benzodiazepine receptors are coupled to a subpopulation of γ-aminobutyric acid (GABA) receptors: Evidence from a quantitative autoradiographic study, *J. Pharmacol. Exp. Ther.* **218:**797–803.

Venault, P., Chapouthier, G., Simiand, J., Dodd, R. H., and Rossier, J., 1987, Enhancement of performance by β-carboline in learning and memory tasks, *Brain Res. Bull.* **19**(4):(in press).

Wang, J. K., Taniguchi, T., and Spector, S., 1980, Properties of ^{3}H diazepam binding sites on rat blood platelets, *Life Sci.* **27:**1881–1888.

White, W. F., Dichter, M. A., and Snodgrass, S. R., 1981, Benzodiazepine binding and interactions wih the GABA receptor complex in living cultures of rat cerebral cortex, *Brain Res.* **215:**162–176.

Willow, M., and Johnston, G. A. R., 1980, Enhancement of GABA binding by pentobarbitone, *Neurosci. Lett.* **18:**323–327.

14

Acetylcholine as Transmitter in the Cerebral Cortex

K. Krnjević

1. Introduction

Both longer and more firmly established as a peripheral transmitter than any other agent, acetylcholine (ACh) is by no means well defined as a transmitter in the cerebral cortex. As will be made clear below (and by other contributors to this section), it is unlikely that ACh is a fast-acting transmitter at most synapses in the vertebrate CNS. There is a wide consensus rather that ACh *modulates* synaptic activity by nonconventional mechanisms which tend to suppress outward currents that normally stabilize the membrane potential. In this introductory chapter, salient features of ACh in relation to cortical neurons are briefly reviewed, more detailed descriptions of various actions of ACh being given in the following chapters.

2. Presence and Release of ACh in the Cortex

That ACh can be synthesized in the cortex has been known for many years (Feldberg and Vogt, 1948; Hebb and Silver, 1956). Of special importance was the demonstration that ACh is released in the cortex in a manner consistent with some significant role in neural activity. In the present context, particularly relevant are Celesia and Jasper's (1966) studies of ACh release. Following MacIntosh and Oborin's (1953) pioneering research, they used a technique of superfusion—the "cortical cup" illustrated in Fig. 1—to collect ACh from the surface of the cortex. They found that ACh release varies consistently according to the level of arousal. Stimulation of the brain stem reticular formation in the "encéphale isolé" preparation, which predictably elicits electrographic and other signs of cortical arousal, also enhanced ACh release (Fig. 2). But both ongoing and evoked release were much reduced by a brain stem section that isolates the forebrain from nearly all incoming neural signals. These results have been confirmed by other investigators (Mitchell, 1963; Dudar and Szerb, 1969). But the identity of the relevant cholinergic fibers became evident only after some extensive histo- and immunocytochemical investigations.

K. Krnjević • Departments of Anaesthesia Research and Physiology, McGill University, Montreal, Quebec H3G 1Y6, Canada.

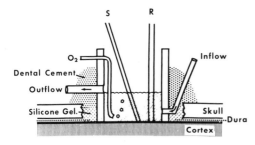

Figure 1. Cross-sectional diagram of chamber used to collect ACh from cortical surface. Superfusing solution was a mammalian Ringer containing an anti-cholinesterase agent to prevent ACh breakdown. ACh was assayed on a sensitive smooth muscle preparation. S and R: stimulating and recording electrodes. (From Celesia and Jasper, 1966.)

These investigations first demonstrated numerous acetylcholinesterase (AChE)-containing cells in the basal forebrain, where fibers project to all regions of the cortex, forming a widely distributed net of presumed cholinergic terminals (Shute and Lewis, 1963, 1967; Krnjević and Silver, 1965, 1966). In more recent studies, antibodies for choline acetyltransferase have confirmed the cholinergic nature of these neurons, and horseradish peroxidase has been used to obtain more detailed information about their cortical projections (see Mesulam, this volume). How ACh is synthesized and stored in cholinergic nerve endings, and then released, is discussed by Collier (this volume).

3. Actions of ACh on Cortical Neurons

Two prominent features have been known for over 20 years: ACh has a relatively slow and prolonged excitatory or facilitatory effect that is mediated predominantly by muscarinic receptors (Krnjević and Phillis, 1963a,b). In both respects, this is typical of actions of ACh in the vertebrate CNS, where so far very few examples of quick, nicotinic actions have been identified. Since the early discovery of the motor axon collateral–Renshaw cell pathway in the spinal cord (Eccles *et al.*, 1954), convincing evidence of a nicotinic junction has been obtained at only one other site: in the retina, between starburst amacrine cells and the dendrites of ganglion cells (Masland *et al.*, 1984a,b). The suggestion that retinotectal fibers are nicotinic in some lower vertebrates (Oswald *et al.*, 1979) is not supported by more recent findings (Henley *et al.*, 1986). On the other hand, the possibility of a nicotinic action in the medial habenula is discussed by McCormick and Prince (this volume). The slow muscarinic action is particularly effective in enhancing (often also in

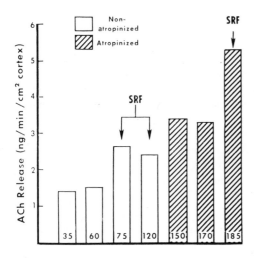

Figure 2. Release of ACh from primary somatosensory cortex of cat by technique described in Fig. 1. The first two columns represent ACh output in normal drowsy animal. Other columns show effect of stimulating midbrain reticular formation (SRF). Numbers on abscissa indicate time in minutes after start of superfusion. Note marked increase in release after i.v. injection of atropine (1 mg/kg). (From Celesia and Jasper, 1966.)

prolonging) fast excitations evoked in various ways, for example by local applications of gluta-mate (Krnjević and Phillis, 1963b; Krnjević *et al.*, 1971) or by sensory inputs (Sillito and Kemp, 1983; Dykes *et al.*, this volume).

4. Cellular Mechanism of ACh Action: Depression of K^+ Conductance

In every respect, the muscarinic effects on cortical neurons proved to be quite "unconven-tional." Numerous studies on the more accessible peripheral junctions had definitively shown that transmitters act by opening ionic channels, thus generating excitation or inhibition according to the nature of the permeant ions and their transmembrane electrochemical gradients. In cortical cells, on the other hand, no increase in conductance could be detected; instead the resistance

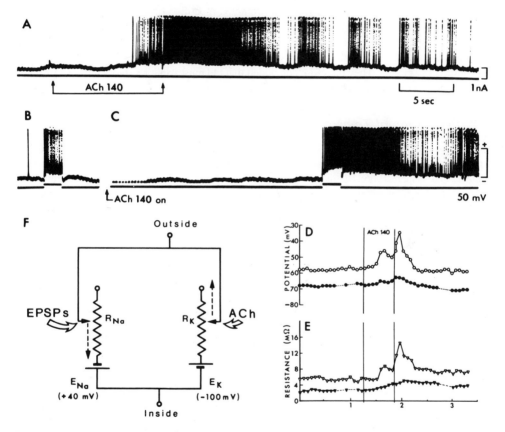

Figure 3. Salient features of prolonged facilitatory action of ACh on cat's cortical neuron *in situ*. Slow and prolonged firing (A) induced by iontophoretic application of ACh (indicated in nA) is contrasted with rapid firing evoked by depolarizing pulse in B. C illustrates voltage dependence of ACh action: after treatment with di-nitrophenol, neuron was hyperpolarized and no longer overtly responsive to ACh; but ACh powerfully enhanced and prolonged the response to a brief depolarizing pulse (identical to that in B). Open symbols in D and E illustrate the slow depolarizing effect induced by ACh in a cortical neuron and accompanying increase in resting resistance. Closed symbols show only minor changes in IPSP characteristics. F, circuit diagram showing the contrast between typical nicotinic effect of ACh, which generates EPSPs by increasing G_{Na} (at left) and, at right, muscarinic effect in the cortex which facilitates inward currents by reducing K^+ outward current. (Mainly from Figs. 5 and 10 in Krnjević *et al.*, 1971.)

tended to *increase* (Krnjević *et al.*, 1971). Because the depolarizing action had a very negative reversal potential (about −90 mV) and was quite unaffected by intracellular injections of Cl⁻, it was concluded that ACh lowers K⁺ conductance (G_K). The main characteristics of the effects of ACh in a cortical neuron are summarized in Fig. 3. The circuit diagram in Fig. 3F indicates how conventional EPSPs—which are generated predominantly by an increase in Na⁺ conductance—would be potentiated by the ACh-mediated depression of K⁺ outward current. That the muscarinic action facilitates neuronal firing in the neocortex and hippocampus by reducing membrane conductance, probably to K⁺, has been repeatedly confirmed (Woody *et al.*, 1978; Dodd *et al.*, 1981; Ben-Ari *et al.*, 1981; Benardo and Prince, 1981; Halliwell and Adams, 1982; Cole and Nicoll, 1984a,b).

4.1. Depression of Afterhyperpolarization (AHP)

In addition to a reduction in basal G_K, Krnjević *et al.* (1971) found evidence of a depression of a postspike repolarization, an effect that promoted repetitive firing. How this might operate became much clearer when Benardo and Prince (1982) demonstrated that the muscarinic action eliminates the Ca²⁺-dependent AHP of hippocampal pyramidal slices. While confirming this finding Cole and Nicoll (1984a) found no evidence that ACh suppresses Ca²⁺ action potentials in the same cells (Fig. 4). They therefore concluded that the muscarinic receptors must act primarily on the Ca²⁺-activated K⁺ channels responsible for the AHP.

4.2. Depression of Transmitter Release

It has long been known that the release of ACh itself, in the cortex, is reduced by muscarinic agonists and facilitated by antagonists (Fig. 2) (MacIntosh and Oborin, 1953; Mitchell, 1963; Celesia and Jasper, 1966; Dudar and Szerb, 1969). The possibility that ACh might prevent the release of other transmitters was first suggested by Yamamoto and Kawai (1967), and confirmed by Hounsgaard's (1978) demonstration that ACh depresses hippocampal IPSPs, evidently by a presynaptic action. According to a more recent study (Rovira *et al.*, 1983), muscarinic and nicotinic agonists have opposite effects at this site, the latter enhancing the hippocampal EPSPs.

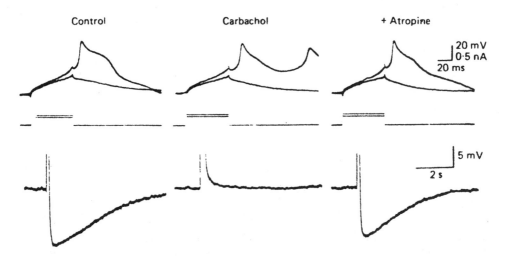

Figure 4. Muscarinic action blocks a Ca²⁺-mediated afterhyperpolarization (AHP) but not Ca²⁺ action potential in hippocampal slice treated with 1 μM tetrodotoxin and 5 mM tetraethylammonium. Traces above show Ca²⁺ action potential evoked by depolarizing pulses and below the corresponding AHP. Only the latter was blocked by carbachol (10 μM). The effect of carbachol was abolished by atropine (1 μM). (From Cole and Nicoll, 1984a.)

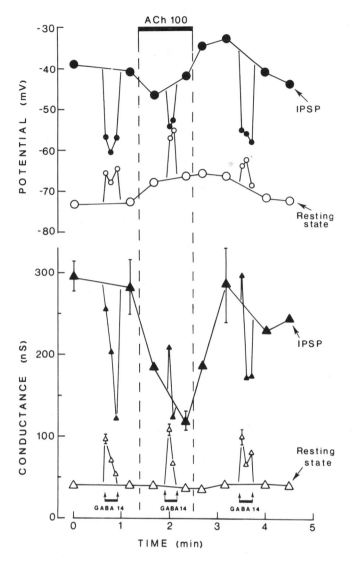

Figure 5. In rat hippocampus *in situ,* ACh greatly diminishes IPSPs. Iontophoretic current of ACh is indicated in nanoamperes. Note especially the markedly reduced IPSP conductance increase, and no depression of effects of GABA (small symbols). (From Ben-Ari *et al.,* 1981.)

Perhaps more significant is a marked depressant action of hippocampal IPSPs (e.g., Ben-Ari *et al.,* 1981; Haas, 1982). Because the action of GABA is not altered (Fig. 5), ACh probably acts via presynaptic receptors, that have both muscarinic and nicotinic properties (Ropert and Krnjević, 1982). A direct action of ACh on GABAergic *terminals* is strongly indicated by a reduction in IPSP quantal *content* (but not *size*) observed in hippocampal cells in culture (Segal, 1983). Thus, ACh must somehow suppress Ca^{2+} influx into nerve endings afferent to hippocampal cells.

Although both EPSPs and IPSPs can be reduced by ACh, the loss of IPSPs functionally is probably more important, because the predominant effect of either ACh applications or activation of a cholinergic input, such as the septohippocampal pathway, is to facilitate CA1 population spikes (Krnjević and Ropert, 1982; Jeantet and Jaffard, 1983; Krnjević *et al.,* 1987).

5. Membrane Mechanisms

The first voltage-clamp study led to a significant reassessment of the comparable mechanism of postsynaptic muscarinic facilitation of sympathetic neurons. According to Brown and Adams (1980), muscarine blocked a low-threshold, voltage- and time-dependent noninactivating K^+ current, which was therefore named the M current. These characteristics of the M current—clearly different from those of other K^+ currents, such as the high-threshold "delayed rectifier" or the low-threshold but fast-adapting A current—helped to explain the powerful facilitatory action of ACh. Finding no evidence of muscarinic effects on Na^{2+} or Ca^{2+} currents, Brown and Adams (1980) concluded that the muscarinic action was exerted directly and exclusively on the M channels. Using a similar approach, Halliwell and Adams (1982) identified a fully comparable M current in hippocampal slices: this was manifested as a slow inward relaxation evoked by hyperpolarizing pulses—starting from a holding potential of about -30 mV where M channels should be fully open—which was reversibly abolished by muscarinic agonists (Fig. 6).

The first hint of a less direct mechanism came from the report of Gähwiler and Dreifuss (1982) that ACh was ineffective in the absence of Ca^{2+}. This suggested that the M current may in fact be a Ca^{2+}-dependent K^+ current (as speculated earlier by Krnjević, 1977). In a more recent voltage-clamp study of rat sympathetic ganglia, Belluzzi et al. (1985) indeed found that muscarine blocks only Ca^{2+} inward current and is quite ineffective in the absence of extracellular Ca^{2+}. Hence, they concluded that M channels are really Ca^{2+}-activated K^+ channels, and that their apparent voltage- and time-dependence reflects the properties of the Ca^{2+} channels. As pointed out by Wanke and Ferroni (this volume), all three known types of neuronal Ca^{2+} currents (Nowycky et al., 1985) can be depressed by muscarine; though different Ca^{2+} currents may be affected in various cells.

The idea that ACh acts primarily on Ca^{2+} channels is attractive because it would provide a simple, unitary explanation for all the muscarinic actions discussed so far, i.e., the block of a noninactivating, voltage-dependent K^+ current (M type), the suppression of the Ca^{2+}-dependent AHP, as well the presynaptic inactivation of IPSPs and EPSPs. The muscarinic inhibitory action in parasympathetic ganglia (Hartzell et al., 1977)—which is mediated by a rise in G_K—may

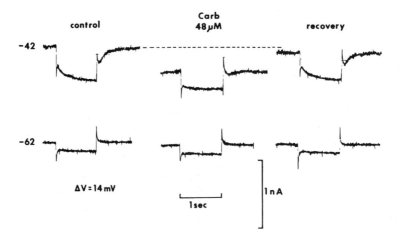

Figure 6. Demonstration of carbachol-sensitive M current in hippocampal slice. Voltage-clamp study shows substantial inward current relaxations evoked by 14-mV hyperpolarizing pulses when initial resting potential was held at -42 mV (above) but not at -62 mV (below). In presence of carbachol, less current is needed to hold cell at -42 mV (note downward displacement of middle trace) and inward relaxation has disappeared. Carbachol has no effect when cell potential is held at -62 mV. (From Halliwell and Adams, 1982.)

perhaps be explained by an *enhancement* of Ca^{2+} current. In any case, there is as yet no compelling evidence that such inhibitory cholinergic synapses exist in the cortex.

6. Internal Messengers

The slow and prolonged character of muscarinic facilitation indicated a possible mediation by some internal messenger system. Though an early favorite for this role, cGMP is no longer viewed as the most likely general messenger of muscarinic actions (because it fails to reproduce consistently the actions of ACh in a variety of neurons; Krnjević *et al.,* 1976; Bernardo and Prince, 1982; Adams *et al.,* 1982), but it may be a second messenger of the cholinergic action in some neocortical (Woody *et al.,* 1978; see also Woody and Gruen, this volume) and hippocampal neurons (Cole and Nicoll, 1984b).

7. Conclusions

The data reviewed here and in the following chapters demonstrate predominantly muscarinic actions of ACh in the cortex, which "modulate" synaptic inputs. These relatively slow and prolonged facilitatory effects may be important in at least two ways: as a mechanism of arousal, essential for awareness and related neural activity; and as part of the learning process that imprints information through a long-term selective enhancement of synaptic efficacy. As emphasized in the chapters by Woody and Gruen and Dykes *et al.,* it appears that a combination of neuronal firing and a local release of ACh may produce very long-lasting changes in excitability. This intriguing phenomenon opens up some fascinating new prospects for the understanding of cerebral mechanisms of learning.

ACKNOWLEDGMENT. The author's research is supported by the Medical Research Council of Canada.

References

Adams, P. R., Brown, D. A., and Constanti, A., 1982, Pharmacological inhibition of the M-current, *J. Physiol. (London)* **332:**223–262.

Belluzzi, O., Sacchi, O., and Wanke, E., 1985, Identification of delayed potassium and calcium currents in the rat sympathetic neurone under voltage clamp, *J. Physiol. (London)* **358:**109–129.

Benardo, L. S., and Prince, D. A., 1981, Acetylcholine induced modulation of hippocampal pyramidal neurons, *Brain Res.* **211:**227–234.

Benardo, L. S., and Prince, D. A., 1982, Cholinergic excitation of mammalian hippocampal pyramidal cells, *Brain Res.* **249:**315–331.

Ben-Ari, Y., Krnjević, K., Reinhardt, W., and Ropert, N., 1981, Intracellular observations on the disinhibitory action of acetylcholine in the hippocampus, *Neuroscience* **6:**2475–2484.

Brown, D. A., and Adams, P. R., 1980, Muscarinic suppression of novel voltage-sensitive K^+ current in a vertebrate neurone, *Nature* **283:**673–676.

Celesia, G. G., and Jasper, H. H., 1966, Acetylcholine released from cerebral cortex in relation to state of activation, *Neurology* **16:**1053–1064.

Cole, A. E., and Nicoll, R. A., 1984a, Characterization of a slow cholinergic postsynaptic potential recorded *in vitro* from rat hippocampal pyramidal cells, *J. Physiol. (London)* **352:**173–188.

Cole, A. E., and Nicoll, R. A., 1984b, The pharmacology of cholinergic excitatory responses in hippocampal pyramidal cells, *Brain Res.* **305:**283–290.

Dodd, J., Dingledine, R., and Kelly, J. S., 1981, The excitatory action of acetylcholine on hippocampal neurones of the guinea pig and rat maintained in vitro, *Brain Res.* **207:**109–127.

Dudar, J. D., and Szerb, J. C., 1969, The effect of topically applied atropine on resting and evoked cortical acetylcholine release, *J. Physiol. (London)* **203**:741–762.

Eccles, J. C., Fatt, P., and Koketsu, K., 1954, Cholinergic and inhibitory synapses in a pathway from motor-axon collaterals to motoneurones, *J. Physiol. (London)* **126**:524–562.

Feldberg, W., and Vogt, M., 1948, Acetylcholine synthesis in different regions of the central nervous system, *J. Physiol. (London)* **107**:372–381.

Gähwiler, B. H., and Dreifuss, J. J., 1982, Multiple actions of acetylcholine on hippocampal pyramidal cells in organotypic explant cultures, *Neuroscience* **7**:1243–1256.

Haas, H. L., 1982, Cholinergic disinhibition in hippocampal slices of the rat, *Brain Res.* **233**:200–204.

Halliwell, J. V., and Adams, P. R., 1982, Voltage-clamp analysis of muscarinic excitation in hippocampal neurons, *Brain Res.* **250**:71–92.

Hartzell, H. C., Kuffler, S. W., Stickgold, R., and Yoshikami, D., 1977, Synaptic excitation and inhibition resulting from direct action of acetylcholine on two types of chemoreceptors on individual amphibian parasympathetic neurones, *J. Physiol. (London)* **271**:817–846.

Hebb, C. O., and Silver, A., 1956, Choline acetylase in the central nervous system of man and some other mammals, *J. Physiol. (London)* **134**:718–728.

Henley, J. M., Lindstrom, J. M., and Oswald, R. E., 1986, Acetylcholine receptor synthesis in retina and transport to optic tectum goldfish, *Science* **232**:1627–1629.

Hounsgaard, J., 1978, Presynaptic inhibitory action of acetylcholine in area CA1 of the hippocampus, *Exp. Neurol.* **62**:787–797.

Jeantet, Y., and Jaffard, R., 1983, Influence of the medial septal nucleus on the excitability of the commissural path–CA1 pyramidal cell synapse in the hippocampus of freely moving mice, *Neuroscience* **8**:291–297.

Krnjević, K., 1977, Control of neuronal excitability by intracellular divalent cations: A possible target for neurotransmitter actions, in: *Neurotransmitter Function: Basic and Clinical Aspects* (W. S. Fields, ed.), Symposia Specialist Press, Miami, pp. 11–26.

Krnjević, K., and Phillis, J. W., 1963a, Acetylcholine-sensitive cells in the cerebral cortex, *J. Physiol. (London)* **166**:296–327.

Krnjević, K., and Phillis, J. W., 1963b, Pharmacological properties of acetylcholine-sensitive cells in the cerebral cortex, *J. Physiol. (London)* **166**:328–350.

Krnjević, K., and Ropert, N., 1982, Electrophysiological and pharmacological characteristics of facilitation of hippocampal population spikes by stimulation of the medial septum, *Neuroscience* **7**:2165–2183.

Krnjević, K., and Silver, A., 1965, A histochemical study of cholinergic fibres in the cerebral cortex, *J. Anat.* **99**:711–759.

Krnjević, K., and Silver, A., 1966, Acetylcholinesterase in the developing forebrain, *J. Anat.* **100**:63–89.

Krnjević, K., Pumain, R., and Renaud, L., 1971, The mechanism of excitation by acetylcholine in the cerebral cortex, *J. Physiol. (London)* **215**:247–268.

Krnjević, K., Puil, E., and Werman, R., 1976, Is cyclic guanosine monophosphate the internal "second messenger" for cholinergic actions on central neurons? *Can. J. Physiol. Pharmacol.* **54**:172–176.

Krnjević, K., Ropert, N., and Casullo, J., 1987, Septo-hippocampal disinhibition, *Brain Res.* (in press).

MacIntosh, F. C., and Oborin, P. E., 1953, Release of acetylcholine from intact cerebral cortex, *Abstr. XIX Int. Physiol. Congr.* pp. 580–581.

Masland, R. H., Mills, J. W., and Cassidy, C., 1984a, The functions of acetylcholine in the rabbit retina, *Proc. R. Soc. Lond. B* **223**:121–139.

Masland, R. H., Mills, J. W., and Hayden, S. A., 1984b, Acetylcholine-synthesizing amacrine cells: identification and selective staining by using radioautography and fluorescent markers, *Proc. R. Soc. Lond. B* **223**:79–100.

Mitchell, J. F., 1963, The spontaneous and evoked release of acetylcholine from the cerebral cortex, *J. Physiol. (London)* **165**:98–116.

Nowycky, M. C., Fox, A. P., and Tsien, R. W., 1985, Three types of neuronal calcium channel with different calcium agonist sensitivity, *Nature* **316**:440–442.

Oswald, R. E., Schmidt, D. E., and Freeman, J. A., 1979, Assessment of acetylcholine as an optic nerve neurotransmitter in *Bufo marinus*, *Neuroscience* **4**:1129–1136.

Ropert, N., and Krnjević, K., 1982, Pharmacological characteristics of facilitation of hippocampal population spikes by cholinomimetics, *Neuroscience* **7**:1963–1977.

Rovira, C., Ben-Ari, Y., Cherubini, E., Krnjević, K., and Ropert, N., 1983, Pharmacology of the dendritic action of acetylcholine and further observations on the somatic disinhibition in the rat hippocampus *in situ*, *Neuroscience* **8**:97–106.

Segal, M., 1983, Rat hippocampal neurons in culture: Responses to electrical and chemical stimuli, *J. Neurophysiol.* **50**:1249–1264.

Shute, C. C. D., and Lewis, P. R., 1963, Cholinesterase-containing systems of the brain of the rat, *Nature* **199:**1160–1164.

Shute, C. C. D., and Lewis, P. R., 1967, The ascending cholinergic reticular system: Neocortical olfactory and subcortical projections, *Brain* **90:**497–520.

Sillito, A. M., and Kemp, J. A., 1983, Cholinergic modulation of the functional organization of the cat visual cortex, *Brain Res.* **289:**143–155.

Woody, C. D., Swartz, B. E., and Gruen, E., 1978, Effects of acetylcholine and cyclic GMP on input resistance of cortical neurons in awake cats, *Brain Res.* **158:**373–395.

Yamamoto, C., and Kawai, N., 1967, Presynaptic action of acetylcholine in thin sections from the guinea pig dentate gyrus *in vitro*, *Exp. Neurol.* **19:**176–187.

15

Central Cholinergic Pathways
Neuroanatomy and Some Behavioral Implications

M.-Marsel Mesulam

Neurons which synthesize and secrete acetylcholine (ACh) for the purpose of neurotransmission are designated as cholinergic. The pioneering work of Otto Loewi established ACh as a neurotransmitter in the peripheral nervous system (Loewi, 1921). Soon thereafter, the suggestion was made that ACh could also serve a similar purpose in central nervous structures (Dale, 1938). Partial support for this possibility was obtained by pharmacological and physiological investigations which showed that ACh, acetylcholinesterase (AChE), choline acetyltransferase (ChAT), and cholinergic receptor sites were widely distributed throughout the neuraxis and that many central neurons were responsive to ACh (for review see Silver, 1974; Fibiger, 1982; Mesulam *et al.*, 1983b). Observations based on AChE histochemistry provided additional information on the anatomical arrangement of cholinergic pathways in the brain stem, diencephalon, limbic system, and neocortex (Krnjević and Silver, 1965; Shute and Lewis, 1967). However, uncertainty has always been associated with conclusions based on AChE histochemistry since this enzyme is also present in many noncholinergic neurons. The production of monoclonal and monospecific antibodies to ChAT by several research groups has now provided new and much more reliable information on the distribution of cholinergic neurons and on the organization of their connections (Rossier, 1984; Wainer *et al.*, 1984). Since the presence of ChAT is necessary and probably also sufficient for the synthesis of ACh, the immunohistochemical demonstration of ChAT currently constitutes the most specific anatomical marker for putative cholinergic neurons and their processes. Although it is not yet known if all neurons that contain ChAT also secrete ACh, this seems like a reasonable assumption to make, but will ultimately need definitive confirmation through a combination of anatomical and physiological approaches.

The contemporary literature on the anatomy of cholinergic neurons is vast and varied. The purpose of this chapter is not to provide a critical review of these developments but to summarize some observations on central cholinergic pathways that my colleagues and I have made in the past 10 years. The papers cited provide additional references to the rich literature on this subject.

M.-Marsel Mesulam • Bullard and Denny-Brown Laboratories, Division of Neuroscience and Behavioral Neurology, Dana Research Institute, Harvard Neurology Department, Beth Israel Hospital, Boston, Massachusetts 02215.

2. Cholinergic Innervation of the Striatal Complex

The striatal complex has four major components: the *caudate* and *putamen*, collectively designated as the neostriatum, and the *olfactory tubercle* and *nucleus accumbens* also known as the limbic striatum. All four components contain cholinergic neurons. In the rhesus monkey, ChAT-positive cholinergic neurons in the caudate and putamen are larger but less densely packed than those in the olfactory tubercle and nucleus accumbens (Mesulam *et al.*, 1984a). The concentration of cholinergic neurons in the limbic striatum is particularly high around the islands of Calleja (Fig. 1). The density of other cholinergic markers (e.g., AChE, muscarinic receptors) also displays patchy variations in the striatum. These patches have been designated as striosomes (Nastuk and Graybiel, 1985).

The striatal complex contains populations of large and small neurons. The cholinergic cells of the striatum belong to the class of large aspiny neurons seen in Golgi preparations (Wainer *et al.*, 1984). Only 1–2% of the striatal perikarya are cholinergic. These neurons do not seem to have projections outside the striatum (Woolf and Butcher, 1981). In fact, the striatal complex

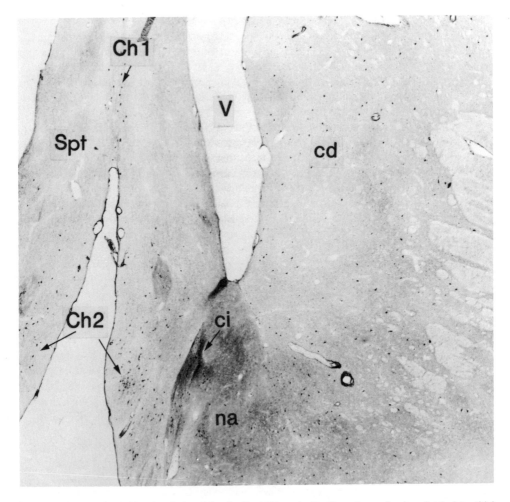

Figure 1. ChAT immunohistochemical staining in the macaque brain. Curved arrowheads point to interstitial elements of Ch4. Magnification is 24×. The photomicrograph is taken from coronal sections that are from progressively more posterior levels of the brain. (From Mesulam *et al.*, 1984a.)

provides the best known example of a telencephalic structure which receives almost all of its cholinergic input from local circuit interneurons. In addition to these local projections, the striatum also receives what is probably a relatively minor cholinergic innervation from the ChAT-positive neurons of the basal forebrain (Arikuni and Kubota, 1984).

3. Source of Cholinergic Innervation for the Hippocampus, Olfactory Bulb, Amygdala, and Cerebral Cortex—The Ch1–Ch4 Cell Groups

In contrast to the striatum, the great majority of the cholinergic innervation for the hippocampus, olfactory bulb, amygdala, and neocortex comes from extrinsic sources located in the basal forebrain. The adult rodent neocortex and hippocampus contain intrinsic ChAT-positive cell bodies which may provide approximately 30% of their cholinergic innervation (Johnston et al., 1981; Eckenstein and Thoenen, 1983: Houser et al., 1983; Levey et al., 1984). Immunohistochemical observations suggest that such neurons are either less conspicuous or perhaps absent in the adult brain of other species including reptiles, carnivores, and primates (Kimura et al., 1981; Mesulam et al., 1984a; Mufson et al., 1984). Extrinsic sources therefore account for as much as 70% of the cortical cholinergic input in the rodent brain and this proportion may be even higher in the adult primate.

The cholinergic innervation of olfactory, limbic, and neocortical regions arises from basal forebrain nuclei which contain cholinergic as well as noncholinergic cells. In order to focus attention on the cholinergic component of these nuclei, we have designated the ChAT-positive cell groups in these regions as Ch1–Ch4 (Mesulam et al., 1983a,b, 1984a). The Ch1–Ch4 nomenclature is based not only on the location of the neurons but also on their connectivity patterns. The following discussion will concentrate on observations in the primate even though comparative information from the rodent brain will also be included.

Ch1–Ch2: The Ch1 and Ch2 cell groups collectively provide (by way of the fornix, fimbria, and perhaps supracallosal fibers) the major cholinergic innervation of the hippocampal formation. In the rhesus monkey as well as in the rat, Ch1 consists of the ChAT-positive neurons within the traditional boundaries of the medial septal nucleus (Fig. 1). These are the smallest of the basal forebrain cholinergic neurons. The proportion of medial septal cells that are ChAT-positive varies from about 50% in the rat brain to even less in the monkey. The boundary between the Ch1 and Ch2 groups is not sharp. In both rat and monkey, approximately 70% of the cell bodies within the vertical nucleus of the diagonal band of Broca are cholinergic and make up the Ch2 cell group (Fig. 1).

Experiments based on the concurrent demonstration of retrogradely transported horseradish peroxidase (HRP) and perikaryal cholinergic markers have shown that only about half of the projections from the septal area to the hippocampal formation arise from cholinergic Ch1–Ch2 neurons (Mesulam et al., 1977, 1983b; Baisden et al., 1984; Wainer et al., 1985). The septohippocampal pathway is therefore not uniformly cholinergic. The transmitter(s) for the other components of the septohippocampal pathway remain unknown. This anatomical arrangement is consistent with physiological observations on hippocampal theta, a rhythm which is dependent on the integrity of the septohippocampal projections. According to these observations, the hippocampal theta rhythm has at least two components only one of which can be abolished by cholinergic antagonists (Rawlins et al., 1979; Vanderwolf, 1983).

Ch3: The Ch3 cell group provides the principal source of cholinergic innervation for the olfactory bulb. In the rhesus monkey, approximately 2% of the cell bodies in the horizontal limb nucleus of the diagonal band of Broca are ChAT-positive. This cell group makes up the major aggregate of cholinergic cells projecting to the olfactory bulb and is designated as Ch3 (Figs. 2 and 3). In the rat, the Ch3 designation fits most appropriately the cholinergic neurons only in the *lateral* portion of the horizontal limb nucleus since this is the component from which the principal connection to the olfactory bulb arises. Approximately 20% of the cell bodies in this lateral

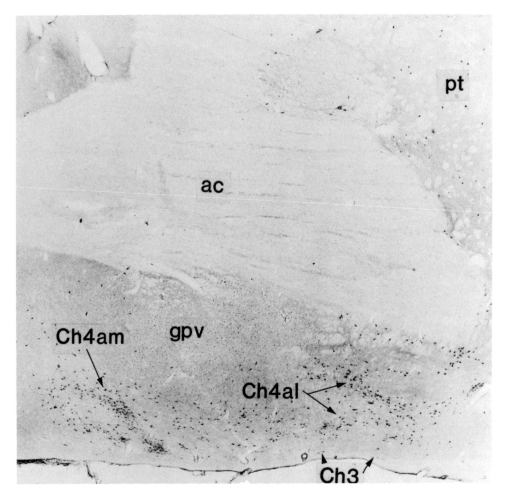

Figure 2. ChAT immunohistochemical staining in the macaque brain. Curved arrowheads point to interstitial elements of Ch4. Magnification is 24×. The photomicrograph is taken from coronal sections that are from progressively more posterior levels of the brain. (From Mesulam *et al.,* 1984a.)

portion of the rodent's horizontal limb nucleus are ChAT-positive. The great majority of projections from the horizontal nucleus of the diagonal band to the olfactory bulb in the rodent as well as in the monkey arise from noncholinergic neurons (Mesulam *et al.,* 1977, 1983b).

Ch4: The Ch4 neurons provide the major cholinergic innervation for the amygdala and all neocortical regions. In keeping with the highly developed cerebral cortex of the primate brain, the Ch4 group is very extensive in monkeys and humans (Figs. 2–6). In the primate brain, the Ch4 complex contains the cholinergic neurons within the nucleus basalis (NB) of the substantia innominata (Mesulam and Van Hoesen, 1976; Parent *et al.,* 1977; Mesulam *et al.,* 1983a). At least 90% of the neurons in the NB are cholinergic and belong to Ch4. For practical purposes, therefore, the NB and Ch4 are coextensive and share an identical topography in the primate brain (Mesulam *et al.,* 1986b). In the rat, however, the Ch4 group (defined as the collection of ChAT-positive forebrain cells which provide the major cholinergic innervation of cortex and amygdala) is more modest in size and less easily confined to any specific nuclear formation (Mesulam *et al.,* 1983b). Studies based on the concurrent demonstration of perikaryal cholinergic markers and retrogradely transported HRP suggest that the Ch4 of the rodent includes ChAT-positive neurons in the *medial* part of the horizontal limb nucleus of the diagonal band and also in a location just medial and ventral to the globus pallidus. It is this latter region that is usually designated as the nucleus basalis in the rat brain. Many ChAT-positive neurons in the lateral portion of the vertical limb nucleus of the rat also project to neocortex and probably belong to the Ch4 group.

The Ch4–NB complex of the primate brain extends from the level of the olfactory tubercle anteriorly to that of the lateral geniculate body posteriorly. In the human, this complex contains approximately 200,000 neurons in each hemisphere (Arendt *et al.*, 1985). This extensive nuclear complex comes into intimate contact with many other cell groups including those of the ventral striatum, the septal area, the ventral globus pallidus, the amygdaloid complex, the preoptic region, and the lateral hypothalamus. In addition to the compact cell group which is coextensive with the NB, Ch4 also contains interstitial elements embedded among the fibers of the diagonal band of Broca, the anterior commissure, the stria terminalis, the ansa peduncularis, the ansa lenticularis, the inferior thalamic peduncle, and the medullary laminae of the globus pallidus. The Ch4 complex can be subdivided into several sectors. The anterior sector of Ch4 is located at the level of the decussation of the anterior commissure. A vascular marking or a rarefaction in cell density divides this into anteromedial (Ch4am) and anterolateral (Ch4al) subsectors (Fig. 2). The passage of the ansa peduncularis through the basal forebrain identifies the intermediate sector of Ch4 which is further subdivided by the ansa into dorsal (Ch4id) and ventral (Ch4iv) subsectors (Fig. 4). Behind the ansa peduncularis lies the extensive posterior sector of Ch4 (Ch4p) (Figs. 5

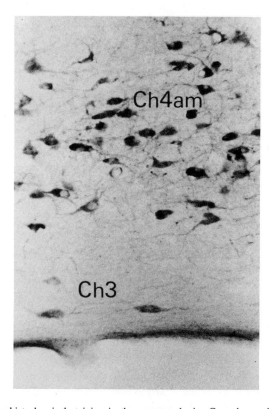

Figure 3. ChAT immunohistochemical staining in the macaque brain. Curved arrowheads point to interstitial elements of Ch4. Magnification is 150×. The photomicrograph is taken from coronal sections that are from progressively more posterior levels of the brain. (From Mesulam *et al.*, 1984a.)

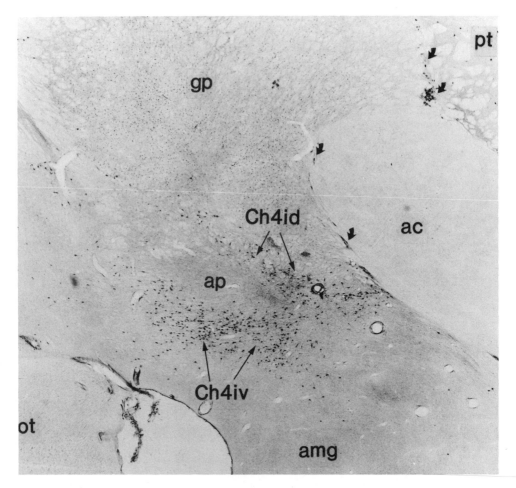

Figure 4. ChAT immunohistochemical staining in the macaque brain. Curved arrowheads point to interstitial elements of Ch4. Magnification is 24×. The photomicrograph is taken from coronal sections that are from progressively more posterior levels of the brain. (From Mesulam *et al.*, 1984a.)

and 6). If the few noncholinergic neurons of the NB are also taken into account, these topographical subdivisions could be designated as NBam, NBal, NBiv, NBid, and NBp. A similar arrangement is present in the human brain (Mesulam *et al.*, 1983a; Arendt *et al.*, 1985).

The three-dimensional reconstruction of the Ch4–NB cell group, even without including its interstitial elements, shows a remarkable structural complexity (Fig. 7A). In the absence of specific cholinotoxins, attempts at destroying Ch4–NB would lead to extensive damage in a large number of additional noncholinergic structures.

4. Topography of Projections from Ch4 to the Amygdala and Cortex

Observations based on 36 rhesus monkeys, each with an HRP injection within a specific brain region, and each prepared for the concurrent visualization of retrogradely transported HRP and perikaryal cholinergic markers, indicated that different cortical regions receive their principal cholinergic innervation from different Ch4 subsectors (Mesulam *et al.*, 1983a, 1986b). Thus,

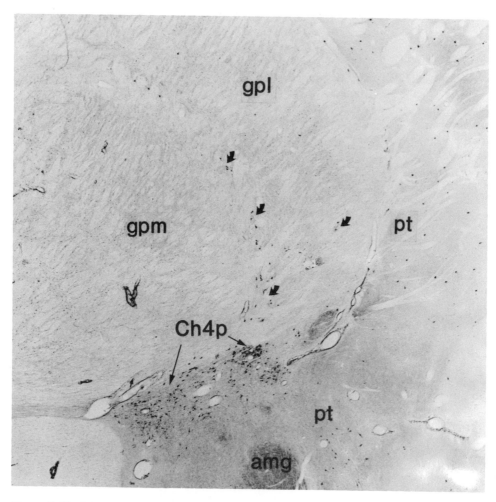

Figure 5. ChAT immunohistochemical staining in the macaque brain. Curved arrowheads point to interstitial elements of Ch4. Magnification is 24×. The photomicrograph is taken from coronal sections that are from progressively more posterior levels of the brain. (From Mesulam *et al.,* 1984a.)

Ch4am is the major source of projections for the dorsomedial surface of the cerebral hemispheres including medial parietal, medial frontal, and cingulate cortex; Ch4al is the major source of cholinergic projections for the frontoparietal operculum and the amygdaloid complex; the Ch4i sector provides the major cholinergic input for lateral prefrontal, parietal, peristriate, midtemporal, and inferotemporal cortex; Ch4p provides the major cholinergic innervation for the superior temporal gyrus and the adjacent temporal pole (Figs. 7B and 8, Table I). Although this topography is not as specific as the arrangement of thalamocortical connections, there is anatomical organization in that each cortical region receives its primary cholinergic input from a circumscribed portion of Ch4. Approximately 96% of the projections from the NB to cortex arise from ChAT-positive cell bodies (Mesulam *et al.,* 1986b). The transmitter for the noncholinergic NB neurons remains unknown. Extremely few (less than 2%) Ch4 neurons have contralateral projections (Mesulam *et al.,* 1983a). Observations in the rat suggest that each Ch4 neuron innervates a small cortical area, approximately 1 mm in diameter, without sending additional collaterals to other cortical regions (Price and Stern, 1983). This question deserves more attention, especially in

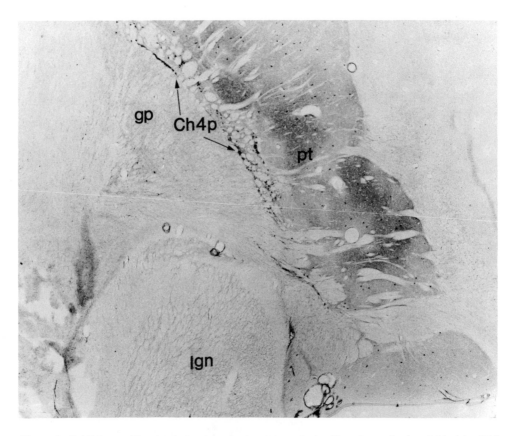

Figure 6. ChAT immunohistochemical staining in the macaque brain. Curved arrowheads point to interstitial elements of Ch4. Magnification is 24×. The photomicrograph is taken from coronal sections that are from progressively more posterior levels of the brain. (From Mesulam *et al.*, 1984a.)

the monkey brain where the total number of Ch4 neurons appears to be too low if each cell is to innervate such a small area of cortex.

5. Sources of Cholinergic Projections for the Thalamus and Some Mesencephalic Structures—The Ch5–Ch8 Groups

Ch5–Ch6: No ChAT-positive thalamic neurons have yet been reported in any animal species. Although this does not prove the absence of such neurons, it raises the possibility that the cholinergic innervation for this region of the brain may be predominantly, if not entirely, extrinsic. Approximately 80% of all cholinergic neurons that project to the thalamus are located within two pontomesencephalic cholinergic cell groups that we have designated as Ch5 and Ch6 (Figs. 9 and 10). The rest of the cholinergic neurons that project to the thalamus are located primarily within the Ch1–Ch4 groups (Mesulam *et al.*, 1983b). The Ch5–Ch6 groups also contain about 10% of cholinergic cell bodies projecting to limbic and cortical regions (Mufson *et al.*, 1982; Mesulam *et al.*, 1983b). Therefore, cortical and limbic regions are under three types of cholinergic influence: (1) a major direct input from Ch1–Ch4; (2) a minor direct input from Ch5–Ch6; (3) an indirect input with a cholinergic relay from Ch5–Ch6 to the thalamus and a noncholinergic relay from the thalamus to cortex.

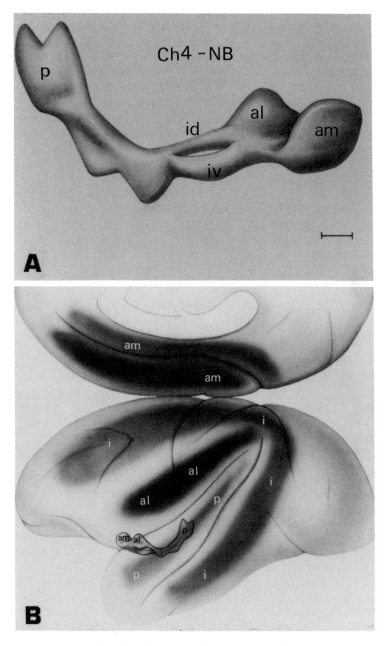

Figure 7. (A) A three-dimensional drawing of the left NB–Ch4 in the macaque brain showing its anteromedial (am), anterolateral (al), intermediodorsal (id), intermedioventral (iv), and posterior (p) sectors. The ansa peduncularis passes through the space between id and iv. Bar ~ 1.3 mm. Dorsal is toward the top. In the primate brain and at the macroscopic level of analysis, Ch4 is coextensive with what is now commonly designated as the nucleus basalis. Therefore, this three-dimensional representation applies equally well to the NB as well as to Ch4. (B) A schematic diagram showing the distribution of cortical areas that receive their major cholinergic input from the am, al, intermediate (i), and p sectors of Ch4. Definitive information is not yet available for the occipital lobe. (From Mesulam *et al.*, 1986b.)

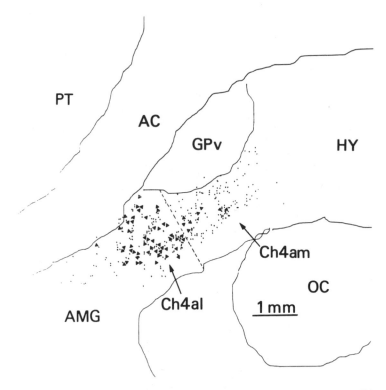

Figure 8. Tracing obtained from an X–Y plotter electronically coupled to the microscope stage. Triangles indicate retrogradely labeled Ch4 neurons after a large HRP injection in frontoparietal opercular cortex of a macaque brain. The dots represent Ch4 neurons not labeled with the retrogradely transported HRP. The dashed line provides an approximate demarcation between Ch4am and Ch4al. (From Mesulam *et al.*, 1986b.)

The Ch5 group is made up of large (75–80 by 40–45 μm in the monkey) ChAT-positive neurons which are aggregated mostly in the pedunculopontine nucleus but which also extend into the nucleus cuneiformis and the parabrachial region (Figs. 9 and 10). In the pedunculopontine region Ch5 has a compact lateral portion which abuts upon the lateral lemniscus and a more diffuse medial component which is largely embedded within the central tegmental tract and the superior cerebellar peduncle (Figs. 9 and 10). Large and small cells are intermingled with each other in the pedunculopontine nucleus. About 75% of the large neurons in the lateral part of this nucleus and 25% of those in the medial part belong to Ch5. The remainder of the neurons in these regions do not stain positively for ChAT.

The Ch6 sector consists of relatively smaller (40–45 by 50–55 μm in the monkey) cholinergic neurons which are located within the boundaries of the laterodorsal tegmental nucleus. The laterodorsal tegmental nucleus contains both large and small cells. Approximately 90% of the larger neurons are ChAT-positive and make up the Ch6 group. The majority of projections from the laterodorsal tegmental nucleus and pedunculopontine nuclei to the thalamus arise from the cholinergic Ch5–Ch6 component of neurons (Mesulam *et al.*, 1983b; Isaacson and Tanaka, 1986).

Ch7: The medial habenular nucleus contains oval, lightly ChAT-positive neurons (30 by 35 μm in the monkey). Although we have not checked this directly by combined transport and immunohistochemical methods, it is reasonable to assume that these neurons send cholinergic projections to the interpeduncular nucleus via the habenulo-interpeduncular tract (Kataoka *et al.*, 1974).

Table I. Percentage of Retrograde Labeling and Number of Retrogradely Labeled Neurons in the Ch Sectors of Two Macaque Hemispheres[a]

	Case I—HRP in frontoparietal operculum								Case II—HRP in superior temporal gyrus							
Percent of total labeling:	Ch1 0%	Ch2 1%	Ch3 0%	Ch4am 11%	Ch4al 52%	Ch4id 12%	Ch4iv 12%	Ch4p 11%	Ch1 4%	Ch2 2%	Ch3 0%	Ch4am 3%	Ch4al 0%	Ch4id 1%	Ch4iv 1%	Ch4p 89%
Level[b]																
1	1	3							3	3						
2	0	2	1	6	25				0	2	1	0	0			
3	0	0	0	9	66				1	0	0	1	0			
4			0	12	83						0	2	0			
5			0	9	18	5	11				0	0	0	0		
6						18	19							1	1	
7						23	14							0	0	
8								15								16
9								16								5
10								9								12
11								1								28
12								0								8
13								0								9
14								0								4

[a]From Mesulam et al. (1986b).
[b]Level 1 is most anterior, level 14 most posterior. The distance between each level is approximately 1 mm. The numbers at each level represent the counts of retrogradely labeled Ch4 neurons. Observations based on 36 macaque cerebra show that these topographical patterns are quite reliable.

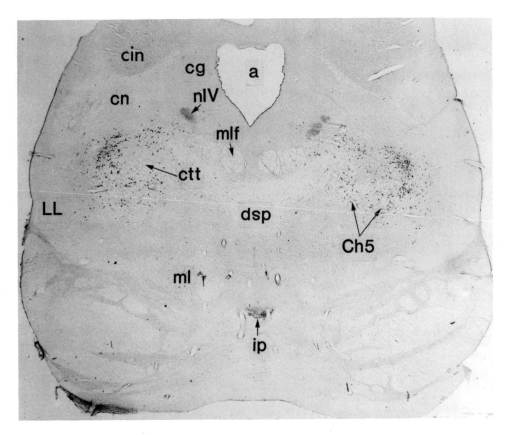

Figure 9. ChAT immunohistochemical staining in the macaque brain stem at the pontomesencephalic level. Magnification 10×. (From Mesulam *et al.*, 1984a.)

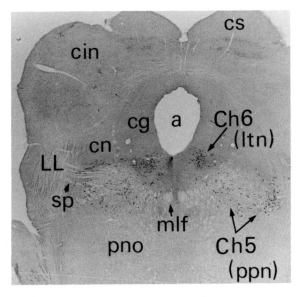

Figure 10. ChAT immunohistochemical staining in the rat brain stem at the pontomesencephalic level. Magnification 17×. (From Mesulam *et al.*, 1983b.)

Ch8: Studies in the mouse show that most of the cholinergic cell bodies which project to the superior colliculus are located in the parabigeminal nucleus (Mufson *et al.*, 1986). Another but smaller contingent of cholinergic cells projecting to the superior colliculus is located in Ch5 and Ch6. About 80–90% of the cell bodies in the parabigeminal nucleus are ChAT-positive and have been designated as Ch8. In keeping with the proportion of cholinergic to noncholinergic neurons, approximately 80% of the parabigeminal neurons that project to the superior colliculus are also ChAT-positive. In contrast to the Ch1–Ch6 projections which are predominantly, if not exclusively, ipsilateral, the projection from Ch8 to the superior colliculus is mostly crossed.

6. Feedback Control of the Ch4–NB in the Monkey Brain

The Ch4 cell group provides the cholinergic innervation for the entire cortical surface and the amygdala. It had been known that the Ch4 region receives neural input from limbic structures such as the amygdala, septal nuclei, and hypothalamus (Saper *et al.*, 1979; Price and Amaral, 1981). As evidence accumulated for an extensive net of projections from Ch4 to the cortical surface, it became important to determine if these cortical regions also sent reciprocal projections back into Ch4. This question was addressed in a study based on 35 rhesus monkeys, each with an injection of tritiated amino acids within a specific cerebral area (Mesulam and Mufson, 1984). These studies showed that virtually none of the primary sensory-motor and association areas in the frontal, parietal, occipital, and temporal lobes projected back to Ch4–NB. The only cortical areas with substantial projections to Ch4–NB were located in the orbitofrontal, anterior insular, temporopolar, and parahippocampal, and probably cingulate regions (Fig. 11). Almost all of these regions that project to Ch4–NB belong to the paralimbic group of cortical regions. These anatomical conclusions have been confirmed by subsequent studies based on HRP injections within the Ch4–NB region (Russchen *et al.*, 1985).

This remarkable selectivity of corticofugal projections into Ch4–NB indicates that primary and association areas have little or no direct feedback upon the cholinergic input that they receive whereas a handful of limbic and paralimbic areas can regulate not only the cholinergic input that they receive but also the cholinergic innervation directed to the rest of the cortical surface. This anatomical arrangement suggests that the Ch4–NB region is in a position to act as a cholinergic relay for modulating the activity of the entire cortical surface according to the prevailing motivational state as encoded by limbic and paralimbic regions (Mesulam and Mufson, 1984).

7. The Cortical Distribution of Cholinergic Innervation

Cortical fibers form a dense and intricate plexus in almost all cortical areas. Observations based on the distribution of ChAT and AChE in the monkey show that these cholinergic markers display marked and statistically significant regional variations (Mesulam *et al.* 1984b, 1986a; Lehmann *et al.*, 1984).

The hippocampus and amygdala contain high levels of the presynaptic cholinergic marker ChAT. This confirms the well-accepted notion that these two limbic structures receive a rich cholinergic input. In addition, we found that the paralimbic (mesocortical) areas of the brain (e.g., parahippocampal, insular, caudal orbitofrontal, temporopolar, and parolfactory cortex) also contain high levels of cholinergic input. In contrast, the concentration of ChAT was much lower (by as much as sevenfold) within all frontal and temporoparietal association areas. As a group, the primary sensory and motor regions contained an intermediate level of ChAT activity. The cingulate gyrus was the only major paralimbic area with a relatively low level of ChAT. Within each paralimbic area, the more primitive nonisocortical sectors tended to have higher levels of cholinergic innervation than the immediately adjacent isocortical regions (Fig. 12, Table II).

As mentioned above, several lines of observation suggest that regional ChAT activity in the adult primate cortex is likely to reflect primarily the density of cholinergic fibers which arise from extrinsic sources located within the Ch4 sectors (Mesulam *et al.*, 1986a). The observations on regional ChAT activities therefore suggest that the projections from Ch4 to the cerebral cortex are not uniformly distributed and that the variations in these projections respect architectonic and functional boundaries. Our preliminary observations on the distribution of cortical AChE axons suggest that a similar pattern of regional variations may be present in the human cerebral cortex (Green *et al.*, 1986). It is not yet known if cortical regions with a more intense cholinergic input

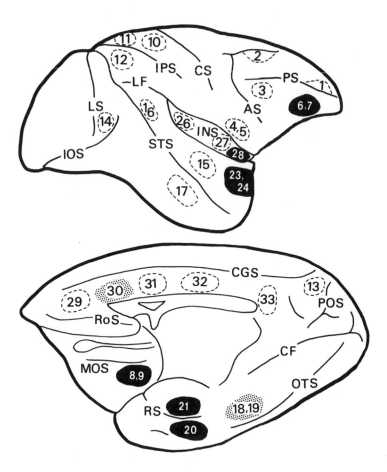

Figure 11. Summary diagram of cortical regions in the macaque that project to the Ch4–NB complex. Each animal involved in this study received a tracer injection in only one of the regions shown in this summary diagram. The dashed circles indicate regions where tritiated amino acid injections did not result in anterograde transport to Ch4–NB. Lightly stippled regions indicate areas that send fibers through the substantia innominata and perhaps also a relatively minor projection to Ch4–NB. Tracer injections within the blackened regions resulted in definite projections to the Ch4–NB complex. The diagram on top shows the lateral surface of the cerebral hemisphere and the one at the bottom, the medial and basal surfaces. The descriptive location of the regions are as follows: 1–3: dorsolateral prefrontal association cortex, 4–5: frontal operculum, 6–7: lateral orbitofrontal cortex, 8–9: caudal orbitofrontal cortex, 10: somatosensory cortex, 11: somatosensory association cortex, 12–13: caudal parietal association cortex, 14: peristriate visual association cortex, 15–16: auditory association cortex, 17: inferotemporal visual association cortex, 18–19: parahippocampal cortex, 20: medial inferotemporal and parahippocampal areas, 21: entorhinal cortex, 23–24: temporopolar cortex, 26: posterior insula, 27: middle insula, 28; anterior insula, 29–30: anterior cingulate gyrus, 31: middle cingulate gyrus, 32: posterior cingulate gyrus, 33: retrosplenial area. Injections 22 and 25 (within the hippocampus and piriform olfactory cortex, respectively) are not shown. Of these two, only the piriform injection showed anterograde transport to Ch4–NB. (From Mesulam and Mufson, 1984.)

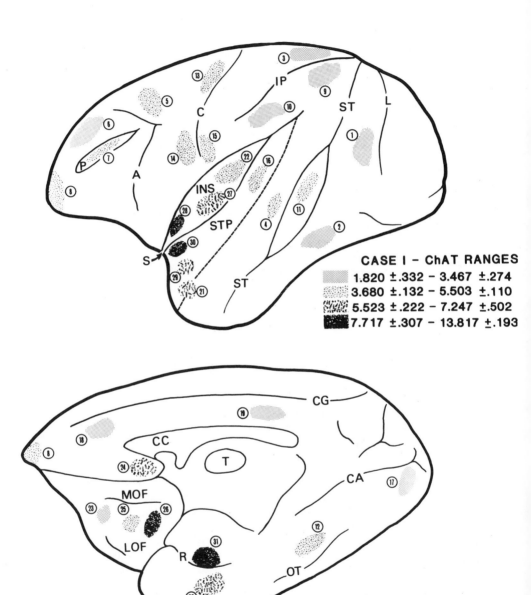

Figure 12. Regional distribution of ChAT activities in the macaque brain (expressed as nanomoles of ACh produced per 15 min per milligram protein). The ChAT activities are divided into four nonoverlapping ranges. The sample numbers correspond to those in Table II which can be consulted for specific values and anatomical descriptions. All assays were performed in triplicate. (From Mesulam *et al.*, 1986a.)

Table II. ChAT Enzymatic Activities and Standard Errors[a,b]

Sample number	Area	ChAT (nmoles/15 min per mg protein)	
		Case I	Case II
	Association areas	**3.465 ± 0.278**	**7.202 ± 0.790**
1	(OA,OB) Peristriate visual association	3.467 ± 0.274	3.938 ± 0.186
2	(TE) Temporal visual association	1.820 ± 0.332	5.560 ± 0.077
3	(PE) Somatosensory association	3.213 ± 0.162	4.327 ± 0.043
4	(TA) Auditory association	4.357 ± 0.047	9.081 ± 0.520
5	(FB) Dorsal premotor association	3.990 ± 0.336	9.708 ± 0.466
6	(FD) Dorsolateral prefrontal	2.740 ± 0.075	6.096 ± 0.208
7	(FD) Principalis cortex (prefrontal)	3.680 ± 0.132	6.758 ± 0.014
8	(FD) Frontopolar cortex	4.157 ± 0.162	5.827 ± 0.290
9	(PG) Caudal inferior parietal lobule	2.070 ± 0.123	4.092 ± 0.225
10	(PF) Rostral inferior parietal lobule	2.867 ± 0.132	11.320 ± 0.144
11	Banks of superior temporal sulcus	4.157 ± 0.113	11.707 ± 0.470
12	(TF) Caudal inferotemporal cortex	5.047 ± 0.283	8.002 ± 0.039
	Primary sensory-motor	**4.394 ± 0.576**	**9.820 ± 3.068**
13	(FA) Dorsal primary motor	4.013 ± 0.084	6.335 ± 0.255
14	(FBA-FA) Ventral primary motor	5.443 ± 0.154	7.191 ± 0.070
15	(PC(3b)) Primary somatosensory	5.503 ± 0.110	10.511 ± 0.480
16	(TC) Primary auditory	4.653 ± 0.177	21.307 ± 1.213
17	(OC) Primary visual	2.367 ± 0.124	3.762 ± 0.078
	Cingulate gyrus	**3.170 ± 0.130**	**7.600 ± 1.440**
18	(LA) Anterior cingulate	3.040 ± 0.310	9.043 ± 0.507
19	(LC) Caudal cingulate	3.300 ± 0.134	6.158 ± 0.126
	Isocortical paralimbic areas	**5.405 ± 0.775**	**14.358 ± 3.166**
20	(TE$_m$) Medial inferotemporal visual association	5.523 ± 0.222	11.268 ± 0.564
21	(STPg-anterior TA) Temporopolar auditory association	7.247 ± 0.502	23.366 ± 0.182
22	(Ig) Granular insula	5.387 ± 0.122	13.870 ± 0.533
23	(OFg) Granular anterior orbitofrontal	3.457 ± 0.156	8.933 ± 0.142
	Nonisocortical paralimbic	**8.686 ± 1.280**	**17.282 ± 2.162**
24	(FL) Parolfactory area	6.670 ± 0.326	9.574 ± 0.311
25	(OFdg) Dysgranular mid-orbitofrontal	5.147 ± 0.135	14.282 ± 0.395
26	(OFap) Agranular caudal orbitofrontal	13.733 ± 1.025	28.754 ± 1.133
27	(Idg) Dysgranular insula	5.703 ± 0.136	15.358 ± 0.683
28	(Iap) Agranular insula	7.717 ± 0.307	22.827 ± 0.675
29	(TPdg) Dysgranular temporopolar	5.767 ± 0.350	18.418 ± 0.233
30	(TPap) Agranular temporopolar	13.817 ± 0.193	16.850 ± 0.442
31	Entorhinal–prorhinal	10.927 ± 0.513	12.206 ± 0.281
	Limbic areas	**21.675 ± 12.795**	**39.730 ± 11.850**
32	Midhippocampus	8.883 ± 0.613	27.878 ± 0.340
33	Amygdala	34.470 ± 2.023	51.582 ± 1.128
	Comparison areas		
	Nucleus basalis	37.527 ± 1.292	41.050 ± 2.555
	Putamen	45.380 ± 1.300	46.477 ± 1.200
	Corpus callosum	1.670 ± 0.071	3.578 ± 0.092
	Cerebellum	0.210 ± 0.150	1.012 ± 0.017

[a]From Mesulam *et al.* (1986a).
[b]The anatomical location of samples 1–31 are shown in Fig. 2. Values in bold type indicate group means. Letters in parentheses indicate the architectonics designation of Mesulam and Mufson (1982) and von Bonin and Bailey (1947).

receive projections from a larger number of Ch4 neurons or if the input from an individual Ch4 neuron in these regions has more ramifications and a greater ChAT content.

The cholinergic receptors in cortex and hippocampus are mostly muscarinic. Although most of these receptors are postsynaptic, some presynaptic receptor sites may also exist and may participate in the autoregulation of ACh secretion. In cortical slices, the effect of ACh upon pyramidal neurons consists of a short-latency inhibition followed by a prolonged increase in excitability (McCormick and Prince, 1985). The inhibitory effect seems to be mediated by GABAergic interneurons whereas the excitatory effect reflects a direct action of ACh upon pyramidal neurons. The increase of excitability in response to ACh appears to be caused by a reduction of membrane K^+ conductance (Krnjević, 1981). Since this effect lasts for a relatively long time, ACh is considered to act, at least in part, as an excitatory neuromodulator upon pyramidal neurons.

Recent observations indicate the existence of more than one type of muscarinic receptor in the CNS (Mash et al., 1985). We examined the regional distribution of cholinergic receptor subtypes within the cortex of the monkey brain (Mash and Mesulam, 1986). The pirenzepine-sensitive M1 subtype (which is also the dominant species of cortical muscarinic receptor) was distributed according to a pattern that approximated the variations of ChAT activity. Thus, both M1 receptor density and ChAT enzyme activity displayed peaks mostly within limbic and para-limbic regions such as the amygdala, hippocampal complex, parahippocampal cortex, orbitofron-tal cortex, and the temporopolar region. However, there were also discrepancies. For example, peak M1 receptor densities were seen in posterior cingulate cortex and in some patches of association cortex even though these areas contain relatively low levels of ChAT activity. Further-more, the insula and the basolateral nucleus of the amygdala contain very high levels of ChAT and AChE but did not display M1 density peaks.

The primate cortex contains substantially fewer M2 than M1 receptor sites. The cortical distribution of M2 receptors displayed a rather unexpected pattern characterized by distinct peaks in the primary areas of all five sensory modalities and in parts of the primary motor cortex. We speculated that these receptors may be associated with cholinergic reticulocortical projections (perhaps emanating from Ch5–Ch6), thus providing a physiological mechanism through which all primary sensory and motor areas can be activated in concert according to the prevailing state of arousal (Mash and Mesulam, 1986).

A closer analysis of muscarinic and nicotinic receptors in the hippocampal complex revealed marked regional variations that reflected cytoarchitectonic subdivisions. Thus, the M1 receptor showed regional density peaks in the dentate gyrus (molecular layer), the CA3, and CA4 hippo-campal sectors and in some parahippocampal regions. The M2 receptor sites showed the highest density in the subiculum, parasubiculum, ventral entorhinal cortex, and the prorhinal region. Nicotinic receptors, although much less dense than either muscarinic subtype, showed a regional peak within the presubicular component of the hippocampal formation. Thus, selective cho-linergic agonists could conceivably be used to selectively influence specific sectors of the hetero-geneous hippocampal formation (Mash et al., 1987).

The lack of a perfect fit between the distribution of ChAT and that of the M1 and M2 receptor subtypes may initially appear surprising since one might have expected the distribution of postsynaptic receptor sites to mirror the distribution of the incoming presynaptic innervation. One possibility for this discrepancy is that we do not yet possess a ligand which reliably binds to all postsynaptic cholinergic receptors and to nothing but these receptors. Alternatively, a very large number of neural membranes may contain sites that will bind to available receptor ligands but these sites may remain physiologically inactive unless coupled to the proper presynaptic innerva-tion. Yet a third possibility is that the distribution of active receptor sites simply does not parallel the distribution of presynaptic fibers (Herkenham, 1987). Perhaps some transmitter systems (e.g., cholinergic, dopaminergic) are distributed not only in the form of traditional neural pathways with spatially coupled pre- and postsynaptic junctional complexes but also in the form of more diffuse arrays within which the transmitter substance acts as a hormone, at much larger distances. These considerations, while they do not alter the implications based on the differential distribution of cortical ChAT, indicate that the organization of central cholinergic pathways contains additional complexities that need to be elucidated.

8. Behavioral Affiliations of Central Cholinergic Pathways

In keeping with their widespread anatomical distribution, a number of behavioral affiliations have been attributed to central cholinergic pathways. These can be divided into four major groups: (1) extrapyramidal motor function, (2) sleep and arousal, (3) mood and affect, and (4) memory and learning.

With respect to motor function, many centrally acting cholinergic agonists are known to be tremorogenic. Especially in parkinsonian patients, cholinergic agents intensify the tremor whereas anticholinergic medication provides effective symptomatic relief. It is thought that the motor deficit in parkinsonism results from an impairment in the balance between cholinergic and dopaminergic innervation within the striatum (Calne, 1978). It is not known if the Ch1–Ch8 cell groups also participate in the cholinergic regulation of extrapyramidal motor function. Several studies indicate that the pedunculopontine nucleus (which contains most of the Ch5 neurons) may have some interaction with the mesencephalic locomotor region and that it may participate in extrapyramidal pathways (Moon-Edley and Graybiel, 1983; Skinner et al., 1985; Isaacson and Tanaka, 1986). Recent anatomical studies, however, have shown that the mesencephalic sites with the most extrapyramidal connections are adjacent to but not overlapping with the pedunculopontine nucleus (Rye et al., 1987).

With respect to the regulation of arousal, cholinergic pathways have traditionally been considered as major components of the ascending reticular activating system (Shute and Lewis, 1967). In keeping with this concept, physiological studies show that cholinergic activation in the thalamus is likely to have a net facilitatory effect upon the thalamocortical transmission of neural impulses (McCance et al., 1968; Dingledine and Kelly, 1977). This activating effect is probably mediated predominantly by the Ch5–Ch6 neurons of the pontomesencephalic reticular formation since they supply most of the thalamic cholinergic innervation.

Behavioral arousal as well as electrical stimulation of the brain stem reticular formation are associated with a low-voltage fast-activity pattern in the neocortical EEG. This EEG pattern, which is largely abolished by cholinergic antagonists and enhanced by cholinergic agonists, also shows a positive correlation with the amount of neocortical ACh release (Kanai and Szerb, 1965; Sie et al., 1965; Steward et al., 1984). This cholinergic influence upon neocortical low-voltage fast activity is thought to be mediated by corticopetal projections from the nucleus basalis (Ch4) rather than by thalamocortical projections (Stewart et al., 1984). The extent to which direct cholinergic projections from Ch5–Ch6 to neocortex (and perhaps to Ch4) also contribute to the regulation of this neocortical low-voltage fast activity has not yet been determined specifically. If the influence of septohippocampal projections (arising from Ch1–Ch2) upon the arousal-related hippocampal theta activity is also taken into consideration, it becomes clear that the cholinergic cell groups in the basal forebrain as well as those in the brain stem participate extensively in the electrophysiological regulation of arousal states. These considerations lend further credence to the suggestion that the nuclei containing the Ch1–Ch4 groups represent, at least in part, a telencephalic extension of the brain stem reticular formation (Ramon-Moliner and Nauta, 1966).

The putative role of cholinergic pathways in emotion and memory is entirely consistent with the preferential association of the Ch1–Ch4 cell groups with the limbic system. As shown above, limbic and paralimbic regions receive a heavier cholinergic input than other cortical areas and also play a more important role in the feedback regulation of the Ch1–Ch4 neurons. With respect to emotion, cholinergic agonists such as physostigmine have, in my experience, produced acute dysphoria in individuals with no evidence of prior mood disturbance. Furthermore, this same agent has been advocated as an effective treatment for acute manic episodes. It has also been suggested that the antidepressant effect of tricyclic substances is partly due to their well-known anticholinergic activity. Conceivably, certain emotional states may represent a balance between cholinergic and monoaminergic innervation within the limbic system (Janowsky *et al.*, 1972).

The relationship of central cholinergic pathways to memory and learning has recently attracted a great deal of attention. For example, young experimental animals and human volunteers show an impairment of new learning when given anticholinergic agents such as scopolamine. The similarity of this scopolamine-induced effect to the memory difficulty that emerges in the course of aging has led to the suggestion that the memory decline of senescence could be caused by an age-related depletion of cholinergic innervation within cortex and limbic structures (Drachman and Leavitt, 1974; Bartus *et al.*, 1982; Mesulam *et al.*, 1987). The importance of cholinergic innervation to memory is further shown by experiments where Ch4 ablations which result in a loss of neocortical AChE and ChAT also result in memory deficits (Flicker *et al.*, 1983). An excessive loss of cortical and limbic cholinergic innervation, above and beyond what is expected on the basis of age alone, has been reported in Alzheimer's disease and this could contribute to the emergence of the severe amnesia (and perhaps some of the other clinical features) seen in this dementing condition (Davies and Maloney, 1976). In keeping with the loss of cortical and limbic cholinergic innervation in Alzheimer's disease, the Ch1, Ch2, and Ch4 regions show marked cell loss in patients with this condition (Whitehouse *et al.*, 1981; Arendt *et al.*, 1985).

The pattern of regional variations in ChAT activity has led us to speculate that cortical cholinergic pathways may participate in memory processes by regulating sensory–limbic interactions (Mesulam *et al.*, 1986a). Sensory–limbic interactions are thought to underlie many important behaviors including the ability to direct drives toward the appropriate object and also the ability to store and retrieve memory traces. Paralimbic areas provide one important avenue for sensory–limbic interactions and these regions have among the highest ChAT activities. It is also known that there are additional multisynaptic pathways for conveying modality-specific information in each of the major sensory modalities into core limbic structures such as the hippocampus and the amygdala (Van Hoesen, 1981; Mishkin, 1982; Mesulam, 1985). An analysis of regional ChAT activities along these pathways shows that this sensory information is likely to come under progressively more intense cholinergic influence as it approaches the limbic system (Fig. 13). Furthermore, single-unit studies in awake and behaving rhesus monkeys have shown that the Ch4–NB neurons which provide this cholinergic influence are particularly responsive to the delivery of reward and to the motivational relevance of sensory events (DeLong, 1971; Rolls *et*

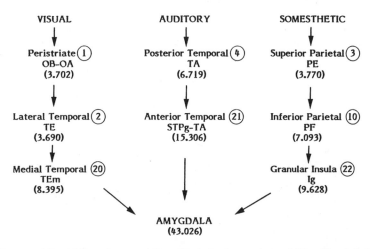

Figure 13. The amygdalopetal flow of sensory information in the three major modalities. The circled numbers and the architectonic designations correspond to those in Table II. The numbers in parentheses show the mean ChAT activity in that area as calculated from values obtained in the two macaque monkeys which were used for the regional enzymatic assays. (From Mesulam *et al.*, 1986a.)

al., 1979). Taken together, these observations lead to the speculation that cortical cholinergic pathways could provide a gating mechanism for channeling motivationally relevant sensory information into and out of the limbic system. Therefore, a dysfunction of these pathways (e.g., by ablations of Ch4, scopolamine administration, or in the course of Alzheimer's disease) could cause a memory impairment by interfering with crucial sensory–limbic interactions (Mesulam *et al.,* 1986a). In partial support for this hypothesis, it has been shown that procaine or GABA injections into the nucleus basalis of the rat inhibit the response of frontal neurons to a sensory cue that signaled the delivery of reward (Rigdon and Pirch, 1984). Thus, cortical cholinergic innervation could be regulating the neuronal response to motivationally relevant sensory stimuli in a way that determines whether or not the pertinent information gets relayed into the limbic system. This gating hypothesis also explains how cholinergic input within sensory and association areas (not particularly known for their involvement in learning) could participate in the overall process of memory storage and retrieval. The gating function of cholinergic pathways is a hypothesis that lends itself to experimental verification.

9. Summary

Although ubiquitous, central cholinergic projections also have a specific topographic organization. The cholinergic innervation of the striatal complex is predominantly intrinsic whereas that of thalamic, limbic, and cortical regions is mostly extrinsic. Four groups of neurons in the basal forebrain (Ch1–Ch4) provide the major cholinergic innervation for limbic, olfactory, and cortical structures; two cell groups in the pontomesencephalic reticular formation (Ch5–Ch6) provide the major cholinergic input for thalamic nuclei; neurons in the medial habenula (Ch7) provide the cholinergic input for the interpeduncular nucleus; and the ChAT-positive cells in the parabigeminal nucleus (Ch8) provide the major cholinergic input for the superior colliculus. The most extensive of these cell groups, the Ch4 complex, innervates the amygdala and the entire cortical mantle. There is further internal topography in the projections from Ch4 to the cortical surface so that each cortical region receives its major cholinergic input from one of the Ch4 subsectors. Furthermore, the Ch4 complex sends a more intense cholinergic projection to limbic and paralimbic structures than to the other portions of the cortical surface. In turn, these limbic and paralimbic areas seem to have a greater feedback influence upon the activity of the Ch4 neurons. These details of anatomical organization are consistent with many of the behavioral affiliations that have been attributed to central cholinergic pathways.

ACKNOWLEDGMENTS. The preparation of this chapter was supported in part by a Javits Neuroscience Investigator Award, the McKnight Foundation, and an Alzheimer's Disease Research Center Grant (AG05134). I am grateful to Leah Christie for expert secretarial assistance.

Abbreviations

A	arcuate sulcus
a	cerebral aqueduct
ac	anterior commissure
al	anterolateral subsector of Ch4
am	anteromedial subsector of Ch4
amg	amygdala
ap	ansa peduncularis
AS	arcuate sulcus
C	central sulcus
CA	calcarine fissure
CC	corpus callosum
cd	caudate nucleus

CF	calcarine fissure
cg	central gray substance
CG(S)	cingulate gyrus
Ch1	first cholinergic cell group
Ch2	second cholinergic cell group
Ch3	third cholinergic cell group
Ch4	fourth cholinergic cell group
Ch5	fifth cholinergic cell group
Ch6	sixth cholinergic cell group
Ch4al	anterolateral subsector of Ch4
Ch4am	anteromedial subsector of Ch4
Ch4id	intermediodorsal subsector of Ch4
Ch4iv	intermedioventral subsector of Ch4
Ch4p	posterior subsector of Ch4
ci	islands of Calleja
cin	inferior colliculus
cn	cuneiform nucleus
CS	central sulcus
cs	superior colliculus
ctt	central tegmental tract
dsp	decussation of the superior cerebellar peduncle
gp	globus pallidus
gpl	lateral globus pallidus
gpm	medial globus pallidus
gpv	ventral globus pallidus
HY	hypothalamus
i	intermediate sector of Ch4
ic	internal capsule
id	intermediodorsal subsector of Ch4
INS	insula
IOS	inferior occipital sulcus
ip	interpeduncular nucleus
IP	intraparietal (sulcus)
iv	intermedioventral subsector of Ch4
L	lunate sulcus
LF	lateral (sylvian) fissure
lgn	lateral geniculate nucleus
LL	lateral lemniscus
LOF	lateral orbitofrontal sulcus
LS	lunate sulcus
ltn	laterodorsal tegmental nucleus
ml	medial lemniscus
mlf	medial longitudinal fasciculus
MOF	medial orbitofrontal sulcus
MOS	medial orbitofrontal sulcus
na	nucleus accumbens
NB	nucleus basalis
nIV	fourth cranial nerve
OC	optic chiasm
ot	optic tract
OT	occipitotemporal (sulcus)
P	principal sulcus

p   posterior sector of Ch4
pno   oral division of the pontine reticular nucleus
POS   parietooccipital sulcus
ppn   pedunculopontine nucleus
PS   principal sulcus
pt   putamen
R   rhinal sulcus
RoS   rostral sulcus
RS   rhinal sulcus
S   sylvian fissure
sp   superior cerebellar peduncle
Spt   septal area
STP   supratemporal plane
ST(S)   superior temporal sulcus
T   thalamus

References

Arendt, T., Bigl, V., Tennstedt, A., and Arendt, A., 1985, Neuronal loss in different parts of the nucleus basalis is related to neuritic plaque formation in cortical target areas in Alzheimer's disease, *Neuroscience* **14**:1–14.

Arikuni, T., and Kubota, K., 1984, Substantia innominata projection to caudate nucleus in macaque monkeys, *Brain Res.* **302**:184–189.

Baisden, R. H., Woodruff, M. L., and Hoover, D. B., 1984, Cholinergic and non-cholinergic septo-hippocampal projections: A double-label horseradish peroxidase–acetylcholinesterase study in the rabbit, *Brain Res.* **290**:146–151.

Bartus, R. T., Dean, R. L., III, Beer, B., and Lippa, A. S., 1982, The cholinergic hypothesis of geriatric memory dysfunction, *Science* **217**:408–417.

Calne, D. B., 1978, Parkinsonism, clinical and neuropharmacological aspects, *Postgrad. Med.* **2**:1457–1459.

Dale, H. H., 1938, Acetylcholine as a chemical transmitter, *J. Mt. Sinai Hosp.* **4**:401–429.

Davies, P., and Maloney, A. J. F., 1976, Selective loss of central cholinergic neurons in Alzheimer's disease, *Lancet* **2**:1403.

DeLong, M. R., 1971, Activity of pallidal neurons during movement, *J. Neurophysiol.* **34**:414–427.

Dingledine, R., and Kelly, J. S., 1977, Brain stem stimulation and the acetylcholine-evoked inhibition of neurons in the feline nucleus reticularis thalami, *J. Physiol. (London)* **271**:135–154.

Drachman, D. A., and Leavitt, J., 1974, Human memory and the cholinergic system—A relationship to aging? *Arch. Neurol. Psychiatry* **30**:113–121.

Eckenstein, F., and Thoenen, H., 1983, Cholinergic neurons in the rat cerebral cortex demonstrated by immunohistochemical localization of choline acetyltransferase, *Neurosci. Lett.* **36**:211–215.

Fibiger, H., 1982, The organization and some projections of cholinergic neurons of the mammalian forebrain. *Brain Res. Rev.* **4**:322–388.

Flicker, C., Dean, R. L., Watkins, D. L., Fisher, S. K., and Bartus, R. T., 1983, Behavioral and neurochemical effects following neurotoxic lesions of a major cholinergic input to the cerebral cortex in the rat, *Pharmacol. Biochem. Behav.* **18**:973–981.

Green, R. C., Moran, M. A., Martin, T. L., Mash, D. C., Mufson, E. J., and Mesulam, M.-M., 1986, Distribution of acetylcholinesterase fiber staining in the human hippocampus and parahippocampal gyrus, *Soc. Neurosci. Abstr.* **12**:356.

Herkenham, M., 1987, Mismatches between receptor and transmitter localizations in the brain: observations and implications, *Neuroscience* **23**:1–38.

Houser, C. R., Crawford, G. D., Barber, R. P., Salvaterra, P. M., and Vaughn, J. E., 1983, Organization and morphological characteristics of cholinergic neurons: An immunohistochemical study with a monoclonal antibody to choline acetyltransferase, *Brain Res.* **266**:97–119.

Isaacson, L. G., and Tanaka, D., Jr., 1986, Cholinergic and non-cholinergic projections from the canine pontomesencephalic tegmentum (Ch5 area) to the caudal intralaminar thalamic nuclei, *Exp. Brain Res.* **62**:179–188.

Janowsky, D. S., Davis, J. M., El-Yousef, M. K., and Sekerke, H. J., 1972, A cholinergic–adrenergic hypothesis of mania and depression, *Lancet* **2**:632–635.

Johnston, M. V., McKinney, M., and Coyle, J. T., 1981, Neocortical cholinergic innervation: A description of extrinsic and intrinsic components in the rat, *Exp. Brain Res.* **43**:159–172.

Kanai, T., and Szerb, J. C., 1965, The mesencephalic reticular activating system and cortical acetylcholine output, *Nature* **205**:80–82.

Kataoka, R., Nakamura, Y., and Hassler, R., 1974, Habenulointerpeduncular tract: A possible cholinergic neuron in the rat brain, *Brain Res.* **62**:264–267.

Kimura, H., McGeer, P. L., Peng J. H., and McGeer, E. G., 1981, The central cholinergic system studied by choline acetyltransferase immunohistochemistry in the cat, *J. Comp. Neurol.* **200**:151–201.

Krnjević, K., 1981, Acetylcholine as a modulator of amino-acid-mediated synaptic transmission, in: *The Role of Peptides and Amino Acids as Neurotransmitters,* Liss, New York, pp. 124–141.

Krnjević, K., and Silver, A., 1965, A histochemical study of cholinergic fibers in the cerebral cortex, *J. Anat.* **99**:711–759.

Lehmann, J., Struble, R. G., Antuono, P. G., Coyle, J. T., Cork, L. C., and Price, D. L., 1984, Regional heterogeneity of choline acetyltransferase activity in primate neocortex, *Brain Res.* **322**:361–364.

Levey, A. I., Rye, D. B., Wainer, B. H., Mufson, E. J., and Mesulam, M.-M., 1984, Choline acetyltransferase-immunoreactive neurons intrinsic to rodent cortex and distinction from acetylcholinesterase-positive neurons, *Neuroscience* **13**:341–353.

Loewi, O., 1921, Uber humorale Ubertragbarkeit der Herznervenwirkung, *Pfluegers Arch. Gesamte Physiol. Menschen Tiere* **189**:239–242.

Mash, D. C., White, F., Mufson, E. J., and Mesulam, M.-M., 1987, Muscarinic and nicotinic acetylcholine receptors in the hippocampal formation of the monkey, *Neurology* **37**(Suppl. 1):194.

Mash, D. C., and Mesulam, M.-M., 1986, Muscarine receptor distributions within architectonic subregions of the primate cortex, *Soc. Neurosci. Abstr.* **12**:809.

Mash, D. C., Flynn, D. D., and Potter, L. T., 1985, Loss of M2 receptors in the cerebral cortex in Alzheimer's disease and experimental cholinergic denervation, *Science* **228**:1115–1117.

McCance, I., Phillis, J. W., and Westerman, R. A., 1968, Acetylcholine-sensitivity of thalamic neurons: Its relationship to synaptic transmission, *Br. J. Pharmacol.* **32**:635–651.

McCormick, D. A., and Prince, D. A., 1985, Two types of muscarinic responses to acetylcholine in mammalian cortical neurons, *Proc. Natl. Acad. Sci. USA* **82**:6344–6348.

Mesulam, M.-M., 1985, Patterns in behavioral neuroanatomy, in: *Principles of Behavioral Neurology* (M.-M. Mesulam, ed.), Davis, Philadelphia, pp. 1–70.

Mesulam, M.-M., and Mufson, E. J., 1982, Insula of the Old World monkey. Part I. Architectonics in the insulo-orbito-temporal component of the paralimbic brain, *J. Compl Neurol.* **212**:1–22.

Mesulam, M.-M., and Mufson, E. J., 1984, Neural inputs into the nucleus basalis of the substantia innominata (Ch4) in the rhesus monkey, *Brain* **107**:253–274.

Mesulam, M.-M., and Van Hoesen, G. W., 1976, Acetylcholinesterase-rich projections from the basal forebrain of the rhesus monkey to neocortex, *Brain Res.* **109**:152–157.

Mesulam, M.-M., Van Hoesen, G. W., and Rosene, D. L., 1977, Substantia innominata, septal area and nuclei of the diagonal band in the rhesus monkey: Organization of efferents and their acetylcholinesterase histochemistry, *Soc. Neurosci. Abstr.* **3**:202.

Mesulam, M.-M., Mufson, E. J., Levey, A. I., and Wainer, B. H., 1983a, Cholinergic innervation of cortex by the basal forebrain: Cytochemistry and cortical connections of the septal area, diagonal band nuclei, nucleus basalis (substantia innominata) and hypothalamus in the rhesus monkey, *J. Comp. Neurol.* **214**:170–197.

Mesulam, M.-M., Mufson, E. J., Wainer, B. H., and Levey, A. I., 1983b, Central cholinergic pathways in the rat: An overview based on an alternative nomenclature (Ch1–Ch6), *Neuroscience* **10**:1185–1201.

Mesulam, M.-M., Mufson, E. J., Levey, A. I., and Wainer, B. H., 1984a, Atlas of cholinergic neurons in the forebrain and upper brainstem of the macaque based on monoclonal choline acetyltransferase immunohistochemistry and acetylcholinesterase histochemistry, *Neuroscience* **12**:669–686.

Mesulam, M.-M., Rosen, A. D., and Mufson, E. J., 1984b, Regional variations in cortical cholinergic innervation: Chemoarchitectonics of acetylcholinesterase-containing fibers in the macaque brain, *Brain Res.* **311**:245–258.

Mesulam, M.-M., Volicer, L., Marquis, J. K., Mufson, E. J., and Green, R. C., 1986a, Systematic regional differences in the cholinergic innervation of the primate cerebral cortex: Distribution of enzyme activities and some behavioral implications, *Ann. Neurol.* **19**:144–151.

Mesulam, M.-M., Mufson, E. J., and Wainer, B. H., 1986b, Three-dimensional representation and cortical projection topography of the nucleus basalis (Ch4) in the macaque: Concurrent demonstration of choline acetyltransferase and retrograde transport with a stabilized tetramethylbenzidine method for HRP, *Brain Res.* **367**:301–308.

Mesulam, M.-M., Mufson, E. J., and Rogers, J., 1987, Age-related shrinkage of cortically projecting cholinergic neurons: A selective effect, *Ann. Neurol.* **22**:31–36.

Mishkin, M., 1982, A memory system in the monkey, *Phil. Trans. R. Soc. London Ser. B* **298**:85–92.

Moon-Edley, S., and Graybiel, A. M., 1983, The afferent and efferent connections of the feline nucleus tegmenti pedunculopontinus, pars compacta, *J. Comp. Neurol.* **217**:187–215.

Mufson, E. J., Levey, A. I., Wainer, B. H., and Mesulam, M.-M., 1982, Cholinergic projections from the mesencephalic tegmentum to neocortex in rhesus monkey, *Soc. Neurosci. Abstr.* **8:**135

Mufson, E. J., Desan, P. H., Mesulam, M.-M., Wainer, B. H., and Levey, A. I., 1984, Choline acetyltransferase-like immunoreactivity in the forebrain of the red-eared pond turtle (*Pseudemys Scripta elegans*), *Brain Res.* **323:**103–108.

Mufson, E. J., Martin, T. L., Mash, D. C., Wainer, B. H., and Mesulam, M.-M., 1986, Cholinergic projections from the parabigeminal nucleus (Ch8) to the superior colliculus in the mouse: A combined analysis of HRP transport and choline acetyltransferase immunohisto-chemistry, *Brain Res.* **370:**144–148.

Nastuk, M. A., and Graybiel, A. M., 1985, Patterns of muscarinic cholinergic binding in the striatum and their relation to dopamine islands and striosomes, *J. Comp. Neurol.* **237:**176–194.

Parent, A., Poirier, L. J., Boucher, R., and Butcher, L. L., 1977. Morphological characteristics of acetylcholinesterase-containing neurons in the CNS of DFP-treated monkeys, *J. Neurol. Sci.* **32:**9–28.

Price, J. L., and Amaral, D. G., 1981, An autoradiographic study of the projections of the central nucleus of the monkey amygdala, *J. Neurosci.* **1:**1242–1259.

Price, J. L., and Stern, R., 1983, Individual cells in the nucleus basalis–diagonal band complex have restricted axonal projections to the cerebral cortex in the rat, *Brain Res.* **269:**352–356.

Ramon-Moliner, E., and Nauta, W. J. H., 1966, The isodendritic core of the brain stem, *J. Comp. Neurol.* **126:**311–335.

Rawlins, J. N. P., Feldon, J., and Gray, J. A., 1979, Septo-hippocampal connections and the hippocampal theta rhythm, *Exp. Brain Res.* **37:**49–63.

Rigdon, G. C., and Pirch, J. H., 1984, Microinjection of procaine or GABA into the nucleus basalis magnocellularis affects cue-elicited unit responses in the rat frontal cortex, *Exp. Neurol.* **85:**283–296.

Rolls, E. T., Sanghera, M. K., and Roper-Hall, A., 1979, The latency of activation of neurons in the lateral hypothalamus and substantia innominata during feeding in the monkey, *Brain Res.* **164:**121–135.

Rossier, J., 1984, On the mapping of the cholinergic neurons by immunocytochemistry, *Neurochem. Int.* **6:**183–184.

Russchen, F. T., Amaral, D. G., and Price, J. L., 1985, The afferent connections of the substantia innominata in the monkey, *Macaca fascicularis, J. Comp. Neurol.* **24:**1–27.

Rye, D. B., Saper, C. B., Lee, H. J., and Wainer, B. H., Pedunculopontine tegmental nucleus of the rat: Cytoarchitecture, cytochemistry, and some extrapyramidal connections of the mesopontine tegmentum, *J Comp. Neurol.* **259:**483–528.

Saper, C. B., Swanson, L. W., and Cowan, W. M., 1979, Some efferent connections of the rostral hypothalamus in the squirrel monkey (*Saimiri sciureus*) and cat, *J. Comp. Neurol.* **184:** 5–242.

Shute, C. C. D., and Lewis, P. R., 1967, The ascending cholinergic reticular system: Neocortical, olfactory and subcortical projections, *Brain* **90:**497–520.

Sie, G., Jasper, H. H., and Wolfe, I., 1965, Rate of ACh release from cortical surface in encephale and cerveau isole preparations in relation to arousal and epileptic activation of the EEG, *Electroencephalogr. Clin. Neurophysiol.* **18:**206.

Silver, A., 1974, *The Biology of Cholinesterases,* Elsevier, Amsterdam.

Skinner, R. D., Garcia-Rill, D., Conrad, C., and Mosley, D., 1985, The mesencephalic locomotor region. II. Ascending and descending projections in the rat, *Anat. Rec.* **211:**180a.

Steward, D. J., MacFabe, D. F., and Vanderwolf, C. H., 1984, Cholinergic activation of the electrocorticogram: Role of the substantia innominata and effects of atropine and quinuclidinyl benzylate, *Brain Res.* **322:**219–232.

Vanderwolf, C. H., 1983, The role of the cerebral cortex and ascending activating systems in the control of behavior, in: *Handbook of Behavioral Neurobiology* (E. Satinoff and P. Teitelbaum, eds.), Plenum Press, New York, pp. 67–104.

Van Hoesen, G. W., 1981, The differential distribution, diversity and sprouting of cortical projections to the amygdala in the rhesus monkey, in: *The Amygdaloid Complex* (Y. Ben-Ari, ed.), Elsevier, Amsterdam, pp. 77–90.

von Bonin, G., and Bailey, P., 1947, *The Neocortex of Macaca Mulatta,* University of Illinois Press, Urbana.

Wainer, B. H., Levey, A. I., Mufson, E. J., and Mesulam, M.-M., 1984, Cholinergic systems in mammalian brain identified with antibodies against choline acetyltransferase, *Neurochem. Int.* **6:**163–182.

Wainer, B. H., Levey, A. I., Rye, D. B., Mesulam, M.-M., and Mufson, E. J., 1985, Cholinergic and noncholinergic septohippocampal pathways, *Neurosci. Lett.* **54:**45–52.

Whitehouse, P. J., Price, D. L., Clark, A. W., Coyle, J. T., and DeLong, M. R., 1981, Alzheimer's disease: Evidence for selective loss of cholinergic neurons in the nucleus basalis, *Ann. Neurol.* **10:**122–126.

Woolf, N. J., and Butcher, L. L., 1981, Cholinergic neurons in the caudate–putamen complex proper are intrinsically organized: A combined Evans blue and acetylcholinesterase analysis, *Brain Res. Bull.* **7:**487–507.

16

The Synthesis and Storage of Acetylcholine in Mammalian Cholinergic Nerve Terminals

B. Collier

1. Introduction

The notion that acetylcholine (ACh) might function as a neurotransmitter in the mammalian CNS was mentioned by Dale in his 1937 William Henry Welch Lectures (Dale, 1938). Almost 50 years later, we have some understanding of this function and of the consequences of dysfunction. The function of ACh in the CNS appears to relate to enhancement of neuronal excitability, and it is significant that the first direct demonstration that increased ACh release in cerebral cortex is associated with increased neuronal activity in unanesthetized animals was made in H. H. Jasper's laboratory (Celesia and Jasper, 1966). The dysfunctions of central cholinergic neurons appear to relate to conditions associated with memory loss, and it is equally significant that Dr. Jasper makes no contribution to the statistics associating these parameters: it is evident that his central cholinergic neurons are fully functional.

My work in the 1960s on ACh release from the brain was my introduction to Jasper. He soon convinced me, without effort on his part, that I was unlikely to learn anything he didn't know, so I turned my attention to other aspects of cholinergic function. In this article, I will summarize some recent work from my laboratory within the framework of a review of the synthesis and storage of ACh in cholinergic neurons. The objectives are to understand the dynamics of these processes as they relate to transmitter release and to develop ways of manipulating ACh release by altering its synthesis or storage. In this way we hope eventually to provide tricks by which function of cholinergic synapses can be altered, in particular to enhance function by increasing ACh release, which would presumably be of use in states of cholinergic hypofunction. Success in this might contribute to the linking of "molecules to mind," but presently we remain with the molecules.

2. ACh Synthesis

ACh is synthesized in neurons by the reaction of choline with acetyl-CoA, choline acetyltransferase (ChAT) being the catalyst. The reaction is reversible:

$$\text{acetyl-CoA} + \text{choline} \rightleftharpoons \text{ACh} + \text{CoA}$$

B. Collier • Department of Pharmacology, McGill University, Montreal, Quebec H3G 1Y6, Canada.

2.1. Intracellular Location of ChAT

Like other proteins, the enzyme ChAT is synthesized in the perikarya of cholinergic cells and moved by axonal transport to the nerve terminals. Thus, the enzyme is present throughout the neuron, and ACh can be synthesized in all parts of the cell; but the only place of known functional importance of ACh synthetic activity is the nerve terminal. Within the nerve terminal, most of the ChAT appears to be a soluble cytoplasmic component (e.g., Fonnum, 1968). Thus, the simple view is that ACh is synthesized in the nerve terminal cytosol from where it is either released, taken up into storage sites, or hydrolyzed in some futile cycle. But, as usual, there are certain observations that belie the simple view. First, ChAT is positively charged and forms ionic bonds with membranes (e.g., Malthe-Sorenssen, 1979); it has been suggested that this association has functional significance and results in an obligatory coupling between choline uptake and choline acetylation (e.g., Barker and Mittag, 1975; Rylett and Colhoun, 1980). Second, a part of nerve terminal ChAT is reportedly nonionically associated with membranes (Benishin and Carroll, 1983; Eder-Colli and Amato, 1985), and this enzyme's properties might differ from those of the soluble enzyme, in particular in its substrate specificity (Benishen and Carroll, 1981, 1983). This last-mentioned point is somewhat intriguing because the soluble enzyme is not well able to acetylate the choline analogue, homocholine, whereas the membrane-bound enzyme can; we, and others, have consistently found that homocholine is acetylated by ChAc *in situ* (e.g., Collier *et al.*, 1977; von Schwarzenfeld, 1979; Boksa and Collier, 1980a,b; Carroll and Aspry, 1981) and the product is released as a false cholinergic transmitter. Taken together, these observations suggest membrane-associated enzyme is likely responsible for the synthesis of releasable transmitter when that transmitter is synthesized from the homocholine. It is tempting to extrapolate this conclusion to include transmitter synthesized from choline, but as yet there is no evidence to support that extrapolation, and further work is needed on the point.

2.2. Source of Choline for ACh Synthesis

It is mostly agreed that choline to support ACh synthesis is transported into the cholinergic neuron from extracellular choline by a choline transport system. Certainly, cholinergic nerve terminals transport choline by both a high- and a low-affinity process (Haga and Noda, 1973; Yamamura and Snyder, 1973); choline delivered by the high-affinity transport process seems to be used preferentially for ACh synthesis under most experimental conditions (for review see Jope, 1979); blockade of choline uptake by drugs like hemicholinium blocks ACh synthesis (e.g., Guyenet *et al.*, 1973); and most of a tissue's endogenous ACh can be labeled from exogenous choline with little loss of specific radioactivity (Collier and MacIntosh, 1969; Potter, 1970). Thus, the simplest interpretation is that choline for ACh synthesis is derived from circulating free choline, i.e., dietary choline supplemented by that synthesized in the liver. However, there is evidence for limited choline production *de novo* by nervous tissue (e.g., Blusztajn and Wurtman, 1981), as well as suggestive evidence that phospholipid-associated choline might be mobilized for ACh synthesis under certain conditions (see Wecker, 1986).

2.3. Activation of Choline Transport by Synaptic Activity

It is now evident that the choline uptake system of cholinergic nerve terminals is a regulated process. The terminal responds to altered states of impulse activity by altered rates of transport activity. The idea, as far as I am aware, arose from experiments made to test the fate of recaptured choline derived from released ACh following its hydrolysis (Collier and Katz, 1974). In that study, we confirmed the earlier observations (e.g., Perry, 1953; Collier and MacIntosh, 1969) that choline efflux from a sympathetic ganglion stimulated through its sympathetic trunk was less than was ACh efflux when the latter was measured in the presence of an esterase inhibitor and the former (i.e., choline efflux) was measured without an esterase inhibitor. That this choline was recaptured for ACh synthesis in sympathetic ganglia was shown by following [³H]choline to [³H]-ACh in the tissue, releasing that ACh to allow hydrolysis back to [³H]choline, and recovering the [³H] on ACh subsequent to the reuptake of the [³H]choline: some 90% of recaptured choline was used for ACh synthesis, clearly indicating its selective capture by preganglionic nerve terminals. However, at rest, there was no selective accumulation of choline by cholinergic terminals of ganglia, suggesting preferential activation of choline uptake by nerve terminals during stimulation. This suggestion was subsequently confirmed directly by experiments using analogues of choline under conditions where their rate of accumulation exceeded their rate of metabolism. With homocholine or triethylcholine, their uptake by sympathetic ganglia was increased during preganglionic activity, and this change was the result of a presynaptic alteration of choline transport activity, not the result of a postsynaptic change due to transmitter release and action (Collier and Ilson, 1977; Collier, 1981; O'Regan and Collier, 1981b). These analogues of choline were used in these studies because they satisfy better the structural requirements of the choline transport system than those of intracellular metabolizing enzymes and, thus, can dissociate uptake from uptake and metabolism, processes that are fairly tightly coupled when the substrate is choline.

Table I summarizes a part of the evidence that was discussed above: it shows the altered uptake by sympathetic ganglia during preganglionic nerve stimulation for five analogues of choline. Only the three that are substrates for the choline uptake mechanism show a positive result.

The mechanism by which impulse activity enhances choline transport activity is not yet clear. The simple explanation would be that intracellular ACh inhibits choline uptake and that ACh release removes that inhibition. But this explanation appears not to be: inhibition of ACh release does not always obtain the stimulus-induced increase in choline uptake activity (Collier and Ilson, 1977; O'Regan and Collier, 1981b; Welner and Collier, 1985). Nerve-terminal depolarization *per se* is not the trigger for increased choline uptake, because potassium- or veratridine-induced depolarization is inhibitory, not facilitatory, to choline uptake (Simon and Kuhar, 1976; Collier and Ilson, 1977; Vaca and Pilar, 1979; O'Regan and Collier, 1981b). A likely possibility remains: that enhanced choline uptake is associated with impulse afterhyperpolarization, maybe some Ca^{2+}-activated outward current, because stimulus-enhanced choline uptake appears Ca^{2+}-dependent (Collier and Ilson, 1977; O'Regan and Collier, 1981b).

That transmitter release activates choline uptake has been concluded from experiments with

Table I. Altered Uptake of Choline Analogues during Synaptic Activity

$$R_2 - \overset{\overset{\displaystyle R_1}{\underset{\displaystyle R_3}{\big|}}}{\overset{+}{N}} - (CH_2)_n - OH$$

R_1	R_2	R_3	n	Trivial name	K_m (μM) uptake	Uptake (stimulated : resting)
C_2H_5	C_2H_5	C_2H_5	2	Triethylcholine	5	2.3
CH_3	CH_3	CH_3	3	Homocholine	3	3.2
CH_3	CH_3	CH_3	4	Butylcholine	N.S.[a]	1.0
CH_3	C_2H_5	C_2H_5	3	Diethylhomocholine	8	4.1
C_2H_5	C_2H_5	C_2H_5	3	Triethylhomocholine	N.S.	1.0

[a]N.S. = not a substrate. K_m uptake measured with synaptosomes. Uptake (stimulated : resting) is accumulation by sympathetic ganglia during preganglionic stimulation divided by resting accumulation.

isolated synaptosomes (e.g., Murrin and Kuhar, 1976; Weiler *et al.*, 1981). In such experiments, synaptosomes were depolarized by K^+ so that they released ACh, they were returned to a normal medium, and choline uptake was shown enhanced during this recovery period. The increased choline uptake activity measured in this test is related to ACh synthesis necessary to replenish the ACh exhausted by the prior stimulation; it remains uncertain whether it is a good model for the physiological situation where synthesis activation is closely time-locked to transmitter release. Whatever its relevance, it is of considerable interest that this poststimulation phenomenon appears to be associated with the appearance of more choline carrier molecules in the nerve-terminal membrane (Rylett, 1986).

The activation of choline transport triggered by impulse activity can last beyond the period of neuronal activity. This has been shown for sympathetic ganglia (Collier *et al.*, 1983) as well as for cholinergic neurons of the rat CNS, where the consequences of *in vivo* changes of neuronal activity survive for the *in vitro* study of choline uptake (e.g., Simon and Kuhar, 1975; Richter *et al.*, 1982). This phenomenon provides a useful trick by which changes of central cholinergic neuronal activity can be inferred from simple postmortem biochemical measures.

2.4. Source of Acetyl-CoA for ACh Synthesis

It is generally accepted that the acetyl groups for ACh synthesis in mammalian cholinergic nerves originate from glucose and pyruvate (see Tuček, 1978). Thus, acetyl-CoA is generated within the mitochondrial matrix and the unsolved issue is its transfer from an intra- to an extramitochondrial location. The inner mitochondrial membrane is considered to be impermeable to acetyl-CoA and, therefore, it is usually presumed that intramitochondrial acetyl-CoA is transformed to some carrier compound which can cross the barrier, become converted back to acetyl-CoA in the extramitochondrial space and, thus, fuel ACh synthesis. There are several possibilities for the identity of such acetyl-carrier molecules (see Tuček, 1983), but no compelling evidence that favors any single intermediate as that responsible. It is tempting to go along with Tuček's analysis that concluded, rather tentatively, that some two-thirds of the acetyl-CoA for ACh synthesis is provided by acetylcarnitine and the rest by citrate. This conclusion was reached from experiments made with a rat brain preparation (Doležal and Tuček, 1981; Říčný and Tuček, 1982). However, at least in sympathetic ganglion, appropriately labeled carbon atoms of citrate or of acetylcarnitine are not efficiently transferred to ACh (results of Tuček and Collier, unpublished, and of Collier, unpublished) as they might be expected to be if these compounds are the important intermediates. The sympathetic ganglion does show the labeling of ACh from glucose and from acetate (see Kwok and Collier, 1982); the former is not surprising, but the labeling from acetate is rather different from results of similar experiments on brain (e.g., Browning and Schulman, 1968; Nakamura *et al.*, 1970; Sollenberg and Sörbo, 1970). Taken together, these results suggest variations in the intermediary metabolism by cholinergic nerve endings of central and peripheral tissue. In the sympathetic ganglion, the labeling of ACh from acetate was equivalent when the acetate was labeled with ^{14}C on the C-1 or the C-2 atom. This result is more compatible with the direct synthesis of acetyl-CoA from acetate by extramitochondrial acetyl-CoA synthetase, than it is with intramitochondrial acetate metabolism with its subsequent transformation to acetyl-CoA; if intramitochondrial metabolism were to be responsible, [2-^{14}C]acetate would retain better its labeled acetyl than would [1-^{14}C]acetate.

The study of Kwok and Collier (1982) showed a second interesting phenomenon and that is the reduced incorporation of labeled acetate into ganglionic ACh during preganglionic nerve stimulation; this contrasts to the enhanced incorporation of labeled atoms from glucose. The transfer of acetate to ACh in this experiment was measured in the presence of unlabeled glucose and, thus, we postulated that during activity, there results increased delivery from the mitochondria of unlabeled acetyl-CoA derived from glucose and that this dilutes the specific radioactivity of acetyl-CoA derived from labeled acetate as the result of cytoplasmic synthesis. If this interpretation is the correct one, the delivery of acetyl-CoA to ChAT, like the delivery of choline, is increased during neuronal activity.

The increased delivery of acetyl-CoA during activity might be the result of increased efflux of whatever acetyl carrier operates the acetyl shuttle from intra- to extramitochondrial compartments, or it might be the result of increased efflux from mitochondria of acetyl-CoA itself. There are reports (Tuček, 1967; Benjamin and Quastel, 1981; Říčný and Tuček, 1983) indicating that mitochondria release acetyl-CoA, and that this output is increased in the presence of increasing Ca^{2+} concentration; of course, one effect of nerve impulses is to increase intraterminal levels of Ca^{2+}.

2.5. The Control of ACh Synthesis

It is generally agreed that the rate of ACh synthesis in cholinergic nerve terminals is regulated such that it is low during periods of rest and is accelerated during periods of stimulation that releases transmitter; in this way, nerve-terminal stores are maintained relatively constant. The mechanism of this control is not known with any certainty.

In general, transmitter synthesis can be controlled by feedback inhibition, by altered enzyme delivery, by altered precursor activity, or by reaction equilibrium.

2.5.1. Feedback Inhibition

This is not thought the most likely mechanism for the control of ACh synthesis because the ChAT is not strongly inhibited by product. The most plausible product to inhibit synthesis by feedback is ACh because it is this product whose intracellular concentration will change to reflect recent release. At the ACh concentration considered likely to exist in the nerve-terminal cytosol (about 200 μM according to Tuček, 1984), its inhibitory effect on ChAT is minimal (e.g., Glover and Potter, 1971).

2.5.2. Enzyme Activity

It has usually been concluded that ChAT activity is not rate limiting to ACh synthesis because the activity that can be measured in a homogenate of tissue is considerably greater than the rate of maximal ACh synthesis measurable on the same tissue left intact. This conclusion might require reevaluation for the following reasons: (1) If there is any value to the notion (see Section 2.2) that membrane-bound ChAT is uniquely associated with ACh synthesis of physiological relevance, the argument that total ChAT activity is in excess (presented above) is irrelevant because this membrane-associated activity is only a small percentage of the total. (2) If endogenous factors described as being capable of inhibiting or of activating ChAT (Cozzari and Hartman, 1983) turn out to be present in cholinergic nerve terminals, activity of enzyme *in situ* might be quite different from activity *in vitro*. (3) ChAT can be phosphorylated by endogenous kinase activity (Bruce and Hersh, 1985) and if this results in altered enzymatic activity, the state of phosphorylation of enzyme *in situ* and *in vitro* might well be different. (4) Vasointestinal polypeptide can increase ACh synthesis by intact tissue and, as yet, this can only be associated with altered ChAT activity (see Collier *et al.*, 1987).

2.5.3. Precursor Delivery

The estimated intracellular concentrations of free choline and of extramitochondrial acetyl-CoA (50 and 5 μM, respectively, according to Tuček, 1984) are below their K_m for ChAT (400–1200 μM for choline and 7–18 μM for acetyl-CoA; see White and Wu, 1973). Thus, it seems that the enzyme *in situ* is not saturated with substrate and altered delivery of precursors should change the amount of product generated. As reviewed above (Sections 2.3 and 2.4), there is evidence for the increased delivery of both precursors during stimulation and this phenomenon is at least conducive to increased ACh synthesis.

It is difficult to ascertain if increased precursor delivery can fully account for increased ACh synthesis. Certainly, in sympathetic ganglia, the provision of only more choline appears not to result in any major change in ACh synthesis (O'Regan and Collier, 1981a). Also, the increased uptake of choline associated with increased neuronal activity does not always result in increased generation of product (Collier and Ilson, 1977; O'Regan and Collier, 1981b; Welner and Collier, 1985). Similarly, in the CNS choline loading does not increase ACh synthesis under normal conditions, although it can when ACh turnover is high (see Wecker, 1986). Overall, these results suggests that choline delivery can become rate limiting to synthesis, but that it is not so limiting under more normal conditions of activity. Thus, if precursor delivery regulates ACh synthesis, that regulation is either via acetyl-CoA delivery or, more likely, synthesis activation requires the simultaneous change in the delivery of both precursors.

2.5.4. Reaction Equilibrium

As already mentioned, the ACh synthetic reaction is reversible. The equilibrium constant has been measured as about 12 by Pieklik and Guynn (1975), and Tuček (1984, 1985) has presented a persuasive argument supporting the notion, originally expressed by Potter et al. (1968), that the ChAT reaction is close to equilibrium under conditions likely to prevail in the nerve terminal. Thus, ACh synthesis could be regulated simply by transmitter release, which would transiently lower the nerve-terminal ACh concentration and bring about the synthesis of new ACh necessary to reestablish the reaction equilibrium. By this hypothesis, the cytosolic ACh level is established by reaction equilibrium, because the cytosol is the site of ACh synthesis. However, ACh release that triggers ACh synthesis occurs not from cytosolic stores, but from synaptic vesicle stores (see Section 3.1). Thus, the stimulus for increased ACh synthesis is not transmitter release *per se,* but the lowering of cytosolic ACh as the result of its translocation from the cytosol to synaptic vesicles: i.e., ACh synthesis is postulated to be regulated by ACh uptake into synaptic vesicles.

This hypothesis became testable when it was shown that ACh uptake into synaptic vesicles could be selectively inhibited by the compound 2(4-phenylpiperidino) cyclohexanol or AH5183 (Anderson et al., 1983; Bahr and Parsons, 1986). The postulate would be that if mass action regulates ACh synthesis, AH5183 would block the activation of ACh synthesis that occurs during activity. When we tested this (Collier et al., 1986), the answer was negative to the hypothesis: ACh synthesis by a sympathetic ganglion was activated to a similar extent in the presence or absence of AH5183. Thus, we make the simplest, but not necessarily correct conclusion that disturbance of reaction equilibrium is not enough to account for the phenomenon of ACh synthesis control.

AH5183 causes inhibition of ACh release (see Section 3.2), and the maintenance of activated synthesis with reduced release causes tissue ACh to increase. We analyzed this increase in tissue content (Collier et al., 1986) in ganglia stimulated in the presence of AH5183 to show the phenomenon appears to be less when Ca^{2+} influx is less and greater when Ca^{2+} influx is increased by 4-aminopyridine. This prompted the conclusion that the activation of ACh synthesis depends, at least partly, on changed intracellular Ca^{2+}, an idea for which there is some complementary evidence (Birks, 1983; Welner and Collier, 1985).

2.5.5. Summary

The evidence at the moment seems to point to several factors being necessary for the activation of ACh synthesis: increased delivery of precursors, both choline and acetyl-CoA, and increased intracellular Ca^{2+} (illustrated by Fig. 1). The role of Ca^{2+} is uncertain; it could simply

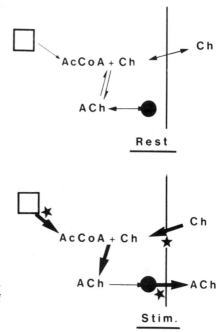

Figure 1. A scheme illustrating the postulated change in precursor delivery considered to be involved in the regulation of ACh synthesis. Asterisks indicate possible sites of Ca^{2+} interaction.

be necessary for the mobilization of acetyl-CoA (see Section 2.4); it could be involved in enzyme phosphorylation (see Section 2.5.2); or it could be involved in some other biochemical event that is necessary for ACh synthesis.

3. ACh Storage and Release

Since the 1930s, it has been clear that tissues now known to release ACh contain an appreciable store of the ester (Chang and Gaddum, 1933). Kinetic analysis of ACh release rates has shown that this ACh store is compartmental, with a part of stored ACh being more readily available for release than the rest (Birks and MacIntosh, 1961). When techniques of subcellular fractionation of tissue were applied to nervous tissue by Gray and Whittaker (1962), it became evident that a part of the nerve-terminal ACh store is occluded within synaptic vesicles and that a part appears not to be so (Whittaker *et al.*, 1964); this nonoccluded ACh is considered to be cytoplasmic. Whether the synaptic vesicles or the cytosol contains that part of nerve-terminal ACh that is readily available for release upon stimulation is still argued.

3.1. Synaptic Vesicles and Releasable Transmitter

The classical view that the quantal release of ACh from cholinergic nerve terminals occurs as the result of the exocytosis of vesicle-stored transmitter (reviewed by Zimmermann, 1979; Ceccarelli and Hurlbut, 1980) has been contested (see reviews by Israël and Manaranche, 1985; Dunant, 1986). These last-named authors argue that ACh is released in response to nerve impulses from the cytoplasmic store of transmitter by its passage through channels in the nerve-terminal membrane that respond to changed intracellular Ca^{2+}. There is considerable experimental evidence to support this notion, including the isolation of a purified protein, termed mediatophore, from cholinergic nerve terminals of *Torpedo* electric organ that, when incorporated into the membrane of liposomes that contain ACh, can mediate a Ca^{2+}-dependent release of that ACh (Israël et al., 1987).

We have attempted to distinguish transmitter release of vesicle-bound stores from the release of cytosolic stores for the mammalian cholinergic nerve terminals by studying the subcellular distribution and the releasability of cholinergic false transmitters. This sort of approach contributes a strong point in favor of exocytosis being the mechanism for the release of the adrenergic nerve transmitter (e.g., Muscholl, 1972; Smith, 1973), and it seemed possible the approach might be similarly popular if applied to the cholinergic nervous system.

The potential false transmitters we have studied are those whose structure is shown in Table II. They are acetyl esters of choline analogues and they were formed in situ by exposing tissue (cerebral cortex or sympathetic ganglia) to the choline analogues. Cholinergic nerve terminals take up the choline analogues via their choline uptake mechanism, and endogenous ChAT can acetylate some of the accumulated choline analogue to form ACh analogues. The subcellular distribution of these false esters was similar to that of ACh when measured for the acetylated derivatives of monoethylcholine, diethylcholine, triethylcholine, pyrrolidinecholine, or homocholine (Boksa and Collier, 1980a,b,c), but that of acetyldiethylhomocholine differed from ACh by being preferentially distributed to nonoccluded transmitter stores (Welner and Collier, 1984). Thus, it appears that the process by which ACh is taken up into synaptic vesicles has a structural specificity such that acetyldiethylhomocholine does not satisfy that requirement.

One might then predict that if transmitter release is from vesicle-bound stores, all the above false esters except the acetyldiethylhomocholine would be releasable. On the other hand, if transmitter were released from cytoplasmic stores, the false esters including acetyldiethylhomocholine might be expected to be released. The results of this test favored the first prediction: acetylmonoethylcholine, acetyldiethylcholine, acetyltriethylcholine, acetylpyrrolidinecholine, and acetylhomocholine all were released in an amount, relative to tissue stores of the ester, that was similar to that of ACh (Collier et al., 1976, 1977; Ilson et al., 1977). But acetyldiethylhomocholine was clearly less available for release than ACh (Welner and Collier, 1984, 1985).

Thus, these experiments with false transmitters (summarized in Table II) are evidently more compatible with the classical hypothesis that synaptic vesicles store releasable ACh than they are

Table II. Characteristics of Esters Formed from Choline Analogues[a]

$$R_2 - \overset{\displaystyle R_1}{\underset{\displaystyle R_3}{\overset{+}{N}}} - (CH_2)_n - O - \overset{\displaystyle O}{\overset{\|}{C}} \diagdown CH_3$$

R_1	R_2	R_3	n	Trivial name	Relative subcellular distribution (cytoplasmic : vesicular)	Fraction store released (10^3 impulses)
CH_3	CH_3	CH_3	2	Acetylcholine	1.0 ± 0.07	8 ± 0.8
C_2H_5	CH_3	CH_3	2	Acetylmonoethylcholine	1.0 ± 0.12	8 ± 0.8
C_2H_5	C_2H_5	CH_3	2	Acetyldiethylcholine	1.1 ± 0.10	7 ± 1.2
C_2H_5	C_2H_5	C_2H_5	2	Acetyltriethylcholine	1.4 ± 0.12	10 ± 2.5
CH_3	CH_3	CH_3	3	Acetylhomocholine	1.5 ± 0.20	9 ± 1.0
C_2H_5	C_2H_5	CH_3	3	Acetyldiethylhomocholine	10.1 ± 0.8	1.7 ± 1.1

[a]Subcellular distribution measured from slices of cerebral cortex; amount of ester in cytoplasmic fraction was divided by amount in vesicle fraction. Release was measured from sympathetic ganglion; values are percent of store released by 1000 impulses.

with the notion that cytoplasmic transmitter is the immediate source of releasable ACh. In this way, the false transmitters augment and complement arguments based on other approaches (see Zimmermann, 1979; Ceccarelli and Hurlbut, 1980).

3.2. Heterogeneity of Releasable ACh Stores and of Synaptic Vesicles

The analysis by Birks and MacIntosh (1961) of ACh release rate from sympathetic ganglia provided the clear evidence that not all stored ACh is equally available for release during preganglionic stimulation. They estimated that some 15% of tissue ACh was unavailable for release, that some 13% of the total store was readily available to be released, and that the rest (72%) could be released but less readily so than that smaller releasable store. The compartments within a nerve terminal that contain these differently releasable stores of ACh have escaped precise analysis. The compound mentioned earlier (Section 2.5.4), AH5183, which apparently selectively blocks the uptake of ACh into synaptic vesicles (Anderson et al., 1983; Bahr and Parsons, 1986), offers the opportunity to measure the amount of ACh that preexists in synaptic vesicles and is available for release therefrom. The idea is that cholinergic nerve terminals will contain a complement of ACh prepackaged in synaptic vesicles, that stimulation will release that store, and that AH5183 will prevent its replenishment from ACh that is newly synthesized outside the vesicles.

We tested the effect of AH5183 on ACh release from sympathetic ganglia (Collier et al., 1986). The drug had no effect on ACh released by up to 500 or so impulses, but with successive trains of impulses, transmitter release was less in the presence of the drug than in its absence. Thus, evoked ACh release was reduced to an unmeasurable amount after some 3500–4000 impulses. The total amount of ACh measured as releasable in such experiments was 194 pmoles, a value that was independent of the frequency of preganglionic nerve stimulation; this represented 14 ± 1% of the total ACh contained in such ganglia. The simplest interpretation of this result is that only a small fraction of the ACh store preexists in synaptic vesicles available to release their content in response to nerve impulses.

The value of 14% of tissue ACh store that is releasable in the presence of AH5183 is most likely the store of almost identical size identified as readily releasable by Birks and MacIntosh (1961). But it is too small to represent only vesicle-bound ACh: after subcellular fractionation, some 50% or more of nerve-terminal ACh can usually be recovered in occluded stores, and this is probably an underestimate of the vesicle-bound ACh considering that vesicles are likely to lose ACh during their preparation. Thus, we suggested that the fraction of transmitter released upon stimulation in the presence of AH5183 represents ACh in a particular population of synaptic vesicles that actively participate in transmitter turnover, and that the ACh that is unreleasable by nerve impulses is contained, in part, outside synaptic vesicles and, in part, within synaptic vesicles that do not actively participate in transmitter turnover. In the absence of AH5183, it is presumed that ACh from the reserve population of vesicles can be mobilized to the releasable store. Clearly, AH5183 blocks this process of mobilization, and if AH5183 has a unique action to block ACh uptake into vesicles, then this process of transmitter mobilization must involve the movement of ACh out of some and into other organelles, rather than the mobilization involving movement of preloaded vesicles. This idea is illustrated by Fig. 2.

The idea that ACh-containing synaptic vesicles are heterogeneous is not new. The matter has been well studied with the electromotor system of *Torpedo* where morphological, biophysical, and metabolic differences have been shown for at least two populations of synaptic vesicles containing ACh (Zimmermann and Denston, 1977a,b; Zimmermann and Whittaker, 1977, Suszkiw et al., 1978; Giompres et al., 1981a,b,c; Giompres and Whittaker, 1984). These vesicle populations from *Torpedo* were called VP_1 and VP_2 and some evidence for their existence in mammalian cholinergic nerve terimnals was presented by Ágoston et al. (1985) from their study with the myenteric plexus of guinea pig ileum. Earlier, an analogous phenomenon was described

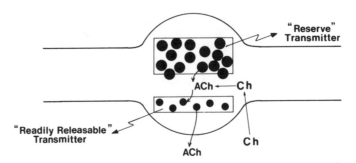

Figure 2. A scheme illustrating the pools of nerve-terminal ACh stores and their relationship to each other.

for cholinergic nerve terminals of mammalian cerebral cortex, from which were isolated two fractions, called D and H, containing synaptic vesicles with a different apparent turnover rate of ACh (Barker *et al.*, 1972; von Schwarzenfeld, 1979; Boksa and Collier, 1980a).

It has usually been concluded that the less metabolically active pool of synaptic vesicles are recruited to become active ones by stimuli that release ACh (see Zimmermann, 1979), and the conclusion reached above that intravesicular movement of ACh represents mobilization of transmitter is not entirely in accord with that view. It is possible that AH5183 acts upon the vesicle mobilization process in addition to blocking ACh uptake into vesicles, and this idea is worth testing. Nevertheless, there are other observations that are compatible with the notion of ACh movement between vesicles. For example, it has long been known that depletion of motor nerve-terminal ACh by stimulation in the presence of hemicholinium is associated with a reduced quantal size and a normal quantal content of transmitter (Elmqvist and Quastel, 1965; Jones and Kwanbunbumpen, 1970). Since hemicholinium blocks ACh synthesis, the reduced amount of ACh per quantum is best taken to indicate that individual vesicles become partly depleted in parallel with the general store of transmitter, rather than some vesicles being depleted and others retaining their full complement of transmitter; i.e., stored ACh is exchangeable between vesicles.

The effect of AH5183 to block mobilization of transmitter during nerve impulses can be overcome if ACh release is evoked by α-latrotoxin, the active component of the venom of the black widow spider. Thus, when ACh release from a sympathetic ganglion during its stimulation in the presence of AH5183 is exhausted, residual ACh is readily released by α-latrotoxin (Cabeza and Collier, 1986). This result supports the argument presented above that ACh not released by nerve impulses in the presence of AH5183 is, in part, stored in vesicles, because α-latrotoxin is well established as an agent that induces exocytosis of transmitters from vesicle stores (see Hurlbut and Ceccarelli, 1979; Ceccarelli and Hurlbut, 1980; Meldolesi *et al.*, 1986).

We have attempted to separate, by subcellular fractionation, the tissue stores of ACh releasable in the presence of AH5183 from those stores that appear not releasable. In this study (Říčný and Collier, 1986), slices of rat striata were stimulated to release ACh by K^+ in the presence or absence of AH5183. The drug inhibited ACh release, as also reported by others (Carroll, 1985; Jope and Johnson, 1986). The amount of ACh recovered in the cytosol fraction prepared from synaptosomes made from the slices was greater when tissue was stimulated in the presence of AH5183 than it was when tissue was stimulated in the drug's absence (see also Jope and Johnson, 1986). In contrast, ACh occluded in synaptic vesicles was less from tissue exposed to AH5183, and separation of vesicles by gradient centrifugation showed appreciable depletion of ACh in D-fraction vesicles, but not in H-fraction vesicles. Thus, this result suggests that the synaptic vesicles that contain readily releasable transmitter can be separated from those that do not. This result also supports the notion discussed above (Section 3.1) that the vesicle ACh store, not the cytosolic one, is the origin of releasable transmitter, because in the presence of AH5183 ACh release was depressed when vesicles were depleted of their ACh and when cytoplasmic ACh was increased in amount.

3.3. Plasticity of ACh Storage and Release

Adaptive changes of synaptic transmission are considered of importance in the functioning of the nervous system, particularly so in the CNS where presynaptic changes in transmitter turnover contribute to such phenomena. This kind of adaptation is not yet well studied for the central cholinergic nervous pathways, but the results from studies on peripheral cholinergic transmission have provided clear evidence that plasticity of ACh storage and release is possible.

The first demonstration that activity-related changes in ACh storage can occur was the measure of increased transmitter content of a cat's sympathetic ganglion following conditioned stimulation of its preganglionic nerve (Rosenblueth *et al.*, 1939). The observation has been repeatedly confirmed (e.g., Friesen and Khatter, 1971; Birks and Fitch, 1974; Bourdois *et al.*, 1975). The increased amount of ACh stored as the result of conditioning is releasable, its formation is associated with an activation of choline uptake, and transmitter release (but not action) during the period of conditioning is required for the phenomenon to be manifest (Collier *et al.*, 1983). A somewhat similar increase in ACh stores and release has been shown to occur during the activation of ganglia by stimulus trains, when the pattern of activity is an important determinant of the magnitude of the change (Birks, 1977, 1978).

Thus, it appears that following activity or during certain patterns of activity, the cholinergic nerve terminal can adapt by increasing its rate of ACh synthesis and by increasing its transmitter store; as the increased store is paralleled by increased release, much of the extra ACh is presumably in the readily releasable fraction.

A slightly different adaptive response has been reported by Briggs and his colleagues on the basis of experiments made with rat sympathetic ganglion. This preparation shows a long-lasting posttetanic potentiation of synaptic transmission (Dunant and Dolivo, 1968; Briggs *et al.*, 1985a); and this is associated with increased ACh release without measurable increased ACh content (Briggs *et al.*, 1985b). Thus, this presumably is an example of adaptation in response to the tetanus whereby the proportion of ACh in the readily releasable store is increased at the expense of that in the reserve pool.

The molecular basis of these plastic changes in ACh storage and release is not yet known with certainty, although a long-term potentiation of transmitter release induced by adrenaline in amphibian sympathetic ganglion appears to involve cyclic nucleotide-dependent processes (Kuba and Kumamoto, 1986). Whether the neuronally induced potentiation is similar in mechanism remains to be established. Endogenously released catecholamines in the sympathetic ganglia can be shown to reach a concentration that can alter ACh release (Araujo and Collier, 1986), but a catecholamine seems not to be the intermediate in the posttetanic potentiation discussed above, because α or β receptor antagonists do not ablate the phenomenon (Briggs *et al.*, 1985a).

3.4. The Spontaneous Release of ACh

Tissues that contain cholinergic nerve terminals release an appreciable amount of ACh in the absence of stimuli that evoke transmitter release. The two processes, spontaneous and depolarization-induced release, differ in several respects. Spontaneous ACh release is mostly independent of extracellular Ca^{2+}, whereas evoked release is clearly Ca^{2+} requiring (e.g., Carroll and Aspry, 1981). Spontaneous ACh release is accompanied by the release of false transmitters in a ratio that suggests a cytoplasmic origin (Boksa and Collier, 1980a; Welner and Collier, 1984), which contrasts with evoked release (see Section 3.1). Thus, spontaneous ACh release measured by neurochemical technique probably is the spontaneous ACh release shown by electrophysiology to be responsible for the H-effect (Katz and Miledi, 1977; Vyskočil and Illés, 1977), rather than that responsible for miniature synaptic potentials.

This nonquantal release of cytoplasmic ACh appears not to simply result from the leakage of transmitter from nerve terminals by efflux down its concentration gradient, because it is now apparent that the ACh transport blocker, AH5183, suppresses this spontaneous release of transmitter (Edwards *et al.*, 1985, Vyskočil, 1985; Říčný and Collier, 1986). Thus, it is possible that the nerve-terminal membrane contains an ACh transporter and it is tempting to speculate that this might be the mediatophore mentioned earlier (Section 3.1). Edwards *et al.* (1985) and Vyskočil (1985) hypothesize that the ACh translocating protein becomes incorporated into the plasma membrane of the nerve terminal during exocytosis; i.e., the component that transports ACh from cytosol to vesicle transports ACh from cytosol to the extracellular space during the time between vesicle fusion and retrieval. Alternatively, the AH5183-sensitive site that contributes to spontaneous ACh release might be an integral membrane component of cholinergic nerve terminals, related to but not necessarily identical with the vesicle ACh transporter.

The functional significance of nonquantal ACh release is not yet clear; the tendency has been to consider it of trivial importance to the process of synaptic transmission. However, the growing evidence that favors a slowly effective, long-lasting, modulating function for ACh at many synapses, suggests that nonquantal release could be of considerable importance.

References

Ágoston, D. V., Kosh, J. W., Lisziewicz, J., and Whittaker, V. P., 1985, Separation of recycling and reserve synaptic vesicles from cholinergic nerve terminals of the myenteric plexus of guinea pig ileum, *J. Neurochem.* **44:**299–305.

Anderson, D. C., King, S. C., and Parsons, S. M., 1983, Pharmacological characterization of the acetylcholine transport system in purified *Torpedo* electric organ synaptic vesicles, *Mol. Pharmacol.* **24:**48–54.

Araujo, D. M., and Collier, B., 1986, Evidence that endogenous catecholamines can regulate acetylcholine release in a sympathetic ganglion, *Eur. J. Pharmacol.* **125:**93–101.

Bahr, B. A., and Parsons, S. M., 1986, Acetylcholine transport and drug inhibition kinetics in *Torpedo* synaptic vesicles, *J. Neurochem.* **46:**1214–1218.

Barker, L. A., and Mittag, T. W., 1975, Comparative studies of substrates and inhibitors of choline transport and choline acetyltransferase, *J. Pharmacol. Exp. Ther.* **192:**86–94.

Barker, L. A., Dowdall, M. J., and Whittaker, V. P., 1972, Choline metabolism in the cerebral cortex of guinea pig, *Biochem. J.* **130:**1063–1080.

Benishin, C. G., and Carroll, P. T., 1981, Acetylation of choline and homocholine by membrane-bound choline-O-acetyltransferase in mouse forebrain nerve endings, *J. Neurochem.* **36:**732–740.

Benishin, C. G., and Carroll, P. T., 1983, Multiple forms of choline-O-acetyltransferase in mouse and rat brain: Solubilization and characterization, *J. Neurochem.* **41:**1030–1039.

Benjamin, A. M., and Quastel, J. H., 1981, Acetylcholine synthesis in synaptosomes: Mode of transfer of mitochondrial acetyl coenzyme A, *Science* **213:**1495–1497.

Birks, R. I., 1977, A long-lasting potentiation of transmitter release related to an increase in transmitter stores in a sympathetic ganglion, *J. Physiol. (London)* **271:**847–862.

Birks, R. I., 1978, Regulation by patterned preganglionic neural activity of transmitter stores in a sympathetic ganglion, *J. Physiol. (London)* **280:**559–572.

Birks, R. I., 1983, Activation of feline acetylcholine synthesis in the absence of release: Dependence on sodium, calcium and sodium pump, *J. Physiol. (London)* **344:**347–357.

Birks, R. I., and Fitch, S. J. G., 1974, Storage and release of acetylcholine in a sympathetic ganglion, *J. Physiol. (London)* **240:**125–134.

Birks, R. I., and MacIntosh, F. C., 1961, Acetylcholine metabolism of a sympathetic ganglion, *Can. J. Biochem. Physiol.* **39:**787–827.

Blusztajn, J. K., and Wurtman, R., 1981, Choline biosynthesis by a preparation enriched in synaptosomes from rat brain, *Nature* **290:**417–418.

Boksa, P., and Collier, B., 1980a, Spontaneous and evoked release of acetylcholine and a cholinergic false transmitter from brain slices: Comparison to true and false transmitter in subcellular stores, *Neuroscience* **5:**1517–1532.

Boksa, P., and Collier, B., 1980b, Acetylation of homocholine by rat brain: Subcellular distribution of acetyl-homocholine and studies on the ability of homocholine to serve as substrate for cholineacetyltransferase in situ and in vitro, *J. Neurochem.* **34:**1470–1482.

Boksa, P., and Collier, B., 1980c, N-ethyl analogues of choline as precursors to cholinergic false transmitters, *J. Neurochem.* **35:**1099–1104.

Bourdois, P. S., McCandless, D. L., and MacIntosh, F. C., 1975, A prolonged after effect of intense synaptic activity on acetylcholine in a sympathetic ganglion, *Can. J. Physiol. Pharmacol.* **53:**155–165.

Briggs, C. A., Brown, T. H., and McAfee, D. A., 1985a, Neurophysiology and pharmacology of long-term potentiation in the rat sympathetic ganglion, *J. Physiol. (London)* **359:**503–521.

Briggs, C. A., McAfee, D. A., and McCamen, R. E., 1985b, Long-term potentiation of synaptic acetylcholine release in the superior cervical ganglion of the rat, *J. Physiol. (London)* **363:**181–190.

Browning, E. T., and Schulman, M. P., 1968, [^{14}C]acetylcholine synthesis by cortex slices of rat brain, *J. Neurochem.* **15:**1391–1405.

Bruce, G., and Hersh, L. B., 1985, Phosphorylation of human choline acetyltransferase, *Soc. Neurosci. Abstr.* **11:**444.

Cabeza, R., and Collier, B., 1986, Acetylcholine mobilization in the presence of AH5183, *Trans. Am. Soc. Neurochem.* **17:**273.

Carroll, P. T., 1985, The effect of the acetylcholine transport blocker 2-(4-phenylpiperidino) cyclohexanol (AH5183) on the subcellular storage and release of acetylcholine in mouse brain, *Brain Res.* **358:**200–209.

Carroll, P. T., and Aspry, J. M., 1981, Spontaneous and potassium-evoked release of acetylcholine from mouse forebrain minces, *Neuroscience* **6:**2555–2559.

Ceccarelli, B., and Hurlbut, W. P., 1980, Vesicle hypothesis of the release of quanta of acetylcholine, *Physiol. Rev.* **60:**396–441.

Celesia, G. G., and Jasper, H. H., 1966, Acetylcholine release from cerebral cortex in relation to state of activation, *Neurology* **16:**1053–1064.

Chang, H. C., and Gaddum, J. H., 1933, Choline esters in tissue extracts, *J. Physiol. (London)* **79:**255–285.

Collier, B., 1981, The structural specificity of choline transport into cholinergic nerve terminals, *J. Neurochem.* **36:**1292–1294.

Collier, B., and Ilson, D., 1977, The effect of preganglionic nerve stimulation on the accumulation of certain analogues of choline by a sympathetic ganglion, *J. Physiol. (London)* **264:**489–509.

Collier, B., and Katz, H. S., 1974, Acetylcholine synthesis from recaptured choline by a sympathetic ganglion, *J. Physiol. (London)* **238:**639–655.

Collier, B., and MacIntosh, F. C., 1969, The source of choline for acetylcholine synthesis in a sympathetic ganglion, *Can. J. Physiol. Pharmacol.* **47:**127–135.

Collier, B., Barker, L. A., and Mittag, T. W., 1976, The release of acetylated choline analogues by a sympathetic ganglion, *Mol. Pharmacol.* **12:**340–344.

Collier, B., Lovat, S., Ilson, D., Barker, L. A., and Mittag, T. W., 1977, The uptake, metabolism and release of homocholine: Studies with rat brain synaptosomes and cat superior cervical ganglion, *J. Neurochem.* **28:**331–339.

Collier, B., Kwok, Y. N., and Welner, S. A., 1983, Increased acetylcholine synthesis and release following presynaptic activity in a sympathetic ganglion, *J. Neurochem.* **40:**91–98.

Collier, B., Welner, S. A., Říčný, J., and Araujo, D. M., 1986, Acetylcholine synthesis and release by a sympathetic ganglion in the presence of 2-(4-phenylpiperidino) cyclohexanol (AH5183), *J. Neurochem.* **46:**822–830.

Collier, B., Araujo, D. M., and Lapchak, P. A., 1987, Presynaptic effects of peptides at cholinergic synapses, in: *Cellular and Molecular Basis of Cholinergic Function* (M. J. Dowdall and J. N. Hawthorn, eds.), Ellis Horwood Press, Chichester, pp. 454–459.

Cozzari, C., and Hartman, B. K., 1983, An endogenous inhibitory factor for choline acetyltransferase, *Brain Res.* **276:**109–118.

Dale, H. H., 1938, Acetylcholine as a chemical transmitter of the effects of nerve impulses, *J. Mt. Sinai Hosp.* **4:**401–429.

Doležal, V., and Tuček, S., 1981, Utilization of citrate, acetylcarnitine, acetate, pyruvate and glucose for the synthesis of acetylcholine in rat brain slices, *J. Neurochem.* **36:**1323–1330.

Dunant, Y., 1986, On the mechanism of acetylcholine release, *Prog. Neurobiol.* **26:**55–92.

Dunant, Y., and Dolivo, M., 1968, Plasticity of synaptic functions in the excised sympathetic ganglion of the rat, *Brain Res.* **10:**271–273.

Eder-Colli, L., and Amato, S., 1985, Membrane-bound choline acetyltransferase in *Torpedo* electric organ, *Neuroscience* **15:**577–589.

Edwards, C., Doležal, V., Tuček, S., Zemková, H., and Vyskočil, F., 1985, Is an acetylcholine transport system responsible for non-quantal release of acetylcholine at the rodent myoneural junction? *Proc. Natl. Acad. Sci. USA* **82:**3514–3518.

Elmqvist, D., and Quastel, D. M. J., 1965, Presynaptic action of hemicholinium at the neuromuscular junction, *J. Physiol. (London)* **177:**463–482.

Fonnum, F., 1968, Choline acetyltransferase binding to and release from membranes, *Biochem. J.* **109:**389–398.

Friesen, A. J. D., and Khatter, J. C., 1971, The effect of preganglionic stimulation on the acetylcholine and choline content of a sympathetic ganglion, *Can. J. Physiol. Pharmacol.* **49:**375–381.

Giompres, P. E., and Whittaker, V. P., 1984, Differences in the osmotic fragility of recycling and reserve vesicles from the electromotor nerve terminals of *Torpedo* and their possible significance for vesicle recycling, *Biochim. Biophys. Acta* **770:**166–170.

Giompres, P. E., Morris, S. J., and Whittaker, V. P., 1981a, The water spaces in cholinergic synaptic vesicles from *Torpedo* measured by changes in density induced by permeating substances, *Neuroscience* **6:**757–763.

Giompres, P. E., Zimmermann, H., and Whittaker, V. P., 1981b, Purification of small dense vesicles from stimulated *Torpedo* electric tissue by glass bead column chromatography, *Neuroscience* **6:**765–774.

Giompres, P. E., Zimmermann, H., and Whittaker, V. P., 1981c, Changes in the biochemical and biophysical parameters of cholinergic synaptic vesicles on transmitter release and during a subsequent period of rest, *Neuroscience* **6:**775–785.

Glover, V. A. S., and Potter, L. T., 1971, Purification and properties of choline acetyltransferase from ox brain striate nuclei, *J. Neurochem.* **18:**571–580.

Gray, E. G., and Whittaker, V. P., 1962, The isolation of nerve endings from brain: An electron microscopic study of cell fragments derived by homogenization and centrifugation, *J. Anat.* **96:**79–87.

Guyenet, P., Lafresne, P., Rossier, J., Beaujouin, J. C., and Glowinski, J., 1973, Inhibition by hemicholinium-3 of [^{14}C]acetylcholine synthesis and [^{3}H]choline high affinity uptake in rat striatal synaptosomes, *Mol. Pharmacol.* **9:**630–639.

Haga, T., and Noda, H., 1973, Choline uptake systems of rat brain synaptosomes, *Biochim. Biophys. Acta* **291:**564–575.

Hurlbut, W. P., and Ceccarelli, B., 1979, Use of black widow spider venom to study the release of neurotransmitters, in *Neurotoxins, Tools in Neurobiology* (B. Ceccarelli and F. Clementi, eds.), Raven Press, New York, pp. 87–115.

Ilson, D., Collier, B., and Boksa, P., 1977, Acetyltriethylcholine: A cholinergic false transmitter in cat superior cervical ganglion and rat cerebral cortex, *J. Neurochem.* **28:**371–381.

Israël, M., and Manaranche, R., 1985, The release of acetylcholine: From a cellular toward a molecular mechanism, *Biol. Cell* **55:**1–14.

Israël, M., Morel, N., Lesbats, B., Birman, S., and Manaranche, R., 1987, Isolation and reconstitution of a synaptosomal membrane protein translocating acetylcholine, in: *Cellular and Molecular Basis of Cholinergic Function* (M. J. Dowdall and J. N. Hawthorn, eds.), Ellis Horwood Press, Chichester, pp. 232–244.

Jones, S. F., and Kwanbunbumpen, S., 1970, Some effects of nerve stimulation and hemicholinium on quantal transmitter release at the mammalian neuromuscular junction, *J. Physiol. (London)* **207:**51–61.

Jope, R. S., 1979, High affinity choline transport and acetyl-CoA production in brain and their roles in the regulation of acetylcholine synthesis, *Brain Res. Rev.* **1:**313–344.

Jope, R. S., and Johnson, G. V. W., 1986, Quinacrine and 2-(4-phenylpiperidino) cyclohexanol (AH5183) inhibit acetylcholine release and synthesis in rat brain slices, *Mol. Pharmacol.* **29:**45–51.

Katz, B., and Miledi, R., 1977, Transmitter leakage from motor nerve endings, *Proc. R. Soc. London Ser.* **196:**59–72.

Kuba, K., and Kumamoto, E., 1986, Long-term potentiation of transmitter release induced by adrenaline in bullfrog sympathetic ganglia, *J. Physiol. (London)* **374:**515–530.

Kwok, Y. N., and Collier, B., 1982, Synthesis of acetylcholine from acetate in a sympathetic ganglion, *J. Neurochem.* **39:**16–26.

Malthe-Sorenssen, D., 1979, Recent progress in the biochemistry of choline acetyltransferase, in: *The Cholinergic Synapse* (S. Tuček, ed.), Elsevier, Amsterdam, pp. 45–58.

Meldolesi, J., Scheer, H., Madeddu, L., and Wanke, E., 1986, Mechanism of action of α-latrotoxin: The presynaptic stimulatory toxin of the black widow spider venom, *Trends Pharmacol. Sci.* **7:**151–155.

Murrin, L. C., and Kuhar, M. J., 1976, Activation of high-affinity choline uptake in vitro by depolarizing agents, *Mol. Pharmacol.* **12:**1082–1090.

Muscholl, E., 1972, Andrenergic false transmitters, *Handb. Exp. Pharmacol.* **33:**618–660.

Nakamura, R., Cheng, S.-C., and Naruse, H., 1970, A study on the precursors of the acetyl moiety of acetylcholine in brain slices, *Biochem. J.* **118:**443–450.

O'Regan, S., and Collier, B., 1981a, Effect of increasing choline in vivo and in vitro on the synthesis of acetylcholine in a sympathetic ganglion, *J. Neurochem.* **36:**420–430.

O'Regan, S., and Collier, B., 1981b, Factors affecting choline transport by the cat superior cervical ganglion during and following stimulation, and the relationship between choline uptake and acetylcholine synthesis, *Neuroscience* **6:**511–520.

Perry, W. L. M., 1953, Acetylcholine release in the cat's superior cervical ganglion, *J. Physiol. (London)* **119:**439–454.

Pieklik, J. R., and Guynn, R. W., 1975, Equilibrium constants of the reactions of choline acetyltransferase, carnitine acetyltransferase, and acetylcholinesterase under physiological conditions, *J. Biol. Chem.* **250**:4445–4450.

Potter, L. T., 1970, Synthesis, storage and release of [^{14}C] acetylcholine in isolated rat diaphragm muscles, *J. Physiol. (London)* **206**:145–166.

Potter, L. T., Glover, V. A. S., and Saelens, J. K., 1968, Choline acetyltransferase from rat brain, *J. Biol. Chem.* **243**:3864–3870.

Richter, J. A., Gormley, J. M., Holtman, J. R., and Simon, J. R., 1982, High affinity choline uptake in the hippocampus: Its relationship to the physiological state produced by administration of barbiturates, *J. Neurochem.* **39**:1440–1445.

Říčný, J., and Collier, B., 1987, Effect of 2-(4-phenylpiperidino) cyclohexanol on acetylcholine release and subcellular distribution in rat striatal slices, *J. Neurochem.* **47**:1627–1633.

Říčný, J., and Tuček, S., 1982, Acetylcoenzyme A and acetylcholine in slices of rat caudate nuclei incubated with (−) hydroxycitrate, citrate and EGTA, *J. Neurochem.* **39**:668–673.

Říčný, J., and Tuček, S., 1983, Ca^{2+} ions and the output of acetylcoenzyme A from brain mitochondria, *Gen. Physiol. Biophys.* **2**:27–37.

Rosenblueth, A., Lissák, K., and Lanari, A., 1939, An explanation of the five stages of neuromuscular and ganglionic synaptic transmission, *Am. J. Physiol.* **128**:31–44.

Rylett, R. J., 1986, Choline mustard: An irreversible ligand for use in studies of choline transport mechanisms at the cholinergic nerve terminal, *Can. J. Physiol. Pharmacol.* **64**:334–340.

Rylett, R. J., and Colhoun, E. H., 1980, Carrier-mediated inhibition of choline acetyltransferase, *Life Sci.* **26**:909–914.

Simon, J. R., and Kuhar, M. J., 1975, Impulse-flow regulation of high affinity choline uptake in brain cholinergic and nerve terminals, *Nature* **255**:162–163.

Simon, J. R. and Kuhar, M. J., 1976, High affinity choline uptake: Ionic and energy requirements, *J. Neurochem.* **27**:93–99.

Smith, A. D., 1973, Mechanisms involved in the release of noradrenaline from sympathetic nerves, *Br. Med. Bull.* **29**:123–129.

Sollenberg, J., and Sörbo, B., 1970, On the origin of the acetyl moiety of acetylcholine in brain studied with a differential labelling technique using ^{3}H–^{14}C-mixed labelled glucose and acetate, *J. Neurochem.* **17**:201–207.

Suszkiw, J. B., Zimmermann, H., and Whittaker, V. P., 1978, Vesicular storage and release of acetylcholine in *Torpedo* electroplaque synapses, *J. Neurochem.* **30**:1269–1280.

Tuček, S., 1967, The use of choline acetyltransferse for measuring the synthesis of acetyl-coenzyme A and its release from brain mitochondria, *Biochem. J.* **104**:749–756.

Tuček, S., 1978, *Acetylcholine Synthesis in Neurons,* Chapman & Hall, London.

Tuček, S., 1983, Acetylcoenzyme A and the synthesis of acetylcholine in neurones: Review of recent progress, *Gen. Physiol. Biophys.* **2**:313–324.

Tuček, S., 1984, Problems in the organization and control of acetylcholine synthesis in brain neurones, *Pro. Biophys. Mol. Biol.* **44**:1–46.

Tuček, S., 1985, Regulation of acetylcholine synthesis in the brain, *J. Neurochem.* **44**:11–24.

Vaca, K., and Pilar, G., 1979, Mechanisms controlling choline transport and acetylcholine synthesis in motor nerve terminals during electrical stimulation, *J. Gen. Physiol.* **73**:605–628.

von Schwarzenfeld, I., 1979, Origin of transmitters released by electrical stimulation from a small, metabolically very active vesicular pool of cholinergic synapses in guinea pig cerebral cortex, *Neuroscience* **4**:477–493.

Vyskočil, F., 1985, Inhibition of non-quantal acetylcholine leakage by 2(4-phenylpiperidine) cyclohexanol in the mouse diaphragm, *Neurosci. Lett.* **59**:277–280.

Vyskočil, F., and Illés, P., 1977, Non-quantal release of transmitter at mouse neuromuscular junction and its dependence on the activity of Na$^+$–K$^+$–ATPase, *Pfluegers Arch.* **370**:295–297.

Wecker, L., 1986, Neurochemical effects of choline supplementation, *Can. J. Physiol. Pharmacol.* **64**:329–333.

Weiler, M. H., Gundersen, C. B., and Jenden, D. J., 1981, Choline uptake and acetylcholine synthesis in synaptosomes: Investigations using two different labelled variants of choline, *J. Neurochem.* **36**:1802–1812.

Welner, S. A., and Collier, B., 1984, Uptake, metabolism and releasability of ethyl analogues of homocholine by rat brain, *J. Neurochem.* **43**:1143–1151.

Welner, S. A., and Collier, B., 1985, Accumulation, acetylation and releasability of diethylhomocholine from a sympathetic ganglion, *J. Neurochem.* **45**:210–218.

White, H. L., and Wu, J. C., 1973, Kinetics of choline acetyltransferase from human and other mammalian central and peripheral nervous tissues, *J. Neurochem.* **20**:297–307.

Whittaker, V. P., Michaelson, I. A., and Kirkland, R. J. A., 1964, The separation of synaptic vesicles from nerve ending particles (synaptosomes), *Biochem. J.* **90**:293–303.

Yamamura, H. I., and Snyder, S. H., 1973, High affinity transport of choline into synaptosomes of rat brain, *J. Neurochem.* **21:**1355–1374.

Zimmermann, H., 1979, Vesicle recycling and transmitter release, *Neuroscience* **4:**1773–1804.

Zimmermann, H., and Denston, C. R., 1977a, Recycling of synaptic vesicles in the cholinergic synapses of *Torpedo* electric organ during induced transmitter release, *Neuroscience* **2:**695–714.

Zimmermann, H., and Denston, C. R., 1977b, Separation of synaptic vesicles of different functional states from the cholinergic synapses of *Torpedo* electric organ, *Neuroscience* **2:**715–730.

Zimmermann, H. and Whittaker, V. P., 1977, Morphology and biochemical heterogeneity of cholinergic synaptic vesicles, *Nature* **267:**633–635.

17

Modulation of Neuronal Excitability by Acetylcholine

E. Wanke and A. Ferroni

1. Introduction

1.1. General

Several substances have been shown to act as neurotransmitters at a synaptic level. These include acetylcholine (ACh), noradrenaline (NA), adrenaline, and γ-aminobutyric acid (GABA) as well as a variety of other amino acids, amines, and peptides [such as serotonin (5-HT), glycine, glutamic acid, dopamine, and luteinizing hormone-releasing factor (LHRH)]. For a review see Krnjević (1974). These transmitters interact with specific chemoreceptor molecules, changing the permeability of the membrane to specific ions, and producing either an excitatory or an inhibitory synaptic potential. Each transmitter substance may control different specific permeability channels.

The binding of neurotransmitters to receptor molecules on the neuronal membrane can result in changes of membrane potential due (1) to the opening of an ion channel which is a part of the receptor molecule [time scale of milliseconds; e.g., nicotinic ACh receptor (AChR)]; (2) to the activation of GTP binding proteins coupled to ion channel proteins (time scale of seconds; e.g., in heart cells the muscarinic activated K^+ channel, Pfaffinger *et al.*, 1985); (3) to the activation of second messenger systems which phosphorylate ion channel proteins via protein kinase activation (time scale of tens of seconds).

1.2. Neurotransmitters and Excitability

Fast and slow synaptic responses can be recorded in different neurons of the brain and in autonomic ganglion cells. If we look into mammalian sympathetic ganglion cells (SCG), we find that they have a variety of synaptic responses. At least four separate synaptic responses can be seen under appropriate experimental conditions (Kuffler, 1980). The characteristics of the four synaptic potentials and the current components underlying the fast and slow responses are summarized in Table I.

E. Wanke and A. Ferroni • Department of General Physiology and Biochemistry, University of Milan, Milan, Italy.

Table I. Synaptic Potentials in Sympathetic Ganglia

	Excitatory fast	Inhibitory slow	Excitatory slow	Excitatory late slow
Time course	0.1 sec	1–5 sec	10–50 sec	300 sec
Current component	Na^+ and K^+	$\uparrow I_K$	$\downarrow I_K$ $\downarrow G_K$ $\downarrow I_{Cl}$ $\downarrow G_{Cl}$ $\uparrow G_m$	?
Transmitter	ACh	ACh	ACh	LHRH
Blocker	Curare	Atropine	Atropine	LHRH analogues

As shown in Table I, three synaptic responses are mediated by ACh interacting with two different specific receptors: nicotinic for the fast EPSP, and muscarinic for the two different slow synaptic responses (excitatory and inhibitory). The fourth is a late slow depolarization and is caused by the release onto the cell of the peptidergic transmitter LHRH. The fast EPSP is analogous to the end plate potential seen in skeletal muscle and to other fast excitatory synaptic potentials. It is produced by an increase in sodium and potassium permeability and is blocked by curare.

The slow excitatory potential appears to be related to a reduction of the potassium conductance (Adams et al., 1982; the M-current hypothesis). Two other components underlie the cholinergic slow EPSP: a simultaneous outward current due to the inhibition of a voltage-dependent resting current carried by Cl^- and an occasional late inward current associated with an increased membrane conductance (Brown and Selyanko, 1985). These actions of ACh are blocked by atropine and not by curare. The slow inhibitory potential is also caused by ACh. It is related to the activation of voltage-dependent potassium channels; their conductance increasing with hyperpolarization. Potassium channels activated by ACh have been recorded in different nerve cells in the CNS (Egan and North, 1986; McCormick and Prince, 1986), in the parasympathetic cardiac ganglion (Hartzell et al., 1977), in sympathetic ganglia (Cole and Shinnick-Gallagher, 1984; Horn and Dodd, 1981), and in pacemaker cells of mammalian heart (Sakmann et al., 1983). Since this action of ACh is blocked by atropine, this also implies that it is mediated through muscarinic cholinergic receptors.

1.3. Neurotransmitters and Voltage-Gated Ca^{2+} Channels

Moreover in SCG neurons and in vertebrate dorsal root ganglion (DRG) neurons, certain neurotransmitters and neuropeptides can modify the shape of neuronal action potentials (APs) even though they do not produce a change in resting membrane potential. The compounds NA, GABA, and 5-HT all reversibly decrease the duration of the AP in embryonic chick DRG neurons (Dunlap and Fischbach, 1978). In addition, NA decreases the duration of rat SCG APs (Horn and McAfee, 1980).

The AP in these neurons is a mixed Na–Ca AP. Inward Ca^{2+} current (I_{Ca}) rises slowly compared to the Na^+ current and it inactivates slowly. A change in AP duration implies a change in Ca^{2+} influx. Dunlap and Fischbach (1981) in chick DRG neurons and Galvan and Adams (1982) in rat SCG neurons have obtained evidence that NA as well as GABA and 5-HT reduce I_{Ca}.

The entry of Ca^{2+} in the cells means more than the transfer of a depolarizing positive charge: Ca^{2+} serves as a chemical message. By controlling Ca^{2+} entry, Ca^{2+} channels act as transducers converting electrical information into a chemical signal for the control of processes such as excitation–contraction coupling, excitation–secretion coupling, and Ca activation of Ca^{2+}-dependent K^+ channels (K_{Ca}).

The first evidence that Ca^{2+} currents can be modulated by neurotransmitters was obtained in cardiac muscle. Both adrenaline and NA increase Ca^{2+} current (Reuter and Scholz, 1977), but in heart cells I_{Ca} can be strongly modulated in either an excitatory or inhibitory direction. Interaction of ACh with muscarinic receptors decreases Ca^{2+} entry (Giles and Noble, 1976; Carmeliet and Mubagwa, 1986).

In neurons, Ca^{2+} currents or Ca^{2+}-dependent AP respond to a wide variety of agents (NA, GABA, 5-HT, dopamine), but so far all the reported effects have been inhibitory (Rane and Dunlap, 1986; Holz et al., 1986; Marchetti et al., 1986), with the exception of extracellular ATP, which enhances membrane Ca^{2+} channel activity of snail neurons (Yatani et al., 1982), and 5-HT, which induces a voltage-dependent Ca^{2+} current in sensitive neurons of Aplysia californica (Pellman and Carpenter, 1980).

1.4. Effect of ACh on Ca^{2+} Currents

The effect of muscarine on Ca^{2+} and Ca^{2+}-activated K^+ currents was examined by Belluzzi et al. (1985b) in SCG neurons. A direct effect on the voltage-sensitive Ca^{2+} channels was demonstrated. Muscarine produces a decrease of I_{Ca} (see Fig. 1). The parallel decrease of the outward K_{Ca} current is consistent with the resulting partial suppression of Ca^{2+} influx. This muscarinic effect indicates that in neurons of the sympathetic ganglia, Ca^{2+} currents are modulated by activation of muscarinic receptors in the same directions as for activation of adrenergic receptors.

Ca^{2+} current modulation can modify neuron excitability by altering the shape of neuronal APs or by changing the time course of the shoulder on the normal AP influencing the depolarizing afterpotential and the hyperpolarizing afterpotential. Two Ca^{2+} conductances, differentiated by a high- and low-threshold voltage, have been recognized in inferior olivary neurons, and the interplay between these two conductances is capable of generating many aspects of the neuron oscillatory behavior (Llinás and Yarom, 1981a,b).

Later on, in embryonic DRG neurons, isolated Ca^{2+} currents were studied using the patch-clamp technique and two components of an inward Ca^{2+} current were observed: a low-voltage-activated I_{Ca} fully inactivating and a high-voltage-activated current partially inactivating (Carbone and Lux, 1984). The properties of the low-voltage-activated current correspond with those of the inward current that has been inferred to exist in central neurons (Llinás and Yarom, 1981b), which produces depolarizing potentials and burst-firing after membrane hyperpolarization.

Three types of neuronal Ca^{2+} channels have been recorded in cultured DRG cells (Nowycky et al., 1985). In addition to the two current components (low and high voltage activated, termed T

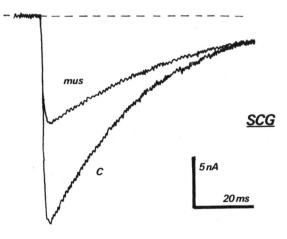

Figure 1. Muscarine modulates Ca^{2+} channels in neurons of the adult rat superior cervical ganglion. Ca^{2+} current traces elicited from a holding potential of -50 mV to a test of -10 mV in an SCG neuron before and after a 2-min application of 10 μM muscarine. The bathing solution contained (mM): Tris, 92; TEA, 50; Ca^{2+}, 10; 37°C. Double electrode voltage-clamp. (Sacchi, Belluzzi, and Wanke, unpublished.)

and L, respectively), a third high-voltage-activated transient current (N) has been recorded. The N current requires a strongly negative potential for complete removal of inactivation and strong depolarization for activation. It is attractive to suggest that the several channels serve different cellular functions. For example, N and L channel types may be important for neurotransmitter release.

1.5. New Data

In the light of these recent results on Ca^{2+} voltage-activated currents, we analyzed membrane I_{Ca} in the whole-cell configuration of the patch-clamp technique (Hamill et al., 1981) on SCG cultured cells. Several lines of evidence indicate that these cells do not possess the low-voltage-activated channels, as observed in cultured DRG neurons (Carbone and Lux, 1984; Fedulova et al., 1985). This is not unreasonable if we consider that the cells come from two different precursors (sensory, S, and autonomic, A). The two precursors arise from a common progenitor (stem cell) in the neural crest, but they then differentiate and migrate to the different sites for gangliogenesis. The neurotransmitter phenotype of neural crest cells is probably selected by the tissue environment during early development (Le Douarin et al., 1985).

In our study, we examined the effects of ACh (muscarinic receptors) on the high-threshold voltage-activated I_{Ca} of SCG neurons and compared these with the ACh effect on high-voltage-activated current in sensory cells. ACh was released onto the neurons in the whole-cell current-clamp configuration, and AP time course and properties were examined. Our results indicate that even though Ca^{2+} currents are modulated in the two different nerve cells (sensory and sympathetic) by the neurotransmitter in the same direction (i.e., decrease of the currents), the effect on the I_{Ca} time course is different. We postulate that ACh produces a selective block of a fast inactivating component of high-voltage-activated currents (N channels) in sympathetic ganglion cells.

2. Methods

SCG neurons were dissociated by treatment with collagenase and trypsin (0.1 and 0.05%, 1 hr, 37°C), then seeded in plastic petri dishes and cultured for 24–72 hr in Leibovitz L15 (Wanke et al., 1987). Ca^{2+} currents were recorded, at 36°C, by the whole-cell configuration of the patch-clamp technique (Hamill et al., 1981). The external standard solution contained (mM): NaCl, 130; $CaCl_2$, 5; KCl, 2; Hepes, 10; glucose, 5; tetrodotoxin (TTX), 0.001; hexamethonium (Hex), 0.5; pH 7.3. The pipette solution contained (mM): CsCl, 120; tetraethylammonium (TEA), 20; $MgCl_2$, 2; Na_2ATP, 2; creatine phosphate, 20; GTP, 0.1; EGTA, 10; Na Hepes, 10; 50 U/ml creatine phosphokinase, pH 7.4. During current-clamp experiments in the pipette solution, Cs and TEA were exchanged with K. Current signals were stored on videotapes and then analyzed with a personal computer.

3. Results and Discussion

3.1. Muscarinic Inhibition of Ca^{2+} Currents in SCG and DRG Neurons

As a rule, neurons after 1–3 days in culture do not show extensive neurite outgrowth. Therefore, they are particularly suitable for voltage clamping because the membrane space constant is small and usually under reasonably good control. In these neurons, Ca^{2+} currents reach an average of 0.5 nA (peak) when bathed in a medium enriched in Ca^{2+} (5 mM) and consequently the clamp error introduced by the pipette resistance is negligible. However, experiments done in fully grown neurons with long neurites (> 500 μm) do not show any detectable differences compared to younger neurons.

In the presence of TTX and Hex (to block the fast voltage-gated and ACh-activated nicotinic currents), it was possible to record the remaining inward currents due to Ca^{2+} channels if K^+ currents are blocked by internal Cs and TEA ions (Fenwick et al., 1982). These currents are stable for 20–30 min, if the repetition rate is slower than 0.03 Hz. They show a reversal potential around +50 or +60 mV which is not the true reversal of Ca^{2+} current (expected at much higher values from the Nernst relation) but the result of a small outward permeability of Cs ions in the Ca^{2+} channels (Fenwick et al., 1982). In contrast to DRG neurons where three types of voltage-gated Ca^{2+} channels can be activated by different protocols (Carbone and Lux, 1984; Nowycky et al., 1985), in SCG neurons only high-voltage-activated Ca^{2+} channels are found (Marchetti et al., 1986; Wanke et al., 1987). In particular, when elicited from −70 mV (in SCG) and −60 mV (in DRG) the current records show a partial and relatively fast (time constant of about 25–30 msec) inactivation which is followed by an incomplete (70–80%) slow inactivation (about 300 msec; Fig. 2, top). The relative contributions of these two current components are highly variable among neurons and we could not find any correlation between morphological characteristics and the relative contributions.

In rat SCG neurons, after 3–4 sec of application of ACh, the transient component of the Ca^{2+} current showed an inhibition (reversible in 15 sec). The effect had an IC_{50} of 2–3 μM and was completely blocked by 1 μM atropine or 100 nM pirenzepine (Fig. 2, top and bottom left). In contrast, in chick DRG neurons, the muscarinic effect of ACh (50 μM) was an inhibition of a stationary component (putative L channel). In fact, the time course of the ACh-inhibited transient current was neither scaled down, nor modified in any obvious way (Fig. 2, bottom right). As a rule, the effects detected in SCG neurons were more pronounced when currents showed a

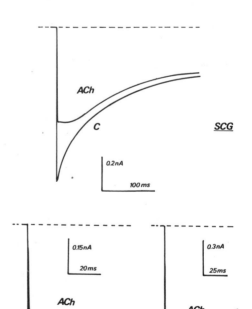

Figure 2. Different mechanisms of ACh-activated muscarinic inhibition of the Ca^{2+} current in SCG (rat; top, bottom left) and DRG (chick; bottom right) neurons. Superimposed Ca^{2+} currents elicited by a depolarizing step to +10 mV from a holding potential of −70 mV. For SCG, note the suppression of the transient component of the current during 50 μM ACh perfusion and −60 mV. For DRG, note the decrease of a stationary component with ACh perfusion. Whole-cell clamp.

significant inactivation. A small fraction (5–8%) of the cells (SCG) did not respond to the transmitter.

The inhibitory effect of ACh in rat SCG neurons was measured at various membrane potentials as shown in the I–V plot (Fig. 3). Measurements were taken at the peak (control and ACh) and after 80 msec. It can be seen that the activation threshold of the current starts at -30 mV but ACh affects the currents over -15 mV where a transient component starts to appear. Moreover, as shown in the plot and in Fig. 2 (top), ACh produces inhibition for a limited time of about 80 msec. This period corresponds to the transient current of the N channel (Nowycky *et al.*, 1985). As will be shown in the following section, this interpretation is consistent with APs recorded under normal conditions.

3.2. ACh Reduces the Duration of the Artificially Long AP in SCG Neurons

When small amounts (5 mM TEA) of K^+ channel blockers are added to the bathing solution, a prolongation of the AP duration occurs. Moreover, if an increased amount of Ca^{2+} is introduced into the extracellular medium, a further modification of the AP can be observed: a brief plateau phase occurs sustained by the increased inward Ca^{2+} current activated at high voltage (Fig. 4, "C" traces). Under these conditions, the application of ACh (in the presence of 0.5 mM Hex) produced a selective modification of the AP consisting of a simple shortening of its duration (Fig. 4, "ACh" traces), without altering appreciably the repolarizing voltage level. It is useful to remember that the repolarization phase of the AP is adjusted by the combination of three K^+ currents: the transient outward A current described by Belluzzi *et al.* (1985a), the delayed rectifier voltage-dependent K_v current, and the Ca^{2+}-activated K_{Ca} current (Belluzzi *et al.*, 1985b). The first channel (not completely developed in these cultured neurons) is inactivated at -50 mV. The third channel (outward current), being Ca^{2+} dependent, is expected to produce, in combination with the Ca^{2+} channel (inward current), different effects according to their relative weights. The presence, in the AP, of a slow declining plateau phase after the fast Na^+ peak is an indication of a reasonably large Ca^{2+} current (due to the high extracellular Ca^{2+} concentration). The partial

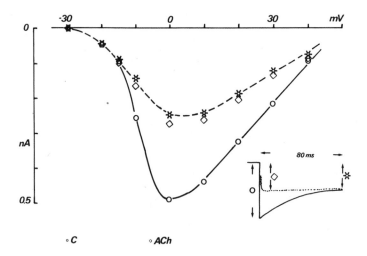

Figure 3. I–V plot of the Ca^{2+} current in rat SCG neurons at different times and during ACh (50 μM) perfusion. Peak control currents (○), control currents after 80 msec (*), and peak currents during ACh administration (◇, 50 μM) are plotted for the same cell, during step depolarizations from a holding potential of -70 mV. Whole-cell clamp.

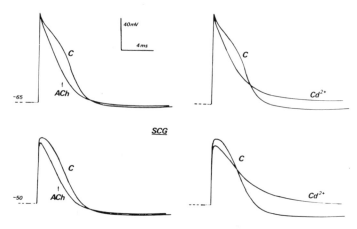

Figure 4. Action potentials in a rat SCG neuron, bathed in a TEA (5 mM) and high-Ca^{2+} (5 mM) solution, elicited from a membrane potential of -65 and -50 mV and perfused with ACh (50 μM) or Cd^{2+} (100 nM). Whole-cell current clamp in the same cell.

ACh-induced Ca^{2+} current inhibition is expected to reduce the slow declining phase of the AP, thus reducing AP duration. This effect is reasonable if the K_{Ca} current is small compared to the Ca^{2+} current.

APs were elicited by short (0.4 msec) but high-current pulses delivered through the patch-clamp pipette. The holding potential ranged from -65 and -50 mV in order to vary the relative importance of Na$^+$ and Ca^{2+} channels in the rising phase of the AP. Na$^+$ channels are almost completely inactivated at -50 mV and the effect of the selective inhibition of the transient Ca^{2+} channels is clearly visible (lower part of Fig. 4). Extracellular application of Cd^{2+} (100 nM), which completely blocks the Ca^{2+} currents (and consequently the K_{Ca} channel), was used to record APs whose repolarization is produced only by the voltage-dependent K_v channels. It can be seen (Fig. 4, right) that the K_{Ca} channels are required to correct the AP duration and time course. Conversely, a comparison with the records, on the left of Fig. 4, clearly demonstrates that the inhibitory action of ACh is truly selective only for a fraction (in time and in amplitude) of the total Ca^{2+} current as expected from Fig. 2 (top records).

3.3. Muscarinic Action on Normal AP in SCG Neurons

As mentioned in the previous section, the action of ACh on the time course of long APs (external TEA and Ca ions added) is in agreement with the data on Ca^{2+} currents previously recorded and measured with K$^+$ blockers inside the cell (Cs and TEA ions), suggesting that ACh influences the Ca^{2+} currents in these cells. By recording APs and membrane currents under normal conditions (outside and inside the cell; see Methods), we have obtained data supporting a physiological role for the muscarinic inhibitory modulation of the N-type Ca^{2+} channel.

As suggested by the experiments of Belluzzi *et al.* (1985b) in adult neurons the amount of inward Ca^{2+} current (studied in normal saline) is negligible compared to the outward K$^+$ currents. It is therefore reasonable to suppose that in cultured neurons the outward currents are not contaminated by inward Ca^{2+} currents by more than 5–8%. In fact, as it can be seen in the left panel of Fig. 5, application of Cd ions (100 nM, thus blocking Ca^{2+} and K_{Ca} current) significantly reduces the amplitude of the outward K$^+$ current (only K_v channels present; the A channels are inactivated at -50 mV and Na$^+$ channels inactivate in a few milliseconds). On the contrary, when ACh (50 μM) was applied in the perfusate, a small decrease of the outward current was

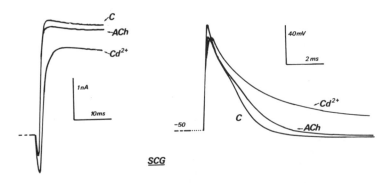

Figure 5. Ionic currents (tested at +10 mV) and action potentials in the same rat SCG neuron, bathed in standard solution, elicited from a holding potential of −50 mV, during perfusion with ACh (50 μM) and Cd^{2+} (100 nM). "C" traces are control curves before and after application of ACh and Cd^{2+}. Whole-cell voltage and current clamp.

found. This is in good agreement with the fact that the inhibitory effect of ACh on I_{Ca} induces a companion inhibitory effect on the K_{Ca} current.

Under these same normal conditions, APs elicited from the same holding potential (in the same cell) show that repolarization are less pronounced in the presence of ACh (50 μM) for a period of 3–4 msec after the AP peak (Fig. 5, right). When Cd^{2+} is applied (100 nM) to block completely Ca^{2+} and K_{Ca} channels, the repolarization is less pronounced due to the weaker K^+ currents. Notice also the reduction of the AP peak in the presence of ACh or Cd^{2+}. This change is consistent with the hypothesis that there is a contribution of Ca^{2+} currents to the depolarizing phase of APs elicited at −50 mV.

4. Conclusions

The data presented above show that the inhibitory effect of ACh is mediated by muscarinic receptors (presumably M_1 high-affinity receptors) but they do not give any indication of the intracellular mechanisms that couple the receptor with the Ca^{2+} channels. As shown elsewhere (Wanke et al., 1987), there is evidence that a GTP binding protein is involved in the transducing mechanism since: (1) the incubation of the cells with pertussis toxin can inhibit ACh action; (2) a nonhydrolyzable GTP analogue, GTPγS, can (when applied intracellularly) by itself inhibit irreversibly the Ca^{2+} channel; a GDP analogue, GDPβS, is able to uncouple the receptor from the final response in the presence of ACh. Other second messenger systems like cAMP, inositol triphosphate, and Ca^{2+}-dependent protein kinase can also be excluded.

A direct connection of G-proteins (Gilman, 1984) with the Ca^{2+} channel or the presence of an unknown messenger are possible coupling mechanisms to be studied in the future. Although some points remain to be resolved, our findings indicate that neurons located in different tissue environments show different Ca^{2+} channel density distributions (N and L in SCG; T, N, and L in DRG) and respond to neurotransmitters (1) through different mechanisms (protein kinase C phosphorylation in DRG; non-protein kinase C dependent in SCG), and (2) with different Ca^{2+} channels (N type in SCG; putative L type in DRG).

ACKNOWLEDGMENTS. We thank Drs. O. Sacchi and O. Belluzzi, Institute of General Physiology, University of Ferrara for permission to report unpublished data, Drs. J. Meldolesi, A. Malgaroli, and A. Ambrosini, Department of Pharmacology, University of Milan, and Dr. T. Pozzan, Department of Pathology, University of Padua for their major collaboration during part of the experiments, Dr. E. Carbone, University of Turin, for helpful suggestions, Dr. F. Franciolini, University of Perugia, and Dr. D. Janigro, University of Washington, Seattle, for comments on the manuscript. Supported in part by grants from MPI (40%) membrane physiology program.

References

Adams, P. R., Brown, D. A., and Constanti, A., 1982, M-currents and other potassium currents in bullfrog sympathetic neurones, *J. Physiol. (London)* **330**:537–572.

Belluzzi, O., Sacchi, O., and Wanke, E., 1985a, A fast transient outward current in the rat sympathetic neurone studied under voltage-clamp conditions, *J. Physiol. (London)* **358**:91–108.

Belluzzi, O., Sacchi, O., and Wanke, E., 1985b, Identification of delayed potassium and calcium currents in the rat sympathetic neurone under voltage-clamp, *J. Physiol. (London)* **358**:109–129.

Brown, D. A., and Selyanko, A. A., 1985, Membrane currents underlying the cholinergic slow excitatory post synaptic potential in the rat sympathetic ganglion, *J. Physiol. (London)* **365**:365–387.

Carbone, E., and Lux, H. D., 1984, A low voltage activated Ca conductance in embryonic chick sensory neurones, *Biophys. J.* **46**:413–418.

Carmeliet, E., and Mubagwa, K., 1986, Changes by acetylcholine of membrane currents in rabbit cardiac Purkinje fibres, *J. Physiol. (London)* **371**:201–217.

Cole, A. E., and Shinnick-Gallagher, P., 1984, Muscarinic inhibitory transmission in mammalian sympathetic ganglia mediated by increased potassium conductance, *Nature* **307**:270–271.

Dunlap, K., and Fischbach, G., 1978, Neurotransmitters decrease the calcium component of sensory neurone action potentials, *Nature* **276**:837–839.

Dunlap, K., and Fischbach, G., 1981, Neurotransmitters decrease the calcium conductance activated by depolarization of embryonic chick sensory neurones, *J. Physiol. (London)* **317**:519–535.

Egan, T., and North, R. A., 1986, Acetylcholine hyperpolarizes central neurones by acting on an M_2 muscarinic receptor, *Nature* **319**:405–407.

Fedulova, S. A., Kostyuk, P. G., and Veselovsky, N. S., 1985, Two types of calcium channels in the somatic membrane of newborn rat dorsal root ganglion neurones, *J. Physiol. (London)* **359**:431–446.

Fenwick, E., Marty, E., and Neher, E., 1982, Sodium and calcium channel in bovine chromaffin cells, *J. Physiol. (London)* **331**:599–635.

Galvan, M., and Adams, P. R., 1982, Control of calcium current in rat sympathetic neurons by norepinephrine, *Brain Res.* **244**:135–144.

Giles, W. R., and Noble, S. J., 1976, Changes in membrane currents in bullfrog atrium produced by acetylcholine, *J. Physiol. (London)* **261**:103–123.

Gilman, A. G., 1984, G proteins and dual control of adenylate cyclase, *Cell* **36**:577–579.

Hamill, P. O., Marty, A., Neher, E., Sakmann, B., and Sigworth, F., 1981, Improved patch-clamp techniques for high resolution current recording from cells and cell-free membrane patches, *Pfluegers Arch.* **391**:85–100.

Hartzell, H. C., Kuffler, S. W., Stickgold, R., and Yoshikami, D., 1977, Synaptic excitation and inhibition resulting from direct action of acetylcholine on two types of chemoreceptors on individual amphibian parasympathetic neurones, *J. Physiol. (London)* **271**:817–846.

Holz, G. G., Rane, S. G., and Dunlap, K., 1986, GTP-binding proteins mediate transmitter inhibition of voltage dependent calcium channels, *Nature* **319**:670–672.

Horn, J. P., and Dodd, J., 1981, Monosynaptic muscarinic activation of K conductance underlies the slow inhibitory postsynaptic potential in sympathetic ganglia, *Nature* **292**:625–627.

Horn, J. P., and McAfee, D., 1980, Alpha-adrenergic inhibition of calcium dependent potentials in rat sympathetic neurones, *J. Physiol. (London)* **301**:191–204.

Krnjević, K., 1974, Chemical nature of synaptic transmission in vertebrates, *Physiol. Rev.* **54**:418–540.

Kuffler, S. W., 1980, Slow synaptic responses in autonomic ganglia and the pursuit of a peptidergic transmitter, *J. Exp. Biol.* **89**:257–286.

Le Dourarin, N. M., Xue, Z. G., and Smith, J., 1985, In vivo and in vitro studies on the segregation of autonomic and sensory cell lineages, *J. Physiol. (Paris)* **80**:255–261.

Llinás, R., and Yarom, Y., 1981a, Electrophysiology of mammalian inferior olivary neurones in vitro: Different types of voltage dependent ionic conductance, *J. Physiol. (London)* **315**:549–567.

Llinás, R., and Yarom, Y., 1981b, Properties and distribution of ionic conductances generating electroresponsiveness of mammalian inferior olivary neurones in vitro, *J. Physiol. (London)* **315**:569–584.

McCormick, D. A., and Prince, D., 1986, Acetylcholine induces burst firing in thalamic reticular neurones by activating a potassium conductance, *Nature* **319:**402–405.

Marchetti, C., Carbone, E., and Lux, H. D., 1986, Effects of dopamine and noradrenaline on Ca channels of cultured sensory and sympathetic neurons of chick, *Pfluegers Arch.* **406:**104–111.

Nowycky, M. C., Fox, A. P., and Tsien, R. W., 1985, Three types of neuronal calcium channel with different calcium agonist sensitivity, *Nature* **316:**440–442.

Pellman, T. C., and Carpenter, D. O., 1980, Serotonin induces a voltage sensitive calcium current in neurons of *Aplysia californica*, *J. Neurophysiol.* **44:**423–439.

Pfaffinger, P. J., Martin, J. M., Hunter, D. D., Hathanson, N. M., and Hille, B., 1985, GTP-binding proteins couple cardiac muscarinic receptors to a K channel, *Nature* **317:**536–538.

Rane, S. G., and Dunlap, K., 1986, C-kinase activator 1,2-oleoylacetylglycerol attenuates voltage dependent calcium current in sensory neurons, *Proc. Natl. Acad. Sci. USA* **83:**184–188.

Reuter, H., and Scholz, H., 1977, The regulation of the calcium conductance of cardiac muscle by adrenaline, *J. Physiol. (London)* **264:**49–62.

Sakmann, B., Noma, A., and Trautwein, W., 1983, Acetylcholine activation of single muscarinic K channels in isolated pacemaker cells of mammalian heart, *Nature* **303:**250–253.

Wanke, E., Ferroni, A., Malgaroli, A., Ambrosini, A., Pozzan, T., and Meldolesi, J., 1986, A novel type of inhibition of voltage gated Ca^{2+} channels via muscarinic receptors in mammalian sympathetic neurons, *Proc. Natl. Acad. Sci. USA* **84:**4313–4317.

Yatani, A., Tsuda, Y., Akaike, N., and Brown, A. M., 1982, Nanomolar concentrations of extracellular ATP activate membrane Ca channels in snail neurones, *Nature* **296:**169–171.

18

Postsynaptic Actions of Acetylcholine in the Mammalian Brain in Vitro

David A. McCormick and David A. Prince

1. Introduction

The central cholinergic system appears to be involved in a number of normal and abnormal behaviors including learning and memory (see Squire and Davis, 1981; Salamone, 1986), sleep (see Sakai, 1985), arousal and attentiveness (Singer, 1977; Steriade, 1981), and Alzheimer's disease (Coyle *et al.*, 1983), to name but a few. Acetylcholine (ACh) is a remarkably versatile neurotransmitter/neuromodulator which is localized in as many as 40 nuclei in the CNS (Kimura *et al.*, 1981; Houser *et al.*, 1983; Mesulam *et al.*, 1983a, 1984). Applications of ACh to central neurons can cause not only rapid and/or slow excitation, but also inhibition (see Krnjević, 1975). Furthermore, these actions are dispersed throughout all levels of the neuraxis (e.g., cerebral cortex, thalamus, hypothalamus, brain stem, spinal cord, and PNS) (see Krnjević, 1975).

Until recently, the study of the ionic mechanisms of these various actions of ACh had been restricted largely to the PNS, where adequate *in vitro* experimental procedures could be performed. The advent of the *in vitro* slice technique and its application to wide regions of the brain has allowed detailed studies to also be performed in the CNS including in the hippocampus (Dodd *et al.*, 1981; Benardo and Prince, 1982a,b; Cole and Nicoll, 1984), and more recently in the cerebral cortex (Constanti and Galvan, 1983; McCormick and Prince, 1985, 1986b), thalamus (McCormick and Prince, 1986a,d, 1987), caudate (Misgeld *et al.*, 1980; Dodt and Misgeld, 1986), hypothalamus (Cobbett *et al.*, 1985), and brain stem (Egan and North, 1985, 1986). These studies have yielded a wealth of information which indicates that every well-documented action of ACh in the PNS is also present in some CNS region (for review see North, 1986). To date, the known postsynaptic actions of ACh in the CNS are sixfold: (1) rapid excitation through an increase in cation conductance mediated through nicotinic receptors; (2) excitation through an increase in membrane cation conductance mediated through muscarinic receptors; (3) slow excitation due to decreases in potassium conductance; (4) block of a particular type of calcium-activated

David A. McCormick and David A. Prince • Department of Neurology, Stanford University School of Medicine, Stanford, California 94305 *Present Address for D. A. McCormick:* Section of Neuroanatomy, Yale University, School of Medicine, New Haven, Connecticut 06510.

potassium conductance; (5) direct inhibition due to an increase in potassium conductance; and (6) decrease in Ca currents.

The different actions of ACh are not only distributed nonhomogeneously in the CNS, but are mediated by at least three (nicotinic and two types of muscarinic), but perhaps as many as six, differing types of cholinergic receptors (Hammer *et al.*, 1980; Birdsall *et al.*, 1984). Furthermore, within a particular region of the CNS (e.g., cerebral cortex) the actions of ACh can differ markedly, depending upon the type of neuron in question (e.g., pyramidal neurons versus GABAergic interneurons).

The regions of the forebrain in which the actions of ACh have been most well studied are the cerebral cortex/hippocampus and the lateral geniculate and reticular nuclei of the thalamus (Krnjević, 1975; Ben-Ari *et al.*, 1976; Dingledine and Kelly, 1977; Woody *et al.*, 1978; Dodd *et al.*, 1981; Cole and Nicoll, 1984; McCormick and Prince, 1985, 1986a,b,d, 1987). We will begin by reviewing the available data on the actions of ACh in the cortical regions and follow this with a discussion of ACh effects in the subcortical areas.

2. Cerebral Cortex

The cerebral cortex is densely innervated by cholinergic axons and terminals which arise from both cells intrinsic to the cerebral cortex and cells located in the basal forebrain (Fibiger, 1982; Mesulam *et al.*, 1983a,b, 1984; Levey *et al.*, 1984; Rye *et al.*, 1984; Saper, 1984). Electron microscopy coupled with immunohistochemical staining of choline acetyltransferase (ChAT) indicates that cholinergic terminals form synaptic contacts with medium- to small-sized dendrites of presumed pyramidal cells and perhaps of cortical interneurons (Wainer *et al.*, 1984; Houser *et al.*, 1985).

Applications of ACh to cortical cells *in vivo* result in both inhibition and slow excitation. Krnjević *et al.* (1971) proposed that the slow excitatory response to ACh was due to the suppression of potassium conductances. Indeed, in the PNS and in the hippocampus, the ACh-induced slow excitation has been found to result from suppression of perhaps three distinct types of potassium currents: (1) a voltage-independent K^+ current (Benardo and Prince, 1982a,b; Morita *et al.*, 1982; Madison *et al.*, 1987), (2) a voltage-sensitive K^+ current, the M current (I_m) (so called because of its sensitivity to muscarine) (Adams and Brown, 1982; Benardo and Prince, 1982a,b; Halliwell and Adams, 1982), and (3) one type of calcium-activated K^+ current—I_{ahp} (Benardo and Prince, 1982; Cole and Nicoll, 1984; Pennefather *et al.*, 1985). Cholinergic inhibition, on the other hand, results both from the excitation of neighboring inhibitory interneurons (Benardo and Prince, 1982a,b; Haas, 1982) as well as from a direct action causing an increase in potassium conductance (Hartzell *et al.*, 1977; Dodd and Horn, 1983).

In the *in vitro* cortical slice, when cortical pyramidal neurons are depolarized to near firing threshold, applications of ACh result in inhibition followed by slow excitation (McCormick and Prince, 1985, 1986b) (Fig. 1B), identical to that reported *in vivo* (Krnjević *et al.*, 1971; Woody *et al.*, 1978). The inhibition both *in vivo* and *in vitro*, is especially prominent in the superficial layers (II–III), while the slow excitation is more prominent in the deeper layers (V–VI). The phenomenological similarities between the responses of cortical neurons in the *in vitro* slice and those found *in vivo* justify the supposition that such *in vitro* experiments will further our understanding of the actions of ACh in the intact animal.

One of the first questions to be addressed in studies of putative neurotransmitter actions is whether the observed effects (in this case ACh-induced inhibition and slow excitation) result from the interaction of the agent in question with receptors directly on the cell studied or indirectly through the stimulated release of other neurotransmitters. When synaptic transmission is blocked with tetrodotoxin, or by substitution of a Ca^{2+} channel blocker (e.g., Mn^{2+}, Co^{2+}, Cd^{2+}) for Ca^{2+} in the bathing medium, the ACh-induced inhibition of pyramidal neurons of the cerebral

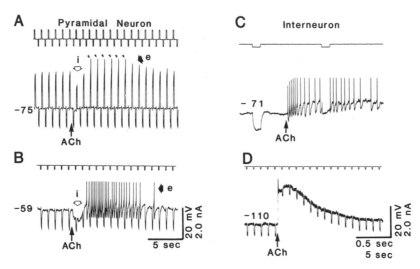

Figure 1. The effects of ACh on physiologically identified cortical pyramidal neurons and interneurons. (A) Applications of ACh to a pyramidal cell at resting membrane potential (V_m −75 mV) initially caused a decrease in the response to the current pulses (i) followed by a selective potentiation of the depolarizing responses without affecting V_m or the response to the hyperpolarizing pulses (e). The potentiated depolarizing pulses reached firing threshold and evoked action potentials (downward arrowheads). (B) Application of ACh to the neuron from A after depolarization to near firing threshold (−59 mV) caused inhibition at a short latency (i) and was followed by a slow depolarization and action potential generation (e). (C) Application of ACh to a typical interneuron at resting V_m (−71 mV) caused robust excitation at short latency. (D) Application of ACh to the interneuron from C after hyperpolarization to −110 mV evoked a large depolarization with short-onset latency. Comparison of responses to hyperpolarizing pulses during ACh-induced depolarization with responses during equivalent direct depolarizations showed that ACh elicited a substantial decrease in input resistance (not shown). The top trace in each set is the current monitor. Action potential amplitudes are truncated. (From McCormick and Prince, 1985.)

cortex and hippocampus is blocked, whereas the slow excitation persists. Thus, the inhibition of pyramidal neurons is indirect (i.e., due to the ACh-induced release of another neurotransmitter) and the slow excitation is direct (Benardo and Prince, 1982a,b; McCormick and Prince, 1985, 1986b). Further pharmacological and electrophysiological analysis indicates that ACh-induced inhibition in the cerebral cortex is due to the relatively rapid excitation of GABAergic interneurons (Fig. 1C,D) (McCormick and Prince, 1985, 1986b). This excitation of GABAergic interneurons is associated with an increase in membrane conductance, and since it is strongly depolarizing in nature, probably represents an increase in membrane conductance to one or more cations (e.g., Na+, Ca2+, K+) (McCormick and Prince, 1985, 1986b).

The possibility that the slow cholinergic excitatory response of cortical pyramidal neurons results from the suppression of voltage-dependent currents has been tested by applying depolarizing and hyperpolarizing current pulses into the neurons before and during exposure to ACh (Fig. 1A). Under these circumstances, ACh selectively enhances the depolarizing current pulses so that a previously subthreshold depolarizing input can become suprathreshold and generate action potentials (Fig. 1A). The resting membrane potential (if it is below approximately −65 mV) and the response to a hyperpolarizing input remain relatively unchanged (Fig. 1A). This type of voltage-dependent action suggests that ACh may be suppressing the M current (I_m) in cortical pyramidal cells. Indeed, a current suppressed by ACh with kinetics very similar to I_m can be recorded in cortical pyramidal cells using single-electrode voltage-clamp techniques in the sensorimotor cortex (Fig. 2; McCormick and Prince, unpublished observations), olfactory cortex (Constanti and Galvan, 1983), hippocampus (Halliwell and Adams, 1982), and in human cortical tissue (Halliwell, 1986).

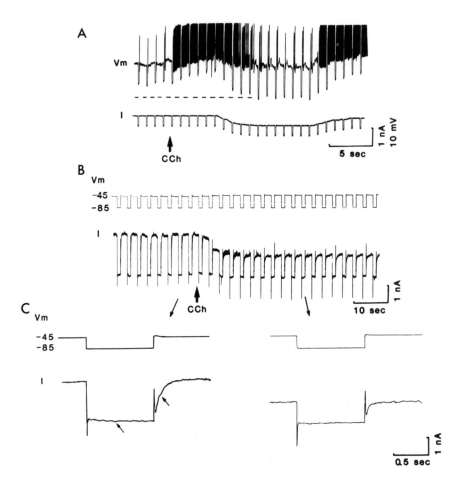

Figure 2. ACh depresses a voltage-dependent current in cortical pyramidal neurons. (A) Application of the cho-linergic agonist, carbachol (CCh) to this cortical pyramidal cell manually depolarized to near firing threshold results in a slow excitatory response. Reducing the membrane potential back to pre-carbachol baseline reveals the response to be associated with a large decrease in membrane conductance. (B) Application of carbachol to the neuron of A while performing voltage clamp causes a large reduction in the amount of current needed to hold the cell at −45 mV, with a much smaller change in current needed to hold the cell at −85 mV. (C) Traces in B expanded for detail. Carbachol suppresses a slow voltage-dependent current which slowly inactivates when the cell is hyperpolarized (first arrow, left) and activates when the cell is depolarized (second arrow, left). This current appears identical to the M current (Adams and Brown, 1982; Halliwell and Adams, 1982).

Another class of potassium currents, called calcium-activated potassium currents, are sen-sitive to a rise in the intracellular concentration of free Ca^{2+} (Meech, 1978; Schwartz and Passow, 1983). Such potassium currents produce an accommodation of spike firing rate during depolarization and a hyperpolarization which follows the train of action potentials (the slow afterhyperpolarization, or ahp). ACh is a potent blocker of one type of calcium-activated po-tassium conductance in both the hippocampus and the cerebral cortex (Benardo and Prince, 1982a,b; Cole and Nicoll, 1984; Pennefather *et al.*, 1985; McCormick and Prince, 1986b). This action together with blockade of I_m greatly enhances the number of action potentials generated by a prolonged depolarizing input (Brown, 1983; Madison and Nicoll, 1984; McCormick and Prince, 1986b).

In addition to the suppression of the M current and the calcium-activated potassium current,

ACh can also suppress a non-voltage-dependent potassium conductance (Benardo and Prince, 1982a,b; Morita et al., 1982; Madison et al., 1987). This effect is particularly prominent in the guinea pig and rat hippocampus (Benardo and Prince, 1982a,b; Madison et al., 1986), and may also occur in cat sensorimotor cortex (Krnjević et al., 1971). Our data indicate that in the guinea pig cingulate cortex, such an effect is small, if present at all (McCormick and Prince, 1986b).

2.1. Cortical ACh Pharmacology

In the past few years a number of pharmacological binding studies have indicated that there are at least two subtypes of muscarinic receptors (termed M_1 and M_2) in the CNS (Hammer et al., 1980). These two subtypes of muscarinic receptors may differ because of differences in their primary amino acid sequence or because the same receptor molecule is placed into different local environments or because it is coupled to different biochemical/electrophysiological effector mechanisms (Birdsall et al., 1984). The best chemical compound presently available for distinguishing between M_1 and M_2 subtypes of muscarinic receptors is the selective antagonist pirenzepine (Hammer et al., 1980). Muscarinic receptors which have a relatively high affinity for pirenzepine are termed M_1, while those which do not are termed M_2. In the PNS, the ACh-induced slow depolarization of ganglion cells is mediated by M_1 receptors. Cholinergic inhibition of these neurons (Ashe and Yarosh, 1984; Newberry et al., 1985) and of cardiac muscle cells (Chassaing et al., 1984) is mediated by M_2 receptors. In both cases the inhibition is produced by an increase in membrane potassium conductance.

In the cerebral cortex, the ACh-induced slow depolarization is selectively blocked by low concentrations of pirenzepine, indicating that this response is mediated by M_1 receptors (Fig. 3) (McCormick and Prince, 1985). The ACh-induced excitation of GABAergic interneurons is blocked only by higher doses of pirenzepine, suggesting that it may be mediated by M_2 receptors (Fig. 3) (McCormick and Prince, 1985).

Egan and North (1985) have also recently reported that ACh can cause a muscarinic excitation in the locus coeruleus associated with an increase in membrane cation conductance and mediated by the M_2 receptors. There is also some preliminary evidence that the muscarinic receptors mediating the slow depolarization in hippocampal pyramidal cells are of the M_1 subtype

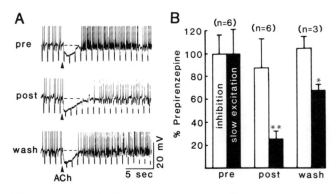

Figure 3. Effect of pirenzepine on the inhibitory and slow excitatory responses to ACh. (A) Application of ACh (upward arrowhead) to this neuron at V_m just above firing threshold evokes the typical inhibitory slow excitatory response (pre). After approximately 1 hr of exposure to pirenzepine, ACh application to the same neuron causes the inhibitory response only (post). Washing out of the pirenzepine for approximately 1 hr partially reinstates the slow excitatory response (wash). (B) Average data for six neurons showing that pirenzepine causes a significant (**, $p < 0.001$) depression of the slow excitatory response without affecting the amplitude of the inhibitory response. Washing out of the pirenzepine caused a significant (*, $p < 0.05$) increase in the slow excitatory response (wash). (From McCormick and Prince, 1985.)

whereas those controlling the suppression of I_{ahp} are of the M_2 subtype (Muller and Misgeld, 1986).

2.2. Endogenous Cortical ACh Responses

One major problem with the present techniques for studying putative neurotransmitter action is that iontophoretic or puffer applications of a neurochemical will activate synaptic as well as extrasynaptic receptors. It is possible therefore that responses evoked by exogenous application of a neurotransmitter may not be activated by the endogenous neurotransmitter system.

Slow cholinergic excitation due to the endogenous release of ACh evoked by electrical stimulation of neural tissue has been shown not only *in vivo* (Krnjević and Ropert, 1981) but also in the *in vitro* hippocampal slice (Cole and Nicoll, 1984) and in cocultures of septal neurons and hippocampal cells (Gahwiler and Brown, 1985). Voltage-clamp analysis in the *in vitro* systems indicates that the slow cholinergic EPSP is due to suppression of a non-voltage-dependent potassium current (Madison *et al.*, 1987) as well as I_m and I_{ahp} (Gahwiler and Brown, 1985; Brown *et al.*, 1986).

An endogenous ACh excitation of cortical GABAergic interneurons has yet to be shown. However, these neurons do appear to receive a cholinergic input (Houser *et al.*, 1985). Furthermore, focal stimulation of cortex elicits inhibition of neighboring pyramidal neurons which can be blocked by atropine, indicating that the inhibition may be due to the release of ACh (Phillis and York, 1968; Jordan and Phillis, 1972).

3. Thalamus

The mammalian thalamus, like the cortex, is the recipient of a substantial innervation of cholinergic axons and terminals which originate from neurons in the brain stem (pedunculopontine and lateral dorsal tegmental nuclei) and possibly from the basal forebrain (Fibiger, 1982; Houser *et al.*, 1983; Mesulam *et al.*, 1983a,b; Woolf and Butcher, 1986). These terminals form classical synaptic contacts both with the dendrites of thalamic relay neurons, presumed GABAergic interneurons, and with the neurons in the GABAergic structure, the nucleus reticularis (Houser *et al.*, 1980; Dolabella de Lima *et al.*, 1985). This ascending cholinergic projection has been implicated in the control of sleep–wake cycles, the maintenance of vigilance, and the gating of information flow through the relay nuclei (see Steriade and Deschenes, 1984). For example, stimulation of some regions of the brain stem gives rise to a facilitatory influence on the transmission of impulses from the optic nerve through the dorsal lateral geniculate to the primary visual cortex (Steriade, 1970; Foote *et al.*, 1974; Francesconi *et al.*, 1984). This facilitation is mimicked in the animal by local iontophoretic application of ACh to neurons of the LGNd and can be blocked by the iontophoretic application of atropine, a potent muscarinic receptor blocker (Francesconi *et al.*, 1984). However, the situation is somewhat more complicated than this since applications of ACh in some of the thalamic nuclei cause inhibition as well as slow excitation, while in others only inhibition is found (Tebecis, 1972; Duggan and Hall, 1975; Ben-Ari *et al.*, 1976; Dingledine and Kelly, 1977). We have recently investigated the mechanisms of ACh action in the nucleus reticularis, the LGNd, and the medial geniculate nuclei of guinea pig and rat using *in vitro* thalamic slices (McCormick and Prince, 1986a,b).

3.1. Nucleus Reticularis

The nucleus reticularis (nRt) is both anatomically and physiologically a very unique thalamic structure. It forms a thin shell over much of the dorsal lateral border of the thalamus and numerous thalamocortical and corticothalamic fibers course through it, giving off excitatory collaterals as they do so (see Steriade and Deschenes, 1984; Kayama, 1985). The axons of the neurons in the nRt project back into the thalamus and synapse on both relay cells and presumed inhibitory interneurons (Steriade et al., 1984). The apparent GABAergic nature of every neuron contained in the nRt (Houser et al., 1980) indicates that this nucleus may function as a feedforward (in the case of a corticothalamic input) as well as a feedback (in the case of a thalamocortical input) inhibitory influence. Indeed, electrical or chemical stimulation of the nRt results in inhibition of neurons in the principal relay nuclei (Mushiake et al., 1984; Kayama, 1985). This inhibition is reduced by iontophoretic application of bicuculline, a GABAergic antagonist (Kayama, 1985).

Functionally, the nRt has been implicated in the synchronization of spindle waves during sleep (Steriade et al., 1985) and possibly in the selective gating of information flow through the thalamus (Crick, 1984). The presence of an ascending cholinergic projection to this nucleus implies that ACh may also have an important modulatory role in regulating these activities. In vivo, iontophoretic applications of ACh to nRt neurons inhibit single spike activity and at the same time increase the occurrence of burst discharges (Ben-Ari et al., 1976; Dingledine and Kelly, 1977). Stimulation of some regions of the brain stem evokes a similar response which can be blocked in some cases by the iontophoretic application of atropine (Dingledine and Kelly, 1977) indicating that it may be mediated by the endogenous ACh projection from the brain stem to the thalamus.

In contrast to the indirect muscarinic inhibition of cortical pyramidal cells, ACh elicits a slow hyperpolarization in nRt neurons which is direct (i.e., not abolished by block of synaptic transmission) (Fig. 4A). This hyperpolarization is associated with an increase in membrane conductance and can be reversed to a slow depolarization if the neuron is hyperpolarized past E_k (Fig. 4A). The reversal potential of the ACh-induced hyperpolarization of nRt neurons obeys the Nernst function for $[K]_o$ (Fig. 4B). Filling the cells with Cl^- does not affect this response (McCormick and Prince, 1986a). These results indicate that the ACh-induced inhibition in nRt cells is caused by an increase in membrane conductance to K ions (McCormick and Prince, 1986a).

Thalamic neurons contain a specialized intrinsic current which allows them to generate a burst of action potentials when they are transiently depolarized from a hyperpolarized membrane potential (i.e., negative to −65 mV) (Jahnsen and Llinas, 1984a,b). This current is known as the

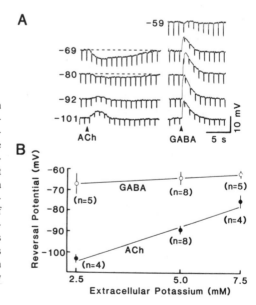

Figure 4. ACh activates a potassium conductance in nucleus reticularis neurons of the thalamus. (A) Application of ACh to this neuron causes a slow hyperpolarization and increase in membrane conductance (−69 mV). Applications at different membrane potentials reveal this response to reverse to a depolarization at approximately −90 mV. Application of GABA causes a depolarization which, in contrast, reverses at approximately −59 mV. (B) Changing the concentration of extracellular potassium $[K]_0$ causes the reversal potential of the ACh-induced hyperpolarization to change as predicted by the Nernst equation. In contrast, responses to GABA changed by only 11 mV per tenfold change in $[K]_0$, indicating that they are not primarily mediated by K^+ ions.

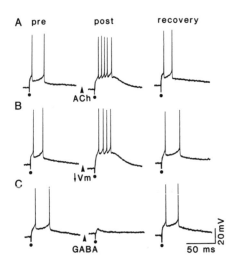

Figure 5. Effect of ACh, GABA, and change in membrane potential on the response of a nucleus reticularis neuron to orthodromic synaptic inputs. (A) Application of ACh between pre and post examples (arrowhead) caused a membrane hyperpolarization and changes the response of the neuron to the synaptic stimulus (dot) from two action potentials (pre) to a burst of five (post). After approximately 15 sec, the response of the neuron returns to normal (recovery). (B) Hyperpolarizing the membrane potential through intracellular injection of current alone has a similar effect on the response of the neuron to the synaptic stimulus. (C) In contrast, application of GABA, which presumably causes an increase in Cl⁻ conductance, depolarizes the membrane potential and inhibits all spike activity. (From McCormick and Prince, 1986a.)

low-threshold calcium current or as the transient calcium current (t-current) (Nowycky *et al.*, 1985). It is completely inactivated at membrane potentials positive to approximately -60 mV and this inactivation is progressively removed by hyperpolarization (i.e., deinactivation) (Jahnsen and Llinas, 1984a,b). Thus, the pattern of spike discharge generated by an excitatory input depends critically upon the membrane potential of the neuron. At relatively depolarized membrane potentials (e.g., -50 mV) the low-threshold calcium current is completely inactivated and a synaptic input or depolarizing current pulse gives rise to single, regularly spaced action potentials only (Fig. 5). On the other hand, if the cell is relatively hyperpolarized (e.g., -70 mV), the low-threshold calcium current will not be completely inactivated and the same synaptic input will evoke a Ca^{2+}-mediated slow spike which elicits a burst of two to eight spikes (Fig. 5B). Thalamic neurons tend to be largely in the burst mode of operation during certain stages of sleep (e.g., slow-wave sleep), and in the single spike firing mode during awake, alert states (Hirsch *et al.*, 1983; McCarley *et al.*, 1983; Steriade and Deschenes, 1984). During periods of sleep in which the thalamic neurons are in the burst-type mode and generating spindling waves, the relaying of information to the cerebral cortex is greatly degraded by the "scrambling" effects of the spontaneous burst discharges in these cells (Livingstone and Hubel, 1981). In contrast, the transfer of information is greatly enhanced when the thalamic neurons move into the single spike mode (Livingstone and Hubel, 1981).

By activating a potassium conductance, ACh can bring the membrane potential within the burst firing range (i.e., below -65 mV). Thus, applications of ACh to nRt neurons whose membrane potential is tonically depolarized into the single spike firing range will hyperpolarize the cells and promote the occurrence of burst discharges (Fig. 5A). This effect of ACh appears to result merely from its effects on the membrane potential and not from changes in the voltage activation/inactivation characteristics of the low-threshold Ca^{2+} current, since the increase in burst probability can be replicated merely by hyperpolarizing the cell to a similar extent after the ACh response is over (Fig. 5B). In contrast, GABA application, which causes a large increase in membrane Cl⁻ conductance in nRt neurons, elicits only inhibition of both single spike and burst firing activities (Fig. 5C).

3.2. Pharmacology of Cholinergic Inhibitory Responses in Thalamic Neurons

The ACh-induced increase in potassium conductance in the nRt is readily blocked with applications of scopolamine (McCormick and Prince, 1986a,c), indicating that it is mediated by muscarinic receptors. The inability of pirenzepine to completely block this response even at high doses indicates that it may be mediated by M_2 receptors (McCormick and Prince, 1986a,c).

ACh also causes an increase in membrane potassium conductance in neurons of the parabrachial nucleus of the brainstem (Egan and North, 1986) and in some parts of the peripheral nervous system (see North, 1986). In all regions so far studied, these responses are mediated by M_2 receptors (see North, 1986).

3.3. Medial and Lateral Geniculate Nuclei

Iontophoretic applications of ACh to presumed relay neurons of the cat LGNd result in excitation which is associated with an increase in cellular responsiveness to other excitatory, as well as inhibitory, inputs (Phillis *et al.*, 1967; Krnjević, 1975; Sillito *et al.*, 1983; Francesconi *et al.*, 1984; Eysel *et al.*, 1986); inhibitory ACh responses are only rarely observed (Phillis *et al.* 1967). In contrast, application of ACh to neurons in the cat MGN causes inhibition about as often as slow excitation and can even occasionally cause both responses in the same neuron (Tebecis, 1972). Analysis of the projection targets of the MGN neurons indicated that those which project to the cerebral cortex are excited by ACh, while those that do not are inhibited (Tebecis, 1972).

To our surprise, application of ACh to neurons in the guinea pig LGNd and MGN resulted in every case in a robust hyperpolarization identical to that found in nRt neurons. This hyperpolarization was followed by a slow depolarization in approximately 25–50% of the cells. Subsequent analysis of the ionic mechanisms underlying the hyperpolarizing ACh response indicated that it was due to activation of a potassium conductance. As in the nRt, this hyperpolarization could inhibit single spike activity and promote the occurrence of burst discharges.

The slow depolarizing response which followed the inhibition was associated with a substantial increase in membrane resistance which was linear (i.e., not effected by changes in membrane potential), indicating that is is probably due to the closing of some type of non-voltage-dependent ionic channel (perhaps potassium channels). This result contrasts with the pronounced voltage dependency of the resistance increases during the ACh-induced slow depolarizations in cortical neurons (Benardo and Prince, 1982a,b; McCormick and Prince, 1986b). The slow depolarizing ACh responses in geniculate neurons inhibited burst discharges, promoted single spike firing, and in general increased the neuronal responsiveness to excitatory inputs, as in the cerebral cortex.

The finding that ACh can cause *both* inhibition and slow excitation in the guinea pig LGN and MGN is difficult to reconcile with observations in the cat LGNd where ACh usually evokes only excitation (Phillis *et al.*, 1967; Eysel *et al.*, 1986). A likely explanation for this discrepancy is that species differences exist. Recent experiments in the rat LGNd show that application of ACh typically causes only slow excitation; inhibition is either completely absent or only very weak (McCormick and Prince, 1986d). These data indicate that there are indeed significant species differences in the types of response of LGNd neurons to ACh. The slow depolarizing response appears to be common to all species so far tested (cat, rat, guinea pig), while the inhibitory responses in LGNd are peculiar to the guinea pig.

Our data from thalamic neurons indicate that ACh can cause both direct inhibition by activation of a potassium conductance, and slow excitation through a linear decrease in membrane conductance. The latter process may be similar to the one seen in the hippocampus (Benardo and Prince, 1982a,b; Madison *et al.*, 1987). Since cholinergic terminals are found on relay neurons, inhibitory interneurons, and nRt neurons, ACh can have diverse and potent modulatory influences on the processing of information in the thalamus.

3.4. Endogenous Thalamic ACh Responses

Ever since Moruzzi and Magoun's (1949) report on the role of the brain stem in the maintenance of arousal, the investigation of ascending "alerting" systems has been a popular one for both anatomists and physiologists. In the cat, rat, and monkey, the ascending cholinergic projections from the brain stem to the thalamus have traditionally been thought to have a facilitating influence on the flow of information through the relay nuclei (see Steriade, 1970; Steriade and Deschenes, 1984). The evidence in favor of such a role rests in part on the result of brain stimulation studies. Electrical or chemical stimulation of some regions of the brain stem greatly facilitates the flow of neuronal activity through the thalamic relay nuclei (Foote et al., 1974; Francesconi et al., 1984). In some cases, this increase in excitability is blocked by application of atropine (Francesconi et al., 1984), indicating a possible role for ACh. In other cases, the response is clearly mediated by the release of norepinephrine (Rogawski and Aghajanian, 1980). Our results show how ACh actions increase the excitability of thalamic relay neurons. Release of ACh onto LGNd relay neurons will result in a direct increase in input resistance and a resultant slow depolarization. Both of these effects increase the likelihood that other, more phasic, EPSPs will reach threshold for action potential generation and therefore ACh will facilitate single spike firing and transfer of information. In contrast, the purely inhibitory action of ACh on the GABAergic nucleus, the nRt, may produce disinhibition of relay neurons to which the nRt projects (Kayama, 1985). The actions of ACh on intrinsic interneurons in the LGNd are at present unknown.

4. Medial Habenula

The medial habenula (MHb) is a collection of closely packed cells on the dorsal medial aspect of the thalamus at the floor of the third ventricle. This structure receives its major input via the stria medularis from the postcommissural septum (Herkenham and Nauta, 1977; Gottesfeld and Jacobowitz, 1979; Contestabile and Fonnum, 1983) and gives rise to a large axonal projection through the fasciculus retroflexus to the interpeduncular nucleus at the base of the brain (Herkenham and Nauta, 1979). Both the afferents and the efferents of the MHb may be cholinergic in nature (Kataoka et al., 1973, 1977; Kuhar et al., 1975; Gottesfeld and Jacobowitz, 1979; Contestabile and Fonnum, 1983; Houser et al., 1983; Woolf and Butcher, 1986). Recent immunohistochemical studies for ChAT show that the ventral portions of the MHb nucleus as well as many fibers in the fasciculus retroflexus are heavily reactive (Houser et al., 1983). Lesions of the septal region, stria medularis, medial habenular nucleus, or fasciculus retroflexus reduce ChAT activity in both MHb and interpeduncular nuclei (Katoaka et al., 1973, 1977; Gottesfeld and Jacobowitz, 1979; Contestabile and Fonnum, 1983). These results imply that the MHb nucleus may receive a cholinergic projection from the diagonal band/posterior septal region, while the interpeduncular nucleus may receive a cholinergic input from this region as well as from the MHb.

Autoradiography of putative cholinergic receptors shows that the MHb nucleus contains a high density of nicotinic, but not muscarinic, receptors (Rotter et al., 1979; Clarke et al., 1985). Furthermore, recent autoradiographic labeling of the presumed α subunit of neural nicotinic receptors shows that the MHb contains a high density of this protein (Boulter et al., 1986). These results indicate that cholinergic transmission in the MHb may be largely nicotinic. Given the relative lack of studies on the nicotinic actions of ACh in the CNS, we decided to investigate the possibility that ACh may have an important nicotinic action in the MHb (McCormick and Prince, 1987).

Extracellular single-unit recordings of MHb neurons in the guinea pig in vitro slice indicated that these neurons are spontaneously active, firing with a very regular frequency of about 2–6 Hz. Application of ACh to these cells resulted in rapid excitation followed by a period of inhibition of spike activity (Fig. 6A). The inhibition is not due to depolarization block since second applications of ACh or glutamate during this period result in additional excitatory–inhibitory sequences.

Neither the excitatory nor inhibitory responses of MHb neurons are abolished by blockade of

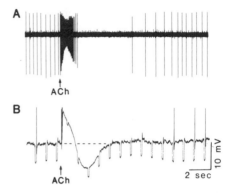

Figure 6. Effect of ACh on neutrons in the medial habenular nucleus. (A) Application of ACh to this MHb neuron recorded extracellularly causes a rapid excitation followed by inhibition. The excitatory response is associated with a transient decrease in spike amplitude. (B) Intracellular recording from another MHb neuron during application of ACh. ACh causes a rapid depolarization followed by a hyperpolarization. Both responses are associated with substantial increases in apparent input conductance.

synaptic transmission, indicating that they are due to direct actions of ACh. Furthermore, pharmacological analysis indicates that both responses are the result of ACh action on nicotinic receptors. Thus, the nicotinic antagonist hexamethonium blocks both responses, while the muscarinic antagonists scopolamine and atropine are completely ineffective. Applications of the muscarinic agonists muscarine and acetyl-β-methacholine evoke very little if any response, while applications of the nicotinic agonists nicotine, cytisine, and 1,1-dimethyl-4-phenylpiperazinium (DMPP) cause robust excitation followed, in the case of DMPP, by prolonged inhibition.

Intracellular recordings have revealed that the rapid excitatory and subsequent inhibitory responses to ACh in the MHb are associated with increases in membrane conductance (Fig. 6B). The reversal potential of the rapid excitatory response (approximately -15 mV) suggests that this response is due to an increase in cation conductance similar to that found in the PNS and muscle (Takeuchi and Takeuchi, 1960; Dennis *et al.*, 1971; Gallagher *et al.*, 1982). The mechanism of the inhibitory response is not known, although it appears to result from an increase in potassium conductance. It may be an indirect response secondary to intense depolarization, since applications of glutamate or direct depolarizations yield almost identical results (i.e., rapid excitation followed by inhibition).

Rapid excitatory responses to ACh due to the activation of nicotinic receptors have been reported in only a few CNS regions, including the interpeduncular nucleus (Brown *et al.*, 1983; Takagi, 1984) and spinal cord (Curtis and Ryall, 1966), and perhaps some regions of the brain stem (Bradley and Dray, 1972), hypothalamus (Cobbett *et al.*, 1986), and caudate (Misgeld *et al.*, 1980). In contrast, autoradiography of putative nicotinic receptors has revealed that they have a widespread distribution in the CNS (Clarke *et al.*, 1985). One possible explanation for this discrepancy may be that many of the putative nicotinic receptors are presynaptic. Indeed, there is evidence for presynaptic nicotinic receptors in the interpeduncular nucleus (Brown *et al.*, 1984) and presynaptic nicotinic–muscarinic receptors in the hippocampus (Rovira *et al.*, 1983).

5. ACh-Induced Decrease in Ca^{2+} Conductance

An ACh-induced decrease in calcium conductance was originally reported in heart cells (Giles and Noble, 1976), and later confirmed in rat sympathetic ganglion cells (Kuba and Koketsu, 1976; North and Tokimasa, 1983; Belluzzi *et al.*, 1985) and locus coeruleus neurons (North, 1986). However, the main difficulty in studying this action of ACh is that there is often a concomitant increase in potassium conductance which may by itself cause a comparable apparent decrease in Ca^{2+} currents. In two studies this problem has apparently been successfully circumvented (Giles and Noble, 1976; Iijima *et al.*, 1985). Iijima *et al.* (1985) obtained whole-cell recordings from dissociated guinea pig atrial cells and used intracellular cesium to block K^+

channels. Under these conditions, ACh could still reduce Ca^{2+} currents, although this reduction was much less than that seen when potassium conductances were not blocked. As noted by these authors, however, the reduction in ACh effects on Ca^{2+} currents could have been due to alterations in an intracellular intermediary caused by establishing a whole-cell recording.

In the CNS, the physiological significance of the ACh-induced decrease in Ca^{2+} currents is not yet known, although this effect may be one mechanism by which ACh causes presynaptic inhibition of transmitter release. The latter effect occurs in a number of CNS regions during interaction with different types of neurotransmitter systems (Yamamoto and Kawai, 1967; Hounsgaard, 1978; Kilbinger, 1984).

6. Conclusion

ACh is a versatile neurotransmitter which is now known to cause six different postsynaptic responses in the CNS: (1) suppression of the voltage-dependent potassium current known as the M current; (2) suppression of at least one type of calcium-activated potassium current; (3) excitation due to an increase in membrane cation conductance, mediated by muscarinic receptors; (4) rapid excitation through an increase in cation conductance, mediated by nicotinic receptors; (5) direct inhibition due to an increase in potassium conductance; and (6) suppression of calcium currents. These different responses to ACh are operational in different types of neurons both within a single region and within different regions of the CNS. Most of the actions (e.g., activation and inactivation of potassium currents, decreases in Ca^{2+} currents) are especially powerful mechanisms by which ACh can modulate the central processing of information.

References

Adams, P. R., and Brown, D. A. 1982, Synaptic inhibition of the M-current: Slow excitatory post-synaptic potential mechanism in bullfrog sympathetic neurones, *J. Physiol. (London)* **332**:263–272.

Ashe, J. H., and Yarosh, C. A., 1984, Differential and selective antagonism of the slow-inhibitory postsynaptic potential and slow-excitatory potential by gallamine and pirenzepine in the superior cervical ganglion of the rabbit, *Neuropharmacology* **23**:1321–1329.

Belluzzi, O., Sacchi, O., and Wanke, E., 1985, Identification of delayed potassium and calcium currents in the rat sympathetic neurone under voltage clamp, *J. Physiol. (London)* **358**:109–129.

Benardo, L. S., and Prince, D. A., 1982a, Cholinergic excitation of hippocampal pyramidal cells, *Brain Res.* **249**:315–333.

Benardo, L. S., and Prince, D. A., 1982b, Ionic mechanisms of cholinergic excitation of mammalian hippocampal pyramidal cells, *Brain Res.* **249**:333–344.

Ben-Ari, Y., Dingledine, R., Kanazawa, I., and Kelly, J. S., 1976, Inhibitory control of acetylcholine on neurones in the feline nucleus reticularis thalami, *J. Physiol. (London)* **261**:647–671.

Birdsall, N. J. M., Hulme, E. C., and Stockton, J. M., 1984, Muscarinic receptor heterogeneity, *Trends Pharmacol. Sci. Suppl.* pp. 4–8.

Boulter, J., Evans, K., Goldman, D., Martin, G., Treco, D., Heinemann, S., and Patrick, J., 1986, Isolation of cDNA clone coding for a possible neural nicotinic acetylcholine receptor alpha-subunit, *Nature* **319**:368–374.

Bradley, P. B., and Dray, A., 1972, Short latency excitation of brain stem neurones in the rat by acetylcholine, *Br. J. Pharmacol.* **45**:100–113.

Brown, D. A., 1983, Slow cholinergic excitation—A mechanism for increasing neuronal excitability, *Trends Neurosci.* **6**:302–307.

Brown, D. A., Docherty, R. J., and Halliwell, J. V., 1983, Chemical transmission in the rat interpeduncular nucleus *in vitro*, *J. Physiol. (London)* **341**:655–670.

Brown, D. A., Docherty, R. J., and Halliwell, J. V., 1984, The actions of cholinomimetic substances on impulse conduction in the habenulointerpeduncular pathway of the rat *in vitro*, *J. Physiol. (London)* **353**:101–109.

Brown, D. A., Gahwiler, B. H., Marsh, S. J., and Selyanko, A. A., 1986, Mechanisms of muscarinic excitatory synaptic transmission in ganglia and brain, *Trends Pharmacol. Sci. Suppl.* pp. 66–71.

Chassaing, C., Dureng, G., Baisset, J., and Buchene-Marullaz, P., 1984, Pharmacological evidence for cardiac muscarinic subtypes, *Life Sci.* **35:**1739–1745.

Clarke, P. B. S., Schwartz, R. D., Paul, S. M., Pert, C. B., and Pert, A., 1985, Nicotine binding in rat brain: Autoradiographic comparison of [^{3}H] acetylcholine, [^{3}H] nicotine, and [^{125}I]-alpha-bungarotoxin, *J. Neurosci.* **5:**1307–1315.

Cobbett, P., Mason, W. T., and Poulain, D. A., 1986, Intracellular analysis of control of rat supraoptic neurone (SON) activity *in vitro* by acetylcholine (ACh), *J. Physiol. (London)* **371:**216P.

Cole, A. E., and Nicoll, R. A., 1984, Characterization of a slow cholinergic post-synaptic potential recorded in vitro from rat hippocampal pyramidal cells, *J. Physiol. (London)* **352:**173–188.

Constanti, A., and Galvan, M., 1983, M-current in voltage-clamped olfactory cortex neurones, *Neurosci. Lett.* **38:**65–70.

Contestabile, A., and Fonnum, F., 1983, Cholinergic and GABAergic forebrain projections to the habenula and nucleus interpeduncularis: Surgical and kainic acid lesions, *Brain Res.* **275:**287–297.

Coyle, J. T., Price, D. L., and DeLong, M. R., 1983, Alzheimer's disease: A disorder of cortical cholinergic innervation, *Science* **219:**1184–1190.

Crick, F., 1984, Function of the thalamic reticular complex: The searchlight hypothesis, *Proc. Natl. Acad. Sci. USA* **81:**4586–4590.

Curtis, D. R., and Ryall, R. W., 1966, The excitation of Renshaw cells by cholinomimetics, *Exp. Brain Res.* **2:**49–65.

Dennis, M. J., Harris, A. J., and Kuffler, S. W., 1971, Synaptic transmission and its duplication by focally applied acetylcholine in parasympathetic neurons in the heart of the frog, *Proc. R. Soc. London Ser. B* **177:**509–539.

Dingledine, R., and Kelly, J. S., 1977, Brain stem stimulation and the acetylcholine-evoked inhibition of neurones in the feline nucleus reticularis thalami, *J. Physiol. (London)* **271:**135–154.

Dodd, J., and Horn, J. P., 1983, Muscarinic inhibition of sympathetic c neurones in the bullfrog, *J. Physiol. (London)* **334:**271–291.

Dodd, J., Dingledine, R., and Kelly, J. S., 1981, The excitatory actions of acetylcholine on hippocampal neurons of guinea pig and rat maintained in vitro, *Brain Res.* **207:**109–127.

Dodt, H. U., and Misgeld, U., 1986, Muscarinic slow excitation and muscarinic inhibition of synaptic transmission in the rat neostriatum, *J. Physiol. (London)* **380:**593–608.

Dolabela de Lima, A., Montero, V. M., and Singer, W., 1985, The cholinergic innervation of the visual thalamus: An EM immunocytochemical study, *Exp. Brain Res.* **59:**206–212.

Duggan, A. W., and Hall, J. G., 1975, Inhibition of thalamic neurons by acetylcholine, *Brain Res.* **100:**445–449.

Egan, T. M., and North, R. A., 1985, Acetylcholine acts on m2-muscarinic receptors to excite locus coeruleus neurones, *Br. J. Pharmacol.* **85:**733–735.

Egan, T. M., and North, R. A., 1986, Acetylcholine hyperpolarizes central neurones by acting on an M2 muscarinic receptor, *Nature* **319:**405–407.

Eysel, U. T., Pape, H. C., and Van Schayck, R., 1986, Excitatory and differential disinhibitory actions of acetylcholine in the lateral geniculate nucleus of cat, *J. Physiol. (London)* **370:**233–254.

Fibiger, H. C., 1982, The organization and some projections of cholinergic neurons of the mammalian forebrain, *Brain Res. Rev.* **4:**327–388.

Foote, W. E., Maciewicz, R. J., and Morden, J. P., 1974, Effect of midbrain raphe and lateral mesencephalic stimulation on spontaneous and evoked activity in the lateral geniculate of the cat, *Exp. Brain Res.* **19:**124–130.

Francesconi, W., Muller, C. M., and Singer, W., 1984, Acetylcholine mediates the effects of mesencephalic reticular formation stimulation in the dorsal lateral geniculate nucleus of the cat, *Neurosci. Lett. Suppl.* **18:**S309.

Gahwiler, B. H., and Brown, D. A., 1985, Functional innervation of cultured hippocampal neurones by cholinergic afferents from co-cultured septal explants, *Nature* **313:**577–579.

Gallagher, J. P., Griffith, W. H., and Shinnick-Gallagher, P., 1982, Cholinergic transmission in cat parasympathetic ganglia, *J. Physiol. (London)* **332:**473–486.

Giles, W., and Noble, S. J., 1976, Changes in membrane currents in bullfrog atrium produced by acetylcholine, *J. Physiol. (London)* **261:**103–123.

Gottesfeld, Z., and Jacobowitz, D. M., 1979, Cholinergic projections from the septal–diagonal band area to the habenular nuclei, *Brain Res.* **176:**291–294.

Haas, H. L., 1982, Cholinergic disinhibition in hippocampal slices of the rat, *Brain Res.* **233:**200–204.

Halliwell, J. V., 1986, M-current in human neocortical neurones, *Neurosci. Lett.* **67:**1–6.

Halliwell, J. V., and Adams, P. R., 1982, Voltage-clamp analysis of muscarinic excitation in hippocampal neurons, *Brain Res.* **250:**71–92.

Hammer, R., Berrie, C. P., Birdsall, N. J. M., Burgen, A. S. V., and Hulme, E. C., 1980, Pirenzepine distinguishes between different subclasses of muscarinic receptors, *Nature* **283:**90–92.

Hartzell, H. C., Kuffler, S. W., Stickgold, R., and Yoshikami, D., 1977, Synaptic excitation and inhibition resulting from direct action of acetylcholine on two types of chemoreceptors on individual amphibian parasympathetic neurones, *J. Physiol. (London)* **271:**817–846.

Herkenham, M., and Nauta, W. J. H., 1977, Afferent connections of the habenular nuclei in the rat: A horseradish peroxidase study, with a note on the fiber-of-passage problem, *J. Comp. Neurol.* **173:**123–146.

Herkenham, M., and Nauta, W. J. H., 1979, Efferent connections of the habenular nuclei in the rat, *J. Comp. Neurol.* **187:**19–48.

Hirsch, J. C., Fourment, A., and Marc, M. E., 1983, Sleep-related variations of membrane potential in the lateral geniculate body relay neurons of the cat, *Brain Res.* **259:**308–312.

Hounsgaard, J., 1978, Presynaptic inhibitory action of acetylcholine in area CA1 of the hippocampus, *Exp. Neurol.* **62:**787–797.

Houser, C. R., Vaughn, J. E., Barber, R. P., and Roberts, E., 1980, GABA neurons are the major cell type of the nucleus reticular thalami, *Brain Res.* **200:**341–354.

Houser, C. R., Crawford, G. D., Barber, R. P., Salvaterra, P. M., and Vaughn, J. E., 1983, Organization and morphological characteristics of cholinergic neurons: An immunocytochemical study with a monoclonal antibody to choline acetyltransferase, *Brain Res.* **266:**97–119.

Houser, C. R., Crawford, G. D., Salveterra, P. M., and Vaughn, J. E., 1985, Immunocytochemical localization of choline acetyltransferase in rat cerebral cortex: A study of cholinergic neurons and synapses, *J. Comp. Neurol.* **234:**17–35.

Iijima, T., Irisawa, H., and Kameyama, M., 1985, Membrane currents and their modification by acetylcholine in isolated single atrial cells of the guinea-pig, *J. Physiol. (London)* **359:**485–501.

Jahnsen, H., and Llinas, R., 1984a, Electrophysiological properties of guinea pig thalamic neurones: An *in vitro* study, *J. Physiol. (London)* **349:**205–226.

Jahnsen, H., and Llinas, R., 1984b, Ionic basis for the electroresponsiveness and oscillatory properties of guinea-pig thalamic neurones *in vitro*, *J. Physiol. (London)* **349:**227–247.

Jordan, L. M., and Phillis, J. W., 1972, Acetylcholine inhibition in the intact and chronically isolated cerebral cortex, *Br. J. Pharmacol.* **45:**584–595.

Kataoka, K., Nakamura, Y., and Hassler, R., 1973, Habenulo-interpeduncular tract: A possible cholinergic neuron in rat brain, *Brain Res.* **62:**264–267.

Kataoka, K., Sorimachi, M., Okuno, S., and Mizuno, M., 1977, Cholinergic and GABAergic fibers in the stria medularis of the rabbit, *Brain Res. Bull.* **2:**461–464.

Kayama, Y., 1985, Ascending, descending and local control of neuronal activity in the rat lateral geniculate nucleus, *Vision Res.* **25:**339–347.

Kilbinger, H., 1984, Presynaptic muscarinic receptors modulating acetylcholine release, *Trends Pharmacol. Sci.* pp. 103–105.

Kimura, H., McGeer, P. L., Peng, J. H., and McGeer, E. G., 1981, The central cholinergic system studied by choline acetyltransferase immunohistochemistry in the cat, *J. Comp. Neurol.* **200:**151–201.

Krnjević, K., 1975, Chemical nature of synaptic transmission in vertebrates, *Physiol. Rev.* **54:**418–540.

Krnjević, K., and Ropert, N., 1981, Septo-hippocampal pathway modulates hippocampal activity by a cholinergic mechanism, *Can. J. Physiol. Pharmacol.* **59:**911–914.

Krnjević, K., Pumain, R., and Renaud, L., 1971, The mechanism of excitation by acetylcholine in the cerebral cortex, *J. Physiol. (London)* **215:**447–465.

Kuba, K., and Koketsu, K., 1976, The muscarinic effects of acetylcholine on the action potential of bullfrog sympathetic ganglion cells, *Jpn. J. Physiol.* **26:**703–716.

Kuhar, M. J., DeHaven, R. N., Yamamura, H. I., Rommel-Spacher, H., and Simon, J. R., 1975, Further evidence for cholinergic habenulo-interpeduncular neurons: Pharmacological and functional characteristics, *Brain Res.* **97:**265–275.

Levey, A. I., Wainer, B. H., Rye, D. B., Mufson, E. J., and Mesulam, M.-M., 1984, Choline acetyltransferase-immunoreactive neurons intrinsic to rodent cortex and distinction from acetylcholinesterase-positive neurons, *Neuroscience* **13:**341–353.

Livingstone, M. S., and Hubel, D. H., 1981, Effects of sleep and arousal on the processing of visual information in the cat, *Nature* **291:**554–561.

McCarley, R. W., Benoit, O., and Barrionuevo, G., 1983, Lateral geniculate nucleus unitary discharges in sleep and waking: State- and rate-specific aspects, *J. Neurophysiol.* **50:**798–818.

McCormick, D. A., and Prince, D. A., 1985, Two types of muscarinic response to acetylcholine in mammalian cortical neurons, *Proc. Natl. Acad. Sci. USA* **82**:6344–6348.

McCormick, D. A., and Prince, D. A., 1986a, Acetylcholine induces burst firing in thalamic reticular neurones by activating a potassium conductance, *Nature* **319**:402–405.

McCormick, D. A., and Prince, D. A., 1986b, Mechanisms of action of acetylcholine in the guinea pig cerebral cortex, *in vitro, J. Physiol. (London)* **375**:169–194.

McCormick, D. A., and Prince, D. A., 1986c, Pirenzepine discriminates among different ionic responses to acetylcholine in guinea pig cerebral cortex and nucleus reticularis of the thalamus, *Trends Pharmacol. Sci. Suppl.* pp. 72–77.

McCormick, D. A., and Prince, D. A., 1986d, Mechanisms of ascending control of thalamic neuronal activities: Acetylcholine and norepinephrine, *Soc. Neurosci. Abstr.* **12**:903.

McCormick, D. A., and Prince, D. A., 1987, Acetylcholine causes rapid nicotinic excitation in the medial habenular nucleus of the guinea pig, *in vitro, J. Neurosci.* **7**:742–752.

Madison, D. V., and Nicoll, R. A., 1984, Control of repetitive discharge of rat CA1 neurones *in vitro, J. Physiol. (London)* **354**:319–331.

Madison, D. V., Lancaster, B., and Nicoll, R. A., 1987, Voltage clamp analysis of cholinergic slow excitation in the hippocampus, *in vitro, J. Neurosci.* **7**:733–741.

Meech, R. W., 1978, Calcium dependent potassium activation in nervous tissue, *Annu. Rev. Biophys. Bioeng.* **7**:1–18.

Mesulam, M.-M., Mufson, E. J., Wainer, B. H., and Levey, A. I., 1983a, Central cholinergic pathways in the rat: An overview based on an alternative nomenclature (Ch1–Ch6), *Neuroscience* **4**:1185–1201.

Mesulam, M.-M., Mufson, E. J., Levey, A. I., and Wainer, B. H., 1983b, Cholinergic innervation of cortex by basal forebrain: Cytochemistry and cortical connections of the septal area, diagonal band nuclei, nucleus basalis (substantia innominata), and hypothalamus in the rhesus monkey, *J. Comp. Neurol.* **214**:170–197.

Mesulam, M.-M., Mufson, E. J., Levey, A. I., and Wainer, B. H., 1984, Atlas of cholinergic neurons in the forebrain and upper brainstem of the macaque based on monoclonal choline acetyltransferase immunohistochemistry and acetylcholinesterase histochemistry, *Neuroscience* **12**:669–686.

Misgeld, U., Weiler, M. H., and Bak, I. J., 1980, Intrinsic cholinergic excitation in the rat neostriatum: Nicotinic and muscarinic receptors, *Exp. Brain Res.* **39**:401–409.

Morita, K., North, R. A., and Tokimasa, T., 1982, Muscarinic agonists inactivate potassium conductance of guinea-pig myenteric neurones, *J. Physiol. (London)* **333**:125–139.

Moruzzi, G., and Magoun, H. W., 1949, Brain stem reticular formation and activation of the EEG, *Electroencephalogr. Clin. Neurophysiol.* **1**:455–473.

Muller, W., and Misgeld, U., 1986, Slow cholinergic excitation of guinea-pig hippocampal neurons is mediated by two muscarinic receptor subtypes, *Neurosci. Lett.* **67**:107–112.

Mushiake, S., Shosaku, A., and Kayama, Y., 1984, Inhibition of thalamic ventrobasal complex neurons by glutamate infusion into the thalamic reticular nucleus in rats, *J. Neurosci. Res.* **12**:93–100.

Newberry, N. R., Priestley, T., and Woodruff, G. N., 1985, Pharmacological distinction between two muscarinic responses on the isolated superior cervical ganglion of the rat, *Eur. J. Pharmacol.* **116**:191–192.

North, R. A., 1986, Muscarinic receptors and membrane ion conductances, *Trends Pharmacol. Sci. Suppl.* pp. 19–22.

North, R. A., and Tokimasa, T., 1983, Depression of calcium-dependent potassium conductance of guinea pig myenteric neurones by muscarinic agonists, *J. Physiol. (London)* **342**:253–266.

Nowycky, M. C., Fox, A. P., and Tsien, R. W., 1985, Three types of neuronal calcium channel with different calcium agonist sensitivity, *Nature* **316**:440–443.

Pennefather, P., Lancaster, B., Adams, P. R., and Nicoll, R. A., 1985, Two distinct Ca-dependent K currents in bullfrog sympathetic ganglion cells, *Proc. Natl. Acad. Sci. USA* **82**:3040–3044.

Phillis, J. W., and York, D. H., 1968, An intracortical inhibitory synapse, *Life Sci.* **7**:65–69.

Phillis, J. W., Tebecis, A. K., and York, D. H., 1967, A study of cholinoceptive cells in the lateral geniculate nucleus, *J. Physiol. (London)* **192**:695–713.

Rogawski, M. A., and Aghajanian, G. K., 1980, Modulation of lateral geniculate neurone excitability by noradrenaline microiontophoresis or locus coeruleus stimulation, *Nature* **287**:731–734.

Rotter, R., Birdsall, N. J. M., Burgen, A. S. V., Field, P. M., Hulme, E. C., and Aisman, G., 1979, Muscarinic receptors in the central nervous system of the rat. I. Technique for autoradiographic localization of the binding of [^{3}H] propylbenzilylcholine mustard and its distribution in forebrain. *Brain Res. Rev.* **1**:141–165.

Rovira, C., Ben-Ari, Y., Cherubini, E., Krnjević, K., and Ropert, N., 1983, Pharmacology of the dendritic action of acetylcholine and further observations on the somatic disinhibition in the rat hippocampus *in situ, Neuroscience* **8**:97–106.

Rye, D. B., Wainer, B. H., Mesulam, M.-M., Mufson, E. J., and Saper, C. B., 1984, Cortical projections arising from the basal forebrain: A study of cholinergic and noncholinergic components employing combined retrograde tracing and immunohistochemical localization of choline acetyltransferase, *Neuroscience* **13**:627–643.

Sakai, K., 1985, Anatomical and physiological basis of paradoxical sleep, in: *Brain Mechanisms of Sleep* (D. J. McGingty, R., Drucker-Colin, A. Morrison, and P. L. Parmaggiani, eds.), Raven Press, New York, pp. 111–137.

Salamone, J. D., 1986, Behavioral functions of nucleus basalis magnocellularis and its relation to dementia, *Trends Neurosci.* **9**:256–258.

Saper, C. F., 1984, Organization of cerebral cortical afferent systems in the rat. II. Magnocellular basal nucleus, *J. Comp. Neurol.* **222**: 313–342.

Schwartz, W., and Passow, H., 1983, Ca^{++}-activated K^+ channels in erythrocytes and excitable cells, *Annu. Rev. Physiol.* **45**:359–374.

Sillito, A. M., Kemp, J. A., and Berardi, N., 1983, The cholinergic influence on the function of the cat dorsal lateral geniculate nucleus (dLGN), *Brain Res.* **280**:299–307.

Singer, W., 1977, Control of thalamic transmission by corticofugal and ascending reticular pathways in the visual system, *Physiol. Rev.* **57**:386–420.

Squire, L. R., and Davis, H. P., 1981, The pharmacology of memory: A neurobiological perspective, *Annu. Rev. Pharmacol. Toxicol.* **21**:323–356.

Steriade, M., 1970, Ascending control of thalamic and cortical responsiveness, *Int. Rev. Neurobiol.* **12**:87–144.

Steriade, M., 1981, Mechanisms underlying cortical activation: Neuronal organization and properties of the midbrain reticular core and intralaminar thalamic nuclei, in: *Brain Mechanisms and Perceptual Awareness* (O. Pompeiano and C. Aimone Marsan, eds.), Raven Press, New York, pp. 327–377.

Steriade, M., and Deschenes, M., 1984, The thalamus as a neuronal oscillator, *Brain Res. Rev.* **8**:1–63.

Steriade, M., Parent, A., and Hada, J., 1984, Thalamic projections of nucleus reticularis thalami of cat: A study using retrograde transport of horseradish peroxidase and fluorescent tracers, *J. Comp. Neurol.* **229**:531–547.

Steriade, M., Deschenes, M., Domich, L., and Mulle, C., 1985, Abolition of spindle oscillations in thalamic neurons disconnected from nucleus reticularis thalami, *J. Neurophysiol.* **54**:1473–1497.

Takagi, M., 1984, Actions of cholinergic drugs on cells in the interpeduncular nucleus, *Exp. Neurol.* **84**:358–363.

Takeuchi, A., and Takeuchi, N., 1960, On the permeability of endplate membrane during the action of transmitter, *J. Physiol. (London)* **154**:52–67.

Tebecis, A., 1972, Cholinergic and non-cholinergic transmission in the medial geniculate nucleus of the cat, *J. Physiol. (London)* **226**:153–172.

Wainer, B. H., Bolam, J. P., Freund, T. F., Henderson, Z., Totterdell, S., and Smith, A. D., 1984, Cholinergic synapses in the rat brain: A correlated light and electron microscopic immunohistochemical study employing a monoclonal antibody against choline acetyltransferase, *Brain Res.* **308**:69–76.

Woody, C. D., Swartz, B. E., and Gruen, E., 1978, Effects of acetylcholine and cyclic GMP on input resistance of cortical neurons in awake cats, *Brain Res.* **158**:373–395.

Woolf, N. J., and Butcher, L. L., 1986, Cholinergic systems in the rat brain. III. Projections from the pontomesencephalic tegmentum to the thalamus, tectum, basal ganglia, and basal forebrain, *Brain Res. Bull.* **16**:603–637.

Yamamoto, C., and Kawai, N., 1967, Presynaptic action of acetylcholine in thin sections from guinea pig dentate gyrus *in vitro*, *Exp. Neurol.* **19**:176–187.

19

Cholinergic Modulation of Neuronal Excitability in Cat Somatosensory Cortex

R. W. Dykes, R. Metherate, and N. Tremblay

1. Introduction

Traditionally, the compounds that influence neuronal excitability have been classified as neurotransmitters, neuromodulators, and trophic substances. If one examines carefully what is meant by these terms, it is apparent that they are based on the time course of the effect produced by a substance as well as on their physiological and biochemical consequences. Thus, neurotransmitter substances are responsible for effects beginning and ending in milliseconds, neuromodulators may provoke changes lasting seconds to hours, and trophic substances provoke changes that may not begin for extended periods but may last indefinitely. Unfortunately for this nomenclature, it has become clear that the same substance may produce both neuromodulatory effects and effects implying a role as a neurotransmitter. In the case of acetylcholine (ACh), it is possible to argue that this substance exerts neurotrophic influences also.

In the spinal cord, ACh is clearly the prototypical synaptic transmitter. However, from the time of the first cortical studies it has been apparent that ACh does not act the same way in the cortex as it does in the spinal cord. The following arguments suggest that, in the somatosensory cortex, ACh serves both as a potent neuromodulator and as a trophic substance which, under certain conditions, permits long-term changes in neuronal excitability.

2. Historical Perspective

From the time that the EEG could be recorded it was clear that cortical electrical activity characteristic of arousal could be provoked by ACh and its analogues (Bonnet and Bremmer, 1937). ACh release, as measured by diffusion from the cortical surface, was used to show that increased levels of cortical activity were correlated with the release of greater quantities of ACh

R. W. Dykes • Departments of Physiology, Neurology, and Neurosurgery, McGill University, Montreal, Quebec H3A 1A1, Canada. *R. Metherate* • Department of Physiology, McGill University, Montreal, Quebec H3A 1A1, Canada. *N. Tremblay* • Departments of Neurology and Neurosurgery, McGill University, Montreal, Quebec H3A 1A1, Canada.

(Elliott *et al.*, 1950; Mitchell, 1963). However, it soon became apparent that ACh release was more likely to be related to activity in the reticular activating system than to activity in specific sensory pathways (Kanai and Szerb, 1965; Phillis and Chong, 1965). Celsia and Jasper (1966) used a continuous cortical perfusion technique to measure ACh release from the somatosensory cortex of unanesthetized cats (Fig. 1A). Also, ACh release could be increased by stimulation of the mesencephalic reticular formation (Fig. 1B).

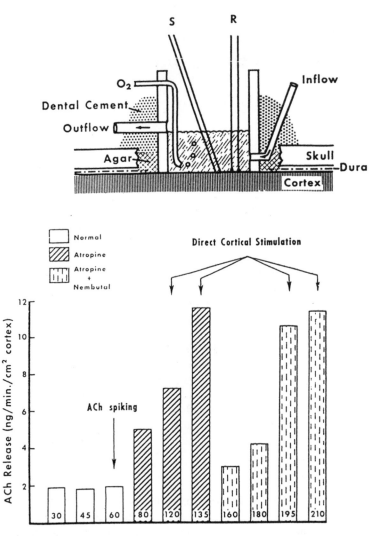

Figure 1. (A) Diagram of the cortical perfusion chamber used by Celsia and Jasper (1966) to measure ACh release. S, stimulating electrodes; R, recording electrodes. (B) Release of ACh from the primary somatosensory cortex of a cat. The first two columns represent the ACh output in the normal, drowsy animal. The next two columns represent the effect of stimulation of the mesencephalic reticular formation. Atropine (1 mg/kg intravenously) elevated the amount of ACh washed out from the cortex during rest and did not prevent the increased liberation due to stimulation of the reticular formation. The numbers on the abscissa represent the time in minutes after the beginning of cortical perfusion with Eliott's solution containing prostigmine. (From Celsia and Jasper, 1966.)

However, the correlation between EEG activity and ACh release did not extend to convulsive states; local cortical epileptiform activity could be induced without a concomitant increase in ACh release. Also, EEG activity could be dissociated from ACh release with atropine. Both of these observations made it difficult to create a general hypothesis that ACh played a central role in cortical arousal.

Studies using direct microiontophoretic administration of ACh to single neurons further complicated the picture. Only 10 to 25% of the neurons examined in early studies could be excited by direct administration of ACh and these effects seemed to be slow in onset and outlasted the period of application (Krnjević and Phillis, 1963; Spehlmann, 1963). Iontophoretic techniques provided no evidence that ACh was an important neurotransmitter in the cortex even though the same techniques had done so in the spinal cord. Thus, ACh has never been considered a major neurotransmitter in the cerebral cortex. From the earliest studies it appeared unsuited as a transmitter for the afferent pathways; most cortical neuronal functions continue even in the presence of muscarinic and nicotinic antagonists. Rather, a neuromodulatory role was suggested (Krnjević, 1974). More recent reports confirm that ACh will depolarize only 20–30% of cortical neurons. Often these effects appear only after a noticeable delay ranging from several seconds to tens of seconds (McCormick and Prince, 1985). Another small proportion of cortical neurons is inhibited.

New perspectives have developed from the introduction of techniques allowing researchers to identify unequivocally cholinergic neurons and fibers. Anatomical studies using antibody stains for choline acetyltransferase (Mesulam and Mufson, 1984; Mesulam et al., 1983; Parent et al., 1981, 1982) have proven the suspicions from earlier work (Krnjević and Silver, 1965; Johnston et al., 1981) that most cholinergic neurons in the rat and perhaps all cholinergic neurons in cats and primates are extrinsic to cortex. With the knowledge recently acquired from studies directed to cholinergic neurons of the basal forebrain, it has been possible to begin to rationalize the role of ACh in the cerebral cortex.

In the area of the basal forebrain, DeLong (1971) and Richardson and DeLong (1986) have recorded from single neurons in behaving monkeys trained to perform motor tasks for a reward. In the latter study of 186 neurons recorded in the nucleus basalis, 26% showed no relation to the task but most of the other neurons responded during the reward period and were highly responsive to events that preceded the reward during movements made to obtain the reward.

Cholinergic inputs seem to be required for cortical neurons to acquire conditioned responses. It has been demonstrated that during Pavlovian conditioning the responses of cortical neurons change to acquire new, enhanced, or attenuated responses. These changes have been observed in motor (Woody and Engel, 1972), auditory (Weinberger and Diamond, 1986), and frontal (Aou et al., 1983) cortex. Rigdon and Pirch (1986) recorded in rat frontal cortex during acquisition of a conditioned neuronal response. The rats learned to associate a tone with a subsequent rewarding stimulus to the medial forebrain bundle. In 22 of 25 cases when the conditioned response was obtained, an intracortical injection of atropine about 0.5 mm away suppressed the conditioned response, showing that the conditioned response was mediated by ACh. Kainic acid lesions of the ipsilateral basal forebrain decreased the probability of finding conditioned cortical neurons from 70% to 25%. In a third experiment, 28 of 38 basal forebrain neurons were shown to change firing rates significantly in response to the conditioned stimulus. Thus, basal forebrain neurons involved in cholinergic circuits behave as if they are involved in reward and motivated behavior, and they release ACh in the cortex. It is also known that the major inputs to the basal forebrain arise from the reticular formation and limbic structures (Russchen et al., 1985; Mesulam and Mufson, 1984). Thus, the appropriate anatomical connections required to release ACh during arousal, wakefulness, and during certain motivated behaviors have been demonstrated. The experiments described below outline efforts to determine how activation of the basal forebrain cells and the subsequent release of ACh in the somatosensory cortex changes the function of neurons.

3. Effects of ACh in the Cerebral Cortex

3.1. ACh as a Neuromodulator

Although the classical studies provided an unequivocal demonstration that ACh is not well suited to serve as a major neurotransmitter in the cortex, it may be well suited for other purposes. If ACh is considered a neuromodulator, then the existing data (such as the slow time course of its effects) begin to make more sense. To explore the possibility that ACh is a neuromodulator rather than a neurotransmitter, the experimental paradigm must be changed so that ACh can be presented to neurons together with putative neurotransmitters or with other sources of excitation so that the neuromodulatory properties of ACh can be observed.

Several studies using such an approach are found in the literature. Each used ACh administration while other excitatory influences drove the cell being studied. The pioneering efforts were those of Woody et al. (1978) who showed that the input resistance of cortical neurons could be increased in awake cats by application of ACh if the cell was being depolarized during the ACh administration. The changed membrane resistance caused the cells to become more excitable. In the same paper Woody et al. (1978) showed that these effects could be produced by intracellular injections of cGMP, implying that the ACh triggered other intracellular processes which in turn mediated the permeability change. Woody et al. (1978) pointed out that these were the kinds of changes in excitability that accompany learned responses (Woody and Engel, 1972).

In the first study of a sensory cortex with this paradigm, Sillito and Kemp (1983) used ACh as a neuromodulator, showing in cat visual cortex that the iontophoretic applications of ACh could enhance the responsiveness of many of the cells to visual stimuli. Using variables such as stimulus orientation and ocular dominance, they demonstrated that cortical neurons typically displayed an enhanced signal-to-noise ratio in the presence of ACh. Subsequent studies have confirmed this observation and have allowed its generalization to other sensory areas.

In somatosensory cortex, Metherate et al. (1987, 1988a,b) showed that ACh is capable of enhancing the responsiveness of cells both to iontophoretically applied glutamate and to natural somatic stimuli. In some cases cortical neurons were driven periodically by iontophoretic pulses of glutamate and the responses to the glutamate applied in the presence of ACh were enhanced severalfold over the response to the same amount of glutamate administered without ACh. In other cases when the neurons were driven by natural somatic stimuli applied to the receptive field, administration of ACh also enhanced those responses. It should be noted that the effects of ACh are complex and in a small fraction of the cases the responses diminished and in other cases no effect at all was observed. Similar observations have been made in rat somatosensory cortex by Lamour et al. (1988). In the hindlimb representation, neurons were shown to become generally more responsive to somatic inputs in the presence of ACh.

3.2. ACh as a Neurotrophic Substance

Another plausible hypothesis is that ACh acts as a trophic substance for cortical neurons. Trophic substances generally have a slow onset and long-lasting effects that may not be dependent upon the continuous presence of the substance in question. Rather, a neurotrophic substance (e.g., nerve growth factor) may be presented intermittently but its periodic presence brings about long-lasting effects in cell morphology and function.

Studies of trophic substances require experimental paradigms allowing the nervous system to be examined days or weeks after an experimental manipulation such as deafferentation. The neuronal plasticity which follows deafferentation and leads to reorganization of the somatosensory map is one example of a sequence of changes in neuronal function potentially attributable to alterations in trophic factors. The changes that produce reorganization of the somatotopic order following deafferentation require changes in neuronal responsiveness that last indefinitely (Kalaska and Pomeranz, 1979; Merzenich *et al.*, 1983a,b; Rasmusson, 1982; Rasmusson and Turnbull, 1983).

In a different experimental situation, Woody and Engel (1972) successfully studied longterm changes in the excitability of single neurons in the motor cortex brought about by learning. These changes were caused by changes in the membrane permeability that seemed to last indefinitely or at least for periods much longer than the several hours which the neurons were studied. Prompted by these observations, ACh was examined in cat somatosensory cortex in an experimental paradigm that would detect long-term changes in neuronal excitability (Metherate *et al.*, 1985). As these studies began, Bear and Singer (1986) demonstrated that removal of ACh and noradrenaline from the visual cortex of young kittens blocked the neuronal plasticity required for shifts in ocular dominance. Thus, ACh has been implicated in long-term changes in the visual cortex in a situation comparable to those described below where ACh has been shown to alter excitability of somatosensory cortical neurons for long periods of time thereby enhancing their responses to signals arising from the skin surface.

The experimental paradigm for studying trophic influences requires monitoring cells for long

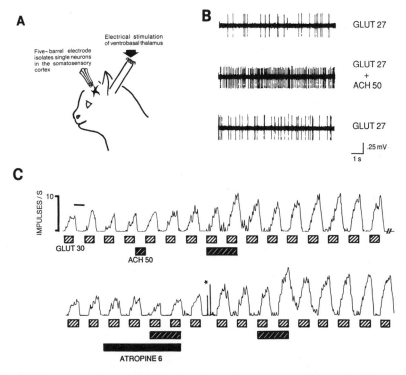

Figure 2. (A) The experimental paradigm for testing ACh as a neuromodulator consists of exciting a neuron with iontophoretically applied glutamate while simultaneously delivering ACh in some of the tests. An indication of the position of the cell in the cortical circuitry can be obtained by activating the thalamocortical input (arrow). (B) The effect of ACh on the glutamate response can be seen as an increase in the response to glutamate in the second trace. (C) Chart recorder records showing the instantaneous frequency of the neuron provide a good visual indication of the response of the cell to repeated pulses of glutamate. After three pulses of 30 nA of glutamate, 50 nA of ACh was delivered between glutamate pulses with no effect. After three more pulses ACh was administered during two glutamate pulses and the subsequent responses to glutamate were augmented for an extended period of time. When the experiment was done in the presence of atropine there was no effect, but after stopping the chart recorder (asterisk) and waiting for the atropine to dissipate, ACh treatment could augment the responses to glutamate, and these remained elevated for as long as the cell was studied. (Modified from Metherate *et al.*, 1988b.)

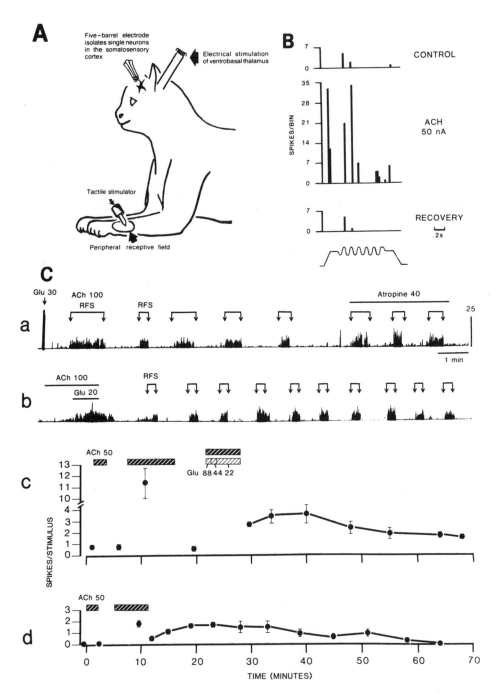

Figure 3. (A) To examine the effects of ACh on cells excited by natural inputs, the experimental paradigm was altered to use somatic stimuli on the cutaneous receptive field as the standard test. (B) The stimulus to the skin was a step with a superimposed sine wave. In the control situation very few impulses were generated by the stimuli, but in the presence of 50 nA of ACh the responses were enhanced several-fold. In this case the effect disappeared when the ACh was stopped. (C) In about one-third of the neurons tested the treatment with ACh caused a prolonged change in responsiveness. (a) This chart recorder record shows the responses of a neuron from rat somatosensory cortex

enough periods of time that changes can be shown to be relatively permanent and that they do not depend directly upon the continued presence of ACh. Single-cell recording is difficult to prolong for these periods but some neurons have been studied for more than 70 min after ACh administration and the population response of somatosensory neurons as reflected in the evoked potential has been recorded for up to 4.5 hr (Rasmusson and Dykes, 1988).

The single-cell studies consist of two manipulations. One used iontophoretically applied glutamate to measure neuronal excitability before, during, and after treatment with ACh. The other, an effort to test the excitability of cells in the context of existing neuronal circuitry, used natural somatic stimuli to examine neuronal responsiveness before, during, and after ACh treatments.

The first experimental paradigm is summarized in Fig. 2A. A fixed amount of glutamate, released at regular intervals from one barrel of a multibarrel pipette, provided a measure of neuronal excitability. After several applications to determine the control level, ACh was administered either together or between glutamate test pulses (Fig. 2B). After this treatment, the excitability of the cell was followed for at least 5 min and if an effect was observed, for up to 1 hr as the time course of the effect was measured by changes in the magnitude of the response to the glutamate pulse (Fig. 2C).

The results of tests like this were obtained for 47 cells. In 34% there was an enhancement of the excitability during or after the ACh treatment that endured more than 5 min after ACh treatment. An example of one of these effects is seen in Fig. 2. The critical event for a prolonged change in excitability seemed to be the presence of ACh during the time that the cell was depolarized.

Figure 3A illustrates the experimental paradigm used to study effects of ACh with natural somatic stimuli. In this paradigm the average response to ten somatic stimuli applied to a cutaneous receptive field was used as the measure of excitability. When this measure had been obtained several times, ACh was administered during or between test stimuli (Fig. 3B). In a sample of 52 neurons so tested, 81% showed changes in responsiveness during ACh administration and in 29% of the cases the changes were long term. Figure 3C illustrates a case in which the effect lasted more than 22 min at which time the cell was lost. Table I summarizes the long-term effects observed in both of these studies.

These observations have also been made in rat somatosensory cortex (Dykes and Lamour, 1988; Lamour *et al.*, 1988). In this case only the paradigm using somatic stimulation was employed. The cells in the latter case tended to show a further growth of the responsiveness to stimulation 3 to 4 min after the ACh treatment was terminated. This suggests that the longest lasting enhancements occurred in those cases when ACh activated some further process in the cell having a delay of 3–4 min. These effects were not observed when the cells were treated with ACh in the presence of atropine.

---

excited by glutamate but lacking an overt receptive field. In the presence of ACh a receptive field appeared and could be used to excite the cell (RFS). After simultaneous stimulation and ACh administration, the receptive field remained and the cell was equally responsive to somatic stimulation even in the absence of ACh. This change was not blocked by 40 nA of atropine. (b) A second rat cortical neuron without a cutaneous receptive field was treated with ACh, glutamate, and somatic stimulation and a receptive field appeared and remained after ACh was stopped. (Modified from Lamour *et al.*, 1988.) (c) Similar studies in cat somatosensory cortex also enhanced the excitability of neurons. In this case a neuron with a very weak response to somatic stimuli could be encouraged to respond more intensely when ACh was given during the test but not with ACh treatment between tests. When glutamate and ACh were combined, the subsequent somatic stimulation tests were enhanced for more than 40 min. (d) When a neuron without a receptive field was tested, no effect was observed with ACh administered between tests, but a receptive field appeared if tested during ACh administration. This combination led to an overt receptive field from which responses could be elicited for about 50 min. (Modified from Metherate *et al.*, 1988b.)

Table I. Effects of Acetylcholine on Cat Somatosensory Cortical Neurons[a]

Treatment	Effect observed	Glutamate test pulse		Somatic test stimulus	
		Number of cells	Percent	Number of cells	Percent
ACh without	Potentiated	7 (2 long-term)	20	4 (2 long-term)	15
excitation	Depressed	2 (1 long-term)	6	0	0
	No effect	25	74	23	85
	Total tested	34	100	27	100
ACh during	Potentiated	30 (16 long-term)	64	42 (15 long-term)	81
excitation	Depressed	4 (1 long-term)	8	0	0
	No effect	13	28	10	19
	Total tested	47	100	52	100

[a]Modified from Metherate et al. (1988b).

4. Implications for the Somatosensory Cortex

If ACh is a neuromodulator as suggested by the data in Section 3.1 and the literature reviewed in Section 2 as well as in other chapters, it can be seen that the responses of some cortical neurons will be dramatically enhanced during the release of ACh, possibly showing doubling or quadrupling of their outputs, markedly lowered thresholds, and enhanced responsiveness to somatic stimuli. (About 10% will be less responsive and as many as one-third will be unaffected.) The reasons that cells are affected differentially have yet to be determined but it is clear that the release of ACh can readily change the excitability of somatosensory neurons, and on balance it seems to enhance the sensory processing capacities of the cortex. Thus, the question of when it is released in the cortex becomes paramount since its presence should augment the outflow of cortical neurons severalfold.

This question remains without detailed answers; however, the early studies of Celsia and Jasper (1966) and others have shown an enhanced release of ACh from the cortex during arousal. However, release studies generally average ACh collection over 15-min epochs and it is not known if the release of ACh in a particular cortical region is (1) periodic, (2) dependent upon direct attention involving that cortical area, or (3) simply a concomitant of alertness. The degree of selectivity with which the basal forebrain neurons can release ACh in one area and not another is unknown. The events which excite these cells are only documented by the few studies reviewed above (DeLong, 1971; Richardson and DeLong, 1986; Rigdon and Pirch, 1986), and much more must be done if we are to understand when and how cortical neurons are presented with ACh.

The potential trophic or more long-lasting influences of ACh also raise questions about where and when ACh is released. ACh could play a crucial role in learning if it were released in the appropriate place at the appropriate time. The temporal and spatial requirements, however, suggest a degree of precision for release of ACh by basal forebrain neurons that has not been documented. The same hypothesis suggests that release of ACh in an inappropriate cortical location or at an inappropriate time could have no effect or could lead to enhancement of neuronal responses that are counterproductive for efficient processing of sensory signals. Clearly more information is needed about the control of basal forebrain neurons and the release of ACh in the cortex.

In the case of cortical reorganization following deafferentation, the role of ACh is equally unclear. It has been shown that the responsiveness to iontophoretically applied ACh is enhanced in deafferented regions (Dykes and Lamour, 1988; Lamour and Dykes, 1988), but a causal relationship between ACh and cortical reorganization has not been established. Potentially, the long-lasting changes in excitability that occur in the presence of ACh may underlie part of the process that leads to cortical reorganization, but much more work remains before a mechanistic explanation of the relationship between ACh and cortical reorganization can be formulated.

5. Conclusion

ACh does not act as a classical neurotransmitter in the somatosensory cortex. However, it has properties that allow it to be considered as a neuromodulator and it produces other effects that could be classified as neurotrophic. Its actions on single neurons in cat and rat somatosensory cortex suggest that ACh could play a very important role by facilitating the processing of somatosensory information during attentive states, that it could play a role in learning in the somatosensory cortex, and that it could facilitate the reorganization of the somatosensory cortex which follows deafferentation.

References

Aou, S., Oomura, Y., and Nishino, H., 1983, Influence of acetylcholine on neuronal activity in monkey orbitofrontal cortex during bar press feeding task, *Brain Res.* **275:**178.

Bear, M. F., and Singer, W., 1986, Modulation of visual cortical plasticity by acetylcholine and noradrenaline, *Nature* **320:**172.

Bonnet, V., and Bremmer, F., 1937, Action du potassium, du calcium et de l'acetylcholine sur les activities electriques, spontanees and provoquees, de l'ecorce cerebrale, *C.R. Soc. Biol.* **126:**1271.

Celsia, G. G., and Jasper, H. H., 1966, Acetylcholine released from cerebral cortex in relation to state of activation, *Neurology* **16:**1053.

DeLong, M. R., 1971, Activity of pallidal neurons during movement, *J. Neurophysiol.* **34:**414.

Dykes, R. W., and Lamour, Y., 1988, An electrophysiological study of single somatosensory neurons in rat granular cortex serving the limbs: A laminar analysis, *J. Neurophysiol.* (in press).

Elliott, K. A. C., Swank, R. L., and Henderson, N. 1950, Effects of anesthetic and convulsants on acetylcholine content of brain, *Am. J. Physiol.* **162:**469.

Jasper, H. H., 1960, Unspecific thalamocortical relations, in: *Handbook of Physiology,* Vol. 2 (N. W. Magoung, ed.), Williams & Wilkins, Baltimore.

Johnston, M. V., McKinney, M., and Coyle, J. T., 1981, Neocortical cholinergic innervation: A description of extrinsic and intrinsic components in the rat, *Exp. Brain Res.* **43:**159.

Kalaska, J., and Pomeranz, B., 1979, Chronic paw denervation causes an age-dependent appearance of novel responses from forearm in "paw cortex" of kittens and adult cats, *J. Neurophysiol.* **42:**618.

Kanai, T., and Szerb, J. C., 1965, Mesencephalic reticular activating system and cortical acetylcholine output, *Nature* **205:**80.

Krnjević, K., 1974, Chemical nature of synaptic transmission in vertebrates, *Physiol. Rev.* **54:**318.

Krnjević, K., and Phillis, J. W., 1963, Pharmacological properties of acetylcholine sensitive cells in the cerebral cortex, *J. Physiol. (London)* **166:**328.

Krnjević, K., and Silver, A., 1965, A histochemical study of cholinergic fibres in the cerebral cortex, *J. Anat.* **99:**711.

Lamour, Y., and Dykes, R. W., 1988, Somatosensory neurons in deafferented rat hindlimb granular cortex subsequent to transection of the sciatic nerve: Effects of glutamate and acetylcholine, *Brain Res.* (in press).

Lamour, Y., Jobert, A., and Dykes, R. W., 1988, An iontophoretic study of single somatosensory neurons in rat granular cortex serving the limbs: A laminar analysis of glutamate and acetylcholine effects on receptive field properties, *J. Neurophysiol.* (in press).

McCormick, D. A., and Prince, D. A., 1985, Two types of muscarinic response to acetylcholine in mammalian cortical neurons, *Proc. Natl. Acad. Sci. USA* **82:**6344.

Merzenich, M. M., Kaas, J. H., Wall, J. T., Nelson, R. J., Sur, M., and Felleman, D., 1983a, Topographic reorganization of somatosensory cortical areas 3b and 1 in adult monkeys following restricted deafferentation, *Neuroscience* **8:**33.

Merzenich, M. M., Kaas, J. H., Wall, J. T., Sur, M., Nelson, R. J., and Felleman, D., 1983b, Progression of change following median nerve section in the cortical representation of the hand in areas 3b and 1 in adult owl and squirrel monkeys, *Neuroscience* **10**:639.

Mesulam, M.-M., and Mufson, E. J., 1984, Neural inputs into the nucleus basalis of the substantia innominata (Ch 4) in the rhesus monkey, *Brain* **107**:253.

Mesulam, M.-M., Mufson, E. J., Levy, A. I., and Wainer, B. H., 1983, Cholinergic innervation of cortex by the basal forebrain: Cytochemistry and cortical connections of the septal area, diagonal band nuclei, nucleus basalis (substantia innominata), and hypothalamus, *J. Comp. Neurol.* **214**:170–197.

Metherate, R., Tremblay, N., and Dykes, R. W., 1985, Changes in neuronal function produced in cat primary somatosensory cortex by the iontophoretic application of acetylcholine, *Soc. Neurosci. Abstr.* **11**:753.

Metherate, R., Tremblay, N., and Dykes, R. W., 1987, Acetylcholine permits prolonged potentiation of neural responsiveness in cat somatosensory cortex, *Neuroscience* **22**:75–81.

Metherate, R., Tremblay, N., and Dykes, R. W., 1988a, The effects of acetylcholine on response properties of cat somatosensory cortical neurons, *J. Neurophysiol.* (in press).

Metherate, R., Tremblay, N., and Dykes, R. W., 1988b, Transient and prolonged effects of acetylcholine on responsiveness of cat somatosensory cortical neurons, *J. Neurophysiol.* (in press).

Mitchell, J. F., 1963, The spontaneous and evoked release of acetylcholine from the cerebral cortex, *J. Physiol. (London)* **207**:1253.

Parent, A., Boucher, R., and O'Reilly-Fromentin, J., 1982, Distribution and morphological characteristics of acetylcholinesterase-containing neurons in the basal forebrain of the cat, *Brain Res. Bull.* **8**:183.

Parent, A., Boucher, R., and O'Reilly-Fromentin, J., 1981, Acetylcholinesterase-containing neurons in cat pallidal complex: Morphological characteristics and projection towards the neocortex, *Brain Res.* **230**:356.

Phillis, J. W., and Chong, G. C., 1965, Acetylcholine release from the cerebral and cerebellar cortices: Its role in cortical arousal, *Nature* **207**:1253.

Rasmusson, D. D., 1982, Reorganization of raccoon somatosensory cortex following removal of the fifth digit, *J. Comp. Neurol.* **205**:313.

Rasmusson, D. D., and Turnbull, B. G., 1983, Immediate effects of digit amputation of SI cortex in the raccoon: Unmasking of inhibitory fields, *Brain Res.* **288**:368.

Rasmusson, D. D., and Dykes, R. W., 1988, Long-term enhancement of evoked potentials in cat somatosensory cortex produced by coactivation of the basal forebrain and sensory receptors, *Exp. Brain Res.* (in press).

Richardson, R. T., and DeLong, M. R., 1986, Nucleus basalis of Meynert neuronal activity during a delayed response task in monkey, *Brain Res.* **399**:364.

Rigdon, G. G., and Pirch, J. H., 1986, Nucleus basalis involvement in conditioned neuronal responses in the rat frontal cortex, *J. Neurosci.* **6**:2535.

Russchen, F. T., Amaral, D. G., and Price, J. L., 1985, The afferent connections of the substantia innominata in the monkey, *Macaca fascicularis, J. Comp. Neurol.* **242**:1.

Sillito, A. M., and Kemp, J. A., 1983, Cholinergic modulation of the functional organization of the cat visual cortex, *Brain Res.* **289**:143.

Spehlmann, R., 1963, Acetylcholine and prostigmine electrophoresis at visual cortex neurons, *J. Neurophysiol.* **26**:127.

Weinberger, N. M., Diamond, D. M., 1987, Physiological plasticity in auditory cortex: rapid induction by learning, *Prog. Neurobiol.* **29**:1–55.

Woody, C. D., and Engel, J., 1972, Changes in unit activity and thresholds to electrical microstimulation at coronal–pericruciate cortex of cat with classical conditioning of different facial movements, *J. Neurophysiol.* **35**:230.

Woody, C. D., Swartz, B. E., and Gruen, E., 1978, Effects of acetylcholine and cyclic GMP on input resistance of cortical neurons in awake cats, *J. Neurophysiol.* **35**:373.

20

Evidence that Acetylcholine Acts in Vivo in Layer V Pyramidal Cells of Cats via cGMP and a cGMP-Dependent Protein Kinase to Produce a Decrease in an Outward Current

C. D. Woody and E. Gruen

1. Introduction

After conditioning of facial reflexes in cats, increases occur in CS (conditional stimulus)-evoked unit activity and excitability of those layer V pyramidal cells of the motor cortex that control production of the specific type of facial movement that is learned (Woody, 1982a,b). The finding of increased excitability to intracellular current in the absence of increased spontaneous rates of discharge or detectable changes in resting membrane potential has been interpreted as suggesting postsynaptic neural changes (Woody and Black-Cleworth, 1973; Brons and Woody, 1980). If the membrane resistance of portions of the dendrites were increased in the cells, this could cause a change in the length constant, governing the spread and weighting of synaptic inputs (as postsynaptic potentials) from these areas to regions of spike initiation (Holmes and Woody, 1983, 1984). The increases in resistance would also be reflected by an increased ease of excitation by intracellularly injected current. Several lines of evidence suggest that a long-lasting decrease in outward current addressable through the cholinergic–cGMP–cGMP-dependent protein kinase system may mediate the excitability increase that supports this type of conditioning.

2. Acetylcholine and cGMP

Increases in input resistance (R_m) can be produced artificially in cells of the pericruciate cortex by extracellular iontophoretic applications of acetylcholine (ACh) (Krnjević et al., 1971). These findings were confirmed in studies in neurons of the motor cortex of awake cats (see Woody et al., 1976, 1978). The later studies disclosed that the increases could be made to persist by pairing iontophoresis of ACh with *intracellular* injection of sufficient depolarizing current to

C. D. Woody and E. Gruen • Mental Retardation Research Center, UCLA Medical Center, Los Angeles, California 90024.

discharge the neuron repeatedly. The increases in R_m did not occur if saline was substituted or if the neurons were simply discharged repeatedly with intracellularly injected current in the absence of extracellular iontophoresis (Woody et al., 1978).

Effects of sequential application of (1) ACh, (2) atropine, (3) repeated ACh, and (4) cGMP (Swartz and Woody, 1979) indicated that the same cells responded to ACh with an increase in input resistance as did to cGMP. The increase to ACh was blocked by atropine, but not the increase in input resistance to cGMP. cGMP was applied intracellularly; the other agents were applied extracellularly. These studies also confirmed that depolarizing current sufficient to produce repeated spike discharge, applied during application of ACh or cGMP, transformed the transient increase in input resistance after these agents into a persistent increase in resistance (Swartz and Woody, 1979).

Further studies of effects of ACh on intracellular K^+ ion concentrations were conducted in single neurons of the motor cortex in awake cats, using ion-sensitive microelectrodes (Woody and Wong, 1981). Cells that responded to ACh with an increased rate of discharge showed small increases in intracellular concentrations of K^+, while cells that did not respond did not show such changes. The hyperpolarizing effect of the small increase in intracellular K^+ would not have been sufficient to overcome the depolarizing effect of the magnitude of associated decrease in K^+ conductance predicted empirically. Concentrations of ACh 10–100 times higher than those applied iontrophoretically were required to produce cross-reactive alterations in the potentials recorded through the K^+-sensitive electrodes (Woody and Wong, 1981).

Horseradish peroxidase (HRP) was pressure injected intracellularly to identify neurons of the motor cortex in which the effects of ACh were studied (Swartz and Woody, 1979). cGMP and HRP were also applied intracellularly by pressure injection (Woody et al., 1986b). Pyramidal cells of layers V and VI were identified that responded to these agents with an increased resistance (Fig. 1). The responsive neurons included those of layer V activated antidromically by pyramidal tract (PT) stimulation. A comparison of the results of pressure-injected cGMP with those of intracellularly iontophoresed cGMP showed similar changes in resistance, but the increase in firing rate after the hyperpolarizing iontophoresis did not occur after pressure injection. The increase in firing rate following application of ACh appears to be a separate effect of this agent, apart from that supported by cGMP as a second messenger. This effect may arise from excitation of surrounding neurons presynaptic to the one recorded or from other, direct conductance effects of ACh acting at the neuronal receptors.

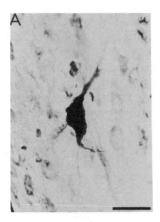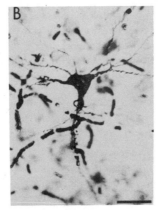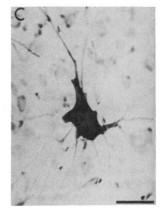

Figure 1. Examples of neurons injected with cGMP and HRP that showed an increase in input resistance. (A) A small pyramidal cell of layer V; (B) an inverted pyramidal cell of layer VI; (C) a large pyramidal (Betz) cell of layer V. Bars = 30 μm (A), 40 μm (B), 50 μm (C). (From Woody et al., 1986b.)

Intracellular injection of specific antibody to cGMP (cGMP-Ab) produced substantial decreases in input resistance selectively in neurons of the motor cortex that had responded with increased resistance to prior application of muscarinic agents (Swartz and Woody, 1984). Intracellular injection of nonspecific immunoglobulins (IgG) did not produce this effect. (Some nonspecific effects on spike production occurred in cells given IgG or cGMP-Ab.) The decrease in R_m may be interpreted as a consequence of reduced baseline levels of active cGMP, due to binding of cGMP with the injected antibody. In cells which demonstrated a prior increase in R_m following extracellular application of the muscarinic agonist, aceclidine, or ACh, injection of cGMP-Ab also resulted in suppression of the increase in R_m to subsequent applications of these muscarinic agents. Increases in firing rate to these agents continued to be observed after injection of cGMP-Ab. The results support the hypothesis that cGMP mediates effects of muscarinic neurotransmission on the conductances of neurons of the motor cortex of awake cats.

3. Calcium and cAMP

Injections of Ca^{2+} ions and HRP were also made intracellularly in neurons of the motor cortex (Wallis *et al.*, 1982). Pressure injection was used to avoid voltage-dependent calcium flux that could arise from currents used for iontophoretic application. Twelve cells with resting potentials averaging -49 mV were injected with 4% HRP in 10^{-3} M $CaCl_2$. Twenty-nine cells injected with HRP without additional calcium had resting potentials averaging -47 mV. Injections with calcium produced an increase in conductance measured by the differential spike height method, that was usually sustained over the course of 3 min. Injections of HRP alone produced no change or significantly smaller conductance increases. HRP solutions were found to contain as much as 10^{-4} M free Ca^{2+}. Cells responding to calcium with a conductance increase were identified as pyramidal cells of layers II, III, and V.

Pressure injection of cAMP and HRP (0.1 mM solution in 4% HRP injected at 60–80 psi for 1–5 sec) into cells of the same cortical region produced results resembling those obtained by injecting Ca^{2+}. Eighty-six percent of injected cells responded to cAMP and HRP with a rapid decrease in input resistance. The decreases in input resistance occurred immediately after injection and began to return toward baseline 2–3 min later. The decreases were significantly greater than the small decreases in input resistance normally seen in uninjected cells held for 2 min or more after penetration and exceeded comparably small decreases in input resistance seen after control injections of 5'-AMP plus HRP. Pyramidal cells of layer V were among those showing these responses. The cells also showed increased rates of discharge after penetration with electrodes containing cAMP, but significant changes in input resistance were not found in association with the increased rates of discharge. After pressure injection of cAMP, the rates of discharge fell toward more normal levels. The results indicate that excitability and membrane resistance are decreased by intracellular cAMP.

4. Calcium–Calmodulin-Dependent Protein Kinase (CaCMPK)

Effects of intracellularly applied CaCMPK were also studied in neurons of the motor cortex of awake cats (Woody *et al.*, 1984a). Intracellular iontophoretic application of CaCMPK was followed by a 30-sec period of steady depolarization (1 nA). These cells showed a transient increase in input resistance in comparison with a control group of 15 cells given depolarization only, without application of CaCMPK, which showed no increases in input resistance (Fig. 2). Postiontophoretic measurements of input resistance in cells given CaCMPK alone were not increased, nor was input resistance increased in cells given equivalent negative currents through electrodes containing only KCl. The results indicate that intracellular injection of CaCMPK,

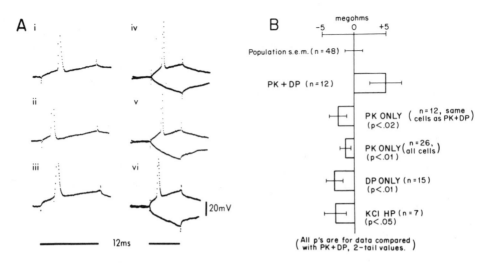

Figure 2. (A) Results of intracellular injection of Ca^{2+}–calmodulin-dependent protein kinase followed by application of depolarizing current. Input resistance: (i, iv) before protein kinase injection; (ii, v) after protein kinase injection; (iii, vi) immediately after subsequent depolarization. (i–iii) show the maintenance of bridge balance to null out changes in electrode resistance. In ii the bridge is slightly out of balance. An increase in resistance is seen in iii and vi. Calibrations are as indicated below and to the right of this portion of the figure. 12 msec applies to both time calibrations and the 20 mV calibration applies to all records. (The tops of the spikes are cut off.) (B) Bar graphs of average change in input resistance before and after protein kinase plus depolarization in responsive cells (PK + DP), after protein kinase only (PK only), after depolarization alone (DP only), and after passage of negative current, i.e., hyperpolarization, without iontophoresis of protein kinase (KCl HP). Standard errors of the means are shown for each different group of cells. (From Woody et al., 1984a.)

followed by depolarization and depolarization-elicited impulse activity, transiently increases input resistance of neurons of the motor cortex of cats for a few seconds. A longer-lasting increase of input resistance can be produced in the type B photoreceptor of *Hermissenda* by applying protein kinase and sufficient depolarization paired with light to increase calcium conductance and internal calcium concentration (Alkon et al., 1983; Connor and Alkon, 1984).

5. cGMP-Dependent Protein Kinase

Intracellular injection of the cGMP-dependent protein kinase into neurons of the precruciate cortex of the awake cat can mimic the actions of extracellularly applied ACh and intracellularly applied cGMP. Purified cGMP-dependent protein kinase produced increases in input resistance (Fig. 3) when injected into neurons of the motor cortex of awake cats (Woody et al., 1986a). Input resistances were measured with 1-nA, 40-msec, rectangular, bridge-balanced, hyperpolarizing and depolarizing pulses. The mean input resistance increased within seconds (as rapidly as measurements could be made) after injection of cGMP-dependent protein kinase and remained elevated for 2 min or longer. In these experiments the cGMP-dependent protein kinase was incubated with 10 µM cGMP 30 min prior to filling the electrodes. Pressure injection of the cGMP-dependent protein kinase without preincubation with cGMP caused smaller increases in R_m that were slower in onset, reaching a maximum value 60–90 sec after injection. "Control cells" injected with heat-inactivated cGMP-dependent protein kinase, with or without preincubation with 10 µM cGMP, did not show such changes in R_m over comparable periods of observation.

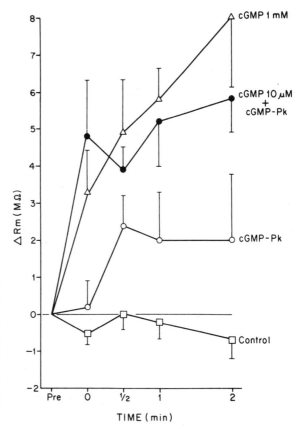

Figure 3. The rate and amplitude of change in input resistance in cortical neurons injected with 1 mM cGMP (△), cGMP-dependent protein kinase activated with 10 μM cGMP (●), cGMP-dependent protein kinase alone (○), and heat-inactivated cGMP-dependent protein kinase (control) (□). Bars are standard errors of the means. All means except that of the cGMP-PK at times 0 and 2 min are significantly different (Student's *t*, 0.001 > *p* > 0.05) from those of the control group. Times shown are before injection (pre), immediately after injection (O), and subsequently in minutes after injection.

6. Cholinergic Effects Mediated by Decreases in an Outward Current

A voltage-dependent, 4-aminopyridine-sensitive, outward current can be measured *in vivo* by single-electrode voltage-clamp techniques in cortical neurons of awake cats (Woody *et al.*, 1985). Studies of neurons of the precruciate cortex disclosed fast, outward currents that increased with increasing, positive step voltage commands from holding potentials set between −60 and −80 mV. Preceding depolarizing pulses reduced the currents while preceding hyperpolarizing pulses potentiated them. Cells pressure injected with 4-aminopyridine showed reduction of the outward current. The degree of reduction varied from cell to cell.

The measurements of changes in current corresponded with previous *in vitro* measurements in other cortical cells (Gustafsson *et al.*, 1982), and in *Tritonia* (see Thompson, 1977). The cable properties of neocortical pyramidal cells are such that an actual voltage clamp is unrealizable with control of but 1–10% of a space constant estimated from previous modeling of theoretical cable properties in cells of known morphology. Also, the fast sodium currents are incompletely controlled. Further, the large number of active synaptic conductances along the cable length results in a kind of counterclamping toward the normal resting potential of the cell. Hence, the potentials are ''squeezed away'' from the normal resting potential and toward the desired holding and command potentials. Nonetheless, the preparation affords qualitative examination of currents and time courses found in the actual *in vivo* state and semiquantitative measurements of sufficient precision and sensitivity to detect changes in outward currents upon administration of pharmacologic blocking agents. Net outward currents of the above type are reduced after application of ACh or cGMP-dependent protein kinase (Woody and Gruen, 1987).

Additional studies assessed possible injury arising from cell penetrations. The response of penetrated neurons to repeated click stimuli was compared with that of unpenetrated (extra-cellularly recorded) units of the same cortical region. Responses obtained from penetrated neu-rons were separated into four groups according to the size of the recorded action potential. The magnitude of the response to click was much the same in cells with action potentials ranging between 50–60 mV, 40–50 mV, and 30–40 mV. The magnitude was slightly greater in the group with action potentials ranging between 20 and 30 mV (suggesting some slight depolarizing injury to some of these cells). The response profiles were comparable to those of extracellularly recorded units (Woody *et al.*, 1970; Woody and Engel, 1972). It appears that whatever injury arose from the penetrations of these cells was minimal and insufficient to impair the ability of most cells to respond with spike activation to natural stimuli such as a weak click (Woody *et al.*, 1984b). In further studies employing pressure injections of HRP, recordings characterized by action poten-tials of amplitudes smaller than the recorded resting potentials were correlated with recoveries of injected dendrites. Penetrations with dendritic recoveries had higher input resistances than did those with recoveries of both somata and dendrites. Increases in spike height during pressure injection were greater in recordings with dendritic recoveries than in recordings with recoveries of both somata and dendritic processes (Woody *et al.*, 1984b).

The outcomes of the above experiments support the hypothesis that ACh acts in layer V pyramidal cells of cats to produce a decrease in an outward membrane current. This action appears to be mediated intracellularly by cGMP and by a cGMP-dependent protein kinase. When a depolarization-induced spike discharge (which likely leads to an increased calcium influx) is associated with application of ACh or cGMP, the duration of the decrease in outward current is transformed from a transient change to a persistent one. This change, or a change like it, may support the increases in excitability of these cells after conditioning that underlie the increased probability of CS-evoked spike discharge that controls the production of the specific movement that is learned (Woody, 1982a,b).

ACKNOWLEDGMENTS. Supported by AFOSR and NICHD HD-05958. I thank all of those (see References) who have collaborated with me in these studies.

References

Alkon, D. L., Acosta-Urquidi, J., Olds, J., Kuzma, G., and Neary, J. 1983, Protein kinase injection reduces voltage-dependent potassium currents, *Science* **219**:303–306.

Brons, J. F., and Woody, C. D., 1980, Long-term changes in excitability of cortical neurons after Pavlovian conditioning and extinction, *J. Neurophysiol.* **44**:605–615.

Connor, J. A., and Alkon, D. L., 1984, Light- and voltage-dependent increases of calcium ion concentration in molluscan photoreceptors, *J. Neurophysiol.* **51**:745–752.

Gustafsson, B., Galvan, M., Grafe, P., and Wigstrom, H., 1982, A transient outward current in a mammalian central neurone blocked by 4-amino pyridine, *Nature* **299**:252–254.

Holmes, W. R., and Woody, C. D., 1983, Effects on input currents of local increases in membrane resistance in cortical pyramidal cell dendrites explored using a passive cable model for determining the transient potential in a dendritic tree of known geometry, *Soc. Neurosci. Abstr.* **9**:603.

Holmes, W. R., and Woody, C. D., 1984, Some effects of tonic afferent activity on input from individual synapses as modeled in a cortical pyramidal cell of known morphology, *Soc. Neurosci. Abstr.* **10**:1073.

Krnjević, K., Pumain, R., and Renaud, L., 1971, The mechanism of excitation by acetylcholine in the cerebral cortex, *J. Physiol. (London)* **215**:247–268.

Swartz, B. E., and Woody, C. D., 1979, Correlated effects of acetylcholine and cyclic guanosine monophosphate on membrane properties of mammalian neocortical neurons, *J. Neurobiol.* **10**:465–488.

Swartz, B. E., and Woody, C. D., 1984, Effects of intracellular antibodies to cGMP on responses of cortical neurons of awake cats to extracellular application of muscarinic agents, *Exp. Neurol.* **86**:388–404.

Thompson, S. H., 1977, Three pharmacologically distinct potassium channels in molluscan neurones, *J. Physiol. (London)* **265**:465–488.

Wallis, R. A., Woody, C. D., and Gruen, E., 1982, Effects of intracellular pressure injections of calcium ions in morphologically identified neurons of cat motor cortex, *Soc. Neurosci. Abstr.* **8**:909.

Woody, C. D., 1982a, Acquisition of conditioned facial reflexes in the cat: Cortical control of different facial movements, *Fed. Proc.* **41**:2160–2168.

Woody, C. D., 1982b, *Memory, Learning, and Higher Function: A Cellular View*, Springer-Verlag, Berlin.

Woody, C. D., and Black-Cleworth, P., 1973, Differences in excitability of cortical neurons as a function of motor projection in conditioned cats, *J. Neurophysiol.* **36**:1104–1116.

Woody, C. D., and Engel, J., Jr., 1972, Changes in unit activity and thresholds to electrical microstimulation at coronal-pericruciate cortex of cat with classical conditioning of different facial movements, *J. Neurophysiol.* **35**:230–241.

Woody, C. D., and Gruen, E., 1987, Acetylcholine reduces net outward currents measured in vivo with single electrode voltage clamp techniques in neurons of the motor cortex of cats, *Brain Res.* **424**:193–198.

Woody, C. D., and Wong, B., 1981, Intracellular recording of potassium in neurons of the motor cortex of awake cats following extracellular applications of acetylcholine, in: *Ion-Selective Microelectrodes and Their Uses in Excitable Tissues* (E. Sykova, P. Hnik, and L. Vyklicky, eds.), Plenum Press, New York, pp. 125–132.

Woody, C. D., Vassilevsky, N. N., and Engel, J., Jr., 1970, Conditioned eye blink: Unit activity at coronal-precruciate cortex of the cat, *J. Neurophysiol.* **33**:851–864.

Woody, C. D., Carpenter, D. O., Gruen, E., Knispel, J. D., Crow, T. W., and Black-Cleworth, P., 1976, Persistent increases in membrane resistance of neurons in cat motor cortex, *AFRRI Scientific Report*, February 1976, pp. 1–31.

Woody, C. D., Swartz, B. E., and Gruen, E., 1978, Effects of acetylcholine and cyclic GMP on input resistance of cortical neurons in awake cats, *Brain Res.* **158**:373–395.

Woody, C. D., Alkon, D. L., and Hay, B., 1984a, Depolarization-induced effects of Ca^{2+}-calmodulin-dependent protein kinase injection, in vivo, in single neurons of cat motor cortex, *Brain Res.* **321**:192–197.

Woody, C. D., Gruen, E., and McCarley, K., 1984b, Intradendritic recordings from neurons of the motor cortex of cats, *J. Neurophysiol.* **51**:925–938.

Woody, C. D., Nenov, V., Gruen, E., and Donley, P., 1985, A voltage-dependent, 4-aminopyridine sensitive, outward current studied in vivo in cortical neurons of awake cats by voltage squeeze techniques, *Soc. Neurosci. Abstr.* **11**:955.

Woody, C. D., Bartfai, T., Gruen, E., and Nairn, A., 1986a, Intracellular injection of cGMP-dependent protein kinase results in increased input resistance in neurons of the mammalian motor cortex, *Brain Res.* **386**:379–385.

Woody, C. D., Gruen, E., Sakai, H., Sakai, M., and Swartz, B., 1986b, Responses of morphologically identified cortical neurons to intracellularly injected cyclic GMP, *Exp. Neurol.* **91**:580–595.

21

Structural Basis of Cortical Monoamine Function

Laurent Descarries, Guy Doucet, Benoît Lemay, Philippe Séguéla, and Kenneth C. Watkins

Can the melody of higher mental processes be played on a keyboard mosaic of modules or cortical columns with rigidly determined functional characteristics? Higher brain functions in the behaving animal or man should require, in addition, that such local functional units be integrated with more widespread neuronal assemblies throughout the neuraxis.

Herbert H. Jasper (1981)

1. Introduction

The title of this chapter suggests that it is possible, in the current state of knowledge, to elaborate meaningful hypotheses regarding the mode of action and function of certain sets of CNS neurons based on the characteristics of their morphological organization. Not so very long ago, such a nosological approach would have been hazardous if not presumptuous. The coherence of physiological and biochemical results ensured their validity and absolved these disciplines from striving for precise cellular localization. On their side, anatomists often relied on purely spatial descriptions of the distribution, configuration, and connectivity of nerve cells to seek some rather primitive understanding of their integrated functioning in mere terms of excitation and inhibition. Nowadays, few neuroscientists would dare to envisage any aspect of a higher neural system without due attention to the varied and interrelated facets of its morphofunctional organization. Herbert H. Jasper has given us leading examples of such broad thinking. The present essay draws heavily on some of his ideas.

    The major morphologic features of central monoamine systems can presently be viewed at three descriptive levels: first, that of the anatomical, overall repartition of these neurons in brain; second, that of the intraregional distribution of their axon terminals within various territories of

Laurent Descarries, Guy Doucet, Benoît Lemay, Philippe Séguéla, and Kenneth C. Watkins • Centre de Recherche en Sciences Neurologiques, Département de Physiologie, Faculté de Médecine, Université de Montréal, Montreal, Quebec, H3C 3J7, Canada.

innervation; and third, that of the fine structural, junctional, and appositional relationships of these nerve endings. From this triple standpoint, it is interesting to consider the main characteristics of the noradrenaline (NA) and serotonin (5-hydroxytryptamine, 5-HT) as opposed to the dopamine (DA) innervations in cerebral cortex.

2. Noradrenaline and Serotonin Innervations of Cerebral Cortex

2.1. Topographic Distribution

As now described with various methods and for various species, the NA and 5-HT projections to mammalian cerebral cortex have several traits in common (for review and detailed references, see Levitt et al., 1984a; Lindvall and Björklund, 1984). Predominantly ipsilateral, they take origin in relatively small nuclei of the brain stem "reticular formation": the locus coeruleus (A-6 in the original nomenclature of Dahlström and Fuxe, 1964), located at the ponto-mesencephalic junction and exclusively composed of NA neurons in the rat, and the nuclei raphe dorsalis and raphe medianus of the midbrain (B-7 and B-8 in the Swedish nomenclature), the cell body composition of which is only partly serotoninergic. Borrowing anatomical pathways that are initially distinct (the so-called dorsal NA and periventricular and transtegmental 5-HT bundles), the NA and 5-HT fibers join at the hypothalamic level to reach the cerebral cortex via branchings of the medial forebrain bundle. These ascending fibers are mostly of fine caliber and unmyelinated, and yet relatively long and extremely ramified. For example, a single coeruleo-cortical axon probably collateralizes from front to back in the cortex, infiltrating its full thickness (Morrison et al., 1981; Nagai et al., 1981; Loughlin et al., 1982). Moreover, recent studies with retrogradely transported fluorescent dyes have convincingly demonstrated that at least some NA or 5-HT neurons can concomitantly innervate the cerebral cortex and other distant CNS regions such as the cerebellum or the spinal cord (Adèr et al., 1980; Nagai et al., 1981; Room et al., 1981; Steindler, 1981). Such is presumably the case also for rapheo-cortical neurons (Fallon and Loughlin, 1982).

In the rat and monkey, the intracortical distributions of the NA and 5-HT systems have now been studied in considerable detail. There are no regions of cerebral cortex without both an NA and a 5-HT innervation. In rat neocortex, the NA axons have been shown to be rather uniformly distributed between the various cytoarchitectonic areas (Fuxe et al., 1968a; Levitt and Moore, 1978). Morrison et al. (1978) have, however, insisted on a certain predominance in layers I and IV of the somatosensory and visual cortices. The overlap with specific thalamic afferents in layer IV has led to the suggestion that the NA system might somehow modulate the response of cortical neurons to thalamic input (see also Morrison et al., 1978; Lidov et al., 1978). In primates, the cortical NA innervation exhibits a greater degree of regional and laminar heterogeneity (Morrison et al., 1982a,b, 1984; Kosofsky et al., 1984; Levitt et al., 1984b). It is the richest in somatosensory cortex, but the least dense in posterior parietal and occipital areas, in sharp contrast with the visual cortex of the rat. A bilaminar pattern of NA input is also noticeable in the monkey, but involving different layers depending upon the area examined and sparing layer IV in visual cortex.

As shown some years ago (Descarries et al., 1975; Beaudet and Descarries, 1976), the 5-HT innervation of cerebral cortex is much more dense and widespread than was initially suspected from fluorescence histochemical studies (Fuxe, 1965; Fuxe et al., 1968b). Early radioautographic studies indicated a tenfold greater number of 5-HT than NA terminals in adult rat frontoparietal cortex (Lapierre et al., 1973; Beaudet and Descarries, 1976). The topographic distribution of the cortical 5-HT input was particularly well documented by subsequent immunohistochemical investigations following the development of specific antibodies against 5-HT–formaldehyde–protein conjugate (Lidov et al., 1980; Steinbusch, 1981; Morrison et al., 1982b, 1984; Takeuchi and Sano, 1983; Kosofsky et al., 1984). The 5-HT terminals were then described as rather equally distributed to all layers in most regions of rat neocortex, except in the posterior cingulate area where clear predilection for laminae I and III was noted (Lidov *et al.*, 1980). In primates, greater differences have again been observed, not only between different cortical regions but also within given cytoarchitectonic areas such as striate cortex (Morrison *et al.*, 1982b).

These data have been taken to indicate that, coincident with the extensive phylogenetic development of the neocortex, there was a parallel elaboration and differentiation of its NA and 5-HT inputs (for review, see Morrison *et al.*, 1984). Eventual quantification of the regional and laminar distribution of these innervations in various species and under various conditions, should help to elucidate their respective roles in cortical function.

2.2. Ultrastructural Features

It is mainly with radioautography that the fine structural features of monoamine terminals have thus far been analyzed in mammalian cerebral cortex (for detailed review, see Beaudet and Descarries, 1984; but see also Molliver *et al.*, 1982). This method takes advantage of the powerful reuptake and storage mechanisms of the monoamine neurons. Radiolabeled NA or 5-HT brought into the immediate vicinity of these cells is concentrated into their varicosities or axon terminals. The accumulated radioactivity is then recorded into a nuclear emulsion superimposed on histological sections for light microscopy or ultrathin sections for electron microscopy.

Systematic examination of hundreds of NA and 5-HT varicosities specifically labeled in adult rat fronto-parietal cortex after topical application of the respective tritiated amine (Descarries *et al.*, 1975, 1977) led us to summarize as follows their main ultrastructural characteristics. These terminals belong to fine unmyelinated axons of small caliber. They are elongated or spherical, averaging 0.7 and 1 μm in diameter in the case of the 5-HT and the NA endings. As defined by the presence of aggregated synaptic vesicles, only a small fraction (< 5%) of these sectional profiles are endowed with the zone of membrane differentiation usually found at synapses (junctional complex). According to probability estimates of seeing these junctions in single thin sections (Beaudet and Sotelo, 1981), it may be assumed that more than 80% of either these NA or 5-HT varicosities do not form true synaptic contacts (Table I).

The notion of nonjunctional innervations has attracted considerable attention since its original formulation with Alain Beaudet in 1975 (Descarries *et al.*, 1975). It has had particular impact on current hypotheses regarding the mode of operation and hence presumed function of the monoamine neurons, not only in cerebral cortex but also in many other brain regions where nonjunctional terminals have subsequently been described (for a review of 5-HT data, see Beaudet and Descarries, 1987). We have proposed that in the cerebral cortex or elsewhere, NA and 5-HT endings might thus be ideally built to act at a distance on vast neuronal ensembles (see Beaudet and Descarries, 1978), perhaps accounting for rather general, sustained and/or indirect

Table I. Incidence of Synaptic Junctions Made by Monoamine Terminals in Adult Rat Cerebral Cortex

	Noradrenaline[a]	Serotonin[b]	Dopamine[c]	
Cortical region	Frontoparietal	Frontoparietal	Mediofrontal	Suprarhinal
Number of profiles	1835	303	121	130
Mean diameter (μm)	1.15	0.7	0.7	0.7
Width of junctions (μm)	0.2–0.4	0.2–0.4	0.23	0.25
Percent showing junction	3.3	4.3	25.6	16.2
Synaptic incidence	10–20%	15–20%	80–85%	50–55%

[a]Based on Descarries *et al.* (1977).
[b]Based on Descarries *et al.* (1975).
[c]See text for explanations.

or mediated effects of these transmitters, often called modulation to distinguish them from classical transmission (Reader et al., 1979). Whatever name is given to such processes, the concept of a diffuse broadcasting of information by nonjunctional terminals might account for various paradoxical findings. For example, it could explain obvious mismatches between the distribution of certain membrane receptors for biogenic amines and that of their respective terminals in cerebral cortex (Wamsley, 1984). Similarly, a widespread action of the biogenic amine would be consistent with the fact that a protein like synapsin, which is phosphorylated through an effect mediated by membrane receptors for NA, is found to be distributed to all nerve endings in cerebral cortex (Mobley and Greengard, 1985). We have also speculated that the rarity of junctional complexes formed by NA or 5-HT terminals in some regions of the CNS could contribute to their particular plasticity and adaptive properties as manifested in various experimental models (e.g., Wiklund et al., 1981).

3. The Dopamine Innervation of Cerebral Cortex

3.1. Topographic Distribution

In dealing with the general topography of this projection, we face a much more compartmentalized organization (for review, see Lindvall and Björklund, 1984). In the rat CNS, the mesocortical DA projection is only one of nine or ten DA subsystems, e.g., meso-striatal, tubero-infundibular, incerto-hypothalamic, diencephalo-spinal (Björklund and Lindvall, 1984). Following demonstration of the origin of these DA afferents in the DA nerve cell body groups of the ventral midbrain tegmentum (Fuxe et al., 1974; Lindvall et al., 1974), numerous biochemical, histo-fluorescence, and immunohistochemical reports have emphasized their restricted distribution in adult rat cerebral cortex (Berger et al., 1974, 1976; Hökfelt et al., 1974a,b, 1977; Lidbrink et al., 1974; Lindvall and Björklund, 1974; Collier and Routtenberg, 1977; Emson and Koob, 1978; Fallon and Moore, 1978a,b; Fallon et al., 1978; Lindvall et al., 1978, 1984; Lewis et al., 1979; Palkovits et al., 1979). The DA innervation of rat cortex has thus usually been described as being confined to the anteromedial or prefrontal, the anterior cingulate or pre- and supragenual, the suprarhinal, the perirhinal, the piriform, and the entorhinal cortex. A recent immuno- and histo-chemical study has revealed the presence of additional DA terminal fields in the motor, visual, and retrosplenial cortex, but it is generally believed that other cortical regions are free of DA varicosities. The compartmentation of the DA system is also manifested by the fact that, in most cortical regions thus far examined, it shows a clear predilection for a restricted number of cortical layers. Moreover, there is increasing suggestive evidence from retrograde fluorescent tracer studies that individual DA neurons innervating the cerebral cortex do not collateralize extensively to other brain regions and have fairly circumscribed intracortical territories of projection (Fallon and Loughlin, 1982; Swanson, 1982; Albanese and Minciacchi, 1983; Loughlin and Fallon, 1984). As yet, few morphological data are available concerning the cortical DA innervation in the monkey. However, there are preliminary indications that, in this species, it may extend throughout the entire motor cortex (Levitt et al., 1984a,b; Berger et al., 1986).

In the last 2 years, in collaboration with Brigitte Berger, we have sought further insights into the topographic distribution of the DA innervation of cerebral cortex by the use of an improved technique for the radioautographic visualization of monoamine terminals in slices of rat whole cerebral hemisphere (Descarries et al., 1987; Doucet et al., 1987). Specific labeling of these DA endings was achieved by in vitro incubation with 10^{-6} M tritiated DA in the presence of a monoamine oxidase inhibitor and of desipramine to prevent cross specific uptake of the tracer in NA and 5-HT terminals (Nguyen-Legros et al., 1981). The slices were fixed, embedded in Epon, and processed for radioautography as large 4-μm-thick sections.

Figure 1 is a camera lucida drawing of one of these light microscope radioautographs

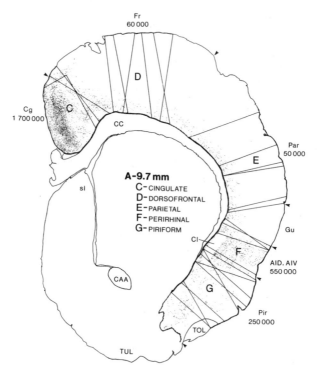

Figure 1. Diagrammatic representation of the topographic distribution and density of cortical DA innervation in a transverse plane across adult rat cerebral hemisphere at the level of the genu of the corpus callosum. The plane of sectioning corresponds approximately to A-10.7 mm in Zilles's (1985) stereotaxic atlas. The labeled varicosities were mapped with a camera lucida, in a light microscope radioautograph from a 4-μm-thick section of a whole hemisphere slice incubated with [³H]-DA as described in the text (for details, see Descarries *et al.*, 1987). The DA innervation shows an obvious predilection for the cingulate (Cg), dorsal and ventral insular agranular (AID, AIV), and piriform (Pir) cortex, but a significant number of terminals are also seen reaching into the mediodorsal frontal area and the deepest layer of the remaining frontal (Fr) and of the parietal (Par) neocortex. Note the sparing of the claustrum (Cl). Counts of the labeled varicosities were obtained from the boxed sectors designated by the letters (C–G), and transformed into number of DA endings per cubic millimeter of tissue (regional innervation density) as also described in the text. (Adapted from Descarries *et al.*, 1987.)

illustrating the overall distribution of DA terminals in a transverse section across the genu of the corpus callosum. In such preparations, the individual labeled varicosities may be clearly distinguished even at relatively low magnification (Fig. 2). As previously shown by histofluorescence studies, the cortical DA innervation at this midfrontal transverse plane shows an obvious predilection for the cingulate, insular agranular, and piriform areas. In addition, however, significant numbers of labeled DA terminals are seen reaching into the mediodorsal frontal agranular area (Berger *et al.*, 1985) as well as in the deepest layer of the entire dorsolateral frontal and parietal neocortex (Descarries *et al.*, 1987).

The DA varicosities labeled *in vitro* were also visualized at the electron microscopic level. In either the cingulate, perirhinal, or deep parietal cortex, they were found to average 0.7 μm in mean caliper diameter. Several were seen to be endowed with junctional complexes of synaptic specialization, such as the one in Fig. 3 coming from the narrow band of innervation overlying the callosal radiations in layer VI of parietal cortex.

As exemplified by Fig. 1, we have now mapped the cortical DA terminals at various levels across the hemisphere. The major advantage of this improved radioautographic approach is that it

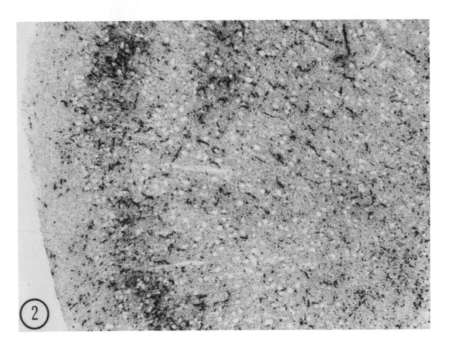

Figure 2. Light microscope radioautograph from the ''supragenual'' anterior cingulate cortex (sector C in Fig. 1) exemplifying the labeling of DA terminals observed in 4-μm-thick sections from whole hemisphere slices. In this region, the DA terminals predominate in layers II and III, but are also numerous in molecular layer I and the deep layers V and VI. Exposure time: 4 weeks. Magnification: 60 ×. Bar = 250 μm.

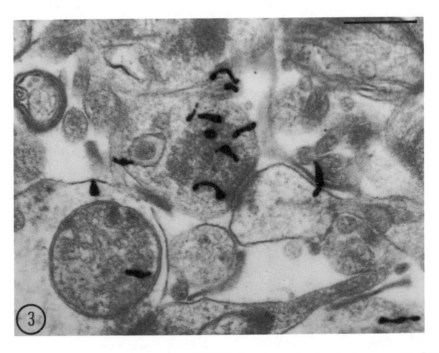

Figure 3. Electron microscope radioautograph of [³H]DA-labeled axonal varicosity from layer VI of parietal cortex. In spite of the relatively poor ultrastructural preservation of incubated tissue, this DA profile clearly exhibits all morphological attributes of a synaptic ending. The junctional complex is made on a dendritic spine but appears rather symmetrical. Round and clear, small synaptic vesicles are aggregated in the ''active zone.'' Para-phenelenediamine development after 4 months of radioautographic exposure; 40,000 ×. Bar = 0.5 μm.

permits quantification of the number of monoamine endings in any region of the rat brain. Conditions can be experimentally established that ensure integral labeling, and their number can be extrapolated to tissue volume by means of standard stereological techniques, provided that their average diameter and depth of detection in the sections are known (Doucet *et al.*, 1987). Using this tool, the density of DA innervation has now been estimated for various cytoarchitectonically and functionally defined regions of adult rat cortex (Descarries *et al.*, 1987). As shown in Fig. 1, the varying densities in different cortical sectors may be expressed in number of DA terminals per cubic millimeter of tissue: 1.7 million in the supragenual cingulate area; half a million in the perirhinal, insular cortex; 60,000 and 50,000, on the average, in the frontal and the parietal neocortex.

The density of DA innervation can also be evaluated in terms of the number of terminals per cubic millimeter of cortical layer to further compare the different anatomical subdivisions of the cortex. The laminar density of DA innervation shows variations, up to fivefold, within neocortical regions with high or moderate innervation densities (mediofrontal, suprahinal, and supragenual cingulate cortex). In layer VI of the dorsofrontal parietal and temporal neocortex, the density of DA innervation is far from negligible when expressed per cubic millimeter of a particular layer rather than per millimeter of whole cortical thickness. These results already allow for fruitful correlations with other measurable parameters of cortical function, albeit electrophysiological, neurochemical, or pharmacological, as illustrated in the following chapters by Reader *et al.* and Ouimet.

3.2. Ultrastructural Features

To examine the ultrastructural features of DA terminals in cerebral cortex, we have recently used immunocytochemistry with the highly specific antiserum against dopamine–glutaraldehyde–lysyl-protein conjugate raised by Geffard *et al.* (1984). The tissue was fixed *in vivo* by perfusion with 3.5% glutaraldehyde, immunostained with the peroxidase–antiperoxidase technique in the presence of saponin, postfixed with osmic acid, and embedded in Epon. Ultrathin sections were obtained from two regions of the cortex known to receive a relatively dense DA input: the deep layers of mediofrontal cortex representing the so-called anteromedian or prefrontal DA field, and, in the same transverse plane, layers IV to VI from the dorsal insular agranular cortex, in the suprarhinal DA field (Séguéla *et al.*, 1986, 1987).

The DA endings were readily identified by their strong and selective immunostaining (Figs. 4 and 5). Most of them showed synaptic vesicles of the small, round, and clear variety, sometimes associated with a few larger electronlucent vesicles and several densely staining ones. In both regions, a considerable proportion of these sectional profiles exhibited well-differentiated complexes of synaptic junction. Such synapses were usually found on dendritic shafts (Fig. 4), but some were also seen on dendritic spines. The junctional complexes were generally symmetrical, but a few asymmetrical ones were encountered on dendritic shafts as well as spines. In either cortical region, the DA terminals rarely came in close contact with neuronal perikarya. In the few such instances thus far observed, the relationship was a mere apposition with no visible membrane thickening, even in series of thin sections (Fig. 5).

A considerable number of these cortical DA varicosities have now been examined in either single or series of thin sections (Table I). As previously observed by radioautography *in vitro*, their mean diameter measured 0.7 μm. Their junctional complexes averaged 0.23 μm in width in the mediofrontal and 0.25 μm in the suprarhinal cortex. Based on these figures, and assuming that all such varicosities engage in synaptic relationships, the probability of seeing the synaptic membrane differentiation in single thin sections could be estimated at 32.4 and 38% in the mediofrontal and the suprarhinal cortex, respectively. This assumption of one synaptic junction per DA varicosity did not seem to be warranted, however, since the observed synaptic incidence in single thin sections amounted to only 25.6% in the mediofrontal and 16.2% in the suprarhinal cortex. From these latter figures, it could be inferred that, in the mediofrontal cortex, a vast

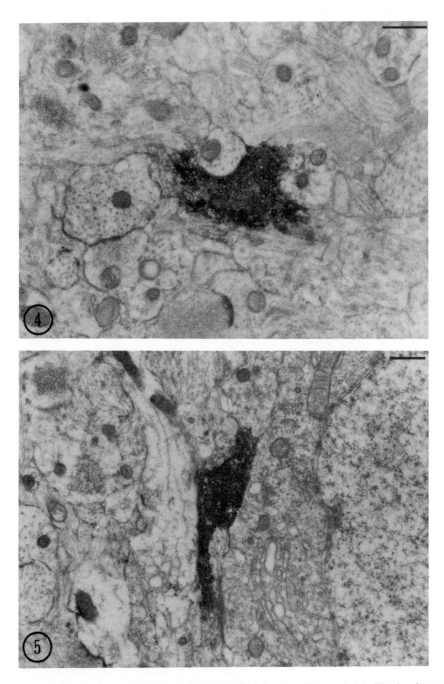

Figures 4 and 5. DA-immunostained endings from mediofrontal cortex. The terminal in Fig. 4 makes a symmetrical synaptic contact with a dendritic shaft. It mostly contains small, round, and clear synaptic vesicles, but several larger electronlucent vesicles as well as a few densely stained ones are also visible. In Fig. 5, the DA varicosity is in direct apposition with a nerve cell body. Such axosomatic contacts were rare, being made with only few cortical neurons within both regions examined. They failed to exhibit membrane differentiations even in serial sections. Further details are reported in Séguéla *et al.* (1987). Magnification: 25,000 × in Fig. 4; 20,000 × in Fig. 5. Bars = 0.5 μm.

majority, i.e., at least 80–85%, of the DA terminals are engaged in morphologically defined synaptic junctions, whereas in the suprarhinal cortex, only 50–55% do make a synaptic contact.

To verify this conclusion, we have further analyzed a fair number of DA-immunostained terminals in series of thin sections. As expected, the proportion of DA varicosities observed to make a synaptic junction was then found to be higher than in single sections in both the medio-frontal and the suprarhinal region. In the mediofrontal cortex, the synaptic incidence ranged from 50 to 92% depending on the number of thin sections in which the varicosities were visualized (from five to ten or more). In the suprarhinal cortex, the incidence of visible junctions also correlated with the number of thin sections, but plateaued at 56% in the longest series of ten sections or more. It is noteworthy that there was little difference between the values extrapolated stereologically from single thin sections and those directly obtained from the longest series sampling the whole thickness of DA varicosities. Interestingly also, the serial sections confirmed the statistically significant difference detected in single thin sections between the mediofrontal and the suprarhinal cortex.

4. Concluding Remarks

As shown in Table I, both mediofrontal and suprarhinal cortex show an incidence of DA junctional varicosities much greater than that previously determined for NA and 5-HT terminals in the frontoparietal cortex. Moreover, while the DA innervation appears to be mostly if not entirely junctional in one cortical region, it is only partly so in another. The functional significance of such differences should become clearer when similar investigations are carried out on more regions, in various species and at various stages of development. Until then, we can only speculate and reiterate a suggestion made several years ago that these structural features might reflect some rather general principle of morphological organization.*

There could be a relation of coherence at stake here, whereby highly anatomically divergent and widespread projection systems, such as the NA or 5-HT innervations of the cortex, would establish rather loose cellular interrelationships at the ultrastructural level as well, whereas more compartmentalized and more focused projections, such as the cortical DA innervation, would be the ones showing precise and perhaps more rigid synaptic connectivity. This theory holds true in view of the recent description of the histamine innervation of cerebral cortex, which also seems to be composed of predominantly nonjunctional axonal varicosities (Takagi *et al.*, 1986). It will certainly need to be refined and will undoubtedly call for adjustments in the light of new data. It is already clear that lumping all NA and 5-HT innervations of different brain regions into a single category is a gross oversimplification. Some NA or 5-HT neuronal subsets are undoubtedly focused and synaptic ones, and we have seen that the DA innervation may show variations in synaptic incidence even within a given CNS region, the cerebral cortex. The principle might hold considerable heuristic value, if only to predict some fundamental properties of the increasing number of chemically identified neuronal subsets nowadays identified in brain, and which really begin to defy the imagination in terms of mode of operation and functional significance.

ACKNOWLEDGMENTS. These investigations were mainly funded by grant MT-3544 from the Medical Research Council of Canada. The dopamine antiserum was kindly donated by Michel Geffard. P.S. was the recipient of a Herbert H. Jasper Fellowship at the Centre de Recherche en Sciences Neurologiques, and G.D. received financial support from Fonds FCAC and l'Équipe de Recherche sur les Neurotransmetteurs du Cerveau (FRSQ). The authors are also indebted to

---

*This hypothesis was first enunciated in the special lecture entitled "Cytological basis of central monoaminergic function" delivered by L.D. at the 6th European Neuroscience Congress, Malaga-Torremolinos, Spain, September 1982.

Sylvia Garcia for technical assistance, Giovanni Battista Filosi and Daniel Cyr for graphic and photographic work, and Lucie Perrault for typing the manuscript.

References

Adèr, J. P., Room, P., Postema, F., and Korf, J., 1980, Bilaterally diverging axon collaterals and contralateral projections from rat locus coeruleus neurons, demonstrated by fluorescent retrograde double labeling and norepinephrine metabolism, *J. Neural Transm.* **49**:207–218.

Albanese, A., and Minciacchi, D., 1983, Organization of the ascending projections from the ventral tegmental area: A multiple fluorescent retrograde tracer study in the rat, *J. Comp. Neurol.* **216**:406–420.

Beaudet, A., and Descarries, L., 1976, Quantitative data on serotonin nerve terminals in adult rat neocortex, *Brain Res.* **111**:301–309.

Beaudet, A., and Descarries, L., 1978, The monoamine innervation of rat cerebral cortex: Synaptic and non-synaptic relationships, *Neuroscience* **3**:851–860.

Beaudet, A., and Descarries, L., 1984, Fine structure of monoamine axon terminals in cerebral cortex, in: *Monoamine Innervation of Cerebral Cortex* (L. Descarries, T. A. Reader, and H. H. Jasper, eds.), Liss, New York, pp. 77–93.

Beaudet, A., and Descarries, L., 1987, Ultrastructural identification of serotonin neurons, in: *Monoaminergic Neurons: Light Microscopy and Ultrastructure* (H. W. M. Steinbusch, ed.), Wiley, Chichester, pp. 265–313.

Beaudet, A., and Sotelo, C., 1981, Synaptic remodeling of serotonin axon terminals in rat agranular cerebellum, *Brain Res.* **206**:305–329.

Berger, B., Tassin, J. P., Blanc, G., Moyne, M., and Thierry, A.-M., 1974, Histochemical confirmation for dopaminergic innervation of the rat cerebral cortex after destruction of the noradrenergic ascending pathways, *Brain Res.* **81**:332–337.

Berger, B., Thierry, A.-M., Tassin, J. P., and Moyne, M. A., 1976, Dopaminergic innervation of the rat prefrontal cortex: A fluorescence histochemical study, *Brain Res.* **106**:133–145.

Berger, B., Verney, C., Alvarez, C., Vigny, A., and Helle, K. B., 1985, New dopaminergic terminal fields in the motor, visual (area 18b) and retrosplenial cortex in the young and adult rat: Immunocytochemical and cate-cholamine histochemical analysis, *Neuroscience* **15**:983–995.

Berger, B., Trottier, S., Verney, C., Gaspar, P., and Alvarez, C., 1986, Major dopamine innervation of the cortical motor areas in the Cynomologous monkey. A radioautographic study with comparative assessment of serotonergic afferents, *Neurosci. Lett.* **72**:121–127.

Björklund, A., and Lindvall, O., 1984, Dopamine-containing systems in the CNS, in: *Handbook of Chemical Neuroanatomy*, Vol. 2 (A. Björklund and T. Hökfelt, eds.), Elsevier/North-Holland, Amsterdam, pp. 55–122.

Collier, T. J., and Routtenberg, A., 1977, Entorhinal cortex: Catecholamine fluorescence and Nissl staining of identical Vibratome sections, *Brain Res.* **128**:354–360.

Dahlström, A., and Fuxe, K., 1964, Evidence for the existence of monoamine-containing neurons in the central nervous system. I. Demonstration of monoamines in the cell bodies of brain stem neurons, *Acta Physiol. Scand.* **62**(Suppl. 232):1–55.

Descarries, L., Beaudet, A., and Watkins, K. C., 1975, Serotonin nerve terminals in adult rat neocortex, *Brain Res.* **100**:563–588.

Descarries, L., Watkins, K. C., and Lapierre, Y., 1977, Noradrenergic axon terminals in the cerebral cortex of rat. III. Topometric ultrastructural analysis, *Brain Res.* **133**:197–222.

Descarries, L., Lemay, B., Doucet, G., and Berger, B., 1987, Regional and laminar density of the dopamine innervation in adult rat cerebral cortex, *Neuroscience* **21**:807–824.

Doucet, G., Descarries, L., Audet, M. A., Garcia, S., and Berger, B., 1987, Radioautographic method for quantifying regional monoamine innervations in the rat brain: Application to the cerebral cortex, *Brain Res.* (in press).

Emson, P. C., and Koob, G. F., 1978, The origin and distribution of dopamine-containing afferents to the rat frontal cortex, *Brain Res.* **142**:249–267.

Fallon, J. H., and Loughlin, S. E., 1982, Monoamine innervation of the forebrain: Collateralization, *Brain Res. Bull.* **9**:295–307.

Fallon, J. H., and Moore, R. Y., 1978a, Catecholamine innervation of the basal forebrain. III. Olfactory bulb, anterior olfactory nuclei, olfactory tubercle and piriform cortex, *J. Comp. Neurol.* **180**:533–544.

Fallon, J. H., and Moore, R. Y., 1978b, Catecholamine innervation of the basal forebrain. IV. Topography of the dopamine projection to the basal forebrain and neostriatum, *J. Comp. Neurol.* **180**:545–580.

Fallon, J. H., Koziell, D. A., and Moore, R. Y., 1978, Catecholamine innervation of the forebrain. II. Amygdala, suprarhinal cortex and entorhinal cortex, *J. Comp. Neurol.* **180**:509–532.

Fuxe, K., 1965, Evidence for the existence of monoamine neurons in the central nervous system. IV. Distribution of monoamine nerve terminals in the central nervous system, *Acta Physiol. Scand.* **64**(Suppl. 247)**:**39–85.

Fuxe, K., Hamberger, B., and Hökfelt, T., 1968a, Distribution of noradrenaline nerve terminals in cortical areas of the rat, *Brain Res.* **8:**125–131.

Fuxe, K., Hökfelt, T., and Ungerstedt, U., 1968b, Localization of indolealkylamines in CNS, in: *Advances in Pharmacology*, Part A (S. Garattini and P. A. Shore, eds.), Academic Press, New York, pp. 235–251.

Fuxe, K., Hökfelt, T., Johansson, O., Jonsson, G., Lidbrink, P., and Ljungdahl, A., 1974, The origin of the dopamine nerve terminals in limbic and frontal cortex: Evidence for meso-cortico dopamine neurons, *Brain Res.* **8:**349–355.

Geffard, M., Buijs, R. M., Séguéla, P., Pool, C. W., and Le Moal, M., 1984, First demonstration of highly specific and sensitive antibodies against dopamine, *Brain Res.* **294:**161–165.

Hökfelt, T., Fuxe, K., Johansson, O., and Ljungdahl, Å., 1974a, Pharmacohistochemical evidence of the existence of dopamine nerve terminals in limbic cortex, *Eur. J. Pharmacol.* **25:**108–112.

Hökfelt, T., Ljungdahl, Å., Fuxe, K., and Johansson, O., 1974b, Dopamine nerve terminals in the rat limbic cortex: Aspects of the dopamine hypothesis of schizophrenia, *Science* **184:**177–179.

Hökfelt, T., Johansson, O., Fuxe, K., Goldstein, M., and Park, D., 1977, Immunohistochemical studies on the localization and distribution of monoamine neuron systems in the rat brain. II. Tyrosine hydroxylase in the telencephalon, *Med. Biol.* **55:**21–40.

Jasper, H. H., 1981, Problems of relating cellular or modular specificity to cognitive functions: Importance of state-dependent reactions, in: *The Organization of the Cerebral Cortex* (F. O. Schmitt, F.-G. Worden, G. Adelman, and S. G. Dennis, eds.), MIT Press, Cambridge, Mass., pp. 375–393.

Kosofsky, B. E., Molliver, M. E., Morrison, J. H., and Foote, S. L., 1984, The serotonin and norepinephrine innervations of primary visual cortex in the cynomolgus monkey (*Macaca fascicularis*), *J. Comp. Neurol.* **230:**168–178.

Lapierre, Y., Beaudet, A., Demianczuk, N., and Descarries, L., 1973, Noradrenergic axon terminals in the cerebral cortex of the rat. II. Quantitative data revealed by light and electron microscope radioautography of the frontal cortex, *Brain Res.* **63:**175–182.

Levitt, P., and Moore, R. Y., 1978, Noradrenergic neuron innervation of the neocortex in the rat, *Brain Res.* **139:**219–231.

Levitt, P., Rakic, P., and Goldman-Rakic, P. S., 1984a, Comparative assessment of monoamine afferents in mammalian cerebral cortex, in: *Monoamine Innervation of Cerebral Cortex* (L. Descarries, T. A. Reader, and H. H. Jasper, eds.), Liss, New York, pp. 41–59.

Levitt, P., Rakic, P., and Goldman-Rakic, P. S., 1984b, Region-specific distribution of catecholamine afferents in primate cerebral cortex: A fluorescence histochemical analysis, *J. Comp. Neurol.* **227:**23–36.

Lewis, M. S., Molliver, M. E., Morrison, J. H., and Lidov, H. G. W., 1979, Complementary of dopaminergic and noradrenergic innervation in anterior cingulate cortex of the rat, *Brain Res.* **164:**328–333.

Lidbrink, P., Jonsson, G., and Fuxe, K., 1974, Selective reserpine-resistant accumulation of catecholamines in central dopamine neurons after dopa administration, *Brain Res.* **67:**439–456.

Lidov, H. G. W., Rice, F., and Molliver, M. E., 1978, The organization of the catecholamine innervation of somatosensory cortex: The barrel field of the mouse, *Brain Res.* **153:**577–584.

Lidov, H. G. W., Grzanna, R., and Molliver, M. E., 1980, The serotonin innervation of the cerebral cortex in the rat: An immunohistochemical analysis, *Neuroscience* **5:**207–227.

Lindvall, O., and Björklund, A., 1974, The organization of the ascending catecholamine neuron systems in the rat brain as revealed by the glyoxylic acid fluorescence method, *Acta Physiol. Scand. Suppl.* **412:**1–48.

Lindvall, O., and Björklund, A., 1984, General organization of cortical monoamine systems, in: *Monoamine Innervation of Cerebral Cortex* (L. Descarries, T. A. Reader, and H. H. Jasper, eds.), Liss, New York, pp. 9–40.

Lindvall, O., Björklund, A., Moore, R. Y., and Stenevi, U., 1974, Mesencephalic dopamine neurons projecting to neocortex, *Brain Res.* **81:**325–331.

Lindvall, O., Björklund, A., and Divac, I., 1978, Organization of catecholamine neurons projecting to the frontal cortex in the rat, *Brain Res.* **142:**1–24.

Lindvall, O., Björklund, A., and Skagerberg, G., 1984, Selective histochemical demonstration of dopamine terminal systems in rat di- and telencephalon: New evidence for a dopaminergic innervation of hypothalamic neurosecretory nuclei, *Brain Res.* **306:**19–30.

Loughlin, S. E., and Fallon, J. H., 1984, Substantia nigra and ventral tegmental area projections to cortex: Topography and collateralization, *Neuroscience* **11:**425–435.

Loughlin, S. E., Foote, S. L., and Fallon, J. H., 1982, Locus coeruleus projections to cortex: Topography, morphology and collateralization, *Brain Res. Bull.* **9:**287–294.

Mobley, P., and Greengard, P., 1985, Evidence for widespread effects of noradrenaline on axon terminals in the rat frontal cortex, *Proc. Natl. Acad. Sci. USA* **82:**945–947.

Molliver, M. E., Grzanna, R., Lidov, H. G. W., Morrison, J. H., and Olschowka, J. A., 1982, Monoamine systems in the cerebral cortex, in: *Cytochemical Methods in Neuroanatomy* (V. Chan-Palay and S. L. Palay, eds.), Liss, New York, pp. 255–277.

Morrison, J. H., Grzanna, R., Molliver, M. E., and Coyle, J. T., 1978, The distribution and orientation of noradrenergic fibers in the neocortex of the rat: An immunofluorescence study, *J. Comp. Neurol.* **181**:17–40.

Morrison, J. H., Molliver, M. E., Grzanna, R., and Coyle, J. T., 1981, The intracortical trajectory of the coeruleocortical projection in the rat: A tangentially organized cortical afferent, *Neuroscience* **6**:139–158.

Morrison, J. H., Foote, S. L., O'Connor, D., and Bloom, F. E., 1982a, Laminar, tangential and regional organization of the noradrenergic innervation of monkey cortex: Dopamine-β-hydroxylase immunohistochemistry, *Brain Res. Bull.* **9**:309–319.

Morrison, J. H., Foote, S. L., Molliver, M. E., Bloom, F. E., and Lidov, H. G. W., 1982b, Noradrenergic and serotonergic fibers innervate complementary layers in monkey primary visual cortex: An immunohistochemical study, *Proc. Natl. Acad. Sci. USA* **79**:2401–2405.

Morrison, J. H., Foote, S. L., and Bloom, F. E., 1984, Regional, laminar, developmental, and functional characteristics of noradrenaline and serotonin innervation patterns in monkey cortex, in: *Monoamine Innervation of Cerebral Cortex* (L. Descarries, T. A. Reader, and H. H. Jasper, eds.), Liss, New York, pp. 61–75.

Nagai, T., Satoh, K., Imamoto, K., and Maeda, T., 1981, Divergent projections of catecholamine neurons of the locus coeruleus as revealed by fluorescent retrograde double labeling techniques, *Neurosci. Lett.* **23**:117–123.

Nguyen-Legros, J., Berger, B., and Alvarez, C., 1981, High resolution radioautography of central dopaminergic fibers labeled in vitro with [³H]dopamine or [³H]norepinephrine, *Brain Res.* **213**:265–276.

Palkovits, M., Zaborszky, L., Brownstein, M. J., Fekete, M. I. K., Herman, J. P., and Kanyicska, B., 1979, Distribution of norepinephrine and dopamine in cerebral cortical areas of the rat, *Brain Res. Bull.* **4**:593–601.

Reader, T. A., Ferron, A., Descarries, L., and Jasper, H. H., 1979, Modulatory role for biogenic amines in the cerebral cortex: Microiontophoretic studies, *Brain Res.* **160**:217–229.

Room, P., Postema, F., and Kort, J., 1981, Divergent axon collaterals of rat locus coeruleus neurons: Demonstration by a fluorescent double labeling technique, *Brain Res.* **221**:219–230.

Séguéla, P., Watkins, K. C., and Descarries, L., 1986, Preliminary data on the ultrastructural features of dopamine terminals in adult rat cerebral cortex, *Soc. Neurosci. Abstr.* **12**:770.

Séguéla, P., Watkins, K. C., and Descarries, L., 1987, Ultrastructural features of dopamine axon terminals in the anteromedial and the suprarhinal cortex of adult rat. *Brain Res.* (in press).

Steinbusch, H. W. M., 1981, Distribution of serotonin in the central nervous system of the rat—Cell bodies and terminals, *Neuroscience* **6**:557–618.

Steindler, D. A., 1981, Locus coeruleus neurons have axons that branch to the forebrain and cerebellum, *Brain Res.* **223**:367–373.

Swanson, L. W., 1982, The projections of the ventral tegmental area and adjacent regions: A combined fluorescent retrograde tracer and immunofluorescence study in the rat, *Brain Res. Bull.* **9**:321–353.

Takagi, H., Morishima, Y., Matsuyama, T., Hayashi, H., Watanabe, T., and Wada, H., 1986, Histaminergic axons in the neostriatum and cerebral cortex of the rat: A correlated light and electron microscopic immunocytochemical study using histidine decarboxylase as a marker, *Brain Res.* **364**:114–123.

Takeuchi, Y., and Sano, Y., 1983, Immunohistochemical demonstration of serotonin nerve fibers in the neocortex of the monkey (*Macaca fuscata*), *Anat. Embryol.* **166**:155–168.

Wamsley, J. K., 1984, Autoradiographic localization of cortical biogenic amine receptors, in: *Monoamine Innervation of Cerebral Cortex* (L. Descarries, T. A. Reader, and H. H. Jasper, eds.), Liss, New York, pp. 153–174.

Wiklund, L., Møllgård, K., and Descarries, L., 1981, Serotoninergic axon terminals in the rat dorsal accessory olive: Normal ultrastructure and light microscopic demonstration of regeneration after 5,6-dihydroxytryptamine lesioning, *J. Neurocytol.* **10**:1009–1027.

Zilles, K., 1985, *The Cortex of the Rat: A Stereotaxic Atlas,* Springer-Verlag, Berlin.

22

The Heterogeneity of the Catecholamine Innervation of Cerebral Cortex
Biochemical and Electrophysiological Studies

Tomás A. Reader, André Ferron, Laurent Diop, Arlette Kolta, and Richard Brière

1. Introduction

1.1. The Cortical Catecholamine Innervation

The central catecholamine (CA) neurons in the brain stem and their CNS projections were the first to be described in correlative biochemical and histofluorescent investigations as chemically identified neurotransmitter systems. By combining histofluorescent, autoradiographic, and immunocytochemical methods with biochemical determinations of endogenous levels and activities of the enzymes of synthesis, three types of CA neuronal systems were described in the CNS, according to the monoamine they can synthesize and presumably use as their neurotransmitter, i.e., dopamine (DA; Berger *et al.*, 1974; Hökfelt *et al.*, 1974; Lindvall *et al.*, 1974), noradrenaline (NA; Carlsson *et al.*, 1962; Dahlström and Fuxe, 1964; Fuxe, 1965; Fuxe *et al.*, 1968; Ungerstedt, 1971; Lindvall and Björklund, 1974), and adrenaline (AD; Hökfelt *et al.*, 1973; Van der Gugten *et al.*, 1976; Versteeg *et al.*, 1976; Reader, 1981).

In the particular case of the cerebral cortex, the afferent NA-containing nerve fibers and terminals (Carlsson *et al.*, 1962) originate almost entirely in the locus coeruleus (Ungerstedt, 1971) or A6 region (Dahlström and Fuxe, 1964), and supply all regions of the allo- and isocortex of the adult rat (Fuxe *et al.*, 1968; Levitt and Moore, 1978), but with a seemingly sparse and ubiquitous innervation (Lapierre *et al.*, 1973). The NA fibers spread throughout all six cortical layers, with a certain predominance in the outer molecular layer and in layers II and III. Such a laminar repartition has been well documented in autoradiographic surveys for the rat frontoparietal cortex (Descarries and Lapierre, 1973; Descarries *et al.*, 1977, 1987). However, using the immunocytochemical localization of dopamine-β-hydroxylase, the NA-containing axons in

Tomás A. Reader, André Ferron, Laurent Diop, Arlette Kolta, and Richard Brière • Centre de Recherche en Sciences Neurologiques, Département de Physiologie, Faculté de Médecine, Université de Montréal, Montreal, Quebec, H3C 3J7, Canada.

the cerebral cortex do not seem to be distributed diffusely, but form hierarchical and geometrically ordered patterns, which vary from one species to another (Morrison *et al.*, 1979, 1984).

The topographic distribution of the DA cortical innervation appears to be more compartmentalized. For the rat brain, the earlier histofluorescent studies demonstrated DA nerve fibers as having their terminal fields confined only to restricted cortical areas, mainly in the anteromedial or prefrontal, the anterior cingulate or pre- and supragenual, the suprarhinal, perirhinal, piriform, and entorhinal regions (Thierry *et al.*, 1973; Hökfelt *et al.*, 1974; Berger *et al.*, 1974; Lindvall *et al.*, 1974). Although biochemical studies have shown that DA exists in many other cortical regions of both the cat (Reader *et al.*, 1976, 1979b; Jones *et al.*, 1977; Törk and Turner, 1981; Reader and Quesney, 1986) and the rat (Kehr *et al.*, 1976; Versteeg *et al.*, 1976; Palkowitz *et al.*, 1979; Reader, 1981), its presence when determined biochemically cannot warrant a true dopaminergic pathway, since DA is the natural precursor of NA. Because of the technical difficulties of histofluorescence, the existence of DA nerve fibers in areas such as the parietal and occipital cortex of the rat has often been questioned. It is only recently by combined histofluorescence and immunocytochemical approaches that new DA terminals have been visualized in the motor, visual, and retrosplenial cortex of young and adult rats (Berger *et al.*, 1985). This survey has been complemented by the autoradiographic quantification of DA nerve endings in several cortical areas (Descarries *et al.*, 1987, see also Chapter 21).

We thus have very refined anatomical and biochemical descriptions of the cortical afferent CA innervation, but this information has to be related to the sites of action of these putative neurotransmitters at the level of the target cells. Such a perspective is deemed necessary to understand the functional role of CA in the cerebral cortex as well as in the other CNS regions innervated by these systems, and inevitably calls upon the need to investigate their specific receptors.

1.2. The Cortical NA Receptors

The adrenergic receptors have been classified into α and β adrenoceptors according to well-established pharmacological criteria. Ahlquist (1948) differentiated two types of physiological responses to CA, due to the activation of distinct α and β adrenergic receptors. The relative potencies of CA and agonists were then used to define β_1 and β_2 adrenergic receptors (Lands *et al.*, 1967). The α adrenergic receptors were then subclassified by their anatomical location and/or functional properties (Langer, 1974; Starke, 1977). The activation of presynaptic α adrenoceptors reduces NA release by a negative feedback mechanism independent of uptake, and this subtype was coined as α_2. On the other hand, the postsynaptic α adrenoceptors mediating orthodox synaptic neurotransmission were designated as α_1 (Starke, 1981). The possible existence of α_2 adrenoceptors located postsynaptically has led to a purely pharmacological definition (Berthelson and Pettinger, 1977; Timmermans and Van Zwieten, 1982). Presently this classification of α_1 and α_2 subtypes relies upon pharmacological criteria, i.e., their relative affinities for specific agonists and antagonists, and thus is independent of their location and/or function (Bylund and Snyder, 1976; Wood *et al.*, 1979; Starke, 1981; Leibowitz *et al.*, 1982; Bylund and U'Prichard, 1983; Dausse *et al.*, 1984). More recently, a certain heterogeneity of adrenoceptors of the α_2 type has been reported (Bylund, 1985) so that eventually these different subtypes may explain various mechanisms and modes of action underlying NA effects in the CNS and in the periphery. In the cerebral cortex, direct binding studies have shown the existence of α_1 (Miach *et al.*, 1978; Glossmann and Presek, 1979; Hornung *et al.*, 1979; U'Prichard *et al.*, 1979; Reader and Brière, 1983; Reader *et al.*, 1986a, 1987), α_2 (Glossmann and Presek, 1979; U'Prichard *et al.*, 1979; Diop *et al.*, 1983; Pimoule *et al.*, 1983; Gadie *et al.*, 1984; Reader *et al.*, 1986a, 1987), and β adrenoceptors (Alexander *et al.*, 1975; Bylund and Snyder, 1976; Minneman *et al.*, 1979; Sutin and Minneman, 1985). These *in vitro* biochemical assays can be performed with relatively small incubation volumes, and the samples obtained from well-delimited and restricted anatomical regions, thus permitting the mapping of the distribution of receptor sites in the CNS. Such a macroscopic approach provides accurate estimations of binding parameters as well as of some of the biochemical and pharmacological characteristics at a regional level, and thus complements autoradiographic surveys of receptor localization (Young and Kuhar, 1980; Palacios and Kuhar, 1982; Rainbow and Biegon, 1983; Unnerstall *et al.*, 1985; Jones *et al.*, 1985). One of the aims of our investigations was to determine the distribution (receptor number or density) and apparent affinities (dissociation constants) of adrenergic receptors using three antagonists: i.e., [^{3}H]prazosin ([^{3}H]-PRZ) for the α_1 adrenoceptors, [^{3}H]idazoxan ([^{3}H]-IDA; RX-781094) for the α_2 adrenoceptors, and [^{3}H]dihydroalprenolol ([^{3}H]-DHA) for total β-adrenergic binding sites, in five well-defined areas of the rat cerebral cortex. To relate the biochemical mapping of receptor sites to the distribution of endogenous CA levels, the monoamine contents in the different regions were determined by high-performance liquid chromatography (HPLC) coupled to electrochemical detection. The five cortical areas chosen in this study represent distinct functional regions, of relative ease of dissection and for which the CA contents have been documented in previous studies (Kehr *et al.*, 1976; Van der Gugten *et al.*, 1976; Versteeg *et al.*, 1976; Palkovits *et al.*, 1979; Reader, 1980a, 1981, 1983; Slopsema *et al.*, 1982; Westerink and De Vries, 1985).

1.3. Electrophysiology of Cortical CA Receptors

The most frequent and consistent response to the microiontophoretic application of CA on cortical neurons is a depression of firing (Krnjević and Phillis, 1963; Phillis *et al.*, 1973; Stone and Taylor, 1977; Reader *et al.*, 1979a; Armstrong-James and Fox, 1983; for reviews, see Krnjević, 1974, 1984; Reader, 1983; Phillis, 1984). There are very few studies, however, on regional variations or particular characteristics of these responses when the CA are iontophoresed in different anatomical and functional cortical areas. In a first series of electrophysiological studies, we examined the responsiveness of spontaneously active cortical neurons in two different regions: the cingulate cortex, known to be densely innervated by DA and NA afferents, and the somatosensory cortex, where the major CA is NA, and where there are lower levels of endogenous DA. These two areas are only a part of the prefrontal and parietal cortical areas which we dissected out for the biochemical assay of adrenergic receptors and the determinations of monoamine content. Therefore, the aim of this electrophysiological survey was to examine the responsiveness of the cortical neurons to the microiontophoretic application of DA and NA and determine if there are quantitative differences between two differentially innervated areas of the cerebral cortex.

Besides exerting an influence on cortical excitability, the CA have also been proposed to have other effects, such as the relative enhancement of synaptic responses (Waterhouse and Woodward, 1980). In some of the electrophysiological experiments, the use of spontaneously active neurons to study CA effects may sometimes be inadequate, since we do not know why these neurons are actively firing in the first place. A paradigm in which cortical neurons are synaptically activated (synaptically driven) may prove to be more adequate to reveal certain modulatory (Reader *et al.*, 1979a) actions of DA and NA. For example, in the adult cat, the iontophoresis of NA in the visual cortex reduces the firing of a majority of cells stimulated by light flashes (Reader, 1978b). These findings were confirmed by Videen and co-workers, who found that NA mainly inhibited the background ("noise") firing of visually driven neurons in kittens and adult cats, thus enhancing the signal-to-noise (S/N) ratio (Videen *et al.*, 1984). If NA modulates the excitability and background firing of cortical neurons, the types of adrenergic receptors involved have yet to be demonstrated. Preliminary electrophysiological experiments (Kolta *et al.*, 1987) designed to characterize the responses to the microiontophoretic application of NA in the occipital (visual) cortex and to determine a possible participation of the α_2 subtype of adrenoceptors in the mediation of these effects are presented below.

2. Materials and Methods

2.1. Tissue Dissections

Adult male Sprague–Dawley rats (250–300 g) were decapitated and their brains quickly removed and placed on crushed ice. The neocortex was dissected under a binocular stereo-microscope as previously described (Kehr et al., 1976; Reader, 1980b, 1981), with a plastic chamber (Henry and Yashpal, 1984) to perform the coronal sections. All visible white matter, blood clots, and pia were carefully removed. The samples of prefrontal cortex (PF) included the most rostral part of the cerebral cortex, from anterior (A) 10,000 μm (König and Klippel, 1963) as the posterior limit to the poles of the hemispheres. The most rostral portion of the caudate nucleus and the olfactory bulbs were dissected out from this sample. The frontal cortex (FR) was obtained between the planes A 10,000 μm and A 7000 μm. It included all the gray matter dorsal to a horizontal plane situated at H 0.0, and the striatum was carefully removed, using as a landmark the fibers of the corpus callosum. The parietal cortex (PA) extended from A 7000 μm to A 4000 μm, and included all the dorsolateral cortex above H 0.0, and limited internally by the white matter of the corpus callosum. The sample of occipital cortex (OCC) was obtained from A 4000 μm to posterior (P) 500 μm, and included the occipital lobes, which were carefully dissected flat and the hippocampus entirely removed. The temporal cortex (TE; or region R in Kehr et al., 1976) was obtained from the slices used for the PA and OCC areas, and included all the cortical tissue lateral to the hypothalamus (entorhinal and piriform cortices), between A 5000 μm and P 500 μm; lateral (L) 2000 μm to 6000 μm and from H -2600 μm to -4500 μm (Reader, 1980b).

2.2. Monoamine Assays

For monoamine assays, the dissected cortical samples from 14 rats were homogenized in 0.1 N cold $HClO_4$ containing 4 mM Na_2EGTA in a glass homogenizer with a Teflon pestle. These homogenates were centrifuged (20,000g for 45 min at 4°C) and the supernatants used for assays by HPLC with ion-pairing and electrochemical detection, following established procedures (Keller et al., 1976; Mefford, 1981; Debets, 1985; Lakhdar-Ghazel et al., 1986; Reader et al., 1986b). The pellets were dissolved overnight in 1 N NaOH for protein assay (Lowry et al., 1951), using bovine serum albumin as standard.

2.3. Binding Assays

The dissected cortical regions were homogenized in 40 volumes (w/v) of cold 50 mM sodium/potassium phosphate buffer, pH 7.4 (Pimoule et al., 1983; Reader et al., 1986a, 1987) for the assay of α adrenoceptors (i.e., [³H]-PRZ for the α_1 sites and [³H]-IDA for the α_2 sites), using a Polytron (15 sec). These homogenates were centrifuged (49,000g, 15 min at 4°C), the pellets washed twice, and resuspended in the same cold buffer. For the β adrenoceptor assays the membranes were homogenized in a Tris–HCl buffer (5 mM at pH 7.4) containing 250 mM sucrose, washed twice in this buffer, and finally resuspended in an incubation buffer made of Tris–HCl (50 mM, pH 7.4). Such membrane preparations were incubated with the radioligands at 25°C for 30–45 min. At the end of the incubation, the mixtures were diluted in 2 ml of cold buffer followed by rapid filtration (5 sec) under vacuum through Whatman GF/C glass fiber filters. The filters were washed twice with 5 ml of cold buffer. Radioactivity was counted by liquid scintillation (Econofluor, New England Nuclear) in an LKB 1215 Rackbetta II counter (efficiency 55–65%). Nonspecific binding represented $< 20\%$ of total binding for [³H]-PRZ, $< 25\%$ of total binding for [³H]-IDA, and $< 20\%$ of total binding for [³H]-DHA. The unlabeled propranolol HCl and phentolamine HCl used in the receptor binding assays were generous gifts of Ayerst and Ciba Pharmaceuticals, respectively. Protein concentrations were assayed (Lowry et al., 1951) in 100-μl aliquots of membrane preparations, and were usually between 1.5 and 2.0 mg/ml.

Analysis of the binding experiments was performed by the iterative analysis "FIT" (Barlow, 1983), a procedure originally developed by Parker and Waud (1971), which gives a more precise estimate of both the density of receptor sites and the dissociation constant than the conventional Scatchard method (Scatchard, 1949; Klotz, 1982; Zivin and Waud, 1982). To speed execution, the original BASIC program was compiled into machine language code for a 6502-based microprocessor, using TASC (Microsoft, Inc., Bellevue, Wash.), thus reducing by five to ten times the duration for iterations. In addition, the data were also examined using SCAT: i.e., a Scatchard plot (Scatchard, 1949), but with a nonlinear, least-squares curve-fitting iterative procedure based on Feldman's parameter fitting (Feldman, 1972; Munson and Rodbard, 1980; Diop et al., 1987). The statistical analysis to compare "goodness of fit" for one or two classes of binding sites was performed by comparing the residual variance of fits (the ratio of sum of squares of residuals divided by the degrees of freedom) to the data by F statistics (Draper and Smith, 1966). Results are expressed as the mean $\pm$ S.E.M., and the statistical analysis of the data was carried out using the unpaired Student's t-test.

2.4. Microiontophoretic Technique

Adult male Sprague–Dawley rats (250–300 g) were used throughout this study. For the recordings, animals anesthetized with urethane (1.25–1.5 g/kg, i.p.) were placed in a stereotaxic frame. The bone overlying the occipital cortex was removed, the dura mater retracted and the surface of the cerebral cortex covered with 2% agar dissolved in 0.9% NaCl. Standard microiontophoretic and extracellular recording techniques were employed (Curtis, 1964; Krnjević, 1964; Salmoiraghi and Weight, 1967; Reader, 1978a,b). Five- or seven-barrel micropipettes, having an overall tip diameter of 5–8 μm, were filled with the following drugs dissolved in 0.1% ascorbic acid and at pH 4.0: noradrenaline HCl (NA; 0.5 M); dopamine HCl (DA; 0.5 M); apomorphine (APO; 0.1 M); clonidine HCl (CLO; 0.1 M); idazoxan HCl (IDA; 0.01 M); and oxymetazoline HCl (OXY; 0.1 M). The resistance of the recording barrel was 2–6 megohms. The central barrel, filled with 2–3 M NaCl, was used for recording, and one of the side barrels (2 M NaCl) used as a balancing channel in conjunction with the operational amplifier (Geller and Woodward, 1972) of the microiontophoresis programmer (BH-2 Neurophore system, Medical Systems, New York). Backing currents of -10 nA were used when not ejecting drugs. Extracellular unitary activity was amplified (P-511; Grass, Massachusetts) displayed on an oscilloscope, and the spikes discriminated by a voltage amplitude discriminator. The neuronal firing rates were integrated with a linear ratemeter over 10-sec intervals, and only neurons with a relatively stable rate of discharge were studied. For the occipital (visual) cortex, on-line analysis of spontaneously active and of visually driven (VD) cells were performed with an averager and digitized with an A/D converter (Adalab; Interactive Microware, Pennsylvania), so that peristimulus histograms (PSH) could be generated using 128 bins of 0.5 to 10 msec/bin. VD cortical units were characterized by the PSH in response to a Grass P-20 photostimulator (Kolta et al., 1987). Another set of microiontophoretic experiments was performed in cingulate and parietal cortex, and in these studies the responsiveness to the application of DA and NA was assessed by the IT_{50} method: i.e., by calculating the current (in nA) $\times$ time (in sec) required to obtain a 50% depression of the firing rate of the spontaneously active units (de Montigny and Aghajanian, 1978; de Montigny et al., 1980).

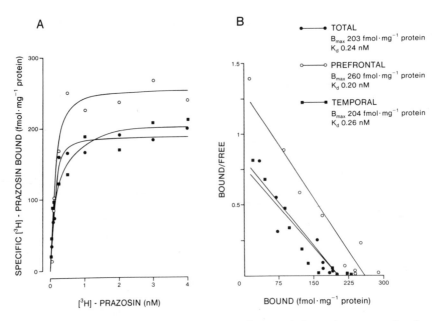

Figure 1. (A) Representative saturation curves obtained with [³H]prazosin in membrane preparations from total (●), prefrontal (○), and temporal (■) cerebral cortex. Membrane preparations were added in 60-μl aliquots to tubes already containing 15 μl of cold buffer, with or without 10 μM phentolamine for nonspecific binding. The saturation experiments were performed at equilibrium with 10–12 dilutions of [³H]prazosin (19.8 or 22.6 Ci/mmole, New England Nuclear; 0.005 to 4 nM, final concentration) and the ligands added in 75-μl aliquots. The final assay volumes were 150 μl, and the tubes incubated at 25°C for 45 min (see Materials and Methods). (B) Scatchard representation of the same saturation curves; the binding parameters B_{max} and K_d were determined by iteration according to Feldman's procedure (see Materials and Methods).

3. Results

3.1. Adrenergic Receptor Distribution

The saturation curves obtained with the tritiated adrenergic antagonists ([³H]-PRZ, [³H]-IDA, and [³H]-DHA) in membrane preparations from total cortex and from the five cortical regions, showed in every case that specific binding was saturable and of high affinity.

3.1.1. Saturation Experiments with [³H]-PRZ

In membrane preparations from total cortex, the saturation curves with [³H]-PRZ revealed by the iterative analysis "FIT" a maximum binding capacity (B_{max}) of about 180 fmoles/mg protein (Fig. 1), and the identification of a single class of binding sites, with a high apparent affinity, as judged by the value of the equilibrium dissociation constant (K_d 25°C) of about 0.16 nM. In addition, the Hill (1910) coefficient confirmed the existence of a single class of α_1 adrenoceptors (Table I). To verify the estimated K_d value, the data were plotted according to the Hill equation, i.e., using the x intercept of the least-square linear-regression analysis of the Hill plot.* The

---

*This analysis is the log ($B/B_{max} - B$) as a function of the log concentration of the radioligand, and where B is the amount bound at each concentration and B_{max} the maximum binding capacity derived by the iterative analysis "FIT". When half the population of available receptors is occupied, then $B/(B_{max} - B) = 1$, and the log is 0, so that the extrapolated x intercept provides the value for the antilog of the K_d (Zivin and Waud, 1982; Reader and Brière, 1983; Reader *et al.*, 1986a, 1987).

Table I. Specific [³H]-Prazosin Binding to Membrane Preparations
from Rat Cerebral Cortex[a]

		Binding capacities (B_{max})		
		SCAT (fmoles/mg protein)	FIT (fmoles/mg protein)	Hill coefficient
Total	(To)	173.6 ± 10.3	181.9 ± 9.3	1.307 ± 0.041
Prefrontal	(PF)	253.0 ± 12.1**	257.7 ± 7.7***	1.221 ± 0.075
Frontal	(FR)	191.2 ± 16.4	191.5 ± 13.5	1.222 ± 0.079
Parietal	(PA)	177.1 ± 21.1	187.3 ± 23.7	1.288 ± 0.064
Occipital	(OCC)	158.8 ± 13.6	165.6 ± 14.9	1.099 ± 0.065
Temporal	(TE)	143.9 ± 12.6	153.2 ± 17.9	0.876 ± 0.074

		Dissociation constants (K_d)		
		SCAT (nM)	FIT (nM)	Hill (nM)
Total	(To)	0.134 ± 0.030	0.160 ± 0.013	0.151 ± 0.013
Prefrontal	(PF)	0.175 ± 0.047	0.167 ± 0.021	0.172 ± 0.014
Frontal	(FR)	0.181 ± 0.050	0.164 ± 0.014	0.182 ± 0.024
Parietal	(PA)	0.198 ± 0.051	0.182 ± 0.020	0.185 ± 0.006
Occipital	(OCC)	0.178 ± 0.055	0.142 ± 0.013	0.150 ± 0.016
Temporal	(TE)	0.201 ± 0.080	0.147 ± 0.040	0.175 ± 0.052

[a]The values represent the mean ± S.E.M. of six separate experiments, performed with six membrane preparations, and in duplicate. Statistical significance was determined using Student's unpaired-t test to compare the homogenates from each region with the total (To) homogenates; **$p < 0.01$ and ***$p < 0.001$.

analysis of the Scatchard plot according to Feldman's method (Draper and Smith, 1966; Feldman, 1972) gave a single straight unbroken line, indicating one class of sites with no evidence of cooperativity. In all experiments, Scatchard plots were better fitted by a one-site than by a two-site model. The values obtained by the "FIT" and the "SCAT" iterations for B_{max} and K_d are given in Table I. The analyses of saturation curves performed by different methods with membrane preparations from the different cortical regions revealed the same values for K_d and Hill coefficients (n_H), but there were differences in the receptor number (B_{max}). In the PF cortex, [³H]-PRZ binding capacity was greater than that measured in the other cortical regions studied.

3.1.2. Saturation Experiments with [³H]-IDA

The specific binding of [³H]-IDA to total cortex membranes was a saturable process, with a maximum binding capacity of 155 ± 10 fmoles/mg protein and an equilibrium dissociation constant (K_d 25°C) between 1.4 and 1.7 nM (Fig. 2). The iterative analyses by either method yielded similar binding parameters (Table II). The Hill coefficients were not significantly different from unity and the Scatchard analysis showed a straight line with no evidence of cooperativity. These results suggest that [³H]-IDA binds to a single class of α_2 adrenoceptors under the present experimental conditions. For the five anatomically defined cortical areas, the values for K_d and n_H were not different from those determined for total cortex (Table II). Again, as was the case for the α_1 sites labeled with [³H]-PRZ, the number (B_{max}) of [³H]-IDA binding sites varied, according to the region examined. The assay of α_2 sites with [³H]-IDA demonstrated a rather uniform density of binding sites in the first four regions examined, i.e., PF, FR, PA, and OCC areas. However, there was a significant difference for the TE region, which showed the highest value for the maximum binding capacity.

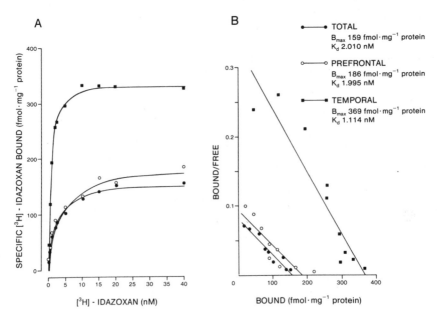

Figure 2. (A) Representative saturation curves obtained with [³H]idazoxan in membrane preparations from total (●), prefrontal (○), and temporal (■) cerebral cortex. Membrane preparations were added in 60-μl aliquots to tubes already containing 15 μl of cold buffer, with or without 10 μM phentolamine for nonspecific binding. The saturation experiments were performed at equilibrium with 10–12 dilutions of [³H]idazoxan (56.1 Ci/mmole, Amersham; 0.05 to 40 nM, final concentration) and the ligands added in 75-μl aliquots. The final assay volumes were 150 μl, and the tubes incubated at 25°C for 45 min (see Materials and Methods). (B) Scatchard representation of the same saturation curves; the binding parameters B_{max} and K_d were determined by iteration according to Feldman's procedure (see Materials and Methods).

Table II. Specific [³H]-Idazoxan Binding to Membrane Preparations from Rat Cerebral Cortex[a]

		Binding capacities (B_{max})		
		SCAT (fmoles/mg protein)	FIT (fmoles/mg protein)	Hill coefficient
Total	(To)	168.4 ± 12.2	153.7 ± 11.3	1.018 ± 0.055
Prefrontal	(PF)	181.0 ± 11.9	177.3 ± 12.2	0.784 ± 0.073
Frontal	(FR)	167.6 ± 16.2	171.3 ± 13.2	0.889 ± 0.048
Parietal	(PA)	158.5 ± 19.3	152.6 ± 16.9	0.748 ± 0.025
Occipital	(OCC)	153.2 ± 16.9	146.9 ± 16.1	0.999 ± 0.046
Temporal	(TE)	376.1 ± 37.6***	374.6 ± 33.9***	0.873 ± 0.046

		Dissociation constants (K_d)		
		SCAT (nM)	FIT (nM)	Hill (nM)
Total	(To)	1.777 ± 0.173	1.453 ± 0.200	1.537 ± 0.187
Prefrontal	(PF)	1.214 ± 0.177	1.283 ± 0.263	1.307 ± 0.256
Frontal	(FR)	1.975 ± 0.225	2.370 ± 0.155	2.350 ± 0.155
Parietal	(PA)	1.819 ± 0.246	1.936 ± 0.286	2.174 ± 0.243
Occipital	(OCC)	2.198 ± 0.433	2.086 ± 0.472	2.067 ± 0.443
Temporal	(TE)	1.196 ± 0.161	1.370 ± 0.282	1.302 ± 0.259

[a]The values represent the mean ± S.E.M. of six separate experiments, performed with six membrane preparations, and in duplicate. Statistical significance was determined using Student's unpaired-t test to compare the homogenates from each region with the total (To) homogenates; ***$p < 0.001$.

3.1.3. Saturation Experiments with [³H]-DHA

[³H]-DHA bound with high affinity and in a saturable manner to membranes for total cortex (Fig. 3). The K_d (25°C) for [³H]-DHA was about 1.5 nM with a maximal number of binding sites of 100 fmoles/mg protein. The values obtained by either FIT or SCAT for the B_{max} and K_d were not significantly different (Table III). The density of total β adrenergic binding sites labeled with [³H]-DHA for the five regions examined was very homogeneous, i.e., the binding parameters (K_d, B_{max}, and n_H) were not significantly different from those found for homogenates of total cortex.

3.2. Cortical Monoamine Contents

The biochemical assays of endogenous monoamines showed that the highest levels were found in the TE region, i.e., the ventral cortex lateral to the hypothalamus, in agreement with previous fluorometric (Kehr et al., 1976) and radioenzymatic (Versteeg et al., 1976; Palkovits et al., 1979; Reader, 1981) studies. In the present determinations, great care was taken to identify the peaks eluted from the column and separate the metabolites, so that they would not interfere and add up to the levels of CA and 5-HT (Fig. 4). The NA concentration was highest in the TE region ($p < 0.01$), but lower and very homogeneous for the other cortical areas (Table IV). The two metabolites of NA [4-hydroxy-3-methoxyphenylglycol (MHPG) and normetanephrine (NMN)] appear to be equally distributed. A slightly higher level of MHPG for the TE region did not attain a statistical level of significance, due to the dispersion in the individual samples. The DA levels were also highest in the TE region ($p < 0.001$), as well as the contents of its three metabolites: 4-hydroxy-3-methoxyphenylacetic acid (HVA), 3,4-dihydroxyphenylacetic acid (DOPAC), and 3-methoxytyramine (3-MT). Traces of adrenaline (AD) and metanephrine (MTN)

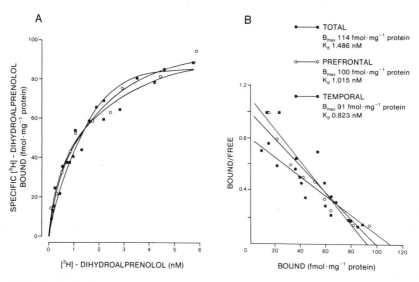

Figure 3. (A) Representative saturation curves obtained with [³H]dihydroalprenolol in membrane preparations from total (●), prefrontal (○), and temporal (■) cerebral cortex. Membrane preparations were added in 150-μl aliquots to tubes already containing 75 μl of cold buffer, with or without 10 μM propranolol HCl for nonspecific binding. The saturation experiments were performed at equilibrium with 10 dilutions of [³H]dihydroalprenolol (82 Ci/mmole, Amersham; 0.2 to 10 nM, final concentration) and the ligands added in 75-μl aliquots. The final assay volumes were 300 μl, and the tubes incubated at 25°C for 30 min (see Materials and Methods). (B) Scatchard representation of the same saturation curves; the binding parameters B_{max} and K_d were determined by iteration according to Feldman's procedure (see Materials and Methods).

Table III. Specific [³H]-Dihydroalprenolol Binding to Membrane Preparations
from Rat Cerebral Cortex[a]

		Binding capacities (B_{max})		
		SCAT (fmoles/mg protein)	FIT (fmoles/mg protein)	Hill coefficient
Total	(To)	102.0 ± 7.6	100.3 ± 4.1	0.967 ± 0.031
Prefrontal	(PF)	96.5 ± 6.9	107.5 ± 10.6	0.875 ± 0.086
Frontal	(FR)	107.1 ± 11.3	112.7 ± 7.8	0.920 ± 0.057
Parietal	(PA)	106.3 ± 13.2	115.9 ± 13.7	0.813 ± 0.020
Occipital	(OCC)	102.8 ± 5.8	111.6 ± 7.0	0.931 ± 0.037
Temporal	(TE)	98.6 ± 11.6	106.7 ± 11.4	0.918 ± 0.041

		Dissociation constants (K_d)		
		SCAT (nM)	FIT (nM)	Hill (nM)
Total	(To)	1.316 ± 0.187	1.549 ± 0.187	1.414 ± 0.194
Prefrontal	(PF)	1.060 ± 0.192	1.234 ± 0.418	1.840 ± 0.404
Frontal	(FR)	0.984 ± 0.109	1.294 ± 0.145	1.265 ± 0.141
Parietal	(PA)	0.985 ± 0.065	1.369 ± 0.195	1.411 ± 0.152
Occipital	(OCC)	1.363 ± 0.229	1.762 ± 0.248	1.734 ± 0.250
Temporal	(TE)	1.397 ± 0.165	1.913 ± 0.370	1.874 ± 0.367

[a]The values represent the mean ± S.E.M. of six separate experiments, performed with six membrane preparations, and in duplicate. There were no statistical differences using Student's unpaired-t test to compare the homogenates from each region with the total (To) homogenates.

were detected in all regions, but since the existence of a defined adrenergic pathway to the neocortex has not been established, these observations do not warrant further speculation. In any case, it was important to be able to detect these compounds to ascertain that they were not contaminating other peaks. The indoleamine 5-HT was more abundant in the TE region ($p <$ 0.001) as compared to the other areas. Its metabolite, 5-hydroxyindole-3-acetic acid (HIAA), appeared slightly higher in the TE and PF regions, although we could not document any significant differences in the present study. There were also traces of 5-hydroxy-1-tryptophan (5-HTP) in all the cortical areas.

3.3. Microiontophoretic Studies

The effects of the microiontophoretic application of DA and NA were examined on spontaneously active cells in the parietal, cingulate, and occipital cortical areas, as well as on VD neurons of the occipital cortex.

For the studies in the cingulate and parietal cortex, in most cases the cells studied were recorded from the same rats with the same pipette, so as to allow for adequate comparisons of eventual sensitivity differences. Most of the data for the parietal cortex were obtained from deep layer neurons. The proportion of spontaneously firing neurons depressed (Reader et al., 1979a) by DA or NA was the same in both the cingulate and the parietal cortex. For DA we recorded from 45 neurons in both cingulate and parietal cortical areas. There were no significant differences in the IT_{50} values for DA in these two regions (cingulate = 1782 ± 208 nC versus parietal = 1363 ± 139 nC). In the case of NA, we recorded from 18 neurons in the cingulate cortex (IT_{50} = 812 ± 131 nC) and from 21 in the parietal area (IT_{50} = 836 ± 106 nC). As was

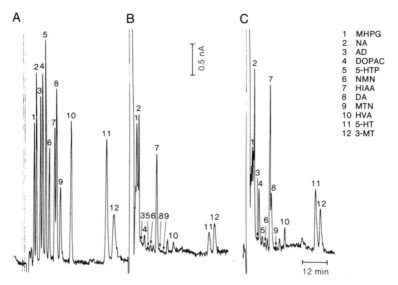

Figure 4. Continuous chromatograms of (A) the external standard solution of monoamines (3.25 ng of each compound) and (B) a sample from the parietal (PA) cortex (flow 0.7 ml/min). (C) Chromatogram of a sample from the temporal (TE) cortex (flow 0.8 ml/min). The peaks are: 1, 4-hydroxy-3-methoxyphenylglycol (MHPG); 2, noradrenaline (NA); 3, adrenaline (AD); 4, 3,4-dihydroxyphenylacetic acid (DOPAC); 5, 5-hydroxy-1-tryptophan (5-HTP); 6, normetanephrine (NMN); 7, 5-hydroxyindole-3-acetic acid (HIAA); 8, dopamine (DA); 9, meta-nephrine (MTN); 10, 4-hydroxy-3-methoxyphenylacetic acid (HVA); 11, serotonin (5-HT); 12, 3-methoxytyramine (3-MT). Briefly, 200-μl aliquots of the HClO₄ extract of the tissue samples, filtered over a 0.2-μm mesh (RC-58, Schleicher and Schuell), were injected into a reversed-phase column (5-μm particles, 250 mm × 4.6 mm Biophase ODS, Bioanalytical Systems; BAS, West Lafayette, Ind.). The mobile phase was composed of 0.15 M mono-chloroacetic acid, containing 750 mg/liter disodium EDTA, 240–280 mg/liter octyl sodium sulfate (Eastman Kodak, Rochester, N.Y.), and 10–14% methanol, adjusted to pH 3.35–3.40 with 1 N NaOH, and degassed under vacuum prior to use. The column was maintained at 32–38°C and the effluent detected at +850 mV using a glassy carbon electrode against the indifferent Ag/AgCl electrode (LC-4B amperometric detector, BAS). The flow was kept at 0.6–0.8 ml/min (PM-30A double piston pump, BAS), the different peaks integrated, and their surfaces compared with external standards of known amounts (100 pg–6.25 ng).

Table IV. Endogenous Monoamine Contents in Five Regions of the Cerebral Cortex[a,b]

		Prefrontal (PF)	Frontal (FR)	Parietal (PA)	Occipital (OCC)	Temporal (TE)
NA	(N = 14)	2.58 ± 0.33	2.58 ± 0.34	2.24 ± 0.28	2.61 ± 0.35	6.49 ± 1.17**
MHPG	(N = 12)	2.43 ± 0.58	2.18 ± 0.48	2.49 ± 0.60	2.60 ± 0.68	4.53 ± 1.33
NMN	(N = 8)	0.20 ± 0.07	0.33 ± 0.07	0.18 ± 0.03	0.23 ± 0.03	0.31 ± 0.04
AD	(N = 14)	0.05 ± 0.01	0.06 ± 0.01	0.07 ± 0.01	0.05 ± 0.01	0.14 ± 0.03
MTN	(N = 8)	0.10 ± 0.02	0.15 ± 0.04	0.19 ± 0.03	0.10 ± 0.02	0.13 ± 0.03
DA	(N = 14)	0.23 ± 0.08	0.21 ± 0.05	0.22 ± 0.06	0.21 ± 0.05	1.52 ± 0.29***
DOPAC	(N = 14)	0.50 ± 0.08	0.40 ± 0.05	0.28 ± 0.06	0.16 ± 0.03	1.78 ± 0.22***
HVA	(N = 14)	0.81 ± 0.15	0.78 ± 0.14	0.45 ± 0.11	0.55 ± 0.12	1.41 ± 0.16**
3-MT	(N = 14)	8.30 ± 0.42	8.52 ± 0.47	8.08 ± 0.48	7.74 ± 0.41	10.09 ± 0.34*
5-HT	(N = 14)	1.46 ± 0.10	1.30 ± 0.10	1.05 ± 0.07	1.17 ± 0.26	2.69 ± 0.20***
HIAA	(N = 14)	5.84 ± 0.75	3.97 ± 0.48	3.12 ± 0.30	3.49 ± 0.39	7.85 ± 1.07
5-HTP	(N = 8)	0.14 ± 0.03	0.15 ± 0.03	0.08 ± 0.02	0.22 ± 0.01	0.20 ± 0.04

[a]Data from Diop et al. (1987).
[b]Results are expressed as the mean contents in ng/mg protein ± S.E.M. The less significant difference between the TE and the other cortical regions was determined by Student's unpaired-t test; *$p < 0.05$, **$p < 0.01$, and ***$p < 0.001$.

the case for DA, there were no significant differences in sensitivity of neurons in these two areas toward NA (Beauregard and Ferron, 1986).

Two populations of cells were sampled in the visual cortex of the rat, i.e., spontaneously active (SA) units and neurons that could be synaptically activated by using a visual stimulation (VD cells). In order to differentiate VD from SA neurons, we used the PSH in response to the photostimulator. However, it cannot be ruled out that some SA units were not also visual neurons, since the stimulus used may not have been adequate to drive them. Furthermore, SA units unresponsive to visual cues could also be participating in information processing by altering the excitability of synaptically driven VD cells. For the majority of cortical neurons (SA and VD) sampled throughout this study, NA and α_2 agonists exerted an inhibitory effect (Fig. 5); excitation was documented in only a few cases. As previously described for the rat frontoparietal cortex (somatosensory area), only in very few instances biphasic responses obtained (Reader *et al.*, 1979a). These results are summarized in Table V.

The microiontophoresis of NA (ejection currents of 10–30 nA for 30–60 sec) on VD neurons induced a long-lasting inhibition of firing in 67 (82%) of the 82 VD cells recorded. This effect started at 15 ± 1.7 sec (mean $\pm$ S.E.M.), attained a maximum effect at 61 ± 5 sec, and had an average duration of 199 ± 14 sec (Fig. 6). Analysis of the PSH showed that NA inhibitory effects first affected the background firing (late components: > 400 msec) and to a lesser degree the specific (earlier components) evoked response (Fig. 6). Since the effects of NA clearly outlasted not only the ejection period but the maximum effect, there was an increase in the S/N ratio of the majority of VD cells, especially evident during the recovery or immediately after recovery to control levels of discharge. In the present series of recordings, only 5 VD cells (5%) were excited while in 7 VD cells (9%) the firing frequency did not change. The excitations appeared during or after NA ejections, reached a maximum at 60 ± 30 sec, and returned progressively to control levels (average duration 133 ± 62 sec). In these cases there were no significant changes in the S/N ratio. Only three cells (2%) in this survey showed biphasic responses: i.e., NA first produced a short period of inhibition, rapidly followed by an increase in firing. Responses to NA were also

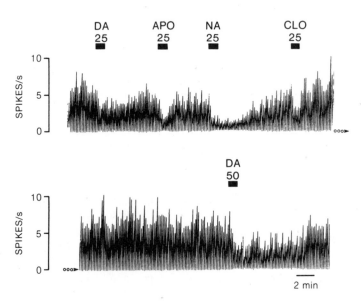

Figure 5. Continuous ratemeter record (integrated over 10-sec intervals) of the firing rate of a spontaneously active cortical neuron. The drugs dopamine (DA), apomorphine (APO), noradrenaline (NA), and clonidine (CLO) were applied for the time and dosage (in nA) indicated by the bars.

Table V. Effects of Adrenergic Drugs on Occipital
Cortex Neurons[a]

	VD neurons		SA neurons	
	N	Percent	N	Percent
Noradrenaline	82		52	
Inhibited	67	82	46	88
Excited	5	6	3	6
Biphasic[b]	3	3	0	0
Unaffected	7	9	3	6
Clonidine	42		31	
Inhibited	26	62	27	87
Excited	3	7	2	6
Unaffected	13	31	2	6
Oxymetazoline	10		6	
Inhibited	7	70	6	100
Excited	1	10	0	0
Unaffected	2	20	0	0

[a]Data from Kolta et al. (1987).
[b]These cells showed an inhibition followed by an excitation.

evaluated on the firing rate of SA neurons (Fig. 5) when encountered, and the effects were similar to the responses documented for the VD units (Fig. 6). Indeed, NA ejections inhibited the spontaneous firing rate of 46 (88%) of 52 SA cells tested, and excited only 3 SA cells (6%). The durations of the inhibitions obtained for SA units were of the same order of magnitude as those documented for VD cells (SA: 158 ± 17 sec; VD: 199 ± 14 sec). In only 3 SA cells (6%), the firing did not change after application of NA.

   The ejection of the α_2 adrenergic agonists (CLO and OXY; ejection currents of 10–30 nA for 10–30 sec) produced long-lasting inhibitions of firing in the majority of the neurons recorded from the visual cortex. For VD cells, CLO inhibited 62% of these neurons (Table V); the responses started at 52 ± 13 sec, attained a maximum at 113 ± 21 sec, and lasted 194 ± 38 sec. Only 3 VD neurons were excited by CLO and the response had a duration of 111 ± 50 sec. In 10 VD cells the agonist OXY was tested, and the inhibitory responses were gradual but of a much longer duration (> 12 min) than those produced by NA or CLO. As was the case for the natural agonist NA, the effects of CLO and OXY seemed to be preferentially exerted on the late components of the PSH (Fig. 5). For SA neurons the main effect of the α_2 agonists was again a reduction in firing. After the microiontophoretic application of CLO, this inhibition of firing rate started at 15 ± 3 sec, attained a maximum at 82 ± 14 sec, and had an average duration of 155 ± 27 sec (Fig. 5). The pattern of the inhibitory effects of selective α_2 agonists was similar to that induced by NA, i.e., a reduction of the firing frequency of discharge. Indeed, CLO and OXY mimicked the effects of neurotransmitter on both SA and VD cortical neurons. These effects of adrenergic agents (NA, CLO, and OXY) could be reduced or blocked by a previous ejection of the specific α_2 antagonist IDA in 50% of cells recorded (Fig. 5). In three neurons during the long-lasting inhibition produced by OXY, the administration of IDA proved to be effective in re-establishing the initial discharge rate.

4. Discussion

   To obtain a cortical topography of the distribution of adrenergic receptors using biochemical assays, the regions analyzed must be dissected both comparably and reproducibly. To this effect,

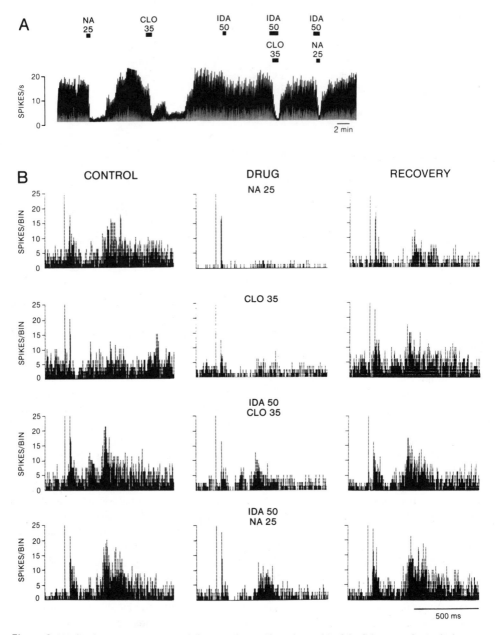

Figure 6. (A) Continuous ratemeter record (integrated over 10-sec intervals) of the firing rate of a cortical neuron in response to the photostimulator. The drugs noradrenaline (NA), clonidine (CLO), and idazoxan (IDA) were applied for the time and dosage (in nA) indicated by the bars. (B) Peristimulus histograms (PSH) of the cell shown in A generated by 60 successive sweeps each of 1024 msec duration. The PSH represent the firing of the neuron before, during the effect of the drugs, and the recovery period for (top to bottom): NA, CLO, IDA + CLO, IDA + NA.

we employed a procedure allowing an easy and exact delimitation of the rat cortex in five distinct areas. This dissection has allowed the characteristics of both NA and DA distributions using fluorometric assays (Kehr *et al.*, 1976). In their original work, Kehr and co-workers had to pool samples of three brains, due to the sensitivity limitations of their assays. In the present study, the use of an HPLC separation method coupled to electrochemical detection allowed us to measure the CA contents without pooling cortical samples. We also used a dissection chamber (Henry and Yashpal, 1984), which has several advantages: (1) the dissections can be carried out very uniformly with unfrozen tissue; (2) the whole procedure is rapid, taking only a few seconds to slice any one brain; and (3) the procedure is extremely reproducible from one rat to another, and this even if different persons perform the dissections.

The binding experiments, using small incubation volumes, were performed with membrane preparations from five different regions of the same animal. The saturation curves with [³H]-DHA, [³H]-PRZ, and [³H]-IDA were in the range of radioligand concentrations where specific binding was saturable, and then analyzed by the iterative method "FIT" (Barlow, 1983). This analysis of binding experiments requires the saturation of the binding isotherms. FIT solves the binding isotherms with equations derived from Taylor's theorem and the maximum binding capacity is calculated by direct fit of the data to the curve (Parker and Waud, 1971). The K_d obtained is derived from the ligand concentration required to occupy 50% of the total available binding sites. In addition, the same data can be used for a Hill-type analysis (Hill, 1910; Zivin and Waud, 1982; Barlow, 1983) a feature of interest since binding experiments could show departures from the law of mass action and/or some forms of allosteric behavior. All the saturation curves were also analyzed by SCAT, i.e., a nonlinear, least-squares curve-fitting iteration of a Scatchard plot (Feldman, 1972; Diop *et al.*, 1987; see also Munson and Rodbard, 1980). The statistical analysis of the comparison between one-site and two-site models allowed us to determine the best fit (Draper and Smith, 1966). In all experiments, the values obtained by the FIT or SCAT program for B_{max} and K_d were not significantly different. For total cortex, B_{max} and K_d were of the same order as those earlier reported in different studies with [³H]-PRZ for α_1 (Miach *et al.*, 1978; Glossmann and Presek, 1979; Hornung *et al.*, 1979; Dausse *et al.*, 1982, 1984; Reader and Brière, 1983; Brière *et al.*, 1986), with [³H]-IDA for α_2 (Pimoule *et al.*, 1983; Lakhdar-Ghazal *et al.*, 1986; Reader *et al.*, 1986a, 1987), and with [³H]-DHA for β adrenoceptors (Bylund and Snyder, 1976; Minneman *et al.*, 1979).

The distribution of the α adrenergic receptors in the five cortical areas examined was heterogeneous and two different patterns could be determined for the two types of α adrenergic binding sites. The highest concentration of α_1 adrenoceptors was located in the PF cortex, where it accounted for more than 60% of the total α adrenergic binding. Since the α_1 sites labeled by [³H]-PRZ are considered to be postsynaptic in the cerebral cortex (Reader and Brière, 1983), this ratio indicates a predominance of postsynaptic α_1 adrenoceptors over α_2 binding sites. The anatomical localization of α_2 adrenoceptors at presynaptic locations has not been proven. The upregulation of α_2 sites after surgical or chemical denervation of NA cortical neurons has been shown and this favors the existence of postsynaptic α_2 sites (U'Prichard *et al.*, 1979; Pimoule *et al.*, 1983). Indeed, α_2 adrenoceptors may not be entirely located on NA terminals. Although the α_2 antagonist radioligand [³H]rauwolscine discriminates two populations of α_2 sites (Diop *et al.*, 1983), and the exact pre- or postsynaptic nature of the α_2 sites recognized by [³H]-IDA may be debatable (U'Prichard *et al.*, 1979; Pimoule *et al.*, 1983; U'Prichard, 1984), it may be surmised that these sites have both pre- and postsynaptic localizations. Since endogenous NA content is moderate in the PF region (2.6 ng/mg protein), it could be considered an area of relatively important NA input, but with a predominance of target receptors of the α_1 subtype. In the FR and PA areas, the density of α_1 adrenoceptors was similar to that of α_2 adrenoceptors. The NA levels of FR, PA, and OCC are about the same as in PF; these cortices appear to have a moderate NA innervation. The densities of α_1 and α_2 adrenoceptors in OCC were lower but not significantly different, with a relative predominance of α_1 adrenoceptors. Thus, the α_1/α_2 ratio was 1.25. In contrast, the TE cortex showed the highest density of α_2 adrenoceptors with an α_1/α_2 ratio of 0.41. Interestingly, this region has the highest NA, DA, and 5-HT concentrations; since α_2 adrenoceptors are involved in the control of NA release, the predominance of the α_2 subtype suggests that a significant proportion of these receptors may have a presynaptic localization in this region.

The distribution of α adrenoceptors in the CNS has been examined using autoradiographic techniques. Among the first such surveys, it was shown that in the cerebral cortex there were moderate to low levels of widely distributed binding sites for the ligands [3H]-WB4101 (α_1 adrenoceptors) and [3H]p-amino-clonidine (α_2 adrenoceptor). For several cortical regions, the α_2 adrenoceptor distribution seems fairly uniform. At the intracortical level there is a slight preponderance of labeling in the more superficial laminae I–IV over that found in the deeper laminae V and VI. Interestingly, there are high levels of [3H]p-amino-clonidine binding sites in the piriform cortex (Young and Kuhar, 1980), which is part of the sample we dissected out as the TE region. This is the cortical area where the highest NA levels were found (Table IV) and where we measured the highest density [3H]-IDA binding sites (Table II).

For adrenoceptors of the α_1 type and employing [3H]-PRZ in autoradiographic surveys, there is a high incorporation in lamina V of the frontoparietal (or motor) cortical area (Rainbow and Biegon, 1983), with somewhat lower amounts for the other laminae in this area. In the somatosensory cortex (a more posterior cortical area), the highest labeling was also found in lamina V, but overall the density of [3H]-PRZ sites was lower than in the more frontal motor area. Based on these data, it has been proposed that the very high level of α_1 adrenoceptors in lamina V of the motor portion of the frontoparietal cortex is indicative of an important target site for the NA afferent innervation. However, the endogenous NA levels in this part of the neocortex are not very different (Table IV) from those measured in other cortical areas (Kehr et al., 1976; Van der Gugten et al., 1976; Versteeg et al., 1976; Palkovits et al., 1979; Reader, 1981; Slopsema et al., 1982; Westerink and De Vries, 1985). In this context it is important to note that the highest incidence of NA varicosities labeled with [3H]-NA in the frontoparietal cortex have been counted in the superficial laminae (Lapierre et al., 1973), and only less than 5% make punctate "classic" synaptic junctions (Descarries and Lapierre, 1973; Descarries et al., 1977; Beaudet and Descarries, 1984). This has led to the suggestion that NA is released in the cortex and diffuses for variable distances before attaining its specific receptors on the target cells. Therefore, perhaps only rough correlations can be made between the afferent NA innervation patterns and the densities of α_1 adrenergic receptors. A better correlation is found when the densities of α_2 adrenoceptors are compared to regional endogenous levels of NA, or with intracortical distributions of [3H]-NA-labeled varicosities. It has also been shown by autoradiography with [3H]-PRZ that human striate (visual) cortex has a high concentration of α_1 adrenoceptors, localized mainly in laminae I and VI, and there are lower densities but with a similar intracortical pattern for the precentral, postcentral, and superior temporal gyri (Wamsley, 1984). These findings suggest a regional heterogeneity and species differences in the distribution of adrenergic receptors, and should caution us when comparisons are made. Another important aspect is the type of ligand used to characterize and quantify the adrenoceptor type. In fact, there are differences in the labeling of α_1 sites when [3H]-PRZ and [3H]-WB4101 are compared (Unnerstall et al., 1985). In such an investigation the differences in labeling could be attributed to two different sites associated with a common α_1-receptor–effector complex. This suggestion was supported by in vitro binding data indicating differences in the equilibrium kinetics and inhibition dissociation constants (displacement experiments) with these two compounds, in contrast to the radioligand data which revealed a similar distribution of binding sites in the different regions examined, including the cerebral cortex. With the reservations due to the use of a different radioligand to label presumptive α_1 sites, it has been shown in in vitro binding assays (Sutin and Minneman, 1985) with [125I]-BE-2254 ([125I]-HEAT) that the highest density of α_1 sites is in the motor cortex, which corresponds in our study to the PF region or prefrontal cortex, in which we also measured the highest density of [^{3}H]-PRZ binding sites. The lowest concentration of α_1 adrenoceptors labeled with [^{125}I]-BE-2254 was found in the visual cortex, with somewhat higher values for the sensory and auditory cortical areas, in close agreement with the B_{max} values measured with [^{3}H]-PRZ in the present study (see Table I), since these areas correspond to the OCC, FR, and PA regions.

A homogeneous distribution of total β adrenoceptors labeled by [^{3}H]-DHA was found in the cortical regions examined here. In this respect the distribution differed markedly from that of NA content and α adrenoceptors, in agreement with previous biochemical in vitro assays using either [^{3}H]alprenolol (Alexander et al., 1975) or [^{125}I]iodocyanopindolol (Sutin and Minneman, 1985), as well as by the autoradiographic localization of [^{3}H]-DHA binding sites (Palacios and Kuhar, 1982). In the present study there was no attempt to discriminate between β_1 and β_2 subtypes. It is possible that some of the β adrenoceptors in the cerebral cortex may be more associated with nonneuronal structures such as blood vessels, pial membranes, or glial cells than with neuronal elements. However, a differential regional distribution of one or another subtype cannot be excluded. In autoradiographic studies with [^{H}]-DHA, β_1 binding sites seem to be concentrated in the superficial laminae (I–III) of rat parietal cortex (Wamsley, 1984), but it is doubtful that even such refined analysis can yield significant differences in distribution for particular areas in the cerebral cortex. In fact, in quantitative autoradiography of β_1 and β_2 adrenergic receptors with [^{125}I]pindolol selectively antagonized by ICI 89.406 or by ICI 118.551, there was no obvious correlation between the known locations of NA and AD terminal fields of innervation and the regions rich in β_1 and β_2 sites (Rainbow et al., 1984).

There are at present no quantitative data on the distribution of NA endings in rat visual cortex, but in the kitten, CA nerve endings are also distributed in all laminae of the visual cortex, and are more dense in laminae II and III (Itakura et al., 1981), in agreement with biochemical determinations of endogenous CA (Reader et al., 1979b). The rat visual cortex (occipital, areas 17 and 18) also receives an important noradrenergic input, as reflected by the endogenous levels of NA, measured by fluorometric (Kehr et al., 1976), radioenzymatic (Palkovits et al., 1979; Reader, 1981), and HPLC procedures (Sutin and Minneman, 1985; Diop et al., 1987). Recent studies suggest that NA may interact with α and β adrenoceptors in the cerebral cortex, and the stimulation of these receptors can regulate the enzymatic activity of adenylate cyclase (Sabol and Nirenberg, 1979; Lefkowitz et al., 1983). Moreover, the existence of both α_1 and β adrenoceptors has been demonstrated by direct receptor labeling experiments in the neocortex in general, as well as in the occipital cortex (Sutin and Minneman, 1985). Our present in vitro data show the presence of α_1, α_2, and β adrenoceptors in the rat visual (occipital) cortex. These biochemical findings would imply that NA could act as a specific neurotransmitter on adrenergic receptors of the target neurons in the visual cortex.

The microiontophoretic results show that NA affects both the spontaneous (i.e., unrelated to the presented stimulus) and evoked activities of neurons in the visual cortex of the rat. For the majority of SA (88%) and VD (82%) cells recorded, the application of NA induced long-lasting inhibitions of cortical neuronal firing, and in only a few cases was it possible to document excitations. These findings are in line with the depressant responses of NA on cortical neurons of adult rats (Jordan et al., 1972; Stone et al., 1975; Reader et al., 1979a; Olpe et al., 1980), kittens (Videen et al., 1984), adult cats (Krnjević and Phillis, 1963; Reader, 1978b; Videen et al., 1984), monkeys (Foote et al., 1975; Sawaguchi et al., 1986), and guinea pigs (Stone and Taylor, 1977). One of the proposed actions of NA, mediated by specific receptor subtypes, is modulation of neuronal excitability through the regulation of the enzymatic activity of the adenylate cyclase which synthesizes cAMP (Greengard and Kebabian, 1974; Stone et al., 1975). Such a mechanism of action requires a biochemical changes in cortical cells, compatible with the long duration of effects of NA on the firing rate, and which could reflect the phosphorylation of postsynaptic proteins involved in synaptic transmission (Dolphin and Greengard, 1981). In the present study the doses of NA used (20–30 nA) were lower than those previously employed (80–100 nA) and which usually produced very pronounced suppressions of neuronal firing (Reader, 1978, 1980a; Reader et al., 1979a). Therefore, the effects on VD cells were not maximal and the analysis of the PSH showed greater effects on the "noise," i.e., the firing unrelated to the stimulus (> 400 msec), than on the specific evoked response. At least two mechanisms can explain this enhancement of the S/N ratio: (1) the neuromodulator increases the specific evoked response without changing background discharge, (2) the evoked response remains constant but the background discharge decreases. It has been shown that NA can enhance the evoked firing of neurons without change of background firing (Woodward et al., 1979; Waterhouse et al., 1980), in support of a modulatory role for NA in the cerebral cortex. In contrast, Videen et al. (1984) working in the cat and kitten visual cortex reported that NA enhanced the S/N ratio, as a consequence of the reduction in the spontaneous activity. In the present study and for some of the VD cells, NA reduced background firing (late firing: > 400 msec), thus supporting the hypothesis that this neuromodulator increases the S/N ratio of a neuron to a stimulus.

Our present in vitro binding studies document three types of adrenergic receptors in the occipital (visual) cortex, and these are all possible candidates for the mediation of NA effects. To determine the involvement of adrenergic receptors of the α_2 subtype in the modulation of the activity in cortical neurons, we applied the agonists CLO and OXY. Previous studies had shown that CLO inhibits the firing of spontaneously active neurons in the locus coeruleus and raphe nucleus in anesthetized (Cedarbaum and Aghajanian, 1976; Freedman and Aghajanian, 1984) as well as unanesthetized animals (Reiner, 1985), and this effect can be blocked by the specific antagonist IDA. These findings not only demonstrated the involvement of α_2 adrenoceptors in the control of firing rate of brain stem neurons, but enabled the authors to conclude that IDA is the first α_2 adrenergic antagonist that allows the resolution of electrophysiological responses of this type (Freedman and Aghajanian, 1984). Pharmacological (Timmermans et al., 1979; Starke, 1981) and biochemical (U'Prichard et al., 1979; Wood et al., 1979; Bylund and U'Prichard, 1983; Lakhdar-Ghazal et al., 1986) studies have also shown specific interactions of CLO and OXY with receptors of the α_2 subtype in the cerebral cortex. In addition, pharmacological studies have shown that OXY is more potent than CLO (Struyker-Baudier et al., 1974; Sakurai et al., 1983), in line with the long duration of inhibitions here obtained by microiontophoresis of this agonist. In the present investigation, the microiontophoretic ejections of CLO and OXY produced long-lasting inhibitions of the firing of both SA and VD neurons. For VD cells, CLO and OXY also enhanced the S/N ratio by reducing the background firing more than the discharge evoked by the stimulus. Similar responses obtained with α_2 adrenergic agonists and the natural CA strengthen the hypothesis that this regulation could be mediated by α_2 adrenoceptors. Finally, and in support of the specificity of the receptor subtype involved, we were able to show that the inhibitory effects of adrenergic agents could be blocked or reduced in duration by microiontophoresis of the selective antagonist IDA (Chapleo et al., 1981; Freedman and Aghajanian, 1984).

The present biochemical survey of CA receptors clearly demonstrates a differential and nonhomogeneous distribution of α_1 and α_2 adrenoceptors in the rat cerebral cortex. In contrast, the β adrenoceptors are distributed relatively homogeneously in the cerebral neocortex. The distribution of α adrenoceptors is only one of the indexes of noradrenergic innervation, but when this information is correlated with the endogenous CA content, it becomes clear that the NA innervation of the mammalian cerebral cortex is hierarchically organized, and this is probably so for the specialized and functionally different cortical areas or regions.

The role of NA as a neuromodulator of neuronal activity, affecting the whole system's efficacy by modifying the S/N ratio, is a valid hypothesis for the visual cortex. Such a regulatory mechanism calls upon the participation of α_2 adrenoceptors, since NA effects are mimicked with α_2 agonists. Although the present demonstration of the involvement of α_2 adrenoceptors contributes to the understanding of some of the NA actions in the visual cortex, we cannot rule out a possible role of α_1 and β adrenergic receptors in the mediation of NA responses.

5. Concluding Remarks

For the past 12 years, the two senior authors have been greatly influenced by the thinking and work of Dr. Herbert H. Jasper. In their first articles with him on CA release and on the microiontophoresis of monoamines, they proposed a modulatory role for these neurotransmitters in the cerebral cortex. This hypothesis still seems valid, and now is even more refined, calling upon distinct receptor subtypes in hierarchically organized cortical areas. It is therefore a great challenge to be able to pursue such studies and a great honor to participate in this monograph. Finally, the best tribute the authors can offer is to continue their scientific endeavors in the domain introduced to them by Dr. Jasper, and while doing so, to guide younger scientists in this pathway of discovery.

ACKNOWLEDGMENTS. The authors' studies referred to in this chapter were funded by grants from the Medical Research Council (MRC) of Canada to T.A.R. (MT-6967) and A.F. (MA-8666). Personal support was provided by the Fonds de la Recherche en Santé du Québec (FRSQ) to T.A.R. (Chercheur-boursier Senior) and R.B. (Studentship). A.F. is an MRC Scholar. L.D. is a Postdoctoral Fellow (Equipe de recherche sur les neurotransmetteurs du cerveau-FRSQ, and Herbert H. Jasper Fellow, Centre de recherche en sciences neurologiques). The expert technical assistance of Miss L. Grondin and that of Miss H. Dussault in typing the manuscript are greatly appreciated. Credit for the graphic work goes to Mrs. G. B. Filosi and D. Cyr.

References

Ahlquist, R. P., 1948, Study of adrenotropic receptors, *Am. J. Physiol.* **153**:586–600.

Alexander, R. W., Davis, J. N., and Lefkowitz, R. J., 1975, Direct identification and characterization of β-adrenergic receptors in rat brain, *Nature* **258**:437–440.

Armstrong-James, M., and Fox, K., 1983, Effects of iontophoresed noradrenaline on the spontaneous activity of neurones in cat primary somatosensory cortex, *J. Physiol. (London)* **335**:427–447.

Barlow, R. B., 1983, Line fitting by least-squares: Expressions solved by iterations, in: *Biodata Handling with Microcomputers,* Elsevier, Amsterdam, pp. 114–185.

Beaudet, A., and Descarries, L., 1984, Fine structure of monoamine axon terminals in cerebral cortex, in: *Monoamine Innervation of the Cerebral Cortex* (L. Descarries, T. A. Reader, and H. H. Jasper, eds.), Liss, New York, pp. 77–93.

Beauregard, M., and Ferron, A., 1986, Neuronal responsiveness to biogenic amines and GABA in rat cingulate vs. parietal cortex: Comparative microiontophoretic study, *Soc. Neurosci. Abstr.* **12**:1517.

Berger, B., Tassin, J.-P., Blanc, G., Moyne, M. A., and Thierry, A. M., 1974, Histochemical confirmation for dopaminergic innervation of the rat cerebral cortex after destruction of the noradrenergic ascending pathway, *Brain Res.* **81**:332–337.

Berger, B., Verney, C., Alvarez, C., Vigny, A., and Helle, K. B., 1985, New dopaminergic terminal fields in the motor, visual (area 18b) and retrosplenial cortex in the young and adult rat: Immunocytochemical and catecholamine histochemical analyses, *Neuroscience* **15**:983–998.

Berthelsen, S., and Pettinger, W. A., 1977, A functional basis for the classification of alpha-adrenergic receptors, *Life Sci.* **21**:595.

Brière, R., Sherwin, A. L., Robitaille, Y., Olivier, A., Quesney, L. F., and Reader, T. A., 1986, α-1 adrenoceptors are decreased in human epileptic foci, *Ann. Neurol.* **19**:26–30.

Bylund, D. B., 1985, Heterogeneity of alpha-2 adrenergic receptors, *Pharmacol. Biochem. Behav.* **22**:835–843.

Bylund, D. B., and Snyder, S. H., 1976, Beta adrenergic receptor binding in membrane preparations from mammalian brain, *Mol. Pharmacol.* **12**:568–580.

Bylund, D. B., and U'Prichard, D. C., 1983, Characterization of α1- and α2- adrenergic receptors, *Int. Rev. Neurobiol.* **24**:343–431.

Carlsson, A., Falck, B., and Hillarp, N.-A., 1962, Cellular localization of brain monoamines, *Acta Physiol. Scand. Suppl.* **196**:1–28.

Cedarbaum, J. M., and Aghajanian, G. K., 1976, Noradrenergic neurons of the locus coeruleus: Inhibition by epinephrine and activation by the α-antagonist piperoxan, *Brain Res.* **112**:413–419.

Curtis, D. R., 1964, Microelectrophoresis, in: *Physical Techniques in Biological Research*, Vol. 5 (W. L. Nastuk, ed.), Academic Press, New York, pp. 144–190.

Dahlström, A., and Fuxe, K., 1964, Evidence for the existence of monoamine-containing neurons in the central nervous system I. Demonstration of monoamines in the cell bodies of brain stem neurons, *Acta Physiol. Scand.* **62**(Suppl. 232):1–55.

Dausse, J. P., Le Quan-Bui, K. H., and Meyer, P., 1982, Effect of neonatal 6-hydroxydopamine treatment on alpha-1 and alpha-2 adrenoceptors in rat cerebral cortex, *J. Cardiovasc. Pharmacol.* **4**:S86–S90.

Dausse, J. P., Guicheney, P., Diop, L., and Meyer, P., 1984, Caractérisation biochimique des récepteurs alpha-adrénergiques centraux, *J. Pharmacol.* **15**(Suppl. 1):23–33.

Debets, H. J. G., 1985, Optimization methods for HPLC, *J. Liq. Chromatogr.* **8**:2725–2780.

Chapleo, C. B., Doxey, J. C., Myers, P. L., and Roach, A. G., 1981, RX81094, a new potent, selective antagonist at α2-adrenoceptors, *Br. J. Pharmacol.* **74**:942p.

de Montigny, C., and Aghajanian, G. K., 1978, Tricyclic antidepressants: Long-term treatment increases responsivity of rat forebrain neurons to serotonin, *Science* **202**:1301–1306.

de Montigny, C., Wang, R. Y., Reader, T. A., and Aghajanian, G. K., 1980, Monoaminergic denervation of the rat hippocampus: Microiontophoretic studies on pre- and postsynaptic supersensitivity to norepinephrine and serotonin, *Brain Res.* **200**:363–376.

Descarries, L., and Lapierre, Y., 1973, Noradrenergic axon terminals in the cerebral cortex of the rat. I. Radio-autographic visualization after topical application of DL-[³H]norepinephrine, *Brain Res.* **51**:141–160.

Descarries, L., Watkins, K. C., and Lapierre, Y., 1977, Noradrenergic axon terminals in the cerebral cortex of rat. III. Topometric ultrastructural analysis, *Brain Res.* **133**:197–222.

Descarries, L., Lemay, B., Doucet, G., and Berger, B., 1987, Regional and laminar density of the dopamine innervation in adult rat cerebral cortex, *Neuroscience* **21**:807–824.

Diop, L., Dausse, J. P., and Meyer, P., 1983, Specific binding of [³H]rauwolscine to alpha2-adrenoceptors in rat cerebral cortex: Comparison between crude and synaptosomal plasma membranes, *J. Neurochem.* **41**:710–715.

Diop, L., Brière, R., Grondin, L., and Reader, T. A., 1987, Adrenergic receptor and catecholamine distribution in rat cerebral cortex: Binding studies with [³H]prazosin, [³H]idazoxan and [³H]dihydroalprenolol, *Brain Res.* **402**:403–408.

Dolphin, C. A., and Greengard, P., 1981, Neurotransmitter and neuromodulator-dependent alterations in phosphorylation of protein I in slices of rat facial nucleus, *J. Neurosci.* **1**:192–203.

Draper, N. R., and Smith, H., 1966, *Applied Regression Analysis*, Wiley, New York.

Feldman, H. A., 1972, Mathematical theory of complex ligand-binding systems at equilibrium: Some methods for parameter fitting, *Anal. Biochem.* **48**:317–338.

Foote, S. L., Freedman, R., and Oliver, A. P., 1975, Effects of putative neurotransmitters on neuronal activity in monkey auditory cortex, *Brain Res.* **86**:229–242.

Freedman, J., and Aghajanian, G. K., 1984, Idazoxan (RX 781094) selectively antagonizes α2-adrenoceptors on rat central neurons, *Eur. J. Pharmacol.* **105**:265–272.

Fuxe, K., 1965, Evidence for the existence of monoamine neurons in the central nervous system. IV. Distribution of monoamine terminals in the central nervous system, *Acta Physiol. Scand.* **64**(Suppl. 247):37–85.

Fuxe, K., Hamberger, B., and Hökfelt, T., 1968, Distribution of noradrenaline nerve terminals in cortical areas of the rat, *Brain Res.* **8**:125–131.

Gadie, B., Lane, A. C., McCarthy, P. S., Tulloch, I. F., and Walter, D. S., 1984, 2-Alkyl analogues of idazoxan (RX 781094) with enhanced antagonist potency and selectivity at central alpha2-adrenoceptors in the rat, *Br. J. Pharmacol.* **83**:707–712.

Geller, H. M., and Woodward, D. J., 1972, An improved constant current source for microiontophoretic drug application studies, *Electroencephalogr. Clin. Neurophysiol.* **33**:430–432.

Glossman, H., and Presek, P., 1979, Alpha-noradrenergic receptors in brain membranes: Sodium, magnesium and guanylnucleotides modulate agonist binding, *Naunyn-Schmiedebergs Arch. Pharmacol.* **306**:67–73.

Greengard, P., and Kebabian, J. W., 1974, Role of cyclic AMP in the mammalian peripheral nervous system, *Fed. Proc.* **33**:1059–1067.

Henry, J. L., and Yashpal, K., 1984, A simple device for rapidly obtaining slices of fresh brain, *Brain Res. Bull.* **13**:195–197.

Hill, A. V., 1910, The possible effects of the aggregation of the molecules of hemoglobins on its dissociation curves, *J. Physiol. (London)* **40**:iv–vii.

Hökfelt, T., Fuxe, K., Goldstein, M., and Johansson, O., 1973, Evidence for adrenaline neurons in the rat brain, *Acta Physiol. Scand.* **89**:286–288.

Hökfelt, T., Fuxe, K., Johansson, O., and Ljundhal, Å., 1974, Pharmacohistochemical evidence for the existence of dopamine nerve terminals in the limbic cortex, *Eur. J. Pharmacol.* **25**:108–112.

Hornung, R., Presek, P., and Glossmann, H., 1979, Alpha adrenoceptors in rat brain: Direct identification with prazosin, *Naunyn-Schmiedebergs Arch. Pharmacol.* **308**:223–230.

Itakura, T., Kasamatsu, T., and Pettigrew, J. D., 1981, Norepinephrine-containing terminals in kitten visual cortex: Laminar distribution in ultrastructure, *Neuroscience* **6**:159–175.

Jones, B. E., Harper, S. T., and Halaris, A. E., 1977, Effects of locus coeruleus lesions upon cerebral monoamine content, sleep–wakefulness states and the response to amphetamine in the cat, *Brain Res.* **124**:473–496.

Jones, L. S., Gauger, L. L., and Davis, J. N., 1985, Anatomy of brain alpha$_1$-adrenergic receptors: In vitro autoradiography with [^{125}I]-Heat, *J. Comp. Neurol.* **231**:190–208.

Jordan, L. M., Lake, N., and Phillis, J. W., 1972, Mechanism of noradrenaline depression of cortical neurones: A species comparison, *Eur. J. Pharmacol.* **20**:381–384.

Kehr, W., Lindqvist, M., and Carlsson, A., 1976, Distribution of dopamine in the rat cerebral cortex, *J. Neural Transm.* **38**:173–180.

Keller, R., Oke, A., Mefford, I., and Adams, R. N., 1976, Liquid chromatographic analysis of catecholamines: Routine assay for regional brain mapping, *Life Sci.* **19**:995–1004.

Klotz, I. M., 1982, Numbers of receptor sites from Scatchard graphs: Facts and fantasies, *Science* **217**:1247–1249.

Kolta, A., Diop, L., and Reader, T. A., 1987, Noradrenergic effects on rat visual cortex: Single-cell microiontophoretic studies of alpha-2 adrenergic receptors, *Life Sci.* **41**:281–289.

König, J. F. R., and Klippel, R. A., 1963, *The Rat Brain: A Stereotaxic Atlas*, Krieger, New York.

Krnjević, K., 1964, Microiontophoretic studies on cortical neurons, *Int. Rev. Neurobiol.* **7**:41–98.

Krnjević, K., 1974, Chemical nature of synaptic transmission in vertebrates, *Physiol. Rev.* **54**:418–540.

Krnjević, K., 1984, Monoamine receptors in cortex: An introduction, in: *Monoamine Innervation of the Cerebral Cortex* (L. Descarries, T. A. Reader, and H. H. Jasper, eds.), Liss, New York, pp. 125–133.

Krnjević, K., and Phillis, J. W., 1963, Actions of certain amines on cerebral cortical neurones, *Br. J. Pharmacol. Chemother.* **20**:471–490.

Lakhdar-Ghazal, N., Grondin, L., Bengelloun, W. A., and Reader, T. A., 1986, Alpha-adrenoceptors and monoamine contents in the cerebral cortex of the rodent *Jaculus orientalis*: Effects of acute cold exposure, *Pharmacol. Biochem. Behav.* **25**:903–911.

Lands, A. M., Arnold, A., McAuliff, J. P., Ludeña, F. P., and Brown, T. G., 1967, Differentiation of receptor systems activated by sympathomimetic amines, *Nature* **214**:597–598.

Langer, S. Z., 1974, Presynaptic regulation of catecholamine release, *Biochem. Pharmacol.* **23**:1793–1800.

Lapierre, Y., Beaudet, A., Demianczuk, N., and Descarries, L., 1973, Noradrenergic axon terminals in the cerebral cortex of rat. II. Quantitative data revealed by light and electron microscope radioautography of the frontal cortex, *Brain Res.* **63**:174–182.

Lefkowitz, R. J., Stadel, J. M., and Caron, M. G., 1983, Adenylate cyclase-coupled beta-adrenergic receptors: Structure and mechanisms of activation and desensitization, *Annu. Rev. Biochem.* **52**:159–186.

Leibowitz, S. F., Jhanwar-Uniyal, M., Dvorkin, B., and Makman, H. M., 1982, Distribution of alpha-adrenergic, beta-adrenergic and dopaminergic receptors in discrete hypothalamic areas of rat, *Brain Res.* **233**:97–114.

Levitt, P., and Moore, R. Y., 1978, Noradrenaline neuron innervation of the neocortex in the rat, *Brain Res.* **139**:219–231.

Lindvall, O., and Björklund, A., 1974, The organization of the ascending catecholamine neuron systems in the rat brain as revealed by the glyoxylic acid fluorescence method, *Acta Physiol. Scand. Suppl* **412**:1–48.

Lindvall, O., Björklund, A., Moore, R. Y., and Stenevi, U., 1974, Mesencephalic dopamine neurons projecting to neocortex, *Brain Res.* **81**:325–331.

Lowry, O. H., Rosebrough, N. J., Farr, A. L., and Randall, R. J., 1951, Protein measurements with Folin phenol reagent, *J. Biol. Chem.* **193**:265–275.

Mefford, I. N., 1981, Application of high performance liquid chromatography with electrochemical detection to neurochemical analysis: Measurement of catecholamines, serotonin and metabolites in rat brain, *J. Neurosci. Methods* **3**:207–224.

Miach, P. J., Dausse, J. P., and Meyer, P., 1978, Direct biochemical demonstration of two types of alpha-adrenoceptor in rat brain, *Nature* **274**:492–494.

Minneman, K. P., Hegstrand, L. R., and Molinoff, P. B., 1979, Simultaneous determination of beta-1 and beta-2-adrenergic receptors in tissues containing both receptor subtypes, *Mol. Pharmacol.* **16**:34–46.

Morrison, J. H., Molliver, M. E., Grzanna, R., and Coyle, J. T., 1979, Noradrenergic innervation patterns in three regions of medical cortex: An immunofluorescence characterization, *Brain Res. Bull.* **4**:849–857.

Morrison, J. H., Foote, S. L., and Bloom, F. E., 1984, Regional, laminar, developmental and functional characteristics of noradrenaline and serotonin innervation patterns in monkey cortex, in: *Monoamine Innervation of the Cerebral Cortex* (L. Descarries, T. A. Reader, and H. H. Jasper, eds.), Liss, New York, pp. 61–75.

Munson, P. J., and Rodbard, D., 1980, LIGAND: A versatile computerized approach for characterization of ligand-binding systems, *Anal. Biochem.* **107**:220–239.

Olpe, H.-R., Glatt, A., Laszlo, J., and Schellenberg, A., 1980, Some electrophysiological and pharmacological properties of the cortical noradrenergic projection of the locus coeruleus in the rat, *Brain Res.* **186:**9–19.

Palacios, J. M., and Kuhar, M. J., 1982, Beta adrenergic receptor localization in rat brain by light microscopic autoradiography, *Neurochem. Int.* **4:**473–490.

Palkovits, M., Zaborsky, L., Brownstein, M. J., Fekete, M. I. K., Herman, J. P., and Kanyicska, B., 1979, Distribution of norepinephrine and dopamine in cerebral cortical areas of rat brain, *Brain Res. Bull.* **4:**593–601.

Parker, R. B., and Waud, D. R., 1971, Pharmacological estimation of drug-receptor dissociation constants: Statistical evaluation. I. Agonists, *J. Pharmacol. Exp. Ther.* **177:**1–12.

Phillis, J. W., 1984, Microiontophoretic studies of cortical biogenic amines, in: *Monoamine Innervation of the Cerebral Cortex* (L. Descarries, T. A. Reader, and H. H. Jasper, eds.), Liss, New York, pp. 175–194.

Phillis, J. W., Lake, N., and Yarbrough, G., 1973, Calcium mediation of the inhibitory effects of biogenic amines on cerebral cortical neurones, *Brain Res.* **53:**465–469.

Pimoule, C., Scatton, B., and Langer, S. Z., 1983, [^{3}H] RX 781094: A new antagonist ligand labels α_2-adrenoceptors in the rat brain cortex, *Eur. J. Pharmacol.* **95:**79–85.

Rainbow, T. C., and Biegon, A., 1983, Quantitative autoradiography of [^{3}H]prazosin binding in rat forebrain, *Neurosci. Lett.* **40:**221–226.

Rainbow, T. C., Parsons, B., and Wolfe, B. B., 1984, Quantitative autoradiography of α1- and α2-adrenergic receptors in rat brain, *Proc. Natl. Acad. Sci. USA* **81:**1585–1589.

Reader, T. A., 1978a, A simplified method of preparing and filling multibarrelled glass microelectrodes, *Brain Res. Bull.* **3:**719–720.

Reader, T. A., 1978b, The effects of dopamine, noradrenaline and serotonin in the visual cortex of the cat, *Experientia* **34:**1586–1587.

Reader, T. A., 1980a, Microiontophoresis of biogenic amines on cortical neurons: Amounts of NA, DA and 5-HT ejected, compared with tissue content, *Acta Physiol. Lat. Am.* **30:**291–304.

Reader, T. A., 1980b, Serotonin distribution in rat cerebral cortex; radioenzymatic assays with thin-layer chromatography, *Brain Res. Bull.* **5:**609–613.

Reader, T. A., 1981, Distribution of catecholamines and serotonin in the rat cerebral cortex: Absolute levels and relative proportions, *J. Neural Transm.* **50:**13–27.

Reader, T. A., 1983, The role of cortical catecholamine in neuronal excitability, in: *Basic Mechanisms of Neuronal Hyperexcitability* (H. H. Jasper and N. M. van Gelder, eds.), Liss, New York, pp. 281–321.

Reader, T. A., and Brière, R., 1983, Long-term unilateral noradrenergic denervation; Monoamine content and [^{3}H]-prazosin binding sites in rat neocortex, *Brain Res. Bull.* **11:**687–692.

Reader, T. A., and Quesney, L. F., 1986, Dopamine in the visual cortex of the cat, *Experientia* 42:1242–1244.

Reader, T. A., De Champlain, J., and Jasper, H. H., 1976, Catecholamines released from cerebral cortex in the cat: Decrease during sensory stimulation, *Brain Res.* **111:**95–103.

Reader, T. A., Ferron, A., Descarries, L., and Jasper, H. H., 1979a, Modulatory role for biogenic amines in the cerebral cortex: Microiontophoretic studies, *Brain Res.* **160:**217–229.

Reader, T. A., Masse, P., and De Champlain, J., 1979b, The intracortical distribution of endogenous biogenic amines in the cerebral cortex of the cat, *Brain Res.* **177:**499–513.

Reader, T. A., Brière, R., and Grondin, L., 1986a, Alpha-1 and alpha-2 adrenoceptor binding in cerebral cortex; role of disulfide and sulfhydryl groups, *Neurochem. Res.* **11:**9–27.

Reader, T. A., Brière, R., and Grondin, L., 1987, Alpha-1 and alpha-2 adrenoceptor binding in cerebral cortex: Competition studies with [^{3}H]prazosin and [^{3}H]idazoxan, *J. Neural Transm.* **68:**79–95.

Reader, T. A., Brière, R., Grondin, L., and Ferron, A., 1986c, Effects of p-chlorophenylalanine on cortical monoamines and on the activity of noradrenergic neurons, *Neurochem. Res.* **11:**1025–1035.

Reiner, P. B., 1985, Clonidine inhibits central noradrenergic neurons in unanesthetized cats, *Eur. J. Pharmacol.* **115:**249–257.

Sabol, S. L., and Nirenberg, M., 1979, Regulation of adenylate cyclase of neuroblastoma–glioma hybrid cells by α-adrenergic receptors, *J. Biol. Chem.* **254:**1913–1920.

Sakurai, S., Wada, A., Izumi, F., Kobayashi, H., and Yanagihara, N., 1983, Inhibition by α_2-adrenoceptor agonists of the secretion of catecholamines from isolated medullary cells, *Naunyn-Schmiedebergs Arch. Pharmacol.* **324:**15–19.

Salmoiraghi, G. C., and Weight, F. F., 1967, Micromethods in neuropharmacology: An approach to the study of anesthetics, *Anesthesiology* **28:**54–64.

Sawaguchi, T., Matsumura, M., and Kubota, K., 1986, Catecholamine sensitivities of motor cortical neurons of the monkey, *Neurosci. Lett.* **66:**135–140.

Scatchard, G., 1949, The attractions of proteins for small molecules and ions, *Ann. N.Y. Acad. Sci.* **51:**660–672.

Slopsema, J. S., Van der Gugten, J., and De Bruin, J. P. C., 1982, Regional concentrations of noradrenaline and dopamine in the frontal cortex of the rat: Dopaminergic innervation of the prefrontal subareas and lateralization of prefrontal dopamine, *Brain Res.* **250**:197–200.

Starke, K., 1977, Regulation of noradrenaline release by presynaptic receptor systems, *Rev. Physiol. Biochem. Pharmacol.* **77**:1–124.

Starke, K., 1981, Alpha-adrenoceptor subclassification, *Rev. Physiol. Biochem. Pharmacol.* **88**:199–236.

Stone, T. W., and Taylor, D. A., 1977, The nature of adrenoceptors in the guinea pig cerebral cortex: A microiontophoretic study, *Can. J. Physiol. Pharmacol.* **55**:1400–1404.

Stone, T. W., Taylor, D. A., and Bloom, F. E., 1975, Cyclic AMP and cyclic GMP may mediate opposite neuronal responses in the rat cerebral cortex, *Science* **187**:845–846.

Struyker-Baudier, H. A. J., Sweets, G., Browner, G., and van Rossum, J. H., 1974, Central and peripheral adrenergic activity of imidazoline derivatives, *Life Sci.* **15**:887–899.

Sutin, J., and Minneman, K. P., 1985, α1- and β-adrenergic receptors are coregulated during both noradrenergic denervation and hyperinnervation, *Neuroscience* **14**:973–980.

Thierry, A. M., Blanc, G., Sobel, A., Stinus, L., and Glowinski, J., 1973, Dopaminergic terminals in the rat cortex, *Science* **182**:499–501.

Timmermans, P. B. M. W. M., and Van Zwieten, P. A. 1982, α_2-Adrenoceptors: Classification, localization, mechanisms and targets for drugs, *J. Med. Chem.* **25**:1389–1401.

Timmermans, P. B. M. W. M., Lam, E., and Van Zwieten, P. A., 1979, The interaction between prazosin and clonidine at α-adrenoceptors in rats and cats, *Eur. J. Pharmacol.* **55**:57–65.

Törk, I., and Turner, S., 1981, Histochemical evidence for a catecholaminergic (presumably dopaminergic) projection from the ventral mesencephalic tegmentum to visual cortex in the cat, *Neurosci. Lett.* **24**:215–219.

Unnerstall, J. R., Fernandez, I., and Oressanz, L. M., 1985, The alpha adrenergic receptor: Radiohistochemical analysis of functional characteristics and biochemical differences, *Pharmacol. Biochem. Behav.* **22**:859–874.

Ungerstedt, U., 1971, Stereotaxic mapping of the monoamine pathways in the rat brain, *Acta Physiol. Scand.* **82**(Suppl. 367):1–48.

U'Prichard, D. C., 1984, Biochemical characterization and regulation of brain alpha2-adrenoceptors, *Ann. N.Y. Acad. Sci.* **430**:55–75.

U'Prichard, D. C., Bechtel, W. D., Rouot, B. M., and Snyder, S. H., 1979, Multiple apparent alpha-noradrenergic receptor binding sites in rat brain: Effect of 6-hydroxydopamine, *Mol. Pharmacol.* **16**:47–60.

Van der Gugten, J., Palkovits, M., Wijnen, H. L. J. M., and Versteeg, D. H. G., 1976, Regional distribution of adrenaline in rat brain, *Brain Res.* **107**:171–175.

Versteeg, D. H. G., Van der Gugten, J., De Jong, W., and Palkovits, M., 1976, Regional concentrations of noradrenaline and dopamine in rat brain, *Brain Res.* **113**:563–574.

Videen, T., Daw, N., and Rader, R., 1984, The effect of noradrenaline on visual cortical neurons in kittens and adult cats, *J. Neurosci.* **4**:1607–1617.

Wamsley, J. K., 1984, Autoradiographic localization of cortical biogenic amine receptors, in: *Monoamine Innervation of the Cerebral Cortex* (L. Descarries, T. A. Reader, and H. H. Jasper, eds.), Liss, New York, pp. 153–174.

Waterhouse, B. D., and Woodward, D. J., 1980, Interaction of norepinephrine with cerebrocortical activity evoked by stimulation of somatosensory afferent pathways in the rat, *Exp. Neurol.* **67**:11–34.

Waterhouse, B. D., Moises, H. C., and Woodward, D. J., 1980, Noradrenergic modulation of somatosensory cortical neuronal responses to iontophoretically applied putative neurotransmitters, *Exp. Neurol.* **69**:30–49.

Westerink, B. H. C., and De Vries, J. B., 1985, On the origin of dopamine and its metabolite in predominantly noradrenergic innervated brain areas, *Brain Res.* **330**:164–166.

Wood, C. L., Arnett, C. D., Clarke, W. R., Tsai, B. S., and Lefkowitz, R. J., 1979, Subclassification of alpha-adrenergic receptors by direct binding studies, *Biochem. Pharmacol.* **28**:1277–1282.

Woodward, D. J., Moises, H., Waterhouse, B., Hoffer, B., and Freedman, R., 1979, Modulatory actions of norepinephrine in the CNS, *Fed. Proc.* **38**:2109–2116.

Young, W. S., III, and Kuhar, M. J., 1980, Noradrenergic α-1 and α-2 receptors: Light microscopic autoradiographic localization, *Proc. Natl. Acad. Sci. USA* **77**:1696–1700.

Zivin, J. A., and Waud, D. R., 1982, How to analyse binding, enzyme and uptake data: The simplest case, a single phase, *Life Sci.* **30**:1407–1422.

23

Cerebrocortical Neurons Containing DARPP-32, a Dopamine- and Adenosine 3':5'-Monophosphate-Regulated Phosphoprotein

Charles C. Ouimet

1. Introduction

Many of the biological effects of neuronal activity are mediated by the sequential activation of first, second, third (etc.) messengers (for review, see Nestler and Greengard, 1984). First messengers, such as neurotransmitters and neurohormones, work through second messengers such as cAMP, cGMP, and calcium to activate protein kinases that in turn phosphorylate third messenger phosphoproteins. The final messengers in this cascade are the effector molecules that directly alter cell metabolism and/or physiology. DARPP-32 (dopamine- and cAMP-regulated phosphoprotein of molecular weight 32,000) is a third messenger phosphoprotein in this cascade. It is regulated by the first messenger dopamine (DA) and by the second messenger cAMP. The possibility exists that other first messengers that increase intracellular cAMP in DARPP-32-containing neurons may also regulate DARPP-32 phosphorylation. In this paper, neurons in the cerebral cortex that contain DARPP-32 are examined.

1.1. Biochemical Characterization and Localization of DARPP-32

DARPP-32 is a cytosolic, acid-soluble protein (Hemmings *et al.*, 1984a). It is an elongated molecule whose sequence of 202 amino acids is known (Williams *et al.*, 1986); its apparent molecular weight (as shown on polyacrylamide gels) is 32,000 (Walaas *et al.*, 1983; Walaas and Greengard, 1984). Early biochemical studies showed that DARPP-32 is enriched in the caudate–putamen (CP) and in the substantia nigra (SN) (Walaas and Greengard, 1984). To examine the possibility that DARPP-32 is contained in projection neurons in either region, the fiber pathways reciprocally connecting the CP to the SN were severed, and the DARPP-32 concentration was measured in both structures. In animals that had received lesions, the levels of DARPP-32 in the CP were essentially unchanged whereas in the SN, the levels of DARPP-32 were substantially reduced (Walaas and Greengard, 1984). This suggested that DARPP-32 was present in the

Charles C. Ouimet • The Rockefeller University, New York, New York 10021.

striatonigral projection but absent from the nigrostriatal projection. Furthermore, it indicated that DARPP-32 was highly enriched in neurons in the CP, a nucleus which receives a massive DA input (Carlsson, 1959).

1.2. DARPP-32, the D-1 Receptor, and Dopaminoceptive Brain Regions

The D-1 dopamine receptor, which increases intracellular cAMP levels by activating adenylate cyclase (Kebabian and Calne, 1979), is associated with the dopaminoceptive cells in the CP (Cross and Waddington, 1981; McGeer et al., 1976; Schwarcz and Coyle, 1977). The D-2 receptor, which inhibits adenylate cyclase (in the striatum) (Onali et al., 1984), is primarily associated with dopaminergic nigrostriatal neurons and with the corticostriatal neurons (Murrin et al., 1979; Schwarcz et al., 1978). In experiments designed to examine a possible relationship between the D-1 receptor and DARPP-32, the application of either DA or cAMP to slice preparations of the rat CP resulted in phosphorylation of DARPP-32 (Walaas et al., 1983; Walaas and Greengard, 1984). Hence, this study strongly supported the concept that in the CP, DARPP-32 was present in dopaminoceptive neurons containing the D-1 receptor.

The concept that DARPP-32 is present in dopaminoceptive cells containing the D-1 receptor is also consistent with immunocytochemical data (Ouimet et al., 1984). In brain regions receiving a DA input from the SN and ventral tegmental area (VTA), DARPP-32 was localized in cell bodies and dendrites. Thus, neuronal somata and dendrites were immunostained for DARPP-32 in the CP, nucleus accumbens, olfactory tubercle, bed nucleus of the stria terminals, and portions of the amygdaloid complex. Immunoreactive axons were traced from the DARPP-32-containing somata to their target regions in the globus pallidus, entopeduncular nucleus, ventral pallidum, and SN. Once these axons reached their target nuclei, they gave rise to dense aggregations of immunoreactive nerve terminals.

Certain regions that are dopaminoceptive, however, do not contain DARPP-32. One of these regions is the anterior pituitary (Walaas and Greengard, 1984; C. Ouimet and P. Greengard, unpublished observations), which contains the D-2 but not the D-1 receptor (Kebabian and Calne, 1979). Other regions that are dopaminoceptive but contain little DARPP-32 are the olfactory bulb and the hypothalamus. One working hypothesis is that these regions, like the anterior pituitary, contain the D-2 but not the D-1 receptor, and accordingly may not contain DARPP-32. DARPP-32 is absent from the dopaminergic neurons of the SN and VTA, which also have the D-2 but not the D-1 receptor.

It should also be noted that DARPP-32 is most closely related to those brain regions that receive their DA input from the SN and VTA (e.g., the basal ganglia); dopaminoceptive areas that lack DARPP-32, such as the olfactory bulb and hypothalamus, do not receive major projections from the SN and VTA. At the present time, however, an exclusive association between D-1 receptors and neurons postsynaptic to the SN and VTA projections, has not been established.

Some brain regions that may lack a DA input contain DARPP-32. One such region is the cerebellum. This structure contains the D-1 receptor (Dolphin et al., 1979), but dopaminergic afferents have not been demonstrated by anatomical methods.

1.3. DARPP-32 and the Cerebral Cortex

The cerebral cortex contains DARPP-32 (Hemmings and Greengard, 1986; Ouimet et al., 1984) and there is recent evidence that it receives a widespread DA input. Early studies suggested that the DA input was restricted primarily to the prefrontal and anterior cingulate cortex (Divac et al., 1975; for reviews, see Lindvall and Björklund, 1984; Thierry et al., 1984). More recent studies, however, suggest that in addition to the relatively concentrated DA input to the "prefrontal cortex," there is a lesser projection to a broader area of the neocortex (Berger et al., 1985; Descarries et al., 1987). It would be interesting, therefore, to see if there is a relationship between the distribution of cortical DARPP-32-containing neurons and the recently identified cortical DA projection. It would also be interesting to compare the distribution of DARPP-32-positive neurons in the cortex to projections that use transmitter agents other than DA to generate cAMP in postsynaptic neurons; these transmitter agents may also regulate DARPP-32 phosphorylation. Noradrenaline, for example, elevates cortical cAMP levels (Kakiuchi and Rall, 1968).

Monoaminergic fibers projecting to the cortex show a marked degree of convergence with the thalamic projection. In the cerebral cortex of the rat, there is a convergence of monoaminergic and thalamic fibers on target neurons in specific laminae (Lidov *et al.*, 1980). This is also true in the reptilian forerunner to the neocortex, where there is a striking overlap, in both laminar and areal distribution, of the projections from the locus coeruleus and thalamus upon the cortex (Ouimet *et al.*, 1985). It is also of interest, then, to compare the distribution of DARPP-32-containing cells in the cortex that may be "monoaminoceptive," to that of the thalamic afferents.

1.4. The Function of DARPP-32

Recent studies have shown that DARPP-32, in its phosphorylated form, is a potent inhibitor of protein phosphatase-1 (Hemmings *et al.*, 1984b). Phosphatases are enzymes that convert phosphoproteins to their dephosphorylated state and can be considered to have a function directly opposed to that of the protein kinases. Protein phosphatase-1 dephosphorylates many of the substrate proteins for cAMP-dependent protein kinase and those of other protein kinases as well (Ingebristen *et al.*, 1983). If DARPP-32 is in a group of several proteins phosphorylated by cAMP-dependent protein kinase, it could amplify the effect of cAMP by preserving the phosphorylation state of other proteins (Hemmings *et al.*, 1984b). Phospho-DARPP-32 could also preserve the phosphorylation state of proteins phosphorylated by kinases other than cAMP-dependent kinase. Phospho-DARPP-32, therefore, prevents the dephosphorylation of certain (as yet unidentified) proteins and thereby prolongs the effects of the first and second messengers they subserve.

Calcineurin (Stewart *et al.*, 1982) is a phosphatase for which phospho-DARPP-32 is an excellent substrate (King *et al.*, 1984; Hemmings *et al.*, 1984b), but since phospho-DARPP-32 does not inhibit this phosphatase it cannot thereby prevent its own dephosphorylation (Hemmings *et al.*, 1984b). Calcineurin is activated by calcium/calmodulin (Stewart *et al.*, 1983) and it is therefore probable that first messengers (such as nerve impulses), using calcium as a second messenger, attenuate DARPP-32 activity (Hemmings *et al.*, 1984b). Thus, it is likely that calcium influx tends to bring about the dephosphorylation of DARPP-32 whereas elevated cAMP levels do the opposite. The final effector molecules in the cascade from D-1 receptor activation to biological effect have not yet been identified. The data suggest, however, that DA, working through DARPP-32, changes the neuron's response to certain first messengers that also regulate phosphoproteins.

1.5. DARPP-32 and Diffusely Organized Projections

Nuclei that project diffusely upon the cortex may alter the responsiveness of their target neurons to input from pathways characterized by "point to point" projections. The projecting fibers from monoaminergic nuclei to the cortex exemplify the highly branched, diffusely organized type of projection that can "influence" large populations of target neurons. The anatomy of these diffusely projecting neurons suggests that this "influence" may be more closely related to "state-dependent" functions than to "stimulus-dependent" functions (e.g., Jasper, 1981). This is consistent with the growing evidence that monoamines may act as neuromodulators (Reader *et al.*, 1979a; Bunney and Chiodo, 1984).

The population of neurons influenced by such a diffusely organized neuromodulatory input are difficult to identify anatomically because these neurons may respond to monoamines diffusing from distant release sites (Reader *et al.*, 1979b). At the same time, certain neurons may also receive monoaminergic inputs via classical synaptic contacts (for discussion, see Beaudet and Descarries, 1984). The response of these neurons to monoamines (whether the monoamines are released synaptically or diffusely) will be determined by the specific molecular machinery that is mobilized by the activation of specific receptors. DARPP-32 is part of the molecular machinery postsynaptic to transmitter agents that increase intracellular cAMP levels, and its immunocytochemical localization can be used to identify a subpopulation of cortical neurons whose responsiveness to other inputs may be altered by this potent phosphatase inhibitor. The purpose of the present study is to identify the DARPP-32-containing neurons in the cortex that could be involved in such a mechanism, and to compare their distribution to that of known cortical afferent systems.

2. Technical Considerations

DARPP-32 was localized in the cortex by an immunocytochemical method employing biotin and avidin–horseradish peroxidase. Because of the sensitivity of this method, it was possible to examine in detail the cortical DARPP-32-containing neurons, which were only weakly labeled in a previous study using fluorescent antibodies (Ouimet et al., 1984). The method in brief is as follows. Male and female Sprague–Dawley rats (100–250 g) are transcardially perfused with 250 ml of sodium phosphate buffer (0.1 M, pH 7.4) followed by 500 ml of 4% formaldehyde (freshly depolymerized from paraformaldehyde) in the same buffer. After a postfixation period of 1 hr, brains are removed and sliced coronally into 3-mm slabs, which are then cut into sections 50–100 μm thick on a vibratome. The sections are washed (3 × 10 min in buffer) and incubated with normal horse serum (1%, 10 min) followed by incubation (18 hr) with a mixture of three monoclonal antibodies against DARPP-32 (as described by Ouimet et al., 1984). These antibodies were diluted to 1 : 30,000–1 : 800,000 in order to increase the staining specificity by utilizing high-affinity binding sites. It is noteworthy that the staining intensity for DARPP-32 actually increases with decreasing concentration of primary antibody, so that staining is more intense with dilutions of 1 : 30,000 than dilutions of 1 : 1000. Staining intensity in the cortex drops off, however, at dilutions greater than 1 : 100,000. Following incubation with antibodies to DARPP-32, the sections are then incubated in biotinylated horse anti-mouse IgG followed by avidin–biotin–horseradish peroxidase complex as per the instructions in the Vector ABC kit (Vector Laboratories). All antibody solutions contain 1% normal horse serum in phosphate-buffered saline (PBS) (0.01 M phosphate, pH 7.5). All antibody incubations are followed by 3 × 10-min washes in PBS. Sections are then briefly washed with 0.1 M phosphate buffer (pH 7.4), incubated in 3,3′-diaminobenzidine (25 mg/50 ml phosphate buffer) and hydrogen peroxide (20 μl/50 ml) for 2–5 min, washed with phosphate buffer, mounted on glass microscope slides, and examined in a Zeiss Photomicroscope III. Cobalt chloride (50 μl/50 ml) was added to the chromogen solution in several cases to provide greater contrast. All steps are carried out at room temperature.

Preparation of low-power photomicrographs: Microscope slides are placed in the negative holder of a Durst enlarger and briefly illuminated to expose photographic paper and produce the low-power images shown in Fig. 1. These photographs, therefore, are negative images and the immunostained regions appear white, similar to the image seen with standard immunofluorescence microscopy. This technique allows greater resolution and contrast than more conventional methods.

3. The Distribution of DARPP-32 in the Cortex

The nomenclature of Zilles (1985) is used in this paper to name the cortical regions. Cortical areas were delineated by cytoarchitectural criteria in cresyl violet-stained sections that were adjacent to sections immunostained for DARPP-32, and by reexamination of immunostained sections that were photographed and subsequently stained with cresyl violet.

In all cortical regions, there was a gradient of neuronal labeling intensity, such that some neurons were faintly stained, some moderately stained, and some strongly stained. These differences existed to some extent within laminae. But in general, cells were most heavily immunostained in layer VI. In Layer IIIb, cells were moderately stained and in the remainder of layer III and in layer II, cells were more lightly stained. Layer IV contained many cells that were very faintly immunoreactive. When the primary antibody solution was diluted to 1 : 800,000, the layer VI staining remained, but the superficial staining was eliminated. This suggests that the DARPP-32 is most heavily concentrated in layer VI somata.

3.1. Cingulate and Retrosplenial Cortex

In the cingulate cortex, very heavily labeled neurons were present throughout layer VI (Figs. 1A–C, 2A). Most of these neurons sent apical dendrites toward the pial surface. Many of the dendrites were bundled in fascicles, which branched profusely in layer I creating a band of faint staining (Fig. 2A). Very faintly stained neurons were present in layer II but their staining was only slightly above background level. Layer VI neurons were also intensely labeled in the retrosplenial cortex (Figs. 1D–F, 2B). In this region, the haze produced by the branching of layer VI apical dendrites was most intense in layer II (Figs. 1D–F, 2B) and layer II somata were more lightly labeled than in the anterior cingulate cortex. In addition, in the retrosplenial granular cortex (RSG), but not in the retrosplenial agranular cortex (RSA), a band of heavily labeled neurons was also present at the border between layers VI and V (Figs. 1D–F, 2B). These neurons were similar in morphology to the cells in deep layer VI and also sent apical dendrites toward the pial surface. Many neurons just superficial to the white matter were oriented horizontal to the pial surface in both the anterior cingulate and the retrosplenial cortex.

3.2. Frontal Cortex

In the frontal cortex, layer VI neurons were heavily labeled (Figs. 1A–D, 2C, D, 3B). The great majority of these neurons had ovoid cell bodies and sent a dendrite toward the pial surface (Fig. 3B). Some neurons, however, were inverted and sent their main dendrites toward the white matter (Fig. 3B). Other neurons, typically just superficial to the white matter, were horizontally oriented (Fig. 3C). As in the cingulate cortex, many of the dendrites ascended in fascicles (Fig. 3B). Ascending dendrites could be traced through layer V. The density of labeled layer VI neurons was much greater in the rostral half (Fig. 1A) than in more caudal regions (Fig. 1B,C) of the frontal cortex. Occasionally, labeled neurons could be found in lower layer V. Very lightly labeled neurons were present in layers II–III.

3.3. Parietal Cortex

As in other cortical regions, heavily labeled neurons were found in layer VI in the parietal cortex (Figs. 1A–E, 4A,B). Most of the labeled neurons were present in layer VIa. Dendrites could be traced from these neurons to the border between layers IV and V. At this point, the dendrites branched profusely in layer IV and possibly layer IIIb. Many of the neurons in layer VIa were vertically stacked. The few layer VIb neurons that were labeled did not send an apical dendrite to layer IV, and were usually oriented horizontal to the surface of the white matter. Immunolabeled neurons were more common in layer VIb of the primary parietal cortex than in the same layer of secondary parietal cortex.

As a general rule, in the granular cortex the most strongly labeled neurons of the superficial layers were present at the border between layers IIIb and IV. The majority of the immunoreactive

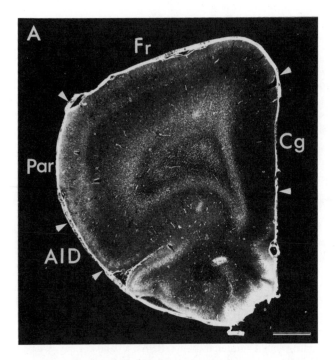

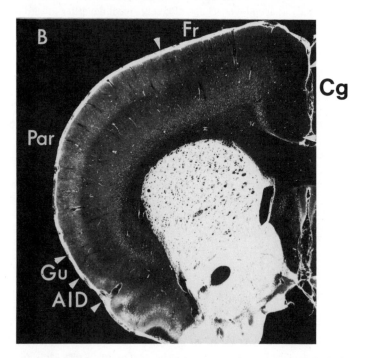

Figure 1. Photomicrographs of coronal sections through representative areas of the brain immunostained for DARPP-32. These photomicrographs are negative images that were produced by inserting microscope slides (tissue side down) in the negative carrier of an enlarger to expose prints that were then developed normally. Thus, these are negative images and immunoreactive areas appear white as with immunofluorescence. The arrowheads indicate borders between cortical regions. AID, anterior dorsal insular cortex; AIP, anterior posterior insular cortex; Cg,

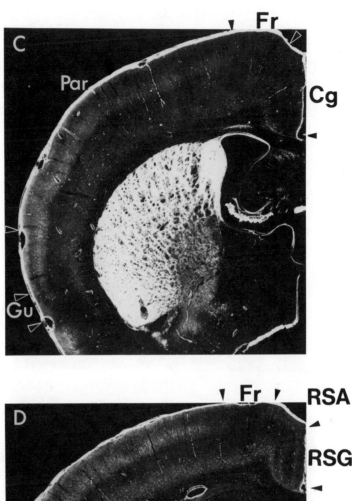

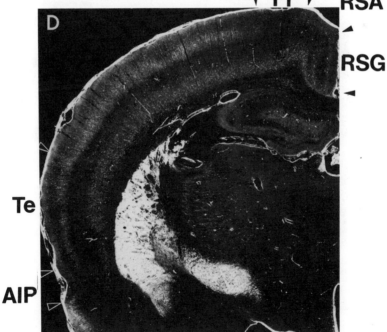

Figure 1. (continued)   cingulate cortex; Fr, frontal cortex; Gu, gustatory cortex; Oc, occipital cortex; Par, parietal cortex; PRh, perirhinal cortex; RSA, retrosplenial agranular cortex; RSG, retrosplenial granular cortex; Te, temporal cortex. Magnification is the same for A–F. Bar in A = 1 mm.

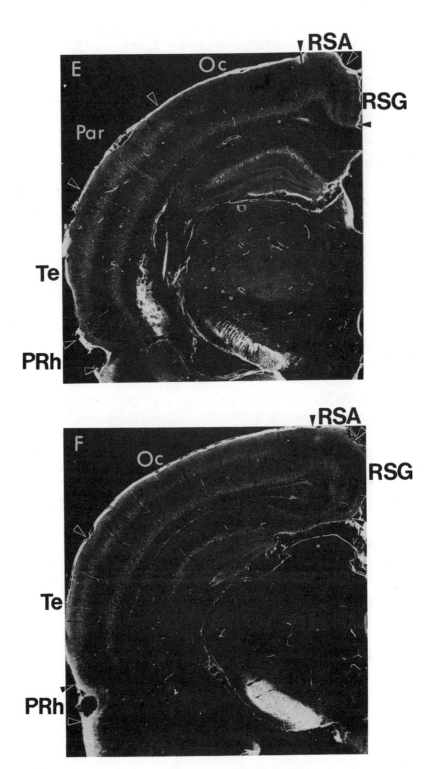

Figure 1. (continued)

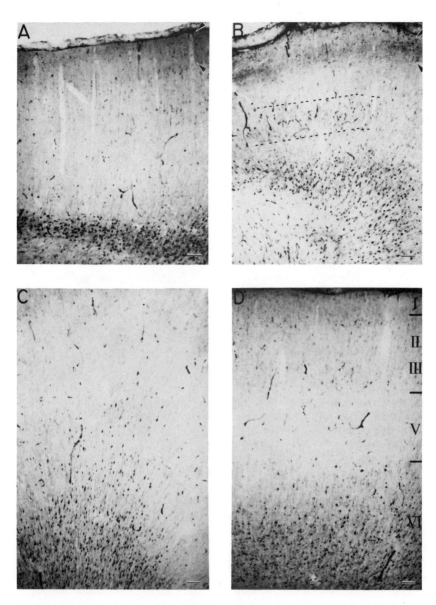

Figure 2. Photomicrographs of the cingulate, retrosplenial, and frontal cortex. In this and subsequent figures, the pial surface is toward the top edge of the photomicrographs. (A) Anterior cingulate cortex on the medial wall of the hemisphere. Note the diffuse staining in layer I (between the arrowheads). Neurons in layer VI (bottom) are heavily immunoreactive. (B) Retrosplenial cortex. Diffuse staining is present in layer II (between arrowheads). In addition to the heavily labeled neurons in layer VI, there is also a band of neurons (between the dotted lines) at the border between layers VI and V. (C) Medial agranular frontal cortex (Fr2). Strongly labeled neurons are present in layer VI (bottom). A light haze of immunoreactivity is present in layer I (top edge of photomicrograph). (D) Lateral agranular frontal cortex. In addition to the heavy labeling in layer VI, there is a diffuse labeling in layers III–I. Many labeled neurons can be seen in layers III–II. Bars = 100 μm.

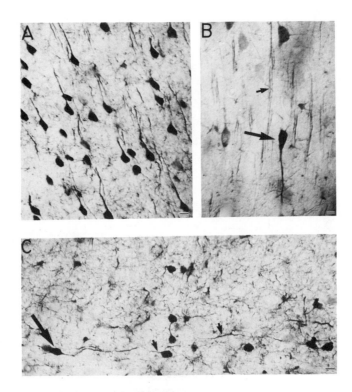

Figure 3. Photomicrographs of cell types in the frontal cortex (Fr1). (A) Most of the neurons in layer VI were ovoid and sent an apical dendrite toward the pial surface. (B) At the junction between layers VI and V, inverted pyramidal cells could occasionally be found (large arrow). Dendrites frequently ascended toward the pial surface in fascicles (small arrow). (C) In layer VIb, fewer cells were present than in layer VIa. Most of the layer VIb cells, in which dendrites were immunostained, were horizontally oriented (large arrow). Dendritic processes could be seen coursing through layer VIb parallel to the white matter (small arrows). Bars = 10 μm.

layer IV neurons were only weakly stained, and layer IV was typically characterized by the presence of a fine network of branching immunolabeled dendrites.

Neurons at the border between layers III and IV often formed vertical stacks, and horizontally oriented neurons were frequently present in layer IIIb (Fig. 5A). Most of the labeled neurons in the parietal cortex, however, were of the pyramidal type and were present throughout layers II and III. In layer IV, a surprising number of pyramidal neurons were weakly labeled. The majority of the layer IV cells, however, did not display an apical dendrite and appeared as round neurons of small diameter. It was difficult to identify these neurons as stellate cells because their staining was so weak that their dendrites were difficult to visualize. Examination of layer IV at high magnification revealed that the staining was due primarily to the branching of dendrites that originated in layer VI neurons. Likewise, the staining in layer I was due to branching dendrites that originated in somata in layers II–III (Fig. 5B). No dendrites were traced from layer VI somata to layer I, but the depth of immunostaining is very shallow (1–3 μm) and DARPP-containing dendrites may be unstained if they are deep in the section where immunoreagent penetration is poor. The staining in layers IV–I grew faint in dysgranular zones.

In the parietal regions exclusive of Par1 [primary parietal cortex as defined in the atlas of Zilles (1985)], the staining was more narrowly restricted to layers IIIb and IV such that a band of reduced staining intensity intervened between layer IIIb and layer I (Fig. 1C,D). Moreover, the

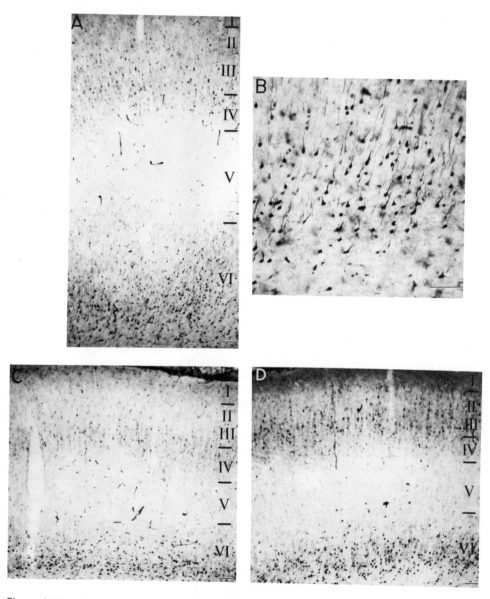

Figure 4. Photomicrographs of the primary parietal (Par1), occipital (Oc1), and temporal (Te1) cortex. (A) Par1. Strongly labeled neurons are present in layer VI. Moderately labeled neurons are also present in layers IV–II. Most of the moderately labeled neurons in layer IV are present in its upper half. Layer I contains labeled dendrites. (B) Neurons in layer VI of Par1. These neurons often showed vertical organization. The main dendrites of these cells could be traced to layer IV, where they branched into smaller processes. (C) Primary visual cortex OC1. The labeled neurons in layer VI are strongly immunoreactive. On the other hand, the labeled neurons in layers IV and III are less immunoreactive than in other cortical regions. Immunoreactivity is relatively weak in layers IIIa and II. (D) Primary temporal cortex Te1. Strongly labeled cells are present in layer VI. Moderately labeled neurons are present in layers II–III and a few are present in layer IV. Dendritic processes in layer I are moderately labeled. Bars = 100 μm.

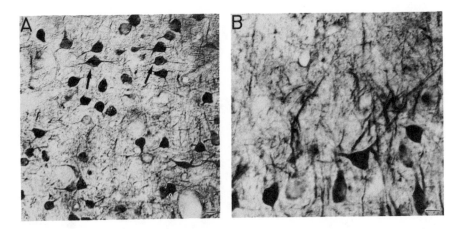

Figure 5. Photomicrographs of primary parietal cortex (Par1). (A) In layer III, neurons (arrows) were found that were oriented parallel to the pial surface. (B) Photomicrograph of the border between layers I and II in Par1. Note the dendritic branching in layer I. Bars = 10 μm.

intensity of staining in layer I was somewhat lessened in the hindlimb and forelimb areas of Par1 (Fig. 1C,D).

3.4. Occipital and Temporal Cortex

In these regions, the lamina of immunostained neurons in layer VI was more compact than it was in the frontal or parietal cortex (Figs. 1E,F, 4C,D). Similarly, the lamina of labeled cells in layer IIIb are more compact in the occipital and temporal cortex than in Par1 (Fig. 1C–F). Thus, in the occipital and temporal cortex, a band of lesser staining intervenes between layer IIIb and layer I (Figs. 1E,F, 4C,D). As in the other granular cortical regions, dendrites can be traced from layer VI somata to the layer IV/V border where the dendrites branch profusely in layer IV. There was a greater number of labeled neurons in layer VIb in the occipital and temporal cortex than in the parietal and frontal regions. Most of these neurons were oriented horizontal to the white matter.

3.5. Perirhinal and Anterior Insular Cortex

DARPP-32 staining was very similar in the perirhinal cortex (Figs. 1E,F) and anterior insular cortex. Labeled somata were concentrated in layer II/III and in layer VI. In the latter, there were far fewer neurons than in adjacent neocortical regions (Fig. 1E,F).

4. The Relationship between the Distribution of DARPP-32-Containing Neuronal Somata and Dendrites in the Cortex, and That of Afferent Inputs to the Cortex

Throughout the neocortex, DARPP-32-containing neurons are concentrated in layers VI and IIIb. DARPP-32-positive neurons are also scattered throughout the remainder of layers II and III, especially in Par1. In all regions, there is a plexus of immunoreactive dendrites in layer I, and in the granular cortex, there is a plexus of immunoreactive dendrites in layer IV. The layer IV dendritic plexus seems to arise primarily from immunolabeled neurons in layer VI.

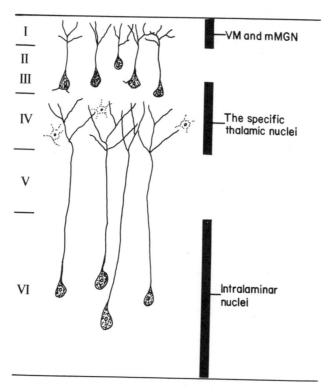

Figure 6. Summary diagram showing in a schematic fashion the overlap between DARPP-32-containing cell bodies and dendrites and the input to the cortex from the thalamus. The neurons represent DARPP-32-containing cells in layers II–III and VI. The dotted cells in layer IV represent weakly labeled neurons that are probably stellate cells. The heavy black bars on the right represent the major zones of thalamic afferent fiber termination (Herkenham, 1980). The intralaminar input to layer V, which is lighter than that to layer VI, is not represented. DARPP-32-containing somata in layer VI are in a position to receive afferents from the intralaminar nuclei. DARPP-32-containing somata in layers IV–III are in a position to receive afferents from the specific thalamic nuclei. The apical dendrites of the layer VI cells are also in a position to receive afferents from the specific thalamic nuclei. DARPP-32-containing dendrites in layer I may receive afferents from the ventromedial thalamic nucleus (VM) and in auditory cortex, from the magnocellular portion of the medial geniculate nucleus (mMGN).

4.1. DARPP-32-Containing Cortical Neurons and the Cortical Dopaminergic Innervation

The cortical neurons that stain most strongly for DARPP-32 reside in layer VI, the layer containing DA afferents (Berger *et al.*, 1985; Descarries *et al.*, 1987) and at least in some regions, the D-1 receptor (Dawson *et al.*, 1985). On the other hand, regional variations in the intensity of DARPP-32 staining do not follow the regional variations in the density of the dopaminergic innervation of the cortex. Thus, neurons in the DA-rich "prefrontal" cortex (Divac *et al.*, 1975; Thierry *et al.*, 1984) were not especially more immunoreactive for DARPP-32 than were neurons in other cortical regions. Moreover, there is a discrepancy between the layers in the cingulate cortex that receive the greatest DA input (the superficial layers) (for review, see Lewis *et al.*, 1979), and the layers that contain the strongest staining DARPP-32 neurons (primarily layer VI). In addition, DARPP-32 staining is not pronounced in perirhinal areas. In agreement with previous observations (Ouimet *et al.*, 1984), this suggests that DARPP-32 is not enriched in all dopaminoceptive regions. One working hypothesis is that in dopaminoceptive areas, DARPP-32 is present in those neurons (or in a subset of those neurons) that contain the D-1 receptor and may be absent from neurons containing the D-2 receptor (but not the D-1 receptor) (Walaas et al., 1983; Ouimet et al., 1984; Walaas and Greengard, 1984). The discrepancy between the laminar pattern formed by DARPP-32-containing somata and that formed by DA afferent fibers is difficult to interpret, however, because the DA fibers may interact with DARPP-32-positive dendrites at any point throughout the depth of the cortex; although DARPP-32 somata are restricted to certain layers, the dendrites from these cells are present in all layers.

There is no evidence, on the other hand, that there is a DA input to layers II–III in the neocortex. Yet these layers contain many DARPP-32-labeled somata. As is possible elsewhere, the DARPP-32 in these neurons may be associated with first messengers other than DA. It is possible that DARPP-32 phosphorylation can be regulated by any first messenger that increases cAMP in a DARPP-32-containing neuron. One candidate for such a first messenger is noradrenaline, which is present in moderate concentrations in the supragranular layers, especially in layer I (for review, see Lindvall and Björklund, 1984).

4.2. The Relationship between DARPP-Containing Somata and Dendrites, and the Thalamic Input to the Cortex

There is a striking degree of overlap between the distribution of DARPP-32-positive somata and dendrites in the cortex and the distribution of thalamic afferents to the cortex. Layer VI receives afferent fibers from the intralaminar nuclei, layers IV and IIIb from sensory relay nuclei (lateral geniculate nucleus, medial geniculate nucleus, and the ventrobasal complex), and layer I from the ventromedial nucleus (VM) and the magnocellular portion of the medial geniculate nucleus (mMGN) (Herkenham, 1980). Layers I and IIIb, IV, and VI all contain moderately labeled DARPP-32 neurons or their dendrites. Although layer V receives some afferent fibers from the intralaminar nuclei (Herkenham, 1980), it contains few DARPP-32-labeled somata.

The strongest staining for DARPP-32 is seen in layer VI. This layer receives a convergent input from the intralaminar nuclei and from dopaminergic nuclei, a characteristic it shares in common with the CP. It is not known whether phospho-DARPP-32 alters the response of neurons to intralaminar input, but it is interesting that both regions stain strongly for DARPP-32.

Consistent with a previous suggestion (Ouimet et al., 1984), there is now preliminary evidence that many of the DARPP-32-positive neurons in layer VI project back upon the thalamus (Ouimet, unpublished observations). The apical dendrites of the layer VI DARPP-32-positive neurons branch profusely in layer IV and are therefore in a position to receive direct afferent fibers from the specific thalamic nuclei. This raises the possibility that layer VI DARPP-32-containing neurons integrate information arriving on their apical dendrites (in layer IV) from the specific thalamic nuclei with information arriving on dendrites closer to the cell body or on the cell body itself from diffusely projecting nuclei (intralaminar nuclei, such as the central medial nucleus, and dopaminergic nuclei). One recipient of this integrated information would be the thalamus. A subset of layer VI neurons in the cat visual cortex (area 17) have recently been described (Katz et al., 1984) that, like the DARPP-32-containing neurons in layer VI of the rat cortex, also have apical dendrites branching in layer IV and axons that project upon the thalamus.

Many neurons in layer IV were weakly positive for DARPP-32 and many neurons in layers II–III were strongly positive. Basal dendrites and somata of the neurons in layer IIIb are also in a position to receive afferents from the unspecific thalamic nuclei. The apical dendrites of layer II–III neurons could be followed into layer I, which receives afferent fibers from the VM and mMGN (Herkenham, 1980), and the locus coeruleus (for review, see Lindvall and Björklund, 1984). Hence, the layer IIIb neurons are in a position to integrate inputs from the specific thalamic nuclei, from diffusely projecting thalamic nuclei (VM and mMGN), as well as from the locus coeruleus (in addition to the other afferents reaching these layers, such as those from the contralateral cortex). The relationship between the laminar distribution of DARPP-32-containing somata and dendrites is summarized in Fig. 6. The demonstration that converging inputs actually form synapses on DARPP-32-containing somata and dendrites will have to be done at the electron microscopic level; it is possible that neurons reside in the same layers as do afferent fibers and that the two are not in synaptic contact.

5. Concluding Remarks

In the CP, dopamine is the first messenger that regulates DARPP-32 phosphorylation. In the cortex, additional first messengers that increase intracellular cAMP levels in DARPP-32-containing neurons may also regulate DARPP-32 phosphorylation. Such transmitter agents are contained in the diffuse projections of monoaminergic neurons to the cerebral cortex. The laminar distribution of DARPP-32-containing somata and dendrites shows that these neurons are in a position to receive convergent inputs from monoaminergic nuclei and thalamic nuclei, and raises the possibility that DARPP-32 plays a role in modulating the cortical response to thalamic input.

ACKNOWLEDGMENTS. The author thanks Drs. Paul Greengard and Hugh C. Hemmings, Jr., for the gift of antibodies against DARPP-32, and Drs. John Donoghue and Ford Ebner for their helpful comments, and Vicki Wells for her expert technical assistance.

References

Beaudet, A., and Descarries, L., 1984, Fine structure of monoamine axon terminals in cerebral cortex, in: *Monoamine Innervation of the Cerebral Cortex* (L. Descarries, T. A. Reader, and H. H. Jasper, eds.), Liss, New York, pp. 77–93.

Berger, B., Verney, C., Alvarez, C., Vigney, A., and Helle, K. B., 1985, New dopaminergic terminal fields in the motor, visual (area 18b) and retrosplenial cortex in young and adult rat: Immunocytochemical and catecholamine histochemical analyses, Neuroscience **15**:983–998.

Bunney, B. S., and Chiodo, L. A., 1984, Mesocortical dopamine systems: Further electrophysiological and pharmacological characteristics, in: *Monoamine Innervation of the Cerebral Cortex* (L. Descarries, T. A. Reader, and H. H. Jasper, eds.), Liss, New York, pp. 263–277.

Carlsson, A., 1959, The occurrence, distribution and physiological role of catecholamines in the nervous system, *Pharmacol. Rev.* **11**:490–493.

Cross, A. J., and Waddington, J. L., 1981, Kainic acid lesions dissociate [3H] spiperone and [3H] cis-flupenthixol binding sites in rat striatum, *Eur. J. Pharmacol.* **71**:327–332.

Dawson, T. M., Gehlert, D. R., Yamamura, H. I., Barnett, A., and Wamsley, J. K., 1985, D-1 dopamine receptors in the rat brain: Autoradiographic localization using [3H]SCH 23390, *Eur. J. Pharmacol.* **108**:323–325.

Descarries, L., Lemay, B., Doucet, G., and Berger, B., 1986, Regional and laminar density of the dopamine innervation in adult rat cerebral cortex, *Neuroscience* **21**:807–824.

Divac, I., Lindvall, O., Björklund, A., and Passingham, R. E., 1975, Converging projections from the mediodorsal thalamic nucleus and mesencephalic dopaminergic neurons to the neocortex in three species, *J. Comp. Neurol.* **180**:59–72.

Dolphin, A., Hamont, M., and Bockaert, J., 1979, The resolution of dopamine and B-1- and B-2-adrenergic-sensitive adenylate cyclase activities in homogenates of cat cerebellum, hippocampus and cerebral cortex, *Brain Res.* **179**:305–317.

Hemmings, H. C., Jr., and Greengard, P., 1986, DARPP-32, a dopamine- and adenosine 3′:5′-monophosphate-regulated phosphoprotein: Regional, tissue and phylogenetic distribution, *J. Neurosci.* **6**:1469–1481.

Hemmings, H. C., Jr., Nairn, A. C., Aswad, D. W., and Greengard, P., 1984a, DARPP-32, a dopamine and adenosine 3′:5′-monophosphate-regulated phosphoprotein enriched in dopamine innervated brain regions. II. Purification and characterization of the phosphoprotein from bovine caudate nucleus, *J. Neurosci.* **4**:99–110.

Hemmings, H. C., Jr., Greengard, P., Lim Tung, H. Y., and Cohen, P., 1984b, DARPP-32, a dopamine-regulated neuronal phosphoprotein, is a potent inhibitor of protein phosphatase-1, *Nature* **310**:503–508.

Herkenham, M., 1980, Laminar organization of the thalamic projections to the rat neocortex, *Science* **207**:532–535.

Ingebristen, T. S., Foulkes, J. G., and Cohen, P., 1983, The protein phosphatases involved in cellular regulation. 4. Glucogen metabolism, *Eur. J. Biochem.* **132:**263–274.

Jasper, H. H., 1981, Problems of relating cellular or modular specificity to cognitive functions: Importance of state-dependent reactions, in: *The Organization of the Cerebral Cortex: Proceeding of a Neurosciences Research Program Colloquium* (F. O. Schmitt, F. G. Worden, G. Edelman, and S. G. Dennis, eds.), MIT Press, Cambridge, Mass., pp. 375–393.

Kakiuchi, S., and Rall, T. W., 1968, Studies on adenosine 3'5'-phosphate in rabbit cerebral cortex, *Mol. Pharmacol.* **4:**379–388.

Katz, L. C., Burkhalter, A., and Dreyer, W. W., 1984, Fluorescent latex microspheres as a retrograde neuronal marker for *in vivo* and *in vitro* studies of visual cortex, *Nature* **310:**498–500.

Kebabian, J. W., and Calne, D. B., 1979, Multiple receptors for dopamine, *Nature* **277:**93–96.

King, M. M., Huang, C. Y., Chock, P. B., Nairn, A. C., Hemmings, H. C., Jr., Chan, K.-F. J., and Greengard, P., 1984, Mammalian brain phosphoproteins as substrates for calcineurin, *J. Biol. Chem.* **259:**8080–8083.

Lewis, M. S., Molliver, M. E., Morrison, J. H., and Lidov, H. G. W., 1979, Complementarity of dopaminergic and noradrenergic innervation in anterior cingulate cortex of rat, *Brain Res.* **164:**328–333.

Lidov, H. G. W., Grzanna, R., and Molliver, M. E., 1980, Serotonin innervation of the cerebral cortex in the rat— An immunohistochemical analysis, *Neuroscience* **5:**207–227.

Lindvall, O., and Björklund, A., 1984, General organization of cortical monoamine systems, in: *Monoamine Innervation of the Cerebral Cortex* (L. Descarries, T. A. Reader, and H. H. Hasper, eds.), Liss, New York, pp. 9–40.

McGeer, E. G., Innanen, V. T., and McGeer, P. L., 1976, Evidence on the cellular localization of adenyl cyclase in the neostriatum, *Brain Res.* **118:**356–358.

Murrin, L. C., Gale, K., and Kuhar, M. J., 1979, Autoradiographic localization of neuroleptic and dopamine receptors in the caudate putamen and substantia nigra: Effects of lesions, *Eur. J. Pharmacol.* **60:**229–235.

Nestler, E. J., and Greengard, P., 1984, *Protein Phosphorylation in the Nervous System,* Wiley, New York.

Onali, P., Olinias, M. C., and Gessa, G. L., 1984, Selective blockade of dopamine D-1 receptors by SCH 23390 discloses striatal dopamine D-2 receptors mediating the inhibition of adenylate cyclase in rats, *Eur. J. Pharmacol.* **99:**127.

Ouimet, C. C., Patrick, R. L., and Ebner, F. F., 1985, The projection of three extrathalamic cell groups to the cerebral cortex of the turtle *Pseudemys, J. Comp. Neurol.* **237:**77–84.

Ouimet, C. C., Miller, P. E., Hemmings, H. C., Jr., Walaas, S. I., and Greengard, P., 1984, DARPP-32, a dopamine- and adenosine 3':5'-monophosphate-regulated phosphoprotein enriched in dopamine-innervated brain regions. III. Immunocytochemical localization, *J. Neurosci.* **4:**114–124.

Reader, T. A., Ferron, A., Descarries, L., and Jasper, H. H., 1979a, Modulating role for biogenic amines in the cerebral cortex: Microiontophoretic studies, *Brain Res.* **160:**217–229.

Reader, T. A., Masse, P., and DeChamplain, J., 1979b, The intracortical distribution of norepinephrine, dopamine, and serotonin in the cerebral cortex of the cat, *Brain Res.* **177:**499–513.

Schwarcz, R., and Coyle, J. T., 1977. Striatal lesions with kainic acid: Neurochemical characteristics, *Brain Res.* **127:**235–249.

Schwarcz, R., Creese, I., Coyle, J. T., and Snyder, S. H., 1978, Dopamine receptors localized on cerebral cortical afferents to rat corpus striatum, *Nature* **271:**766–768.

Stewart, A. A., Ingebristen, T. S., Manalan, A., Klee, C. B., and Cohen, P., 1982, Discovery of a calcium and calmodulin-dependent protein phosphatase, *FEBS Lett.* **137:**80–84.

Stewart, A. A., Ingebristen, T. S., and Cohen, P., 1983, The protein phosphatases involved in cellular regulation. 5. Purification and properties of a calcium/calmodulin-dependent protein phosphatase (2B) from rabbit skeletal muscle, *Eur. J. Biochem.* **132:**289–295.

Thierry, A.-M., Tassin, J.-P., and Glowinski, J., 1984, Biochemical and electrophysiological studies of the mesocortical dopamine system, in: *Monoamine Innervation of the Cerebral Cortex* (L. Descarries, T. A. Reader, and H. H. Jasper, eds.), Liss, New York, pp. 233–261.

Walaas, S. I., and Greengard, P., 1984, DARPP-32, a dopamine- and adenosine-3':5'-monophosphate-regulated phosphoprotein enriched in dopamine-innervated brain regions. I. Regional and cellular distribution, *J. Neurosci.* **4:**84–98.

Walaas, S. I., Aswad, D. W., and Greengard, P., 1983, A dopamine- and cyclic AMP-regulated phosphoprotein enriched in dopamine-innervated brain regions, *Nature* **301:**69–71.

Williams, K. R., Hemmings, H. C., Jr., LoPresti, M. B., Konigsberg, W. H., and Greengard, P., 1986, DARPP-32, a dopamine- and cyclic AMP-regulated neuronal phosphoprotein, *J. Biol. Chem.* **261:**1890–1903.

Zilles, K., 1985, *The Cortex of the Rat: A Stereotaxic Atlas,* Springer-Verlag, Berlin.

24

Synaptic Regulation of Locus Coeruleus Neuronal Activity

Kenneth C. Marshall and Paul G. Finlayson

1. Introduction

The noradrenergic innervation of the cerebral cortex, including both the neocortex (Moore and Card, 1984) and the hippocampus (Loy *et al.*, 1980), appears to originate exclusively in the locus coeruleus (LC), a small nucleus in the pons. The release of noradrenaline (NA) in the cerebral cortex, and its ensuing actions, should therefore be governed by activity of the LC neurons, with the qualifications that NA might be releasable from axonal varicosities in the absence of action potentials, and that release of this transmitter may be modulated by several other neurotransmitters and biologically active substances (Weiner, 1979). An understanding of the control of activity of LC neurons might, then, provide some insight into the role of noradrenergic neurotransmission in the cerebral cortex, and in other areas. It is our purpose, therefore, to briefly review the factors which influence LC neuronal activity, including afferent pathways, neurotransmitters, and intrinsic activity. For the analysis of some of these factors, we will refer particularly to our recent work using intracellularly recorded LC neurons grown in explant cultures.

The LC is a small, compact nucleus located near the lateral edge of the fourth ventricle, in the pons. In rodents and primates, it appears to be composed almost exclusively of NA-containing neurons, while in the cat, these cells are mixed with nonadrenergic neurons. A more ventrally located group of more dispersed NA-containing neurons is often referred to as the nucleus subcoeruleus. The efferent projections of the LC are very widespread, including the spinal cord, cerebellum, brain stem, diencephalon, hippocampus, and neocortex. The details will not be given here, as they have been extensively described in reviews (e.g., Amaral and Sinnamon, 1977; Moore and Bloom, 1979; Foote *et al.*, 1983). It has been demonstrated that the same LC neuron can give rise to axonal projections to such dispersed target areas as the cerebellum, hippocampus, and neocortex (e.g., Nakamura and Iwama, 1975; Steindler, 1981). Because the rat has been the species used in most studies of the LC, and because of difficulties for anatomical and physiological work on the nonhomogeneous LC of the cat, most of the research referred to here is from the rat. Because of space limitations, the literature referenced is in some cases restricted to more recent citations, which in turn refer to earlier work.

Kenneth C. Marshall and Paul G. Finlayson • Department of Physiology, Faculty of Health Sciences, University of Ottawa, Ottawa, Ontario, K1H 8M5, Canada.

2. Afferents to the LC

Sources of afferents to the LC have been studied with several anatomical techniques. Retrograde labeling of cell bodies following administration of horseradish peroxidase (HRP) into the LC has indicated projections from the prefrontal and insular cortex, central nucleus of the amygdala, preoptic area, bed nucleus of stria terminalis, some hypothalamic areas, raphe nuclei, vestibular nuclei, reticular formation, periaqueductal gray, nucleus of the solitary tract, lateral reticular nucleus, cerebellar nuclei, parabrachial regions, the contralateral LC, and the areas of other catecholamine cell groups (A_1, A_2, A_5) and the dorsal horn of the spinal cord (Cedarbaum and Aghajanian, 1978b; Clavier, 1979). Some additional sources have been described in studies using degeneration of nerve terminals in the LC following lesions of other nuclei, and using autoradiographic labeling in the LC following injections of tritiated amino acids in other centers (for references and further detail, see Palkovits and Brownstein, 1983).

Physiological studies have indicated that LC neurons are responsive to electrical stimulation of many other brain areas and peripheral nerves. In anesthetized animals, LC neurons are primarily responsive to nociceptive stimulation (e.g., Korf et al., 1974), although orthodromic responses to electrical stimulation of several CNS structures (Takigawa and Mogenson, 1977) and visceral afferents (e.g., Elam et al., 1986) have also been demonstrated. In unanesthetized rats, LC neurons respond not only to nociceptive stimulation, but to stimuli for apparently all sensory modalities (Aston-Jones and Bloom, 1981b). Widespread responses of LC neurons to sensory stimuli have also been demonstrated in anesthetized neonatal rats (Kimura and Nakamura, 1985). It should be noted that the physiological studies have generally not discriminated between mono- and polysynaptic pathways, and therefore give little information on the *direct* source of afferents to the LC.

A recent preliminary report of afferents to the LC is of interest because it indicates a much more restricted set of afferents than proposed in earlier studies. Aston-Jones et al. (1985) administered wheat germ agglutinin conjugated to HRP, from fine-tipped glass microelectrodes, into the LC. The potential advantage of this approach is the use of small injections within the LC, and the use of a tracer substance which is characterized by anterograde and retrograde transport, by more discrete injection sites than with free HRP, and by higher rates of internalization and greater sensitivity as a tracing probe (Sawchenko and Gerfen, 1985). The study by Aston-Jones et al. demonstrated retrogradely labeled neurons in ipsilateral parabrachial and vestibular nuclei, ventrolateral and parafascicular medullary reticular formation, and in cervical spinal gray matter. Retrograde labeling was *not* observed in central amygdaloid nucleus, nucleus tractus solitarius, or spinal dorsal horn cell columns, areas which had been reported as labeled in the earlier HRP studies. It is puzzling that raphe nuclei were not reported as being labeled in this study, since other studies based on retrograde labeling with HRP (Morgane and Jacobs, 1979), anterograde amino acid labeling and degeneration (Conrad et al., 1974; Bobillier et al., 1978), and detection of serotoninergic terminals within the LC (Léger and Descarries, 1978; Pickel et al., 1977) have all indicated such projections. While caution must be exercised in the acceptance of negative results in such tracing studies, the report by Aston-Jones et al. (1985) may represent a major change in our concepts of the diversity of *direct* afferents to the LC, and we look forward to a full description of this study. As pointed out by Grant and Redmond (1981), the possibility of influences on LC activity by factors in the vascular system or in the CSF of the adjacent fourth ventricle, must also be considered.

3. Neurotransmitters in the LC

Rapid advances in the localization of neurotransmitter substances or their synthetic enzymes within specific brain regions have followed the development of immunohistochemical techniques. In view of evidence for axon collaterals of LC neurons terminating within the LC (Swanson,

1976; Aghajanian *et al.*, 1977; Shimizu *et al.*, 1979) and for dendrodendritic synaptic contacts between LC neurons (Shimizu *et al.*, 1979; Groves and Wilson, 1980a,b), neurotransmitters contained within LC neurons as well as in afferent nerve terminals must be considered as potentially active controllers of LC activity.

3.1. Catecholamines

The demonstration of NA in the neurons of the LC (A6 group) by Dahlström and Fuxe (1964) has been confirmed by biochemical measurements of NA (e.g., Koslow and Schlumpf, 1974) as well as by histochemical localization of the synthetic enzyme dopamine-β-hydroxylase (Swanson and Hartman, 1975; Grzanna and Molliver, 1980). Noradrenergic nerve terminals have been shown in the LC by dopamine-β-hydroxylase staining (Cimarusti *et al.*, 1979). Catecholamine-containing nerve terminals are also indicated by the presence of small dense-core vesicles following 5-hydroxydopamine treatment (Groves and Wilson, 1980b).

The synthetic enzyme for adrenaline, phenylethanolamine-*N*-methyl transferase, has been found in nerve terminals within the LC, but not in cell somata, indicating an afferent input which is thought to originate in the cell groups of the medulla oblongata characterized by this enzyme (Hökfelt *et al.*, 1974). While dopamine and the synthetic enzyme tyrosine hydroxylase have been found in the LC, these might simply reflect the precursor of NA or adrenaline synthetic systems, rather than an independent dopaminergic innervation. However, such a dopaminergic path has been proposed to arise from the A10 group of the ventral mesencephalic tegmentum (Simon *et al.*, 1979; McRae-Degueurce and Milon, 1983).

3.2. Other Neurotransmitters

The presence of acetylcholinesterase in noradrenergic LC neurons has been described (e.g., Albanese and Butcher, 1980), although this does not in itself demonstrate cholinergic neurotransmission at that site. Biochemical measurements have shown the presence of moderate levels of acetylcholine in the LC (Cheney *et al.*, 1975) as well as low levels of the synthetic enzyme choline acetyltransferase (ChAT) (Kobayashi *et al.*, 1975). However, ChAT immunoreactivity has apparently not been observed in the LC of the rat in recent immunohistochemical studies (e.g., Wainer *et al.*, 1984). The case for cholinergic pathways to the LC is therefore not strong, though evidence of functional cholinergic influences on LC neurons exists (see below).

There are strong indications that serotonin (5-HT)-containing nerve terminals are present in the LC, originating from cells in the raphe nuclei. Immunocytochemical studies have shown nerve terminal staining for the synthetic enzyme tryptophan hydroxylase (Pickel *et al.*, 1977), and small numbers of nerve terminals and cell bodies show reaction product using 5-HT antibodies (Steinbusch, 1981). Terminals in the LC have also been demonstrated to take up labeled 5-HT (Léger and Descarries, 1978) and to be labeled following administration of tritiated amino acids into the raphe nuclei (Morgane and Jacobs, 1979). As indicated earlier, raphe nuclei have been reported by some workers to be labeled following HRP injections into the LC (Cedarbaum and Aghajanian, 1978b; Clavier, 1979). Neurochemical measurements in the LC have also indicated moderate levels of both 5-HT (Palkovits *et al.*, 1974) and tryptophan hydroxylase (Brownstein *et al.*, 1975). The biochemical measurement of moderate levels of histamine methyltransferase (Saavedra *et al.*, 1976) suggests a role for histamine in the LC. Innervation of the LC by GABA-containing fibers is indicated by nerve terminals which stain for glutamic acid decarboxylase (Fuxe *et al.*, 1978).

3.3. Neuropeptides

A recent advance in knowledge of neurotransmitters related to the LC has resulted from the immunocytochemical demonstration of various peptides associated with nerve fibers or neuronal somata in this nucleus. Enkephalins have been observed in nerve terminals of the LC (e.g., Sar *et al.*, 1978; Pickel *et al.*, 1979; Khachaturian *et al.*, 1983). Using colchicine to retard axoplasmic transport, Khachaturian *et al.* (1983) observed occasional enkephalin immunoreactivity in LC cell bodies in the rat. Using a similar technique in the cat, however, Charnay *et al.* (1982) demonstrated that *most* LC neurons staining for tyrosine hydroxylase were also stained for enkephalin. Melander *et al.* (1986) have reported that the "vast majority" of cells in the LC and some cells in the subcoeruleus displayed immunoreactivity for galanin. Other peptides have also been found to be contained within LC cell bodies, including vasopressin (Caffe *et al.*, 1985; Sofroniew, 1985), neurotensin (Uhl *et al.*, 1979), corticotropin-releasing factor (CRF) (Swanson *et al.*, 1983; Merchenthaler, 1984), neuropeptide Y (Everitt *et al.*, 1984), and somatostatin (Morley, 1985). Reports of avian pancreatic polypeptide immunoreactivity in LC neurons now appear to be attributable to neuropeptide Y or similar substances (Everitt *et al.*, 1984). The unavoidable conclusion from this is that most LC neurons must contain not only NA, but also at least one and perhaps two or more peptides. Again, this has potential significance for the control of LC activity in view of the descriptions of locally terminating axon collaterals and dendrodendritic junctions between LC neurons.

Several other peptides appear to be localized within nerve terminals in the LC, though not prominently in cell bodies. Such a pattern is presumed to reflect peptide-containing afferent systems terminating within the LC. Substance P-like immunoreactivity is present in moderate numbers of fibers, but only in a few cell bodies (Ljungdahl *et al.*, 1978; Pickel *et al.*, 1979; Shults *et al.*, 1984). Angiotensin II reactivity is also found in moderate numbers of nerve terminals in the LC (Fuxe *et al.*, 1976), while β-lipotropin, a component of the opiocortin complex, is present in high density (Watson *et al.*, 1977). Other peptides have been demonstrated in nerve terminals within the LC in lower densities, e.g., ACTH (Watson *et al.*, 1978), cholecystokinin (Vanderhaeghen *et al.*, 1980), and somatostatin (Finley *et al.*, 1981).

In many cases the results of these immunohistochemical studies are supported by biochemical measurements of low to moderate levels of the peptides in the LC (see Palkovits and Brownstein, 1983).

4. Neurotransmitter Receptors and Responsiveness in the LC

4.1. Receptor Binding

A currently active area of research, and one directly relevant to the topic of this chapter, is the autoradiographic localization of neurotransmitter binding sites within the brain (e.g., Chapters 35 and 36). Perhaps because of its discrete localization and density of neurons, the LC has been noted to exhibit moderate to high binding for several ligands. One of the best characterized is the α_2-adrenergic binding site, which is present in high concentration in the LC, while α_1 binding is low (e.g., Young and Kuhar, 1980). This apparently reflects the presence of "autoreceptors" for NA on the noradrenergic LC neurons. Also present, in very high levels, are binding sites for opiates (e.g., Atweh and Kuhar, 1977), which appear to be largely of the mu subtype (Quirion *et al.*, 1983). High-density binding has also been observed for substance P (Shults *et al.*, 1984), angiotensin II (Mendelsohn *et al.*, 1984), and somatostatin (Leroux *et al.*, 1985). Moderate levels of binding in the LC have been reported for histamine (H_1) receptors (Palacios *et al.*, 1981) and muscarinic receptors (Rotter *et al.*, 1979) while lower levels are seen for 5-HT receptors (Meibach, 1984), vasoactive intestinal peptide (Shaffer and Moody, 1986), CRF (Wynn *et al.*, 1984), and atrial natriuretic factor (Quirion *et al.*, 1984). An apparent parallelism in neurotransmitter presence and in receptor binding therefore exists for NA, enkephalins, substance P, angiotensin II, somatostatin, CRF, and 5-HT (see Table I).

Table I. Transmitters: Presence, Receptors, and Actions in the LC[a,b]

Neurotransmitter	Presence in LC		Receptor binding	Action
	Cell bodies	Terminals		
NA	**8,16	**1,15,47,48,50	α_2 **59 α_1 *21	(−)1,4,10,57
Adrenaline		*(PNMT)20		(−)5
Histamine		**42	**36	
Adenosine				(−)45
Acetylcholine		*(ChAT)23	**41	(+)9,18
Serotonin		*25,37,49	*28	(−)43a
Glutamate				(+)18,19
Glycine				(−)5
GABA		*(GAD)14		(−)5,18
Galanin	**29			
Vasopressin	**3,48			(+)34
Enkephalins	**(cat)6	**22,38,43	**2,39	(−)18,24,33
Substance P	*46	**27,38,46	**46	(+)7,17,18
Somatostatin	*32	*12	**26	
CRF	*31,51		*58	(+)53
Neurotensin	*52	*52		(−)60
Neuropeptide Y	*11			
Angiotensin II		**13	**30	
ACTH		*56		(+)35
Cholecystokinin		*54	**55	
Atrial natriuretic factor			*40	
VIP		*44		

[a]Symbols: *, low levels; **, moderate to high levels. −, inhibitory; +, excitatory.

[b]References: 1, Aghajanian et al. (1977); 2, Atweh and Kuhar (1977); 3, Caffe et al. (1985); 4, Cedarbaum and Aghajanian (1976); 5, Cedarbaum and Aghajanian (1978a); 6, Charnay et al. (1982); 7, Cheeseman et al. (1983); 8, Dahlström and Fuxe (1964); 9, Egan and North (1985); 10, Egan et al. (1983); 11, Everitt et al. (1984); 12, Finley et al. (1981); 13, Fuxe et al. (1976); 14, Fuxe et al. (1979); 15, Groves and Wilson (1980b); 16, Grzanna and Molliver (1980); 17, Guyenet and Aghajanian (1977); 18, Guyenet and Aghajanian (1979); 19, Henderson et al. (1982); 20, Hökfelt et al. (1974); 21, Jones et al. (1985a); 22, Khachaturian et al. (1983); 23, Kobayashi et al. (1975); 24, Korf et al. (1974); 25, Léger and Descarries (1978); 26, Leroux et al. (1985); 27, Ljungdahl et al. (1978); 28, Meibach (1984); 29, Melander et al. (1986); 30, Mendelsohn et al. (1984); 31, Merchenthaler (1984); 32, Morley (1985); 33, North and Williams (1983); 34, Olpe and Baltzer (1981); 35, Olpe and Jones (1982); 36, Palacios et al. (1981); 37, Pickel et al. (1977); 38, Pickel et al. (1979); 39, Quirion et al. (1983); 40, Quirion et al. (1984); 41, Rotter et al. (1979); 42, Saavedra et al. (1976); 43, Sar et al. (1978); 43a, Segal (1979); 44, Shaffer and Moody (1986); 45, Shefner and Chiu (1986); 46, Shults et al. (1984); 47, Shimizu et al. (1979); 48, Sofroniew (1985); 49, Steinbusch (1981); 50, Swanson (1976); 51, Swanson et al. (1983); 52, Uhl et al. (1979); 53, Valentino et al. (1983); 54, Vanderhaegen et al. (1980); 55, Van Dijk et al. (1984); 56, Watson et al. (1978); 57, Williams et al. (1985); 58, Wynn et al. (1984); 59, Young and Kuhar (1980); 60, Young et al. (1978).

4.2. Effects on Neuronal Excitability

The effects of several neurotransmitter substances on LC neurons have been tested using electrophysiological methods. Problems with mechanical stability have prevented reliable intracellular recording in the brain stem of living animals, so most of the electrophysiological studies have been carried out using either extracellular recordings in animals or intracellular recordings in an *in vitro* brain slice preparation. NA and the opiates have been most carefully studied, while less complete tests have been made for other substances. NA depresses the activity of LC neurons, and in intracellular studies is found to hyperpolarize the cells by increasing membrane conductance to potassium ions (Williams et al., 1985). The receptor type mediating this effect is the α_2 adrenergic receptor (Cedarbaum and Aghajanian, 1977; Williams et al., 1985). The actions and mechanisms of opiates are mediated largely by mu receptors (North and Williams, 1983) and appear to be very similar to those of NA (Korf *et al.*, 1974; Pepper and Henderson, 1980). NA and the opiates appear to use the same ionic channels (North and Williams, 1985) and to involve similar mechanisms by which intracellular cAMP levels are reduced (Andrade and Aghajanian, 1985; Aghajanian and Wang, 1986).

Adrenaline, dopamine, and isoproterenol (a β adrenergic agonist) and phenylephrine (an α_1 agonist) all gave inhibitions similar to those of NA, when applied iontophoretically. It seems quite possible, however, that these effects are mediated by actions on α_2 receptors on the basis of tests with receptor-binding drugs (Cedarbaum and Aghajanian, 1977).

Acetylcholine has an excitatory action on LC neurons (Guyenet and Aghajanian, 1977, 1979), mediated by muscarinic receptors, apparently of the M_2 type (Egan and North, 1985). It is interesting that in the slice preparation, the excitatory actions of acetylcholine were enhanced by treatment with acetylcholinesterase inhibitors (Egan and North, 1985). In the same study, it was shown that LC neurons could also be depolarized by nicotine, and this effect was blocked by the nicotinic antagonist hexamethonium. 5-HT has also been tested iontophoretically on LC neurons, and was found to cause a depression of spontaneous activity which could be antagonized by methysergide (Segal, 1979). As might be expected, the amino acid neurotransmitters have been found to exert their usual effects in the LC. Glutamate excites LC neurons (Guyenet and Aghajanian, 1979; Henderson *et al.*, 1982; Marshall *et al.*, 1984), while inhibitory responses are seen with GABA and glycine (Cedarbaum and Aghajanian, 1978a). Recently, it has also been reported that adenosine depresses activity of most LC neurons in the slice preparation (Shefner and Chiu, 1986).

Several peptides have been tested for effects on excitability of LC neurons. Excitatory actions have been reported for substance P (Guyenet and Aghajanian, 1977; Cheeseman *et al.*, 1983), ACTH (Olpe and Jones, 1982), CRF (Valentino *et al.*, 1983), and vasopressin (Olpe and Baltzer, 1981), while in limited tests, no effect was found for iontophoretically applied bradykinin, neurotensin, or thyrotropin-releasing hormone (Guyenet and Aghajanian, 1977). In another study, however, neurotensin was reported to have inhibitory effects (Young *et al.*, 1978). It should be noted that most of these tests of peptide actions have been conducted in anesthetized animals. It is possible that stronger effects would be seen in unanesthetized or *in vitro* preparations.

5. Bursting Activity of LC Neurons

The activity of LC neurons in anesthetized rats is characterized by a slow and rather regular firing of single spikes, usually at a rate of 1–5 per second (e.g., Korf *et al.*, 1974). In such preparations noxious stimuli typically evoke a brief series of action potentials, followed by a prolonged period of inhibition (e.g., Aghajanian *et al.*, 1977). Steady rates of resting discharge are also observed in LC neurons in brain slice preparations (Williams *et al.*, 1984). In the lightly anesthetized or unanesthetized rat, however, irregular patterns of discharge, higher rates, and increased responsiveness to sensory stimulation are observed (Korf *et al.*, 1974; Akaike, 1982). It has also been suggested that the bursting activity observed in these preparations or in response to noxious stimulation reflects the synchronous activation of many LC neurons (Akaike, 1982).

An additional type of preparation which has recently been used to advantage is the behaving animal (rat, cat, or monkey) which has chronically implanted electrodes for recording single-unit activity within the LC (Jacobs, 1986). Because of the nonhomogeneous composition of the LC in cats, physiological and pharmacological criteria have been used to identify noradrenergic neurons. In these chronic experiments, LC neurons are generally found to exhibit slow rates of firing with patterns less regular than in anesthetized animals, and to exhibit brief bursts of activity related to changes in behavioral state or to stimulation of almost any sensory modality (Foote *et al.*, 1980; Aston-Jones and Bloom, 1981a,b). It has also been observed in these studies that the magnitude of the sensory responses is closely related to the level of vigilance of the animal and to the degree of arousal associated with the stimulus. Synchronous activation of large numbers of LC neurons is another characteristic of sensory responses in this preparation (Aston-Jones and Bloom, 1981a,b). The synchronous activation of LC neurons is particularly interesting, because of the implication that it will cause NA to be released almost simultaneously throughout the widespread target areas of the LC.

A potential model for the study of mechanisms of synchronous activation of LC neurons is the explant culture of LC cells (Hendelman *et al.*, 1982). These cultures are prepared from the brains of newborn mice and permit visual identification of LC neurons in the living culture, and electrophysiological and pharmacological testing of them. We have observed that in more than half of the cultures studied, LC neurons exhibit bursting activity (Fig. 1). In a small number of cultures, steady rates of discharge are observed, while in the remainder, there is no spontaneous activity. We have also found that in those cultures in which LC neurons are bursting, almost all of the LC neurons recorded exhibit similar bursting patterns. In addition, simultaneous intracellular recordings from two LC neurons show that there is a very high degree of synchrony between bursts in different cells (Finlayson and Marshall, 1985).

This preparation offers the particular advantages of an *in vitro* system for the study of mechanisms, i.e., possibilities for stable intracellular recordings, introduction of drugs in known, minimal concentrations, and alteration of ionic constituents of the bathing medium. Because the LC slice preparation is characterized by tonic discharge of LC neurons, this culture preparation is also the only *in vitro* model available for study of bursting activity in these cells.

The frequency of bursting observed in the cultured neurons varies widely, from several per minute, to one every 20 min. Their duration may be as short as 1 sec, or even less, but is frequently 10 or more sec, with usual spiking frequencies of 10–30 per sec within the burst. These bursts are thus often more prolonged than those seen in the behaving animal (rat), which have been described to have typical frequencies of 10–20 per sec in a burst of two to six impulses, in response to sensory stimulation (Aston-Jones *et al.*, 1980). Another feature of the bursts in the cultured neurons is the appearance of spontaneous depolarizing events at the time of the bursts. The action potentials seem generated by summations of these events, which generally continue throughout the burst and for some period following the spiking activity (Fig. 2).

The most frequently cited mechanisms of synchronous bursting activity in neurons are (1) electrical coupling by low-resistance electrical junctions between cells, (2) field effects generated by nearby activated neurons, and (3) a common excitatory synaptic input to the population of neurons. The depolarizing events we have observed (Fig. 2) could, in turn, be chemical or electrical synaptic potentials, field potentials spread from activated neurons, or electrotonically conducted dendritic spikes which have failed to activate a somatic action potential.

In order to test for electrical coupling between neurons, we have carried out simultaneous

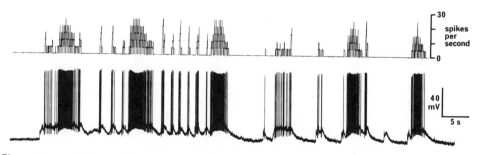

Figure 1. Intracellular recording (lower trace) of a spontaneously bursting locus coeruleus neuron in an explant culture. Upper trace shows ratemeter output, indicating firing frequencies achieved during bursts.

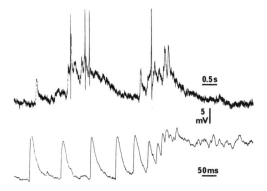

Figure 2. Chart recording of spontaneous potentials in cultured LC neurons. Top trace: spontaneous depolarizing potentials precede and evoke a short burst of activity. Lower trace: example of spontaneous depolarizations which initially occur individually, and subsequently summate to produce a sustained depolarization similar to the depolarizations associated with bursts of activity. Voltage calibration applies to both traces.

intracellular recordings from several pairs of LC neurons. Though highly synchronized bursting was observed in most of these pairs, no evidence for electrical junctions was observed in any pair. Depolarizing and hyperpolarizing current pulses were injected into one cell of the pair while recording from the second neuron. In a few cells, very small (300 μV or less) depolarizing potentials were observed in the second cell, only when spikes were evoked by depolarizing pulses in the first cell. However, these were correlated in time with the afterhyperpolarization of the spike, suggesting that they might be generated by localized increases in extracellular potassium released by the activated neuron (Yarom and Spira, 1982). In addition, the amplitude of these potentials was not consistent with the large depolarizing events observed in association with the bursts.

As a second test for electrical coupling, we have injected lucifer yellow into cultured LC neurons. This fluorescent dye is reported to cross low-resistance junctions between cells and can thus indicate electrical coupling if more than one cell is stained following injection into a single neuron. We found no evidence for electrical coupling in these tests, supporting the negative results of the electrophysiological experiments.

An important test for the discrimination of electrically mediated transmission from chemical transmission is whether the event is calcium-dependent. Our most conclusive experiments for calcium dependency of the bursts involved the exchange of the normal 1.8 mM Ca^{2+}-containing bathing medium with one containing 0.5 mM Ca^{2+} and 2.0 mM manganese. During perfusion with this solution, which blocks chemical synaptic transmission, the bursts were abolished, but returned with restoration of the normal bathing solution. Excitability of the neurons remained constant or was slightly increased (i.e., decreased spike threshold) during perfusion with the test solution, suggesting that the absence of bursting was related to decreased chemical transmission.

In an additional test, we investigated the potential-dependency of the depolarizing events observed in LC neurons. These were found to be progressively increased in amplitude by injection of hyperpolarizing current and decreased by depolarizing currents, suggesting that they are chemically mediated synaptic potentials rather than potentials electrotonically conducted from remote parts of the neuron, or electrically transmitted from other active neurons.

The remaining puzzle is the source of these potent excitatory synaptic inputs. In the living cultures, frequently the only neurons visible in the LC area are the large ones which we have characterized as LC neurons (Hendelman *et al.*, 1982). With Nissl staining, however, we have now observed that in most cultures there is also a limited number of small neurons within or in the periphery of the cluster of LC neurons. This raises the possibility that there is a group of small neurons which lie within or nearby the LC in neonates, which are taken with the LC neurons in our explanting procedure. There are several observations by other workers which might be consistent with this idea. Shimizu *et al.* (1979) have observed small neurons within the LC which do not contain the type of vesicles which appear to characterize the larger noradrenergic neurons.

It is possible that these could be interneurons which mediate the type of excitation we have observed. Aston-Jones and Bloom (1981a) have observed that during most phases of the sleep–waking cycle, phasic discharges of LC neurons are associated with field potentials in the LC. In paradoxical sleep, however, when the LC neurons are quite inactive, the field potentials are still observed. These authors have proposed that the field potentials reflect "intense, concerted excitatory postsynaptic potentials" in LC neurons.

We have considered it unlikely that the excitation is spread by collaterals of the noradrenergic LC neurons themselves. We have never, during intracellular recordings from more than 100 LC neurons, observed a cell whose spikes preceded the barrages of EPSPs, and which might thus "trigger" the bursting activity. In addition, the primary action of NA on LC neurons is inhibitory, and appears to be exclusively inhibitory in LC neurons of older cultures and older animals (see below). Since the bursts are observed in mature animals and older cultures, it is unlikely that they are mediated by NA. We have also observed that in cultures treated with the α_1 adrenergic antagonist prazosin, bursting of LC neurons can still be observed. Since any excitatory actions of NA on LC neurons appear to be mediated by α_1 receptors, this also argues against noradrenergic mediation of the bursts. Nakamura et al. (1980) have reported a recurrent facilitation of LC neurons following electrical stimulation of LC target areas, and found that NA was involved in the mediation of this facilitation. It seems quite possible, however, that this effect is relayed through excitatory neurons to the recorded LC neurons. While the possibility that the depolarizing events are mediated by corelease of excitatory transmitters from LC neurons has not been completely eliminated, it seems unlikely, in the absence of any evidence for excitatory influence from one LC neuron to another.

We feel that the bursting activity of LC neurons has implications for the physiological actions of these neurons on cells in their widespread target areas. The first has been discussed by Aston-Jones et al. (1980). The occurrence of a brief burst of action potentials in LC neurons is likely to result in a higher-frequency burst of potentials at the nerve terminals of these cells, because the first several impulses of such a spike train exhibit progressively shorter conduction times along the axon. This in turn could enhance transmitter release at the terminals due to synaptic facilitation (Aston-Jones et al., 1980). This second implication is that bursts of the type described for LC neurons may preferentially release peptide neurotransmitters. This condition has been described for peripheral noradrenergic neurons by Lundberg et al. (1986). In view of the probable presence of peptide cotransmitters in most LC neurons (see Section 3.3), bursting activity could be an important factor for qualitative as well as quantitative effects of LC activity on target areas.

6. Mechanisms of Postactivation Inhibition

One of the earliest described and most characteristic features of LC neuron activity is a burst of activation in response to sensory or antidromic stimulation followed by a prolonged period of inactivation (e.g., Cedarbaum and Aghajanian, 1976; Aghajanian et al., 1977). This inhibition was proposed to be mediated by adrenergic actions of locally terminating axon collaterals of the LC neurons (Aghajanian et al., 1977). The demonstration of adrenergic inhibitory postsynaptic potentials produced by focal stimulation in the slice preparation (Egan et al., 1983) was consistent with this proposal. In recent work, however, Aghajanian et al. (1983) and Andrade and Aghajanian (1984a) have demonstrated a calcium-dependent potassium conductance $G_K(Ca)$ which is generated following spike activation in LC neurons, and which is capable of potently inhibiting subsequent action potentials in the activated neuron.

In a discriminating experiment, Andrade and Aghajanian (1984b) compared the inhibitions in single LC neurons following perithreshold stimulation of the LC axon bundle, which did or did not evoke an antidromic spike in the recorded neuron. They reported that a significant inhibition was only observed following stimuli which evoked an antidromic spike. Further, increasing the stimulus intensity beyond the level required for consistent activation of the recorded cell (which should evoke activity in other LC neurons) significantly increased the duration of the inhibition in only about half of the tested cells. It was concluded that the postactivation inhibition observed in LC neurons is mainly attributable to the $G_K(Ca)$. In a similar experiment, with a larger number of tests, Ennis and Aston-Jones (1986) have reported evidence for a significant component of poststimulus inhibition which is independent of spike activation following antidromic or sensory nerve stimulation, and which may be blocked by the α adrenergic antagonist piperoxane. Their conclusion was that the $G_K(Ca)$ and collateral noradrenergic inhibition may be about equal in their contributions to the postactivation inhibition.

It appears, therefore, that these mechanisms represent quite potent controls of LC neuron activity, which would serve to limit the rates of firing of LC neurons. It is interesting that a similar $G_K(Ca)$ in hippocampal neurons has been found to be depressed by neurotransmitters such as NA (β-receptor mediated) (Madison and Nicoll, 1986), acetylcholine (Cole and Nicoll, 1984), and histamine (Haas and Konnerth, 1983). If such neurotransmitter effects are active on LC neurons, they would provide a mechanism for controlling at least one component of the postactivation inhibition and thereby permitting higher rates of activation in LC neurons.

7. Developmental Changes in Responsiveness of LC Neurons

In addition to the studies of bursting activity in LC neurons in culture, we have tested neuronal responsiveness to adrenergic drugs, and have found an interesting change during development (Finlayson and Marshall, 1984, 1986). If NA is applied iontophoretically to the LC neurons, with tetrodotoxin in the perfusate to avoid indirect responses, two types of response are observed. In some cells, simple hyperpolarizing responses are observed, while in others, an initial hyperpolarization is succeeded by a later depolarization, giving a biphasic response (Fig. 3). Because the responses of different cells were usually similar within any single culture, correlations were sought between the type of response and the properties of the culture. The only correlation discovered was with the duration of the time the tissue had been in culture. Since all cultures are prepared from the brains of neonatal mice (within 24 hr of birth), the time in culture is related to the postnatal age of the tissue. It was found that in cultures which were 16–19 days old, all LC neurons exhibited the biphasic responses to NA, while in cultures older than 26 days, all cells gave simple hyperpolarizing responses. In cultures in the age range of 20–26 days, responses of either type were observed. This age relationship remains valid after testing more than 100 cells, with a minimum of 16 in each of these three age categories.

Pharmacological investigations have revealed that the simple hyperpolarizing responses and the hyperpolarizing phase of the biphasic responses are mediated by α_2 adrenergic receptors, while the depolarizing component of the biphasic responses is dependent on α_1 receptors (Finlayson and Marshall, 1986). This has been demonstrated both by selective blocking of the

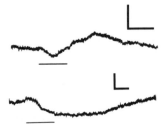

Figure 3. Intracellular recordings of responses of cultured LC neurons to iontophoretically applied noradrenaline (horizontal bars) during tetrodotoxin intoxication. Top trace: a biphasic response to NA in a "young" culture. Bottom trace: a simple hyperpolarizing response to NA in an "older" culture. Calibration bars 5 mV × 10 sec.

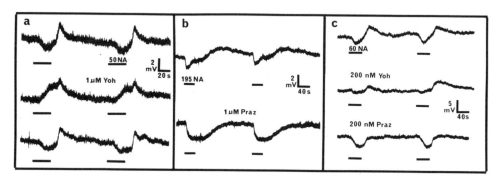

Figure 4. Application of adrenergic antagonists by bath perfusion during recording of biphasic responses to iontophoretically applied NA. Iontophoretic applications are indicated by bars below recording traces. (a) Biphasic response to NA (upper trace); during perfusion of 1 μM yohimbine, hyperpolarizing phase is blocked leaving only a depolarizing response (middle trace); the effect is reversed after washing by control perfusate (lower trace). (b) Upper trace shows control biphasic response to NA; prazosin (1 μM) selectively blocks the depolarizing phase of the response (lower trace). (c) Biphasic response to NA shown in upper trace shows selective reduction of hyperpolarizing phase during perfusion with 200 nM yohimbine (middle trace); subsequent perfusion with 200 nM prazosin resulted in selective loss of the depolarizing phase of the response (lower trace). (From Finlayson and Marshall, 1986.)

responses by antagonists for α_1 (prazosin) and α_2 (yohimbine) receptors (Fig. 4), and by mimicking the depolarization and hyperpolarization using α_1 and α_2 agonists (Fig. 5).

It would appear, therefore that an α_1 adrenergic excitatory responsiveness is present in a period corresponding to early postnatal development, but disappears during subsequent development. In order to determine whether this transient α_1 responsiveness also occurs in the intact, developing animal, tests have been made in LC neurons in brain slices from young rats. In earlier studies, it had been reported that the α_1 agonist phenylephrine was ineffective on LC neurons in brain slices from adult rats, except that in high concentrations, it evoked small hyperpolarizations (Williams *et al.*, 1985). In comparable tests on slices from rats of 8–26 days, however, about 80% of the LC neurons exhibited depolarizing or excitatory responses to phenylephrine (Marshall and Williams, 1986). The demonstration of this transient α_1 responsiveness in two very different *in vitro* preparations, from different species, strongly suggests that this is a phenomenon that occurs normally during development of the LC. It cannot be determined from studies of this type whether the lost responsiveness might be due to a loss of α_1 receptors from the neurons, or uncoupling of the receptor–ionophore interaction. An earlier autoradiographic study of adrenergic receptor binding in the LC of adult rats indicated dense binding of an α_2 ligand, while binding of an α_1 antagonist seemed little higher than background levels (Young and Kuhar, 1980). Using a different α_1 ligand, however, Jones *et al.* (1985a) have demonstrated binding in the LC. It is particularly interesting, however, that they have also shown that in some brain locations, α_1 binding reaches high levels in early postnatal periods, but is very much reduced later in development (Jones *et al.*, 1985b). To clarify whether there are developmentally transient α_1 receptors in the LC, it would be desirable to use high-resolution autoradiography with tritiated prazosin, since this is the antagonist used in our studies to discriminate the age-related response differences.

Is there a functional role for these developmentally transient responses? The effect of excitatory adrenergic responses at this period might be to increase responsiveness of LC neurons to afferent pathways in developing animals. In fact, a recent study of LC neurons in anesthetized neonatal rats has indicated that these neurons are much more responsive to sensory stimulation than are those in adult rats (Kimura and Nakamura, 1985). In view of several suggestions that the LC may play a role in development of neurons in target areas (e.g., Felten *et al.*, 1982; Robain *et*

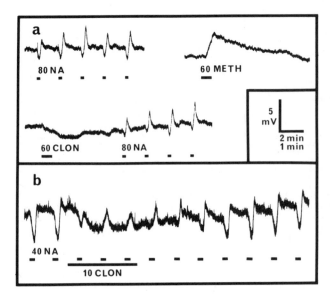

Figure 5. Iontophoretic application of NA and adrenergic agonists to LC neurons. (a) NA evokes biphasic response (upper left) while methoxamine gives a depolarization with no evident hyperpolarizing phase (upper right); clonidine application results in slow hyperpolarization with no apparent depolarizing phase. (b) Application of clonidine during continuing series of NA applications; response to clonidine is a slow hyperpolarization; NA responses appear as simple depolarizations during maximal clonidine response and gradually return to control biphasic pattern. Time calibration bar (inset) represents 2 min for (a) and 1 min for (b). (From Finlayson and Marshall, 1986.)

al., 1985), it is possible that enhanced activity of LC neurons in early postnatal periods could be an important factor in any influence by this nucleus on development of target areas.

8. Summary and Conclusions

It can be concluded that there are several factors which are potentially important for the control of neuronal activity in the LC. Two intrinsic mechanisms are capable of limiting rates of activity in LC neurons: a long afterhyperpolarization due to calcium-dependent potassium conductance increase, and a noradrenergic collateral and/or dendrodendritic inhibition. These may partly underlie the relatively low rates of firing (10–20 per sec) of LC neurons during burst discharges, in comparison with many other types of neurons.

While there is a recent suggestion that the number of afferent fiber systems is lower than previously indicated, the variety of types of synaptic terminations on LC neurons (Groves and Wilson, 1980a) and the reports of afferent fiber systems containing distinct neurotransmitters/neuropeptides suggest considerable diversity of afferent pathways. Conversely, the similarity of LC responses to stimulation of the various sensory systems suggests that there may be convergence of such systems at some other center, with subsequent relay to the LC. It is conceivable that the more direct responses to environmental stimuli are relayed through common paths, but that several modulatory systems also impinge on the LC and are capable of altering its responsiveness.

Evidence has been presented for the colocalization of several peptides within NA-containing LC neurons. Since these peptides are capable of altering neuronal excitability, it is possible that they also modify LC neuronal activity by release from axon collaterals or at dendrodendritic junctions. Since receptor binding sites or electrophysiological responses in the LC have not been demonstrated for some of the colocalized peptides, such a role remains speculative.

Studies of synchronous bursting in cultured LC neurons suggest that such bursts are generated by barrages of excitatory synaptic potentials from neurons which are located in or around the LC, at least at birth. Electrical coupling does not appear to contribute significantly to the generation of bursts. Brief burst responses to various stimuli are common in LC neurons of unanesthetized animals, and a high degree of synchrony has been observed in the responses of different LC neurons. Such bursting patterns of activity may be particularly effective for release of transmitter in target areas, and could also enhance the relative amounts of peptide transmitter released from LC axon terminals.

A transient excitatory responsiveness to NA has been found in developing LC neurons in both tissue culture and brain slices from young rats. Such a mechanism could result in different levels or patterns of LC neuronal activity at different stages of postnatal development and may be a novel example of developmental changes in neuronal responsiveness.

ACKNOWLEDGMENTS. Our research has been supported by a grant from the Medical Research Council of Canada (to K.C.M.). We are grateful to Danielle Richer for technical assistance and to Anita Bouchard for typing the manuscript.

References

Aghajanian, G. K., and Wang, Y.-Y., 1986, Pertussis toxin blocks outward currents evoked by opiate and α_2-agonists in locus coeruleus neurons, *Brain Res.* **371**:390–394.

Aghajanian, G. K., Cedarbaum, J. M., and Wang, R. Y., 1977, Evidence for norepinephrine-mediated collateral inhibition of locus coeruleus neurons, *Brain Res.* **136**:570–577.

Aghajanian, G. K., Vandermaelen, C. P., and Andrade, R., 1983, Intracellular studies on the role of calcium in regulating the activity and reactivity of locus coeruleus neurons in vivo, *Brain Res.* **273**:237–243.

Akaike, T., 1982, Periodic bursting activities of locus coeruleus neurons in the rat, *Brain Res.* **239**:629–633.

Albanese, A., and Butcher, A. L., 1980, Acetylcholinesterase and catecholamine distribution in the locus coeruleus of the rat, *Brain Res. Bull.* **5**:127–134.

Amaral, D. G., and Sinnamon, H. M., 1977, The locus coeruleus: Neurobiology of a central noradrenergic nucleus, *Prog. Neurobiol.* **9**:147–196.

Andrade, R., and Aghajanian, G. K., 1984a, Locus coeruleus activity in vitro: Intrinsic regulation by a calcium-dependent potassium conductance but not α_2-adrenoceptors, *J. Neurosci.* **4**:161–170.

Andrade, R., and Aghajanian, G. K., 1984b, Intrinsic regulation of locus coeruleus neurons: Electrophysiological evidence indicating a predominant role for autoinhibition, *Brain Res.* **310**:401–406.

Andrade, R., and Aghajanian, G. K., 1985, Opiate- and α_2-adrenoceptor-induced hyperpolarizations of locus coeruleus neurons in brain slices: Reversal by cyclic adenosine $3':5'$-monophosphate analogues, *J. Neurosci.* **5**:2359–2364.

Aston-Jones, G., and Bloom, F. E., 1981a, Activity of norepinephrine-containing locus coeruleus neurons in behaving rats anticipates fluctuations in the sleep-waking cycle, *J. Neurosci.* **1**:876–886.

Aston-Jones, G., and Bloom, F. E., 1981b, Norepinephrine-containing locus coeruleus neurons in behaving rats exhibit pronounced responses to non-noxious environmental stimuli, *J. Neurosci.* **1**:887–900.

Aston-Jones, G., Segal, M., and Bloom, F. E., 1980, Brain aminergic axons exhibit marked variability in conduction velocity, *Brain Res.* **195**:215–222.

Aston-Jones, G., Ennis, M., Nickell, W. T., and Shipley, M. T., 1985, The nucleus locus coeruleus: Extensive efferents but restricted afferents as revealed by transport of discretely injected peroxidase-labelled wheat germ agglutinin, *Soc. Neurosci. Abstr.* **11**:829.

Atweh, S. F., and Kuhar, M. J., 1977, Autoradiographic localization of opiate receptors in rat brain. II. The brain stem, *Brain Res.* **129**:1–12.

Bobillier, P., Lewis, B. D., Seguin, S., and Pujol, J. F., 1978, Evidence for direct anatomical connections between the raphe system and other aminergic groups of the central nervous system as revealed by autoradiography, in:

Interactions between Putative neurotransmitters in the Brain (S. Garattini, J. F. Pujol, and R. Samanin, eds.), Raven Press, New York, pp. 343–354.

Brownstein, M. J., Palkovits, M., Saavedra, J. M., and Kizer, J. S., 1975, Tryptophan hydroxylase in the rat brain, *Brain Res.* **97:**163–166.

Caffe, A. R., van Leuwen, F. W., Buijs, R. M., de Vries G. J., and Geffard, M., 1985, Coexistence of vasopressin, neurophysin and noradrenaline immunoreactivity in medium-sized cells of the locus coeruleus and subcoeruleus in the rat, *Brain Res.* **338:**160–164.

Cedarbaum, J. M., and Aghajanian, G. K., 1976, Noradrenergic neurons of the locus coeruleus: Inhibition of epinephrine and activation by the α-antagonist piperoxane, *Brain Res.* **112:**413–419.

Cedarbaum, J. M., and Aghajanian, G., 1977, Catecholamine receptors on locus coeruleus neurons: Pharmacological characterization, *Eur. J. Pharmacol.* **44:**375–385.

Cedarbaum, J. M., and Aghajanian, G. K., 1978a, Activation of locus coeruleus neurons by peripheral stimuli: Modulation by a collateral inhibitory mechanism, *Life Sci.* **23:**1383–1392.

Cedarbaum, J. M., and Aghajanian, G. K., 1978b, Afferent projections to the rat locus coeruleus as determined by a retrograde tracing technique, *J. Comp. Neurol.* **178:**1–16.

Charnay, Y., Léger, L., Dray, F., Berod, A., Jouvet, M., Pujol, J. F., and Dubois, P. M., 1982, Evidence for the presence of enkephalin in catecholaminergic neurones of cat locus coeruleus, *Neurosci. Lett.* **30:**147–151.

Cheeseman, H. J., Pinnock, R. D., and Henderson, G., 1983, Substance P excitation of rat locus coeruleus neurones, *Eur. J. Pharmacol.* **94:**93–99.

Cheney, D. L., LeFevre, H. F., and Racagni, G., 1975, Choline acetyltransferase activity and mass fragmentographic measurement of acetylcholine in specific nuclei and tracts of rat brain, *Neuropharmacology* **14:**801–809.

Cimarusti, D. L., Saito, K., Vaughn, J. E., Barber, R., Roberts, E., and Thomas, P. E., 1979, Immunohistochemical localization of dopamine-β-hydroxylase in rat locus coeruleus and hypothalamus, *Brain Res.* **162:**55–67.

Clavier, R. M., 1979, Afferent projections to the self-stimulation regions of the dorsal pons, including the locus coeruleus, in the rat as demonstrated by the horseradish peroxidase technique, *Brain Res. Bull.* **4:**497–504.

Cole, A. E., and Nicoll, R. A., 1984, Characterization of a slow cholinergic post-synaptic potential recorded *in vitro* from rat hippocampal pyramidal cells, *J. Physiol. (London)* **352:**173–188.

Conrad, L. C. A., Leonard, C. M., and Pfaff, D. W., 1974, Connections of the median and dorsal raphe nuclei in the rat: An autoradiographic and degeneration study, *J. Comp. Neurol.* **156:**129–206.

Dahlström, A., and Fuxe, K., 1964, Evidence for the existence of monoamine-containing neurons in the central nervous system. I. Demonstration of monoamines in the cell body of brain stem neurons, *Acta Physiol. Scand.* **62**(Suppl. 232):1–55.

Egan, T. M., and North, R. A., 1985, Acetylcholine acts on m_2-muscarinic receptors to excite rat locus coeruleus neurones, *Br. J. Pharmacol.* **85:**733–735.

Egan, T. M., Henderson, G., North, R. A., and Williams, J. T., 1983, Noradrenaline-mediated synaptic inhibition in rat locus coeruleus neurones, *J. Physiol. (London)* **345:**477–488.

Elam, M., Thoren, P., and Svensson, T. H., 1986, Locus coeruleus neurons and sympathetic nerves: Activation by visceral afferents, *Brain Res.* **375:**117–125.

Ennis, M., and Aston-Jones, G., 1986, Evidence for self- and neighbor-mediated postactivation inhibition of locus coeruleus neurons, *Brain Res.* **374:**299–305.

Everitt, B. J., Hökfelt, T., Terenius, L., Tatemoto, K., Mutt, V., and Goldstein, M., 1984, Differential coexistence of neuropeptide Y (NPY)-like immunoreactivity with catecholamines in the central nervous system of the rat, *Neuroscience* **11:**443–462.

Felten, D. L., Hallman, H., and Jonsson, G., 1982, Evidence for a neurotrophic role of noradrenaline neurons in the postnatal development of rat cerebral cortex, *J. Neurocytol.* **11:**119–135.

Finlayson, P. G., and Marshall, K. C., 1984, Hyperpolarizing and age-dependent depolarizing responses of cultured locus coeruleus neurons to noradrenaline, *Dev. Brain Res.* **15:**167–175.

Finlayson, P. G., and Marshall, K. C., 1985, Synchronous bursting of locus coeruleus neurons in tissue culture: A common excitatory input or electrotonic coupling of neurons? *Soc. Neurosci. Abstr.* **11:**1081.

Finlayson, P. G., and Marshall, K. C., 1986, Locus coeruleus neurons in culture have a developmentally transient α_1-adrenergic response, *Dev. Brain Res.* **25:**292–295.

Finley, J. C. W., Maderbrut, J. L., Roger, L. J., and Petrusz, P., 1981, The immunocytochemical localization of somatostatin-containing neurons in the rat central nervous system, *Neuroscience* **6:**2173–2192.

Foote, S. L., Aston-Jones, G., and Bloom, F. E., 1980, Impulse activity of locus coeruleus neurons in awake rats and monkeys is a function of sensory stimulation and arousal, *Proc. Natl. Acad. Sci. USA* **77:**3033–3037.

Foote, S. L., Bloom, F. E., and Aston-Jones, G., 1983, Nucleus locus coeruleus: New evidence of anatomical and physiological specificity, *Physiol. Rev.* **63**:844–914.

Fuxe, K., Ganten, D., Hökfelt, T., and Bolme, P., 1976, Immunohistochemical evidence for the existence of angiotensin II-containing nerve terminals in the brain and spinal cord of rat, *Neurosci. Lett.* **2**:229–234.

Fuxe, K., Hökfelt, T., Agnati, L. F., Johansson, M., Goldstein, M., Perez de la Mora, M., Passanti, L., Tapia, R., Teran, L., and Palacios, J., 1978, Mapping out central catecholamine neurons: Immunohistochemical studies on catecholamine-synthesizing enzymes, in: *Psychopharmacology: A Generation of Progress* (M. A. Lipton, A. DiMascio, and K. F. Killam, eds.), Raven Press, New York, pp. 67–95.

Grant, S. J., and Redmond, D. E., Jr., 1981, The neuroanatomy and pharmacology of the nucleus locus coeruleus, in: *Psychopharmacology of Clonidine* (H. Lal and S. Fielding, eds.), Liss, New York, pp. 5–27.

Groves, P. M., and Wilson, C. J., 1980a, Fine structure of rat locus coeruleus, *J. Comp. Neurol.* **193**:841–852.

Groves, P. M., and Wilson, C. J., 1980b, Monoaminergic presynaptic axons and dendrites in rat locus coeruleus seen in reconstructions of serial sections, *J. Comp. Neurol.* **193**:853–862.

Grzanna, R., and Molliver, M. E., 1980, The locus coeruleus in the rat: An histochemical delineation, *Neuroscience* **5**:21–40.

Guyenet, P., and Aghajanian, G. K., 1977, Excitation of neurons in the nucleus locus coeruleus by substance P and related peptides, *Brain Res.* **136**:178–184.

Guyenet, P., and Aghajanian, G., 1979, ACh, substance P and met-enkephalin in the locus coeruleus: Pharmacological evidence for independent sites of action, *Eur. J. Pharmacol.* **53**:319–328.

Haas, H. L., and Konnerth, A., 1983, Histamine and noradrenaline decrease calcium-activated potassium conductance in hippocampal pyramidal cells, *Nature* **302**:432–434.

Hendelman, W. J., Marshall, K. C., Ferguson, R., and Carrière, S., 1982, Catecholamine neurons of the central nervous system in organotypic culture, *Dev. Neurosci.* **5**:64–76.

Henderson, G., Pepper, C. M., and Shefner, S. A., 1982, Electrophysiological properties of neurones contained in the locus coeruleus and mesencephalic nucleus of the trigeminal nerve *in vitro*, *Exp. Brain Res.* **45**:29–37.

Hökfelt, T., Fuxe, K., Goldstein, M., and Johansson, O., 1974, Immunohistochemical evidence for the existence of adrenaline neurons in the rat brain, *Brain Res.* **66**:255–257.

Jacobs, B. L., 1986, Single unit activity of locus coeruleus neurons in behaving animals, *Prog. Neurobiol.* **27**:183–194.

Jones, L. S., Gauger, L. L., and Davis, J. N., 1985a, Anatomy of brain alpha$_1$-adrenergic receptors: In vitro autoradiography with [^{125}I]-HEAT, *J. Comp. Neurol.* **231**:190–208.

Jones, L. S., Gauger, L. L., Davis, J. N., Slotkin, T. A., and Bartolome, J. V., 1985b, Postnatal development of brain alpha$_1$-adrenergic receptors: In vitro autoradiography with [^{125}I]Heat in normal rats and rats treated with alphadifluoromethylornithine, a specific, irreversible inhibitor of ornithine decarboxylase, *Neuroscience* **15**:1195–1202.

Khachaturian, H., Lewis, M. E., and Watson, S. J., 1983, Enkephalin systems in diencephalon and brainstem of the rat, *J. Comp. Neurol.* **220**:310–320.

Kimura, F., and Nakamura, S., 1985, Locus coeruleus neurons in the neonatal rat: Electrical activity and responses to sensory stimulation, *Dev. Brain Res.* **23**:301–305.

Kobayashi, R. M., Brownstein, M., Saavedra, J. M., and Palkovits, M., 1975, Choline acetyltransferase content in discrete regions of the rat brain stem, *J. Neurochem.* **24**:637–640.

Korf, J., Bunney, B. S., and Aghajanian, G. K., 1974, Noradrenergic neurons: Morphine inhibition of spontaneous activity, *Eur. J. Pharmacol.* **25**:165–169.

Koslow, S. H., and Schlumpf, M., 1974, Quantitation of adrenaline in rat brain nuclei and areas by mass fragmentography, *Nature* **251**:530–531.

Leǵer, L., and Descarries, L., 1978, Serotonin nerve terminals in the locus coeruleus of adult rat: A radioautographic study, *Brain Res.* **145**:1–13.

Leroux, P., Quirion, R., and Pelletier, G., 1985, Localization and characterization of brain somatostatin receptors as studied with somatostatin-14 and somatostatin-28 receptor radioautography, *Brain Res.* **347**:74–84.

Ljungdahl, Å, Hökfelt, T., and Nilsson, G., 1978, Distribution of substance P-like immunoreactivity in the central nervous system of the rat. I. Cell bodies and nerve terminals, *Neuroscience* **3**:861–943.

Loy, R., Koziell, D. A., Lindsey, J. D., and Moore, R. Y., 1980, Noradrenergic innervation of the adult rat hippocampal formation, *J. Comp. Neurol.* **189**:699–710.

Lundberg, J. M., Rudehill, A., Sollevi, A., Theodorsson-Norheim, E., and Hamberger, B., 1986, Frequency- and reserpine-dependent chemical coding of sympathetic transmission: Differential release of noradrenaline and neuropeptide Y from pig spleen, *Neurosci. Lett.* **63**:96–100.

McRae-Degeurce, A., and Milon, H., 1983, Serotonin and dopamine afferents to the rat locus coeruleus: A biochemical study after lesioning of the ventral mesencephalic tegmental–A10 region and the raphe dorsalis, *Brain Res.* **263**:344–347.

Madison, D. V., and Nicoll, R. A., 1986, Actions of noradrenaline recorded intracellularly in rat hippocampal CA1 pyramidal neurones, *in vitro, J. Physiol. (London)* **372**:221–244.

Marshall, K. C., and Williams, J. T., 1986, Rhythmic activity and adrenergic responses in locus coeruleus neurons from young rats, *Soc. Neurosci. Abstr.* **12**:1390.

Marshall, K. C., Garber, C. B., and Finlayson, P. G., 1984, Noradrenergic actions of Purkinje and locus coeruleus neurons in culture, *Prog. Neuropsychopharmacol. Biol. Psychiatry* **8**:515–520.

Meibach, R. C., 1984, Serotonergic receptors, in: *Handbook of Chemical Neuroanatomy,* Vol. 3 (A. Björklund, T. Hökfelt, and M. J. Kuhar, eds.), Elsevier, Amsterdam, pp. 304–324.

Melander, T., Hökfelt, T., and Rökaeus, A., 1986, Distribution of galaninlike immunoreactivity in the rat central nervous system, *J. Comp. Neurol.* **248**:475–517.

Mendelsohn, F. A. O., Quirion, R., Saavedra, J. M., Aguilera, G., and Catt, K., 1984, Autoradiographic localization of angiotensin II receptors in rat brain, *Proc. Natl. Acad. Sci. USA* **81**:1575–1579.

Merchenthaler, I., 1984, Corticotrophin releasing factor (CRF)-like immunoreactivity in the rat central nervous system, extrahypothalamic distribution, *Peptides* **5**(Suppl. 1):53–69.

Moore, R. Y., and Bloom, F. E., 1979, Central catecholamine neuron systems: Anatomy and physiology of the norepinephrine and epinephrine systems, *Annu. Rev. Neurosci.* **2**:113–168.

Moore, R. Y., and Card, J. P., 1984, Noradrenaline-containing neuron systems, in: *Handbook of Chemical Neuroanatomy,* Vol. 2 (A. Björklund and T. Hökfelt, eds.), Elsevier, Amsterdam, pp. 123–156.

Morgane, P. J., and Jacobs, M. S., 1979, Raphe projections to the locus coeruleus in the rat, *Brain Res. Bull.* **4**:519–534.

Morley, B. J., 1985, The localization and origin of somatostatin-containing fibers in an auditory brainstem nucleus, *Peptides* **6**(Suppl. 1):165–172.

Nakamura, S., and Iwama, K., 1975, Antidromic activation of the rat locus coeruleus neurons from hippocampus, cerebral and cerebellar cortices, *Brain Res.* **99**:372–376.

Nakamura, S., Tsai, C., and Iwama, K., 1980, Recurrent facilitation of locus coeruleus neurons of the rat, in: *The Reticular Formation Revisited* (J. A. Hobson and M. A. B. Brazier, eds.), Raven Press, New York, pp. 303–315.

North, R. A., and Williams, J. T., 1983, μ-Type opiate receptors on single locus coeruleus neurones, *Br. J. Pharmacol.* **79**:423P.

North, R. A., and Williams, J. T., 1985, On the potassium conductance increased by opioids in rat locus coeruleus, neurones, *J. Physiol. (London)* **364**:265–280.

Olpe, H. R., and Baltzer, V., 1981, Vasopressin activates noradrenergic neurons in the rat locus coeruleus: A microiontophoretic investigation, *Eur. J. Pharmacol.* **73**:377–378.

Olpe, H. R., and Jones, R. S. G., 1982, Excitatory effects of ACTH on noradrenergic neurons of the locus coeruleus of the rat, *Brain Res.* **251**:177–179.

Palacios, J. M., Wamsley, J. K., and Kuhar, M. J., 1981, The distribution of histamine H_1-receptors in the rat brain: An autoradiographic study, *Neuroscience* **6**:15–37.

Palkovits, M., and Brownstein, M. J., 1983, Locus coeruleus, *Adv. Cell. Neurobiol.* **4**:81–103.

Palkovits, M., Brownstein, M., and Saavedra, J. M., 1974, Serotonin content of the brain stem nuclei in the rat, *Brain Res.* **80**:237–249.

Pepper, C., and Henderson, G., 1980, Opiates and opioid peptides hyperpolarize locus coeruleus neurones *in vitro, Science* **209**:394–396.

Pickel, V. M., Joh, T. H., and Reis, D. J., 1977, A serotonergic innervation of noradrenergic neurons in nucleus locus coeruleus: Demonstration by immunocytochemical localization of the transmitter specific enzymes tyrosine and tryptophan hydroxylase, *Brain Res.* **131**:197–214.

Pickel, V. M., Joh, T. H., Reis, D. J., Leeman, S. E., and Miller, R. J., 1979, Electron microscopic localization of substance P and enkephalin in axon terminals related to dendrites of catecholaminergic neurons, *Brain Res.* **160**:387–400.

Quirion, R., Zajac, J. M., Morgat, J. L., and Roques, B. P., 1983, Autoradiographic distribution of mu and delta opiate receptors in rat brain using highly selective ligands, *Life Sci.* **33**(Suppl. I):227–230.

Quirion, R., Dalpe, M., DeLean, A., Gutkowska, J., Cantin, M., and Genest, J., 1984, Atrial natriuretic factor (ANF) binding sites in brain and related structures, *Peptides* **5**:1167–1172.

Robain, O., Lanfumey, L., Adrien, J., and Farkas, E., 1985, Developmental changes in the cerebellar cortex after locus coeruleus lesion with 6-hydroxydopamine in the rat, *Exp. Neurol.* **88**:150–164.

Rotter, A., Birdsall, N. J. M., Field, P. M., and Raisman, G., 1979, Muscarinic receptors in the central nervous system of the rat. II. Distribution of binding of [³H]propylbenzilylcholine mustard in the midbrain and hindbrain, *Brain Res. Rev.* **1**:167–183.

Saavedra, J. M., Brownstein, M. J., and Palkovits, M., 1976, Distribution of catechol-*O*-methyltransferase, histamine-*N*-methyltransferase and monoamine oxidase in specific areas of the rat brain, *Brain Res.* **118:**152–156.

Sar, M., Stumpf, W. E., Miller, R. J., Chang, K. J., and Cuatrecasas, P., 1978, Immunohistochemical localization of enkephalin in rat brain and spinal cord, *J. Comp. Neurol.* **182:**17–38.

Sawchenko, P. E., and Gerfen, C. R., 1985, Plant lectins and bacterial toxins as tools for tracing neuronal connections, *Trends Neurosci.* **8:**378–384.

Segal, M., 1979, Serotonergic innervation of the locus coeruleus from the dorsal raphe and its action on responses to noxious stimuli, *J. Physiol. (London)* **286:**401–415.

Shaffer, M. M., and Moody, T. W., 1986, Autoradiographic visualization of CNS receptors for vasoactive intestinal peptide, *Peptides* **7:**283–288.

Shefner, S. A., and Chiu, T. H., 1986, Adenosine inhibits locus coeruleus neurons: An intracellular study in a rat brain slice preparation, *Brain Res.* **366:**364–368.

Shimizu, N., Katoh, Y., Hida, T., and Satoh, K., 1979, The fine structural organization of the locus coeruleus in the rat with special reference to noradrenaline contents, *Exp. Brain Res.* **37:**109–148.

Shults, C. W., Quirion, R., Chronwall, B., Chase, T. N., and O'Donohue, T. L., 1984, A comparison of the anatomical distribution of substance P and substance P receptors in the rat central nervous system, *Peptides* **5:**1097–1128.

Simon, H., Le Moal, M., Stinus, L., and Calas, A., 1979, Anatomical relationships between the ventral mesencephalic tegmentum–A10 region and the locus coeruleus as demonstrated by anterograde and retrograde tracing techniques, *J. Neural Transm.* **44:**77–86.

Sofroniew, M. V., 1985, Vasopressin- and neurophysin-immunoreactive neurons in the septal region, medial amygdala and locus coeruleus in colchicine-treated rats, *Neuroscience* **15:**347–358.

Steinbusch, H. W. M., 1981, Distribution of serotonin-immunoreactivity in the central nervous system of the rat—Cell bodies and terminals, *Neuroscience* **6:**557–618.

Steindler, D. A., 1981, Locus coeruleus neurons have axons that branch to the forebrain and cerebellum, *Brain Res.* **223:**367–373.

Swanson, L. W., 1976, The locus coeruleus: A cytoarchitectonic Golgi and immunohistochemical study in the albino rat, *Brain Res.* **110:**39–56.

Swanson, L. W., and Hartman, B.K., 1975, The central adrenergic system: An immunofluorescence study of the location of cell bodies and their efferent connections in the rat utilizing dopamine-β-hydroxylase as a marker, *J. Comp. Neurol.* **163:**467–506.

Swanson, L. W., Sawchenko, P. E., Rivier, J., and Vale, W. W., 1983, Organization of ovine corticotropin-releasing factor immunoreactive cells and fibers in the rat brain: An immunohistochemical study, *Neuroendocrinology* **36:**165–186.

Takigawa, M., and Mogenson, G. J., 1977, A study of inputs to antidromically identified neurons of the locus coeruleus, *Brain Res.* **135:**217–230.

Uhl, G., Goodman, R. R., and Snyder, S. H., 1979, Neurotensin-containing cell bodies, fibers and nerve terminals in the brain stem of the rat: Immunohistochemical mapping, *Brain Res.* **167:**77–91.

Valentino, R. J., Foote, S. L., and Aston-Jones, G., 1983, Corticotropin-releasing factor activates noradrenergic neurons of the locus coeruleus, *Brain Res.* **270:**363–367.

Vanderhaeghen, J. J., Lotstra, E., DeMay, J., and Gilles, C., 1980, Immunohistochemical localization of cholecystokinin- and gastrin-like peptides in the brain and hypophysis of the rat, *Proc. Natl. Acad. Sci. USA* **77:**1190–1194.

Van Dijk, A., Richards, J. G., Trzeciak, A., Gillessen, D., and Mohler, H., 1984, Cholecystokinin receptors: Biochemical demonstration and autoradiographic localization in the rat brain and pancreas using ^{3}H-cholecystokinin as radioligand, *J. Neurosci.* **4:**1021–1033.

Wainer, B. H., Levey, A. I., Mufson, E. J., and Mesulam, M.-M., 1984, Cholinergic systems in mammalian brain identified with antibodies against choline acetyltransferase, *Neurochem. Int.* **6:**163–182.

Watson, S. J., and Barchas, J. D., and Li, C. H., 1977, β-Lipotropin: Localization of cells and axons in rat brain by immunohistochemistry, *Proc. Natl. Acad. Sci. USA* **74:**5155–5158.

Watson, S. J., Richard, C. W., III, and Barchas, J. C., 1978, Adrenocorticotropin in rat brain: Immunocytochemical localization in cells and axons, *Science* **200:**1180–1182.

Weiner, N., 1979, Multiple factors regulating the release of norepinephrine consequent to nerve stimulation, *Fed. Proc.* **38:**2193–2202.

Williams, J. T., North, R. A., Shefner, S. A., Nishi, S., and Egan, T. M., 1984, Membrane properties of rat locus coeruleus neurones, *Neuroscience* **13:**137–156.

Williams, J. T., Henderson, G., and North, R. A., 1985, Characterization of α_2-adrenoceptors which increase potassium conductance in rat locus coeruleus neurones, *Neuroscience* **14:**95–101.

Wynn, P. C., Hauger, R. L., Holmes, M. C., Millan, M. A., Catt, K. J., and Aguilera, G., 1984, Brain and pituitary receptors for corticotropin releasing factor: Localization and differential regulation after adrenalectomy, *Peptides* **5**:1077–1084.

Yarom, Y., and Spira, M. E., 1982, Extracellular potassium ions mediate specific neuronal interaction, *Science* **216**:80–82.

Young, W. S., III, and Kuhar, M. J., 1980, Noradrenergic alpha 1 and alpha 2 receptors: Light microscopic autoradiographic localization, *Proc. Natl. Acad. Sci. USA* **77**:1696–1700.

Young, W. S., III, Uhl, G. R., and Kuhar, M. J., 1978, Iontophoresis of neurotensin in the area of the locus coeruleus, *Brain Res.* **150**:431–435.

25

Cortical Monoamines and Injured Brain

Hanna M. Pappius

1. Introduction

It is well established that brain injury which causes gross damage to vascular elements results in opening of the blood–brain barrier and an extravasation of fluid, giving rise to vasogenic edema (Katzman and Pappius, 1973). The edema has been generally accepted as the underlying cause of functional disturbances in conditions in which it occurs, although this assumption has not been validated and has been questioned (Pappius and McCann, 1969; Sutton *et al.*, 1980; Pappius and Wolfe, 1984). On the other hand, brain injury is associated with many other events all of which can be envisaged as leading to disturbances of neuronal function independently of the development of cerebral edema (Pappius and Wolfe, 1984). These include release of arachidonic acid from membrane phospholipids and formation of prostaglandins and thromboxanes (Wolfe, 1982), release of neurotransmitters (Fenske *et al.*, 1976; Bareggi *et al.*, 1975; Vecht *et al.*, 1975) and possibly the generation of free radicals (Demopoulos *et al.*, 1972). In the context of this symposium, effects of injury on neurotransmitter systems are of particular interest.

Until a few years ago, lack of a good method for assessing cerebral function in animals was a major obstacle to the study of mechanisms underlying functional disturbances in traumatized brain (Pappius, 1980). This difficulty was overcome by the development of the deoxyglucose technique for measurement of local cerebral glucose utilization (LCGU) (Sokoloff *et al.*, 1977; Nelson *et al.*, 1986) and the validation of its use for mapping of cerebral functional activity in awake animals (Sokoloff, 1977, 1981).

In recent years my studies have concentrated on the mechanisms by which injury to the brain causes functional neurological disturbances, using a focal freezing lesion in the rat as a model of cerebral injury and the deoxyglucose method as developed and described by Sokoloff (1977, 1981) to assess the functional state of the traumatized brain (Pappius, 1981, 1982; Pappius and Wolfe, 1983a,b).

Initial studies indicated that with time after a focal freezing lesion, a depression of LCGU developed which although widespread was not uniformly distributed throughout the brain (Pappius, 1981). Figure 1 shows [^{14}C]deoxyglucose autoradiographs from a normal and two lesioned animals. In the normal animal, heterogeneous optical densities are seen but no side-to-side

Hanna M. Pappius • The Goad Unit of The Donner Laboratory of Experimental Neurochemistry, Montreal Neurological Institute, McGill University, Montreal, Quebec, H3A 2B4, Canada.

Normal

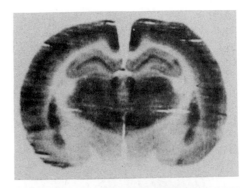

Freezing lesion
24 hours

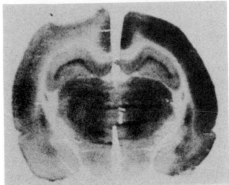

Freezing lesion
72 hours

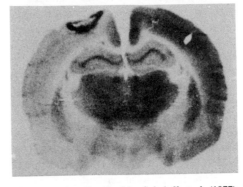

Figure 1. [^{14}C]-Deoxyglucose autoradiographs prepared as described by Sokoloff *et al.* (1977). Representative sections from a normal animal and lesioned animals at 24 and 72 hr after lesion. Note side-to-side differences in the density of the autographs in cortical areas of the lesioned animals, especially at 72 hr. (From data of Pappius, 1981.)

differences are present. In contrast, as a result of a small focal freezing lesion in the left parietal area, in the traumatized hemisphere optical density was obviously decreased 24 hr after the lesion, and was even lower 72 hr after the lesion. A return toward normal was demonstrated at 5 days (data not shown). The effect was not restricted to areas surrounding the lesion or overlying edematous white matter, but involved the whole lesioned hemisphere from frontal to visual cortex. It is important to stress that the exact location of the lesion is not important. The same results, i.e., a widespread cortical depression, were obtained with lesions placed more frontally or toward the visual cortex (Colle *et al.*, 1986).

   Quantitation of glucose utilization in various structures showed that the cortical areas throughout the lesional hemisphere were the most affected although some depression in subcortical structures was also noted, but will not be discussed further here. Figure 2 shows average glucose utilization with time after a lesion in five cortical areas in injured brain expressed as percent of normal. The cortical areas averaged were frontal, somatosensory, parietal, auditory, and visual. It will be seen that in the lesioned hemisphere the maximum depression occurred at 72 hr after the lesion when cortical glucose utilization was about 50% of normal. In the contralateral hemisphere the depression was much less pronounced but was statistically significant at 3 days.

On the basis of these studies it was concluded that focal lesions induce a widespread but nonuniform depression of glucose utilization. Since blood flow was not affected (Pappius, 1981), there was no evidence that direct effects on metabolism were involved. The demonstrated depression of glucose utilization was therefore interpreted as being a manifestation of cerebral dysfunction. In other words, the energy needs of cortical areas in injured brain were thought to be diminished because of a functional depression. Recently, evidence supporting this interpretation has been obtained: it was demonstrated that the degree of somatosensory deficit in animals with standardized freezing lesions was significantly correlated with the extent of the depression of glucose utilization in the cortical areas of the lesioned hemisphere (Colle *et al.*, 1986).

In the search for mechanisms involved in the postulated functional depression resulting from injury, it seemed reasonable to hypothesize that the observed changes in traumatized brain may be mediated through a neurotransmitter system or systems (Pappius and Wolfe, 1983b,c, 1984). The serotoninergic and noradrenergic systems appeared to be good potential candidates for such a role because both innervations are widely distributed to rat cerebral cortex (Beaudet and Descarries, 1976; Descarries *et al.*, 1977; Levitt and Moore, 1978; Lidov *et al.*, 1980), the area most affected in traumatized brain, and because changes in both systems have been reported in association with brain injury (e.g., Bareggi *et al.*, 1975; Fenske *et al.*, 1976; Vecht *et al.*, 1975). Preliminary experiments which showed that inhibition of both the serotonin (5-HT) and the catecholamine synthesis ameliorated the depression of glucose utilization which occurs in lesioned brain (Pappius and Wolfe, 1983c) were compatible with involvement of these neurotransmitter systems in the chain of events envisaged as leading from injury to functional disturbances.

As the first step in elucidating the possible role of biogenic amines in functional disturbances associated with injury, 5-HT, its metabolite 5-hydroxyindoleacetic acid (5-HIAA), norepinephrine (NE), dopamine (DA), and its metabolites were measured with time after a focal unilateral freezing lesion in frontoparietal cortical areas of both hemispheres (Pappius and Dadoun, 1986, 1987). Further, to examine the possibility that 5-HT was involved in the postulated functional depression, the effect of modifying 5-HT levels with *p*-chlorophenylalanine (PCPA), a known inhibitor of 5-HT synthesis (Koe and Weissman, 1966), on glucose utilization in lesioned brain was also studied (Pappius, in preparation).

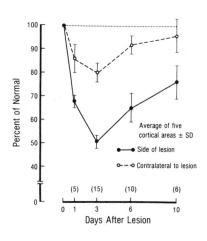

Figure 2. Cortical glucose utilization with time after a freezing lesion. Average of local cerebral glucose utilization, determined by the deoxyglucose method of Sokoloff *et al.* (1977), in five cortical areas (frontal, sensory-motor, parietal, auditory, and visual) expressed as percent of normal. Bars are S.D. Number of animals in parentheses. (Calculated from data of Pappius, 1981, and unpublished.)

2. Materials and Methods

2.1. General Procedure

Freezing lesions standardized to produce superficial focal cortical injury were made in the left parietal region of halothane-anesthetized Sprague–Dawley male rats (280–320 g) by applying a freezing probe (−50°C) to the dura for 5 sec through a 4 × 4-mm opening in the skull. After the lesion was made the wound was sutured and the animals allowed to awaken. Biogenic amine determinations or [^{14}C]deoxyglucose studies were carried out as described below at intervals of up to 10 days after the lesion.

PCPA (methyl ester HCl; Sigma Chemical Co.) was given i.p. 50, 100, or 200 mg/kg as a single dose 24 hr before the lesion was made or the animal was decapitated.

2.2. Determination of Biogenic Amines

In all of the studies presented here, frontoparietal cortex was analyzed. The area of the lesion, clearly visible to the naked eye, was always discarded. Biogenic amines and their metabolites were measured by HPLC with electrochemical detection using a method adapted from Mefford (1981). The experimental conditions are summarized in Table I.

The analyses were performed with a liquid chromatograph equipped with a pump (model 590, Waters Associates) and a reverse-phase Nova-pack C_{18} column (Waters Assoc.). After the extraction procedures, usually 40-μl samples of the supernatant were injected by an automatic injector (WISP 710B, Waters Assoc.) and the results were quantified by an integrator (Data module 730, Waters Assoc.). The mobile phase was pumped at a flow rate of 1 ml/min. A model LC-4B (Bioanalytical Systems) with a glassy carbon amperometric detector (TL3) was used.

2.3. Measurement of LCGU

LCGU was determined by the [^{14}C]deoxyglucose method of Sokoloff et al. (1977) as originally described. Briefly, a pulse of about 40 μCi (1.5 MBq) of 2-deoxy-D-[1-^{14}C]glucose [specific activity, 50 to 56 μCi/mmole (1.85–2.05 MBq); New England Nuclear] was injected via a venous catheter into partially restrained, awake rats. Timed arterial sampling for assay of [^{14}C]deoxyglucose and glucose concentration in the plasma was begun with the injection and

Table I. Summary of Experimental Procedures for Measurement of Biogenic Amines and Their Metabolites by HPLC-EC[a]

	Procedure	
	A	B
Substances measured	Norepinephrine, epinephrine, dopamine	5-HT, 5-HIAA, DOPAC, HVA, tryptophan
Column	5 μC_{18} Nova-pack 15 cm (Waters Assoc.)	
Mobile phase	0.1 M sodium acetate	0.1 M sodium acetate
	0.02 M citric acid	0.1 M citric acid
	150 mg/liter octylsulfate	6.5% (v/v) methanol
	50 mg/liter EDTA	
	7.5% (v/v) methanol	
Applied potential	0.60 V	0.85 V
Internal standard	Dihydroxybenzylamine	4-Hydroxy-3-methoxyphenethyl alcohol

[a]Tissue dissected immediately at room temperature and rapidly frozen. Frozen samples extracted with 0.2 M perchloric acid. For procedure A, aliquot of extract absorbed on and eluted from alumina (recovery 70–75%). (Method adapted from Mefford, 1981.)

continued for 45 min, at which time the animals were killed by decapitation. The brain was immediately removed and frozen. Brain sections 20 μm thick were cut in a cryostat (American Optical Co.) at −22°C. Autoradiographs were made from the dried sections, the local tissue concentrations of ^{14}C were determined from the optical densities of the specific anatomical structures and of appropriately calibrated [^{14}C]methyl methacrylate standards (New England Nuclear) included in each of the autoradiographs. The densitometric measurements were made with a Densichron densitometer (model PPD, Sargent–Welch Scientific Co.) equipped with a 0.1-mm aperture. Final values for LCGU were calculated using a PDP-12 computer (Digital Equipment Corp.).

In each experiment LCGU was determined in 30 areas or structures. In this chapter, data obtained in five cortical areas (visual, auditory, parietal, sensorimotor, and frontal) will be considered; the results for each area are expressed as percent of normal and averaged to give "cortical LCGU."

3. Results

3.1. Validation of the Dissection Method

Although 5-HT is thought to be reasonably stable in postmortem brain because of the vesicular nature of its storage, the question of the stability of indoleamines in injured brain had to be established. The results summarized in Table II show quite clearly that the cortical 5-HT and 5-HIAA content was the same whether the dissection was carried out at room temperature or in frozen state in both normal and lesioned brain 24 hr after the injury. It was assumed that the usually more stable catecholamines are also unaffected and in all subsequent work dissection was carried out at room temperature.

3.2. Effect of Halothane

The results of studies of the effects of halothane anesthesia on cortical 5-HT and 5-HIAA content are summarized in Table III. In anesthetized unlesioned animals, cortical content of the neurotransmitter was significantly increased after 15 min of anesthesia, while the content of the

Table II. Comparison of 5-HT and 5-HIAA Content in Tissue Samples of Rat Cerebral Cortex Dissected at Room Temperature or in Frozen State[a,b]

	5-HT (pmoles/g)	5-HIAA (pmoles/g)
Normal		
Dissected at room temperature[c] (11)	1962 ± 345	867 ± 150
Dissected in frozen state[d] (7)	2057 ± 327	802 ± 101
24 hr after freezing lesion[e]		
Dissected at room temperature (18)	1569 ± 242	1670 ± 668
Dissected in frozen state (12)	1610 ± 391	1918 ± 918

[a]Data from Pappius and Dadoun (1986, 1987).
[b]Averages ± S.D.; number of animals in parentheses.
[c]Animals were decapitated, brain rapidly removed and dissected, and samples then frozen.
[d]Animals were decapitated into liquid nitrogen and cortex samples chiseled out in frozen state.
[e]Lesioned hemisphere was sampled 24 hr after a focal freezing lesion was made.

Table III. Effect of Halothane Anesthesia on 5-HT and 5-HIAA Content of Rat Cerebral Cortex[a,b]

	5-HT (pmoles/g)		5-HIAA (pmoles/g)	
Anesthesia[c]	−	+	−	+
Normal (6)	1983 ± 221	2410 ± 263[d]	906 ± 51	1003 ± 91
Lesioned hemisphere[e] (4)	−	2545 ± 372	−	1260 ± 268

[a]Data from Pappius and Dadoun (1986, 1987).
[b]Averages ± S.D.; number of animals in parentheses.
[c]Animals unanesthetized (−) or subjected to 2.5% halothane for 15 min (+).
[d]Statistically significantly different from unanesthetized, $p < 0.05$.
[e]Animals decapitated exactly 1 min after freezing lesion was made in the parietal cortex.

metabolite was not changed significantly. Immediately after traumatization, the content of 5-HT in lesioned anesthetized animals exactly 1 min after the lesion was not different from the 5-HT content of anesthetized animals. However, a small but not significant increase in 5-HIAA was noted. Thus, there was no immediate effect of the lesion on the cortical content of 5-HT. An earlier observation of an increase in 5-HT (Pappius and Wolfe, 1983c) was probably an artifact of the anesthesia. At all other time intervals, beginning at 4 hr after injury, unanesthetized animals were studied following decapitation.

3.3. Indoleamines in Injured Brain

The time course of changes in 5-HT and its metabolite, 5-HIAA, in rat frontoparietal cerebral cortex of both hemispheres after a standardized, unilateral freezing lesion in the parietal region, is summarized in Table IV.

It is seen that in the lesioned hemisphere there was a statistically significant decrease in 5-HT content only at 24 hr after lesion. This subsequently returned to normal levels. The increase in 5-HIAA lasted longer, with statistically significant differences from normal demonstrable at 4 hr as well as 1, 3, and 6 days after lesion. In contrast, in the contralateral hemisphere, no changes were seen in either 5-HT or 5-HIAA at any time up to 10 days.

When these results were expressed as a ratio of the metabolite to the neurotransmitter (5-

Table IV. 5-HT and 5-HIAA Content (pmoles/g) of Rat Frontoparietal Cerebral Cortex with Time after a Focal Freezing Lesion[a,b,c]

	Lesioned hemisphere		Contralateral hemisphere	
	5-HT	5-HIAA	5-HT	5-HIAA
Normal (13)	1964 ± 316	895 ± 140	—	—
Time after lesion				
4 hr (5)	1901 ± 351	1314 ± 328*	2001 ± 253	892 ± 114
1 day (18)	1569 ± 242**	1670 ± 668**	1976 ± 251	980 ± 172
3 days (21)	1971 ± 405	1366 ± 436**	2160 ± 465	921 ± 192
6 days (8)	1996 ± 230	1144 ± 120*	2122 ± 300	967 ± 163
8 days (3)	2035 ± 81	827 ± 70	2114 ± 634	793 ± 192
10 days (7)	1745 ± 178	871 ± 126	1867 ± 213	804 ± 162

[a]Data from Pappius and Dadoun (1986, 1987).
[b]Averages ± S.D.; number of animals in parentheses.
[c]Statistically significantly different from normal; *$p < 0.05$; **$p < 0.01$.

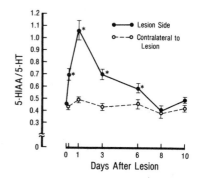

Figure 3. Ratio of 5-hydroxyindoleacetic acid to serotonin with time after a freezing lesion. Average ± S.D. Number of animals in Table IV. Asterisks indicate values significantly different from normal: $p <$ 0.01 at 4 hr and 1 day; $p < 0.05$ at 3 and 6 days. (From data of Pappius and Dadoun, 1986, 1987.)

HIAA/5-HT) (Fig. 3), an indirect measure of 5-HT turnover, significant increases became apparent on the traumatized side. The actual turnover rate of 5-HT cannot be determined from the data since the transport of the metabolite out of the brain was not inhibited, but it was likely greater than indicated by these results. The 5-HIAA/5-HT ratio remained within normal limits in the contralateral hemisphere. It is clear from these results that the 5-HT system is unilaterally affected in injured brain.

3.4. Catecholamines in Injured Brain

The results of the determination of catecholamines in injured brain are summarized in Table V. Surprisingly, cortical norepinephrine levels were decreased in both hemispheres with lowest levels seen at 24 hr, indicating that there were bilateral effects on this catecholamine as a result of a unilateral injury. Dopamine and its metabolites were not affected (data for DOPAC not shown).

3.5. Effects of PCPA in Injured Brain

By themselves, these results do not necessarily indicate that the observed changes in the content of the two biogenic amines are related to the changes in glucose utilization. The 5-HT content of brain was modified with PCPA, to test the hypothesis that 5-HT is involved in the postulated functional depression of injured brain. Glucose utilization in the lesioned brain was determined as a measure of functional depression. The results summarized in Table VI show that

Table V. Norepinephrine, Dopamine, and Homovanillic Acid Content (pmoles/g) of Rat Frontoparietal Cerebral Cortex with Time after a Focal Freezing Lesion[a,b,c]

	Lesioned hemisphere			Contralateral hemisphere		
	NE	DA	HVA	NE	DA	HVA
Normal (9)	1585 ± 198	164 ± 53	112 ± 24	—	—	—
Time after lesion						
4 hr (4)	1284 ± 251	268 ± 150	154 ± 49	1416 ± 174	173 ± 174	146 ± 58
1 day (9)	951 ± 101**	177 ± 52	193 ± 130	1087 ± 125**	160 ± 102	84 ± 30
3 days (9)	1279 ± 129**	185 ± 73	160 ± 100	1326 ± 77**	161 ± 43	104 ± 40
6 days (8)	1346 ± 204*	178 ± 128	152 ± 57	1395 ± 220	151 ± 83	125 ± 44
10 days (8)	1598 ± 273	145 ± 61	159 ± 54	1670 ± 308	132 ± 47	105 ± 45

[a]Data from Pappius and Dadoun (1986).
[b]Averages ± S.D.; number of animals in parentheses.
[c]Statistically significantly different from normal: *$p < 0.05$; **$p < 0.01$.

Table VI. Effect of p-Chlorophenylalanine on Cortical Glucose Utilization and 5-HT and Norepinephrine Content in Rat Brain[a,b]

	LCGU					
	Unlesioned: Percent of normal	72 hr after lesion: Percent of corresponding control		5-HT NE Unlesioned: Percent of normal		
		Lesion side	Contralateral			
Untreated	100 (13)	51 ± 3 (17)	82 ± 4 (17)	100	100	(7)
PCPA						
50 mg/kg	—	55 ± 7 (5)	80 ± 3 (5)	84	105	(2)
100 mg/kg	101 ± 5 (8)	53 ± 4 (4)	74 ± 5 (4)	69	87	(4)
200 mg/kg	89 ± 7 (5)	89 ± 12[c] (6)	102 ± 8[c] (6)	39	79	(3)

[a]Data from Pappius (in preparation).
[b]PCPA given 24 hr before lesion was made or animals were decapitated for determination of biogenic amines.
[c]Statistically significantly different from untreated, $p < 0.05$.

PCPA in doses up to 100 mg/kg had no effect on cortical glucose utilization in unlesioned animals. At 200 mg/kg, however, a 10% depression was noted.

At 50 and 100 mg PCPA/kg given 24 hr before lesioning, there was no effect on glucose utilization in either the lesioned or the contralateral hemisphere, as compared to untreated animals. At 200 mg/kg, PCPA had bilateral effects on cortical glucose utilization in injured brain, with nearly normal rates on the lesioned side and ones within normal limits in the contralateral hemisphere. Results of preliminary experiments in which 5-HT and norepinephrine were measured in unlesioned animals 24 hr after PCPA administration, hence corresponding to levels of these biogenic amines present at the time the lesion was made, are also included in Table VI. It is seen that there was a dose-dependent decrease in 5-HT content of rat brain in animals treated with PCPA, but that the 5-HT level in the cortex had to be considerably diminished (39% of normal) before depression of glucose utilization could be demonstrated. However, at 200 mg PCPA/kg, norepinephrine levels were also affected (79% of normal). Thus, at this point it is not clear whether the effectiveness of the higher dose of PCPA bilaterally on cortical glucose utilization is related only to the significant inhibition of 5-HT synthesis or whether its effects on norepinephrine levels in cortical tissue also play a role in modulation of the metabolic, hence the postulated functional, depression.

4. Discussion and Conclusions

On the basis of the studies on cortical biogenic amine content following a freezing lesion, it can be concluded that in focally injured brain the serotoninergic system is altered unilaterally, and the norepinephrine levels are decreased bilaterally while dopamine and its metabolites are not affected.

The effects of injury on the cortical serotoninergic system are not immediate but develop gradually, reaching a peak at 24 hr. They persist for up to 6 days. 5-HT turnover is increased throughout the lesioned hemisphere of a focally injured brain, although the effect diminishes in extent and duration with greater distance from the lesion (Pappius and Dadoun, 1987). The change in norepinephrine content cannot be interpreted in terms of the turnover of this neurotransmitter until the corresponding level of its major cortical metabolite in the rat, 3-methoxy-4-hydroxyphenylglycol (Schanberg et al., 1968), is also known. These studies are in progress.

The question to be answered is whether the unilateral increase in 5-HT turnover and the bilateral changes in norepinephrine content in injured brain are related to the depression of glucose utilization and hence of functional significance. It is clear that increased metabolism of 5-HT is not necessarily synonymous with its increased release (Kuhn *et al.*, 1986; Lookingland *et al.*, 1986) and the same probably applies to norepinephrine (Commissiong, 1985). 5-HT is thought to be an inhibitory transmitter in the cerebral cortex (Bloom *et al.*, 1972; Sastry and Phillis, 1977; Taylor and Stone, 1981) and is envisaged as exerting profound and global influences on cortical function in general (Lidov *et al.*, 1980), possibly not only as neurotransmitter but also as a modulator of neuronal activity in a nonsynaptic fashion (Beaudet and Descarries, 1978; Reader *et al.*, 1979; Taylor and Stone, 1981). Intracarotid administration of 5-HT in the presence of monoamine inhibition has been shown to decrease cortical glucose utilization and these results were interpreted as supporting the depressive action of 5-HT on cortical neuronal activity (Grome and Harper, 1985). The noradrenergic system, because of its anatomical organization, also appears capable of affecting neuronal function over the whole cerebral cortex, cutting across cytoarchitectonic and functionally distinct regions (Bloom, 1981; Morrison *et al.*, 1981). It has been suggested that norepinephrine neuron systems regulate other neuron systems (Moore, 1982) while 5-HT modulation of noradrenergic activity in rat brain has been demonstrated (Pujol *et al.*, 1978; Ferron *et al.*, 1982; Reader *et al.*, 1986; Stockmeier *et al.*, 1985). Thus, the possibility of a reciprocal functional link between the 5-HT and the norepinephrine systems has been considered previously and anatomical pathways for such interactions have been delineated (Stockmeier *et al.*, 1985).

The changes in glucose utilization in traumatized brain are somewhat different in character from the changes in 5-HT metabolism and norepinephrine content. Glucose utilization was depressed bilaterally, although much more so on the side of the lesion. The changes in 5-HT and 5-HIAA were restricted to the lesioned hemisphere while the decrease in the level of norepinephrine bilaterally. The peak of the depression in glucose utilization occurred at 72 hr after lesion while the greatest changes in 5-HT, 5-HIAA, and norepinephrine were demonstrated at 24 hr. Finally, glucose utilization on the side of the lesion was still significantly below normal at 10 days postlesion, when the indoleamine and norepinephrine contents were already back to control levels.

Nevertheless, the effects of PCPA in ameliorating the metabolic depression under conditions which produce a significant depletion of 5-HT, but also some decrease in norepinephrine content, suggest that the changes in 5-HT and norepinephrine are related to the alteration in cortical glucose utilization associated with brain injury. These results are compatible with the conclusion that the depression in cortical glucose utilization, which is bilateral but much more pronounced on the side of the lesion, may represent the additive effects of the changes in the two biogenic amine systems. If so, it is clear that the relationship must be complex. Further work is required to elucidate the anatomical pathways involved and other related neurochemical sequelae of brain damage, as well as their interrelationships, before the role of biogenic amines in functional disturbances associated with injury can be fully understood.

5. Summary

In summary, the data I have presented implicate the serotoninergic system and possibly the noradrenergic system in the cortical metabolic depression which occurs in the rat following brain injury and which we interpret as reflecting a functional depression. The results do not indicate which mechanisms produce these widespread effects of a focal, apparently nonspecific injury, nor the pathways affected, nor whether these are neurotransmitter or modulatory effects of the two biogenic amines. Our data do not rule out the possibility that other transmitter systems are also involved. However, our studies represent a novel approach to problems related to traumatic brain injury and I believe that further work will increase our understanding of the processes underlying functional disturbances in injured brain.

ACKNOWLEDGMENTS. Supported in part by the Medical Research Council of Canada (Grant MT-3021) and by The Canadian Donner Foundation. I am indebted to Hanna Szylinger, Michael McHugh, and Ralph Dadoun for technical help and to Linda Michel for clerical assistance. Continued interest in this work of Dr. L. S. Wolfe is gratefully acknowledged.

References

Bareggi, S. R., Porta, M., Selenati, A., Assael, B. M., Calderini, G., Collice, M., Rossandra, M., and Morselli, P. L., 1975, Homovanillic acid and 5-hydroxyindoleacetic acid in the CSF of patients after severe head injury, *Eur. Neurol.* **13**:528–544.

Beaudet, A., and Descarries, L., 1976, Quantitative data on serotonin nerve terminals in adult rat neocortex, *Brain Res.* **111**:301–309.

Beaudet, A., and Descarries, L., 1978, The monoamine innervation of rat cerebral cortex: Synaptic and nonsynaptic axon terminals, *Neuroscience* **3**:851–860.

Bloom, F. E., 1981, Chemical signaling and cortical circuitry: Integrative aspects, in: *The Organization of the Cerebral Cortex* (F. O. Schmitt, F. G. Worden, G. Adelman, and S. G. Dennis, eds.), MIT Press, Cambridge, Mass., pp. 359–370.

Bloom, F. E., Hoffer, B. J., Siggins, G. R., Barker, J. L., and Nicoll, R. A., 1972, Effects of serotonin on central neurons: Microiontophoretic administration, *Fed. Proc.* **31**:97–106.

Colle, L. M., Holmes, L. J., and Pappius, H. M., 1986, Correlation between behavioral status and cerebral glucose utilization in rats following freezing lesion, *Brain Res.* **397**:27–36.

Commissiong, J. W., 1985, Monoamine metabolites: Their relationship and lack of relationship to monoaminergic neuronal activity, *Biochem. Pharmacol.* **34**:1127–1131.

Demopoulos, H. B., Milvy, R., Kakari, S., and Ransohoff, J., 1972, Molecular aspects of membrane structure in cerebral edema, in: *Steroids and Brain Edema* (H. J. Reulen and K. Schurmann, eds.), Springer-Verlag, Berlin, pp. 29–39.

Descarries, L., Watkins, K. C., and Lapierre, Y., 1977, Noradrenergic axon terminals in the cerebral cortex of rat. III. Topometric ultrastructural analysis, *Brain Res.* **133**:197–222.

Fenske, A., Sinterhauf, K., and Reulen, H. J., 1976, The role of monoamines in the development of cold-induced edema, in: *Dynamics of Brain Edema* (H. M. Pappius and W. Fiendel, eds.), Springer-Verlag, Berlin, pp. 150–154.

Ferron, A., Descarries, L., and Reader, T. A., 1982, Altered neuronal responsiveness to biogenic amines in rat cerebral cortex after serotonin denervation or depletion, *Brain Res.* **231**:93–108.

Grome, J. J., and Harper, A. M., 1985, Serotonin depression of local cerebral glucose utilisation after monoamine oxidase inhibition, *J. Cereb. Blood Flow Metab.* **5**:473–475.

Katzman, R., and Pappius, H. M., 1973, *Brain Electrolytes and Fluid Metabolism*, Williams & Wilkins, Baltimore.

Koe, B. K., and Weissman, A., 1966, p-Chlorophenylalanine: A specific depletor of brain serotonin, *J. Pharmacol. Exp. Ther.* **154**:499–516.

Kuhn, D. M., Wolf, W. A., and Youdim, M. B. H., 1986, Serotonin neurochemistry revisited: A new look at some old axioms. Critiques, *Neurochem. Int.* **8**:141–154.

Levitt, P., and Moore, R. Y., 1978, Noradrenaline neuron innervation of the neocortex in the rat, *Brain Res.* **139**:219–231.

Lidov, H. G. W., Grzanna, R., and Molliver, M. E., 1980, The serotonin innervation of the cerebral cortex in the rat—An immunohistochemical analysis, *Neuroscience* **5**:207–227.

Lookingland, K. J., Shannon, N. J., Chapin, D. S., and Moore, K. E., 1986, Exogenous tryptophan increases synthesis, storage, and intraneuronal metabolism of 5-hydroxytryptamine in the rat hypothalamus, *J. Neurochem.* **47**:205–212.

Mefford, I. N., 1981, Application of high performance liquid chromatography with electrochemical detection to neurochemical analysis: Measurement of catecholamines, serotonin and metabolites in rat brain, *J. Neurosci. Methods* **3**:207–224.

Moore, R. Y., 1982, Catecholamine neuron system in brain, *Ann. Neurol.* **12**:321–327.

Morrison, J. H., Molliver, M. E., Grzanna, R., and Coyle, J. T., 1981, The intracortical trajectory of the coeruleo-cortical projection in the rat: A tangentially organized cortical afferent, *Neuroscience* **6:**139–158.

Nelson, T., Lucignani, G., Goochee, J., Crane, A. M., and Sokoloff, L., 1986, Invalidity of criticisms of the deoxyglucose method based on alleged glucose-6-phosphatase activity in brain, *J. Neurochem.* **46:**905–919.

Pappius, H. M., 1980, Mapping of cerebral functional activity with radioactive deoxyglucose: Application of studies of traumatized brain, *Adv. Neurol.* **28:**271–279.

Pappius, H. M., 1981, Local cerebral glucose utilization in thermally traumatized rat brain, *Ann. Neurol.* **9:**484–491.

Pappius, H. M., 1982, Dexamethasone and local cerebral glucose utilization in freeze-traumatized rat brain, *Ann. Neurol.* **12:**157–162.

Pappius, H. M., and Dadoun, R., 1986, Biogenic amines in injured brain, *Trans. Am. Soc. Neurochem.* **17:**298.

Pappius, H. M., and Dadoun, R., 1987, The effects of injury on the indoleamines in cerebral cortex, *J. Neurochem.* **49:**321–325.

Pappius, H. M., and McCann, W. P., 1969, Effects of steroids on cerebral edema in cats, *Arch. Neurol.* **20:**207–216.

Pappius, H. M., and Wolfe, L. S., 1983a, The effects of indomethacin and ibuprofen on cerebral metabolism and blood flow in traumatized brain, *J. Cereb. Blood Flow Metab.* **3:**448–459.

Pappius, H. M., and Wolfe, L. S., 1983b, Functional disturbances in brain following injury: Search for underlying mechanisms, *Neurochem. Res.* **8:**63–72.

Pappius, H. M., and Wolfe, L. S., 1983c, Involvement of serotonin and catecholamines in functional depression of traumatized brain, *J. Cereb. Blood Flow Metab.* **3**(Suppl. 1)**:**S226–S227.

Pappius, H. M., and Wolfe, L. S., 1984, Effects of drugs on local cerebral glucose utilization in traumatized brain: Mechanisms of action of steroids revisited, in: *Recent Progress in the Study and Therapy of Brain Edema* (G. Go and A. Baethmann, eds.), Plenum Press, New York, pp. 11–26.

Pujol, J. F., Keane, P., McRae, A., Lewis, B. D., and Renaud, B., 1978, Biochemical evidence for serotonergic control of the locus coeruleus, in: *Interactions between Putative Neurotransmitters in the Brain* (S. Garattini, J. F. Pujol, and R. Samanin, eds.), Raven Press, New York, pp. 401–410.

Reader, T. A., Ferrou, A., Descarries, L., and Jasper, H. H., 1979, Modulatory role for biogenic amines in the cerebral cortex: Microiontophoretic studies, *Brain Res.* **160:**217–229.

Reader, T. A., Briere, R., Groudin, L., and Ferrou, A., 1986, Effects of p-di-chlorophenyl-alanine on cortical monoamines and on the activity of noradrenergic neurons, *Neurochem. Res.* **11:**1025–1035.

Sastry, B. S. R., and Phillis, J. W., 1977, Inhibition of cerebral cortical neurones by a 5-hydroxytryptaminergic pathway from median raphé nucleus, *Can. J. Physiol. Pharmacol.* **55:**737–743.

Schanberg, S. M., Schildkraut, J. J., Breese, G. R., and Kopin, I. J., 1968, Metabolism of norepinephrine-H³ in rat brain: Identification of conjugated 3-methoxy-4-hydroxyphenylglycol as the major metabolite, *Biochem. Pharmacol.* **17:**247–254.

Sokoloff, L., 1977, Relation between physiological function and energy metabolism in the central nervous system, *J. Neurochem.* **29:**13–26.

Sokoloff, L., 1981, Localization of functional activity in the central nervous system by measurement of glucose utilization with radioactive deoxyglucose, *J. Cereb. Blood Flow Metab.* **1:**7–36.

Sokoloff, L., Reivich, M., Kennedy, C., Des Rosiers, M. H., Patlak, C. S., Pettigrew, K. D., Sakurada, O., and Shinohara, M., 1977, The [¹⁴C]deoxyglucose method for the measurement of local cerebral glucose utilization: Theory, procedure, and normal values in the conscious and anesthetized albino rat, *J. Neurochem.* **28:**897–916.

Stockmeier, C. A., Martino, A. M., and Kellar, K. J., 1985, A strong influence of serotonin axons on β-adrenergic receptors in rat brain, *Science* **230:**323–325.

Sutton, L. N., Bruce, D. A., Welsh, F. A., and Jaggi, J. L., 1980, Metabolic and electrophysiologic consequences of vasogenic edema, *Adv. Neurol.* **28:**241–254.

Taylor, D. A., and Stone, T. W., 1981, Neurotransmodulatory control of cerebral cortical neuron activity, in: *The Organization of the Cerebral Cortex* (F. O. Schmitt, F. G. Worden, G. Adelman, and S. G. Dennis, eds.), MIT Press, Cambridge, Mass., pp. 347–357.

Vecht, C. J., Van Woerkom, T. C. A. M., Teelken, A. W., and Minderhoud, J. M., 1975, Homovanillic acid and 5-hydroxyindoleacetic acid cerebrospinal fluid levels, *Arch. Neurol.* **32:**792–797.

Wolfe, L. S., 1982, Eicosanoids: Prostaglandins, thromboxanes, leukotrienes, and other derivatives of carbon-20 unsaturated fatty acids, *J. Neurochem.* **38:**1–14.

26

Behavioral and Other Actions of Adenosine in the Central Nervous System

J. W. Phillis

1. Introduction

In recent years it has become evident that the transmission process of central neurons is extraordinarily varied, as is the chemical vocabulary by which neurons communicate. There has been a considerable accumulation of evidence, primarily from histochemical studies, supporting the existence of transmitter-like molecules within certain neurons (Chan-Palay and Palay, 1984). However, the fact that a neuron contains more than one transmitter substance does not establish that each substance is being released as a transmitter (Phillis, 1984). It is possible that some neurons release more than one type of transmitter substance from the same terminal, with one of these serving as the primary transmitter and the others functioning, either pre- or postsynaptically, to modify or *modulate* the action, or further release, of the primary transmitter.

The term *modulator* was introduced to characterize the actions of putative transmitters that were not readily reconcilable with those of the classical neurotransmitters. Thus, a neuromodulator might modify intercellular communication by affecting transmitter synthesis, release, receptor sensitivity, reuptake, or metabolism. The possibility also arises that modulators need not be released exclusively by the calcium-dependent exocytosis of synaptic vesicles, but rather that they may be released from nonvesicular neuronal pools or glial cells and in some instances by a transport-mediated process.

With these concepts in mind, adenosine may be considered to have met a number of the criteria for consideration as a modulator of synaptic activity in the CNS. Adenosine is present in the nervous system; it is released by electrical stimulation or depolarization of nervous tissues by a process which is at least partially calcium-dependent; and it is taken up by nerve cells (Phillis and Wu, 1981). Adenosine and its analogues exert potent depressant effects on the firing of nerve cells at several levels of the neural axis and depress synaptic transmission (Phillis and Wu, 1981). Its depressant effects on neuronal transmission appear to be primarily a result of inhibition of transmitter release from the presynaptic nerve terminal, probably as a result of a blockade of calcium channels (Wu *et al.*, 1982). There is also evidence to suggest that, at higher concentra-

---

J. W. Phillis • Department of Physiology, School of Medicine, Wayne State University, Detroit, Michigan 48201.

tions, adenosine may increase the potassium permeability of neuronal membranes, thus eliciting a hyperpolarization of central neurons (Dunwiddie, 1985).

Associated with the idea that adenosine may be involved in the modulation of synaptic transmission in the nervous system, has been a proposal that a number of centrally acting drugs might exert at least some of their actions through purine-linked mechanisms (Phillis and Wu, 1981, 1982a,b). Thus, for many years it was assumed that caffeine and theophylline act as central stimulants by inhibiting phosphodiesterase, resulting in an accumulation of cAMP in the brain (Rall, 1985). With the recognition that these methylxanthines are potent antagonists of the depressant effects of adenosine on neuronal firing (Phillis and Kostopoulos, 1975) and are able to displace adenosine analogues in binding studies (Snyder *et al.*, 1981), it became apparent that the central stimulant action of these compounds might be related to blockade of central adenosine receptors. It was subsequently suggested that the actions of several therapeutically employed anxiolytic, hypnotic, and anticonvulsant agents might involve a potentiation of the effects of endogenously released adenosine (Phillis and Wu, 1982a,b; Wu and Phillis, 1984).

2. Behavioral Actions of Adenosine Receptor Agonists

In contrast to the electrophysiological and biochemical evidence on the role of adenosine in the brain, there is a relative paucity of information on the behavioral effects of adenosine. When administered by parenteral injection, adenosine and its analogues have been shown to have a variety of behavioral actions including inhibition of spontaneous motor activity, motor incoordination, analgesia, hypnotic activity, changes in respiratory rate, alterations in food intake, and anticonvulsant activity. Parenteral injections of adenosine and its analogues have also been demonstrated to produce decreases in schedule-controlled operant behavior (Coffin and Carney, 1983; Glowa *et al.*, 1985).

A problem arising from all of these studies has been that, when administered parenterally, adenosine and its analogues have pronounced hypotensive actions and it is difficult to determine whether the behavioral responses are central in origin or secondary to peripheral changes, e.g., decreases in blood pressure (Phillis, 1982; Phillis and Wu, 1981, 1983) or heart rate. Recent studies by Dunwiddie and his colleagues have shown that L-phenylisopropyladenosine (L-PIA) and adenosine N'-ethylcarboxamide (NECA) do not cross in pharmacologically active amounts the intact blood–brain barrier in the cerebellar cortex or hippocampus (Bickford *et al.*, 1985; Dunwiddie and Brodie, 1985; Dunwiddie *et al.*, 1986). This suggests that many of the behavioral actions that have been recorded with parenterally administered adenosine analogues may have been indirectly mediated by actions on peripheral sites, so that caution should be exercised in ascribing these effects to effects at central sites. With this in mind, the subsequent sections of this chapter will emphasize those results obtained with direct or intracerebroventricular (icvt) administration of adenosine and its analogues.

2.1. Effects on Locomotor Activity

A decrease in spontaneous locomotor activity following icvt injections of adenosine or ATP was noted in early experiments on cats (Feldberg and Sherwood, 1954). Similar effects were observed with icvt injections in the rat (Buday *et al.*, 1961). Recently (Barraco *et al.*, 1984a), two adenosine analogues, L-PIA and NECA, were administered icvt in rats, and both compounds produced dose-related decreases in locomotor activity, with NECA exhibiting slightly more potent depressant activity. Both analogues also produced dose-related reductions in blood pressure, although the threshold for the hypotensive effects was 10- to 100-fold higher than the dose required for depression of spontaneous locomotor activity. The depression of locomotor activity and hypotensive effects of both compounds were antagonized by parenteral injections of caffeine.

These results demonstrated that the hypoactive and hypotensive effects of adenosine analogues can be dissociated by using the icvt route of administration. Moreover, antagonism by the methylxanthine caffeine indicates that the effects observed were mediated via an adenosine receptor, and not via some other purine-sensitive site.

In an extensive series of experiments on mice, it was possible to investigate the depressant effects on locomotor activity of a series of adenosine analogues, adenosine transport inhibitors, and an adenosine deaminase inhibitor (Fig. 1) (Phillis *et al.*, 1986). NECA was the most potent analogue, with a number of N^6-substituted compounds also being very effective depressants of locomotor activity. Adenosine itself was considerably less active, but this underestimation was undoubtedly due to tissue uptake and metabolism. Evidence for a neuromodulatory role of endogenously released adenosine in the brain was further investigated in experiments using inhibitors of adenosine transport and adenosine deaminase. The action of adenosine appears to be terminated by its removal from the synaptic cleft either by active neuronal uptake, coupled to the intracellular enzyme adenosine kinase, or by deamination to inosine by the enzyme adenosine deaminase. Three potent transport inhibitors—dipyridamole, dilazep (Fig. 2), and papaverine (Fig. 3) (Phillis and Wu, 1982a)—were injected directly into the lateral cerebral ventricle. All three inhibited locomotor activity and the effects of dilazep and papaverine were antagonized by caffeine. The effects of dipyridamole were not antagonized by caffeine and were therefore attributed to some pharmacological action other than a potentiation of the extracellular levels of adenosine. Erythro(hydroxynonyl)adenine (EHNA) was used as an inhibitor of adenosine deaminase. This compound also depressed locomotor activity and its actions were antagonized by caffeine (Fig. 4).

A paradoxical effect was observed when caffeine administration preceded icvt adenosine, in that low doses of adenosine now stimulated locomotor activity. In contrast, when mice were given NECA with caffeine, there were no dose combinations which produced stimulation. The finding that caffeine reversed the depressant action of low doses of adenosine into locomotor stimulation (Fig. 3) is similar to an earlier report showing that a low dose of L-PIA administered after

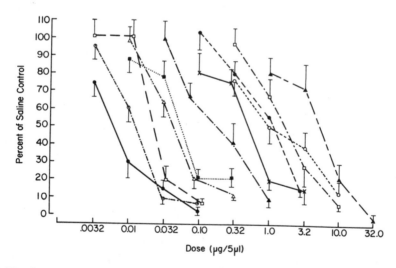

Figure 1. The effect on mouse locomotor activity of icvt injections of 11 adenosine analogues. ●—●, *N*-ethylcarboxamidoadenosine; ⊙– · –⊙, N^6-*S*-1-hydroxy-3-phenyl-2-propyladenosine; □– –□, N^6-3-pentyladenosine; △– ··· –△, N^6-*R*-1-phenyl-2-butyladenosine; ■ ····· ■, N^6-*R*-1-phenylethyladenosine; ▲– · –▲, 2-phenylaminoadenosine; X—X, N^6-*R*-phenylisopropyladenosine; ●– –●, N^6-*S*-1-phenyl-2-butyladenosine; ⊙- - -⊙, 2-chloroadenosine; □– · –□, N^6-*S*-1-phenylethyladenosine; ▲– – –▲, N^6-*S*-phenylisopropyladenosine. Values are expressed as percent of controls (mean ± S.E.M.) receiving saline icvt. (From Phillis *et al.*, 1986.)

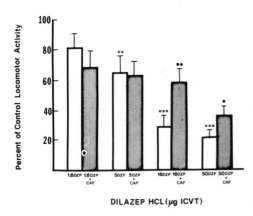

Figure 2. The effect on locomotor activity of icvt injections of dilazep (DZP) and DZP doses in combination with 32 mg/kg of intraperitoneally administered caffeine (CAF). Values are expressed as the percent of controls (mean ± S.E.M.) receiving saline ip and icvt. Individual significance levels were determined by Mann–Whitney U one-tailed comparisons: 5 μg ($p <$ 0.01), 16 μg ($p < 0.001$), and 50 μg ($p < 0.001$) of DZP depressed locomotor activity relative to saline/saline controls (*), and CAF antagonized this depression at 16 μg ($p < 0.01$) and 50 μg ($p < 0.05$) of DZP (●). (From Phillis *et al.*, 1986.)

caffeine, caused a pronounced stimulation (Snyder *et al.*, 1981). This suggests the presence of a heterogeneous population of receptors mediating the behavioral effects of adenosine, some of which produce sedation while others cause stimulation. Caffeine may compete more effectively with adenosine and L-PIA at the receptor subtype responsible for adenosine's depressant actions, thus uncovering effects mediated by the stimulant receptor.

Somewhat paradoxical findings were also observed with isobutylmethylxanthine (IBMX). This methylxanthine depressed locomotor activity in mice when administered into the lateral cerebral ventricle, even though it is an adenosine receptor antagonist. Indeed, IBMX was itself able to antagonize the locomotor depressant effects of adenosine. Its failure to stimulate locomotor activity directly may reflect another activity, perhaps related to phosphodiesterase inhibition, as a variety of other phosphodiesterase inhibitors can cause behavioral depression in mice (Wachtel, 1983) or inhibition of the uptake of adenosine (Phillis and Wu, 1982a). Caffeine reversed the depressant effects of IBMX, producing a behavioral stimulation.

Another type of motor activity sensitive to adenosine modulation is the rotational behavior

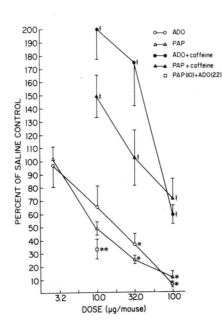

Figure 3. Effects of icvt injections of adenosine and papaverine on spontaneous locomotor activity at four separate doses given alone (ADO, ○; PAP, △) or in combination with a single ip dose (32 mg/kg) of caffeine (ADO, ●; PAP, ▲). □, the effect on locomotor activity of a combined icvt injection of 10 μg PAP + 22 μg ADO. Values represent the mean ± S.E.M. Overall analysis of variance showed dose-related decreases in locomotor activity for ADO alone ($p < 0.01$) and PAP alone ($p < 0.001$). Significances determined by post hoc comparisons with saline controls for individual doses of ADO and PAP are indicated (*$p < 0.001$). Significances determined by post hoc comparisons between doses of ADO and PAP alone and each in combination with ip caffeine are indicated (‡$p < 0.001$). Significance determined by post hoc comparison between saline controls and the combined icvt injection of 10 μg PAP + 22 μg ADO is indicated (**$p < 0.001$). (From Coffin *et al.*, 1984.)

Figure 4. The effect on locomotor activity of icvt injections of erythro-9-(2-hydroxy-3-nonyl)adenine (EHNA), ip injection of 32 mg/kg caffeine (CAF), and EHNA doses in combination with CAF. Values are expressed as the percent of controls (mean ± S.E.M.) receiving saline ip and icvt. Individual significance levels were determined by Mann-Whitney U one-tailed comparisons; the four highest doses of EHNA depressed locomotor activity (all $p <$ 0.001) relative to saline/saline controls (*), and CAF antagonized this depression at 100 μg ($p < 0.05$), 178 μg ($p < 0.001$), and 320 μg ($p < 0.001$) of EHNA (●), although CAF lowered activity relative to saline/saline controls in this experiment ($p < 0.05$). (From Phillis *et al.*, 1986.)

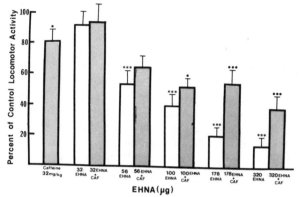

associated with modulation of striatal dopaminergic function. Green *et al.* (1982) showed that local injections of NECA into the striatum induced ipsilateral rotation of rats following systemic apomorphine injection. L-PIA was less effective in this regard than NECA, where 2′,5′-dideoxyadenosine (DDA) antagonized the response to NECA, as did theophylline. Because NECA is a relatively selective agonist for the adenosine receptor site which stimulates adenylate cyclase (Fredholm *et al.*, 1983) and because the activation of adenylate cyclase is inhibited by DDA (a P site agonist; Phillis and Wu, 1981), this may indicate that NECA modulates dopaminergic function by a cAMP mechanism.

2.2. Antinociception

Centrally administered adenosine and its analogues induce analgesia (antinociception) in tail flick latency, hot plate latency, and acetic acid-induced writhing paradigms. When administered intracisternally, adenosine and its analogues caused dose-related increases in hot plate reaction times in mice, with a rank order of potency of NECA > 2-chloroadenosine > adenosine > adenine nucleotides (Yarbrough and McGuffin-Clineschmidt, 1981). Papaverine and EHNA potentiated the analgesic effects of adenosine, whereas caffeine and theophylline antagonized the actions of the adenosine analogues. Adenosine had a similar antinociceptive action when injected into the lateral cerebral ventricle of rats tested with the tail flick latency paradigm (Haulică *et al.*, 1984). Theophylline and DDA antagonized these antinociceptive actions of adenosine.

Antinociceptive effects have been observed following the intrathecal administration of NECA to mice (Post, 1984) and of 2-chloroadenosine to rats (Hedner *et al.*, 1986). In the rat experiments, 2-chloroadenosine, injected at the level of the thoracic spinal cord, enhanced tail flick and hot plate latencies in doses which did not affect blood pressure, heart rate, or body temperature.

2.3. Hypnotic Effects

Intracerebroventricular administration of adenosine has been reported to induce a sleep state in cats, fowl, and dogs (Feldberg and Sherwood, 1954; Marley and Nistico, 1972; Haulică *et al.*, 1973). Parenteral administration of adenosine analogues to rats increased deep slow-wave sleep and rapid eye movement sleep in a dose-related manner (Radulovacki *et al.*, 1984), and these effects were antagonized by caffeine. Parenterally administered deoxycoformycin had very similar effects on deep slow-wave sleep and rapid eye movement sleep (Virus *et al.*, 1983), suggesting that endogenous adenosine has actions similar to peripherally administered analogues.

Intracerebroventricularly administered adenosine, but not the pyrimidine ribonucleosides cytidine and uridine, reduced wakefulness, increased total sleep time and deep slow-wave sleep time in rats (Radulovacki *et al.*, 1985). Adenosine also significantly reduced the time to onset of rapid eye movement sleep. Interestingly, icvt injections of forskolin or DDA failed to alter the amount or quality of sleep in rats, suggesting that generalized stimulation or inhibition of adenylate cyclase is insufficient to mediate sleep in the manner of specific A_1 or A_2 agonists (Glaum *et al.*, 1985). These results with forskolin apparently differ from those observed in mice, in which icvt forskolin depressed locomotor activity in a manner analogous to that observed with adenosine (Barraco *et al.*, 1985).

2.4. Anticonvulsant Activity

Anticonvulsant effects of adenosine and its analogues in intact animals have been described by several groups. Maitre *et al.* (1974) reported that intraperitoneally administered adenosine (130 mg/kg) protected against audiogenic seizures, and Snyder *et al.* (1982) described weak anticonvulsant actions of L-PIA in mice. In an extensive study, Dunwiddie and Worth (1982) compared the actions of several adenosine receptor agonists [CHA, L-PIA, and 2-chloroadenosine [2-ChAd)] and observed moderate anticonvulsant activity in mice and rats against a variety of convulsants. These effects were blocked, for the most part, by theophylline. The anticonvulsant effects of L-PIA were considerably less sensitive to the effects of theophylline, suggesting that the receptors involved in the actions of L-PIA might differ from those mediating the responses to CHA and 2-ChAd. The D isomer of PIA was approximately 20 times less effective than the L isomer in its anticonvulsant effects upon metrozol-induced seizure latency.

The effects of peripherally administered, metabolically stable, adenosine analogues on the threshold for metrazol-induced seizures were observed in rats (Murray *et al.*, 1985). CHA, L- and D-PIA, and 2-ChAd all raised seizure threshold, with L-PIA being 79 times more potent than D-PIA. Theophylline had a proconvulsant action, reducing the seizure threshold for metrazol. Theophylline antagonized the elevation in seizure threshold induced by 2-ChAd. Both adenosine and 2-ChAd have been reported to prolong the refractory time after a seizure produced by maximum electroshock in rats (Burley and Ferrendelli, 1984).

Adenosine antagonizes the electrically evoked after-discharges induced by penicillin in hippocampal slices (Lee *et al.*, 1984). Bath application of adenosine and its analogues reduced the frequency of generation of burst potentials in bicuculline-treated slices. Theophylline increased, and dipyridamole reduced, burst firing in these slices (Ault and Wang, 1986). Further evidence of a role for endogenously released adenosine as a modulator of slice excitability has been obtained in penicillin-treated slices. Both adenosine deaminase (the enzyme which deaminates adenosine to the pharmacologically less active product inosine) and theophylline were found to increase the rate of interictal spiking in penicillin-treated slices (Dunwiddie, 1980) and a series of alkyl-xanthines (theophylline, 8-phenyltheophylline, IBMX) increased interictal spiking with a rank potency order that correlated with the potency of these agents as adenosine antagonists (Dunwiddie *et al.*, 1981).

In the kindling model of epilepsy, adenosine has been shown to have anticonvulsant effects, whether administered peripherally or by the icvt route. Adenosine, adenosine agonists, and the adenosine uptake blocker papaverine reduce the severity and duration of amygdala-kindled seizures (Figs. 5 and 6) (Albertson *et al.*, 1983; Barraco *et al.*, 1984b; Dragunow and Goddard, 1984; Dragunow *et al.*, 1985), and L-PIA prolongs the phase of postictal depression following a seizure (Rosen and Berman, 1985). Conversely, the adenosine antagonists aminophylline, theophylline, caffeine, and IBMX prolong amygdala-kindled seizures (Albertson *et al.*, 1983; Dragunow and

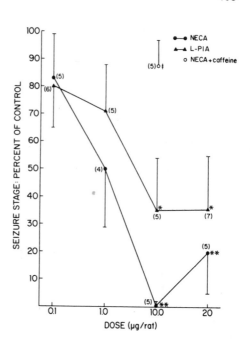

Figure 5. Effects of adenosine analogues on kindled seizure stage at four separate doses. Values represent the mean ± S.E.M. Numbers in parentheses indicate the number of animals tested in each group. The mean ± S.E.M. for saline controls ($N = 10$) was 90.0 ± 9.9%. ANOVA showed significant dose-related reductions in seizure stage for NECA (●) ($p < 0.01$) and L-PIA (▲) ($p < 0.05$). Significances determined by post hoc comparisons with saline controls for individual doses of each analogue are indicated (*$p < 0.05$; **$p \leqslant 0.01$). The effect of caffeine pretreatment on NECA's anticonvulsant activity at the 10-μg dose is shown (○); the significance determined by post hoc comparison between icvt NECA + ip caffeine and icvt NECA alone is indicated (‡$p < 0.05$). (From Barraco et al., 1984b.)

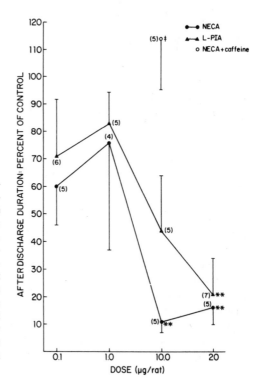

Figure 6. Effects of adenosine analogues on afterdischarge duration at four separate doses. Values represent the mean ± S.E.M. Numbers in parentheses indicate the number of animals tested in each group. The mean ± S.E.M. for saline controls ($N = 10$) was 95.2 ± 16.7%. ANOVA showed significant dose-related reductions in afterdischarge duration for NECA (●) ($p < 0.01$) and L-PIA (▲) ($p < 0.05$). Significances determined by post hoc comparisons with saline controls for individual doses of each analogue are indicated (**$p < 0.01$). ○, the effect of caffeine pretreatment on NECA's anticonvulsant activity at the 10 μg dose; the significance determined by post hoc comparison between icvt NECA + ip caffeine and icvt NECA alone is indicated (‡$p < 0.01$). (From Barraco et al., 1984b.)

Goddard, 1984). Aminophylline and theophylline also facilitate amygdala kindling (Dragunow and Goddard, 1984).

2.5. Adenosine and Food Intake

It is generally accepted that both the central and peripheral nervous systems are involved in the regulation of food intake, with an interplay between multiple neurotransmitter systems regulating the ingestion of food (Deutsch, 1978). Attention was directed to the role of adenosine in feeding behavior because adipocytes, the main metabolic cellular constituents of adipose tissue, have been shown to release adenosine, and since adenosine has a local regulatory effect on the metabolism of adipose tissue, lipolysis is inhibited (Capogrossi et al., 1979). Moreover, adenosine was viewed as providing a potential feedback regulatory signal between adipose tissue and the hypothalamic centers for food intake regulation. It was also shown that adenosine (100 mg/kg), and to a lesser extent inosine, produced significant suppressions of food intake following subcutaneous administration in rats (Capogrossi et al., 1979).

Central (lateral ventricle) administration of adenosine (10 µg), adenine, and 5'-AMP, but not inosine, potently suppressed food intake in rats (Levine and Morley, 1983), while adenosine also decreased water intake. The effect of adenosine was thought to be specific for ingestive behavior, since it did not decrease significantly spontaneous locomotor activity or grooming. The authors commented on their finding that centrally administered adenosine suppressed both food and water intake, in contrast to peripherally administered purines which decreased food intake only, thus suggesting that the peripheral satiety effects of adenosine may be mediated by different mechanisms than the central actions.

2.6. Respiratory Control

Administered intravascularly, adenosine is a respiratory stimulant in man (Watt and Routledge, 1985), rat (Monteiro and Ribeiro, 1986), and rabbit (Buss et al., 1986). In human subjects, this action is manifested as a profound urge to breath deeply or even feelings of suffocation, often associated with neck, chest, and abdominal pain. The site of action of this respiratory stimulant effect is likely to be the carotid body chemoreceptors, the activity of which is enhanced by infusions of adenosine (McQueen and Ribeiro, 1983).

The effects of icvt L-PIA on respiration have been examined in halothane-anesthetized rats (Hedner et al., 1982). Ten micrograms of L-PIA caused a decrease in pulmonary ventilation due to a reduction in respiratory frequency and tidal volume. NECA was ten times more potent in eliciting respiratory depression than was L-PIA. The effects of L-PIA were abolished by theophylline (Wessberg et al., 1985). Wessberg et al. (1985) also showed that intraventricular injections of L-PIA could produce a prolonged depressant effect (> 45 min) on breathing without significantly affecting blood pressure. Similar effects were observed in cats injected in the third ventricle with L-PIA (Eldridge et al., 1985). In a related respiratory study, administration of L-PIA directly onto the exposed surface of the fourth ventricle of anesthetized rabbit neonates produced respiratory depression (Lagercrantz et al., 1984), thus demonstrating that effects of adenosine analogues can be exerted directed on pontobulbar centers.

A physiological effect of endogenously released adenosine was demonstrated by a 10-min exposure to hypoxia of cats that had been glomectomized and vagotomized to avoid stimulation of peripheral receptors (Milhorn et al., 1984). The hypoxia led to depression of respiration, not only during exposure to the hypoxia mixture, but also for more than an hour after the return to hyperoxia. Pretreatment of the animals with theophylline reduced the respiratory depression during hypoxic exposure and prevented the long-lasting depression, indicating an involvement of endogenously released adenosine.

2.7. Body Temperature

Bennet and Drury (1981) demonstrated that adenosine decreased body temperature in dogs. These effects were shown by Green and Stoner (1950) to also occur in the rat and to be shared by ATP. The latter authors also showed that adenosine and ATP caused a fall in oxygen consumption that paralleled the fall in body temperature. The hypothermic effect of adenosine in rats is antagonized by caffeine (Wager-Srdar et al., 1983).

Studies in mice have shown that stable adenosine analogues including L-PIA, CHA, and 2-ChAd, when administered peripherally, also have potent hypothermic effects (Vapaatalo et al., 1975; Dunwiddie and Worth, 1982; Mehta and Kulkarni, 1983; Jonzon et al., 1986). Adenosine and analogues showed the same relative and absolute potencies as hypothermic and as hypotensive agents. Since other vasodilating agents with presumably peripheral sites of action also reduced body temperature (Jonzon et al., 1986), the observations are compatible with the hypothesis that hypothermia is a result of the vasodilatory effect of adenosine.

A suppression of shivering-like muscular activity was observed after the administration of adenosine, NECA, or L-PIA, and this coincided with the temperature reduction (Jonzon et al., 1986). This behavioral change could have been a result of an effect of adenosine on afferent pathways in the CNS or the periphery. In fact, Davies et al. (1983) had previously shown that systemically administered adenosine analogues exert a muscle relaxant effect at doses well below those necessary to inhibit neuromuscular transmission; possibly as a result of central actions.

The hypothermic effects of peripherally administered adenosine are therefore likely to be largely due to peripheral effects of the nucleosides, with the possible involvement of a central component of the shivering response. Intracisternally administered 2-ChAd caused a profound hypothermia and loss of muscle tone in mice (Yarbrough and McGuffin-Clineschmidt, 1981), demonstrating that even when administered centrally, adenosine can elicit falls in body temperature, an action which may further complicate the assessment of other behavioral parameters.

3. Conclusions

The preceding sections have presented a summary of the literature on the actions of centrally administered adenosine and some of its analogues. It becomes apparent that adenosine and its antagonists have a multitude of actions at every level of the neural axis, leaving little doubt that endogenously released adenosine is an important, if rather ubiquitous, regulator of central excitability. The question arises, however, as to the extent to which adenosine-related neuromodulation may reflect a global, as opposed to local, phenomenon. Thus, the sedative, hypnotic, and anticonvulsant effects of adenosine may be a result of a generalized depression of neuronal circuitry and, indeed, a decreased awareness of the environment could explain the anxiolytic and antipsychotic actions that have been attributed to adenosine (Wagner and Katz, 1983; Heffner et al., 1985). Conversely, the stimulant, anxiogenic, and convulsant actions of the methylxanthine adenosine antagonists may result from a generalized and progressive antagonism of adenosinergic tone in the CNS.

There is currently little evidence that adenosine itself is released from an identifiable system of purinergic neurons within the brain. Rather, adenosine efflux from neurons may accompany enhanced levels of neuronal activity, especially where this is associated with a localized or generalized state of hypoxia. Thus, one important function of adenosine may be the maintenance of a balance between neuronal activity and metabolic demand. Ultimately, as has been suggested (Williams, 1984; Newby, 1984), adenosine may act as a homeostatic modulator, preventing tissue damage during insults to the CNS.

Another potential source of extracellular adenosine is represented by the extracellular dephosphorylation of synaptically released ATP (Phillis and Wu, 1981). The literature contains many references to the copackaging of ATP with other neurotransmitters and it is reasonable to assume that ATP release occurs at certain nerve terminals in the CNS (Phillis and Wu, 1981). Indeed, ATP release from depolarized central synaptosomes has been demonstrated (White, 1985). ATP release, with extracellular adenosine formation, at specific nerve terminals may offer the possibility of a circumscribed system in which adenosine could act as a traditional neurotransmitter, in contrast to the more ubiquitous release of adenosine described above.

ACKNOWLEDGMENTS. I thank Mr. R. E. Stair for reading a draft and Ms. L. McCraw for her skill in typing the manuscript. Experiments described were supported by NIH Grant RR-08167-OX and the BRSG program.

References

Albertson, T. E., and Joy, R. M., 1986, Modification of excitation and inhibition evoked in dentate gyrus by perforant path stimulation: Effects of aminophylline and kindling, *Pharmacol. Biochem. Behav.* **24**:85–91.

Albertson, T. E., Stark, L. G., Joy, R. M. and Bowyer, J. F., 1983, Aminophylline and kindled seizures, *Exp. Neurol.* **81**:703–713.

Ault, B., and Wang, C. M., 1986, Adenosine inhibits epileptiform activity arising in hippocampal area CA3, *Br. J. Pharmacol.* **87**:695–703.

Barraco, R. A., Aggarwal, A. K., Phillis, J. W., Moron, M. A., and Wu, P. H., 1984a, Dissociation of the locomotor and hypotensive effects of adenosine and analogues in the rat, *Neurosci. Lett.* **48**:139–144.

Barraco, R. A., Swanson, T. H., Phillis, J. W., and Berman, R. F., 1984b, Anticonvulsant effects of adenosine analogues on amygdaloid-kindled seizures in rats, *Neurosci. Lett.* **46**:317–322.

Barraco, R. A., Phillis, J. W., and Altman, H. J., 1985, Depressant effect of forskolin on spontaneous locomotor activity in mice, *Gen. Pharmacol.* **16**:521–524.

Bennet, D. W., and Drury, A. N., 1931, Further observations relating to the physiological activity of adenine compounds, *J. Physiol. (London)* **72**:288–320.

Bickford, P. C., Fredholm, B. B., Dunwiddie, T. V., and Freedman, R., 1985, Inhibition of Purkinje cell firing by systemic administration by phenylisopropyladenosine: Effect of central noradrenaline depletion by DSP4, *Life Sci.* **37**:289–297.

Buday, P. V., Carr, C. J., and Miya, T. S., 1961, A pharmacologic study of some nucleosides and nucleotides, *J. Pharm. Pharmacol.* **13**:290–299.

Burley, E. S., and Ferrendelli, J. A., 1984, Regulatory effects of neurotransmitters on electroshock and pentylenetetrazol seizures, *Fed. Proc.* **43**:2521–2524.

Buss, D. C., Routledge, P. A., and Watt, A. H., 1986, Intravenous adenosine stimulates respiration in conscious adult rabbits, *Br. J. Pharmacol.* **87**:182P.

Capogrossi, M. C., Francendese, A., and DiGirolamo, M., 1979, Suppression of food intake by adenosine and inosine, *Am. J. Clin. Nutr.* **32**:1762–1768.

Chan-Palay, V., and Palay, S. L., 1984, *Coexistence of Neuroactive Substances in Neurons*, Wiley, New York.

Coffin, V. L., and Carney, J. M., 1983, Behavioral pharmacology of adenosine analogs, in: *Physiology and Pharmacology of Adenosine Derivatives* (J. W. Daly, Y. Kuroda, J. W. Phillis, H. Shimizu, and M. Ui, eds.), Raven Press, New York, pp. 267–274.

Coffin, V. L., Taylor, J. A., Phillis, J. W., Altman, H. J., and Barraco, R. A., 1984, Behavioral interaction of adenosine and methylxanthines in central purinergic systems, *Neurosci. Lett.* **47**:91–98.

Davies, L. P., Baird-Lambert, J., Jamieson, D. D., and Spence, I., 1983, Studies on marine-derived analogs of adenosine, in: *Physiology and Pharmacology of Adenosine Derivatives* (J. W. Daly, Y. Kuroda, J. W. Phillis, H. Shimizu, and M. Ui, eds.), Raven Press, New York, pp. 257–266.

Deutsch, J. A., 1978, The stomach in food satiation and the regulation of appetite, *Prog. Neurobiol.* **10**:135–153.

Dragunow, M., and Goddard, G. V., 1984, Adenosine modulation of amygdala kindling, *Exp. Neurol.* **84**:654–665.

Dragunow, M., Goddard, G. V., and Laverty, R., 1985, Is adenosine an endogenous anticonvulsant? *Epilepsia* **26**:480–487.

Dunwiddie, T. V., 1980, Endogenously released adenosine regulates excitability in the in vitro hippocampus, *Epilepsia* **21**:541–548.

Dunwiddie, T. V., 1985, The physiological role of adenosine in the central nervous system, *Int. Rev. Neurobiol.* **27**:63–139.

Dunwiddie, T. V., and Brodie, M. S., 1985, The effects of systemic and local administration of adenosine analogs on hippocampal evoked responses, *Soc. Neurosci. Abstr.* **11**:576.

Dunwiddie, T. V., and Worth, T., 1982, Sedative and anticonvulsant effects of adenosine analogs in mouse and rat, *J. Pharmacol. Exp. Ther.* **220**:70–76.

Dunwiddie, T. V., Hoffer, B., and Fredholm, B. B., 1981, Alkylxanthines elevate hippocampal excitability: Evidence for a role of endogenous adenosine, *Naunyn-Schmiedebergs Arch. Pharmacol.* **316**:326–330.

Dunwiddie, T. V., Lee, K. S., Fredholm, B. B., and Brodie, M. S., 1986, A comparison of systemic and local administration of adenosine analogs on hippocampal physiology, *Pfluegers Arch.* **402**(Suppl. 1):S41.

Eldridge, F. L., Millhorn, D. E., and Kiley, J. P., 1985, Antagonism by theophylline of respiratory inhibition induced by adenosine, *J. Appl. Physiol.* **59**:1428–1433.

Feldberg, W., and Sherwood, S. L., 1954, Injections of drugs into the lateral ventricle of the cat, *J. Physiol. (London)* **123**:148–167.

Glaum, S. R., Yanik, G. M., Porter, N. M., Chen, E. H., and Radulovacki, M., 1985, Effects of intracerebroventricular administration of forskolin and 2′,5′-dideoxyadenosine on sleep in rats, *Fed. Proc.* **11**:749.

Glowa, J. R., Sobel, E., Malaspina, S., and Dews, P. B., 1985, Behavioral effects of caffeine, (−)N-((R)-1-methyl-2-phenyl)-adenosine (PIA) and their combination in the mouse, *Psychopharmacologia* **87**:421–424.

Green, H. N., and Stoner, H. B., 1950, *Biological Actions of the Adenine Nucleotides,* H. K. Lewis, London.

Green, R. D., Proudfit, H. K., and Yeung, S.-M. H., 1982, Modulation of striatal dopaminergic function by local injection of 5′-N-ethylcarboxamide adenosine, *Science* **218**:58–61.

Haulică, I., Ababei, L., Brănisteanu, D., and Topoliceanu, F., 1973, Preliminary data on the possible hypnogenic role of adenosine, *J. Neurochem.* **21**:1019–1020.

Haulică, I., Nemtu, D., Petrescu, G. H., Frasin, M., Slătineanu, S., and Nacu, C., 1984, The influence of adenosine upon thermoalgesic sensitivity, *Physiologie (Bucarest)* **21**:167–172.

Hedner, T., Hedner, J., Wessberg, P., and Jonason, J., 1982, Regulation of breathing in the rat: Indications for a role of central adenosine mechanisms, *Neurosci. Lett.* **33**:147–151.

Hedner, T., Fredholm, B. B., Hedner, J., Holmgren, M., Nordberg, G., and Sollevi, A., 1986, Intrathecally administered 2-chloroadenosine produces spinal analgesia in the rat, *Pfluegers Arch.* **407**:S43.

Heffner, T. G., Downs, D. A., Bristol, J. A., Bruns, R. F., Harrigan, S. E., Moos, W. H., Sledge, K. L., and Wiley, J. N., 1985, Antipsychotic-like effects of adenosine receptor agonists, *Pharmacologist* **27**:293.

Jonzon, B., Bergquist, A., Li, Y.-O., and Fredholm, B. B., 1986, Effects of adenosine and two stable adenosine analogs on blood pressure, heart rate and colonic temperature in the rat, *Acta Physiol. Scand.* **126**:491–498.

Lagercrantz, H., Yamamoto, Y., Fredholm, B. B., Prabhakar, N. R., and Von Euler, C., 1984, Adenosine analogues depress ventilation in rabbit neonates—Theophylline stimulation of respiration via adenosine receptors, *Pediatr. Res.* **18**:387–390.

Lee, K. S., Schubert, P., and Heinemann, U., 1984, The anticonvulsive action of adenosine: A postsynaptic, dendritic action by a possible endogenous anticonvulsant, *Brain Res.* **321**:160–164.

Levine, A. S., and Morley, J. E., 1983, Effect of intraventricular adenosine on food intake in rats, *Pharmacol. Biochem. Behav.* **19**:23–26.

McQueen, D. D., and Ribeiro, J. A., 1983, On the specificity and type of receptor involved in carotid body chemoreceptor activation by adenosine in the cat, *Br. J. Pharmacol.* **80**:347–354.

Maitre, M., Ciesielski, L., Lehmann, A., Kempf, E., and Mandel, P., 1974, Protective effects of adenosine and nicotinamide against audiogenic seizure, *Biochem. Pharmacol.* **23**:2807–2816.

Marley, E., and Nistico, G., 1972, Effects of catecholamines and adenosine derivatives given into the brain of fowls, *Br. J. Pharmacol.* **46**:619–636.

Mehta, A. K., and Kulkarni, S. K., 1983, Effect of purinergic substances on rectal temperature in mice: Involvement of P_1-purinoceptors, *Arch. Int. Pharmacodyn. Ther.* **264**:180–186.

Milhorn, D. E., Eldridge, F. L., Kiley, J. P., and Waldrop, T. G., 1984, Prolonged inhibition of respiration following acute hypoxia in glomectomized cats, *Respir. Physiol.* **41**:87–103.

Monteiro, E. C., and Ribeiro, J. A., 1986, Adenosine and carotid body chemoreceptor regulation of respiration in the rat, *Pfluegers Arch.* **407**:S56.

Murray, T. F., Sylvester, D., Schultz, C. S., and Szot, P., 1985, Purinergic modulation of the seizure threshold for pentylenetetrazol in the rat, *Neuropharmacology* **24**:761–766.

Newby, A. C., 1984, Adenosine and the concept of 'retaliatory metabolites,' *Trends Biochem. Sci.* **9**:42–44.

Phillis, J. W., 1982, Evidence for an A_2-like adenosine receptor on cerebral cortical neurons, *J. Pharm. Pharmacol.* **34**:453–454.

Phillis, J. W., 1984, A critical evaluation of the evidence for a single transmitter for each nerve cell, in: *Coexistence of Neuroactive Substances in Neurons* (V. Chan-Palay and S. L. Palay, eds.), Wiley, New York, pp. 379–393.

Phillis, J. W., and Kostopoulos, G. K., 1975, Adenosine as a putative transmitter in the cerebral cortex: Studies with potentiators and antagonists, *Life Sci.* **17**:1085–1094.

Phillis, J. W., and Wu, P. H., 1981, The role of adenosine and its nucleotides in central synaptic transmission, *Prog. Neurobiol.* **16**:187–239.

Phillis, J. W., and Wu, P. H., 1982a, The effect of various centrally active drugs on adenosine uptake by the central nervous system, *Comp. Biochem. Physiol.* **72C**:179–187.

Phillis, J. W., and Wu, P. H., 1982b, Adenosine mediates sedative action of various centrally active drugs, *Med. Hypoth.* **9**:361–367.

Phillis, J. W., and Wu, P. H., 1983, Roles of adenosine and adenine nucleotides in the CNS, in: *Physiology and Pharmacology of Adenosine Derivatives* (J. W. Daly, Y. Kuroda, J. W. Phillis, H. Shimizu, and M. Ui, eds.), Raven Press, New York, pp. 219–236.

Phillis, J. W., Barraco, R. A., DeLong, R. E., and Washington, D. O., 1986, Behavioral characteristics of centrally administered adenosine analogs, *Pharmacol. Biochem. Behav.* **24**:261–270.

Post, C., 1984, Antinociceptive effects in mice after intrathecal injection of 5'-N-ethylcarboxamide adenosine, *Neurosci. Lett.* **51**:325–330.

Radulovacki, M., Virus, R. M., Djuricic-Nedelson, M., and Green, R. D., 1984, Adenosine analogs and sleep in rats, *J. Pharmacol. Exp. Ther.* **228**:268–274.

Radulovacki, M., Virus, R. M., Rapoza, D., and Crane, R. A., 1985, A comparison of the dose response effects of pyrimidine ribonucleosides and adenosine on sleep in rats, *Psychopharmacologia* **87**:136–140.

Rall, T. W., 1985, Central nervous system stimulants: The methylxanthines, in: *The Pharmacological Basis of Therapeutics,* 7th ed. (A. G. Gilman, L. S. Goodman, T. W. Rall, and F. Murad, eds.), Macmillan Co., New York, pp. 589–603.

Rosen, J. B., and Berman, R. F., 1985, Prolonged postictal depression in amygdala-kindled rats by the adenosine analog, L-phenylisopropyladenosine, *Exp. Neurol.* **90**:549–557.

Snyder, S. H., Katims, J. J., Annau, Z., Bruns, R. F., and Daly, J. W., 1981, Adenosine receptors and behavioral actions of methylxanthines, *Proc. Natl. Acad. Sci. USA* **78**:3260–3264.

Vapaatalo, H., Onken, D., Neuvonen, P., and Westerman, E., 1975, Stereospecificity in some central and circulatory effects of phenylisopropyladenosine, *Arzneim. Forsch.* **25**:407–410.

Virus, R. M., Djuricic-Nedelson, M., Radulovacki, M., and Green, R. D., 1983, The effects of adenosine and 2'-deoxycoformycin on sleep and wakefulness in rats, *Neuropharmacology* **22**:1401–1404.

Wachtel, H., 1983, Potential antidepressant activity of rolipram and other selective cyclic 3',5'-monophosphate phosphodiesterase inhibitors, *Neuropharmacology* **22**:267–272.

Wager-Srdar, S. A., Oken, M. M., Morley, J. E., and Levine, A. S., 1983, Thermoregulatory effects of purines and caffeine, *Life Sci.* **33**:2431–2438.

Wagner, J. A., and Katz, R. J., 1983, Purinergic control of anxiety: Direct behavioral evidence in the rat, *Neurosci. Lett.* **43**:333–337.

Watt, A. H., and Routledge, P. A., 1985, Adenosine stimulates respiration in man, *Br. J. Clin. Pharmacol.* **20**:503–506.

Wessberg, P., Hedner, J., Hedner, T., Persson, B., and Jonason, J., 1985, Adenosine mechanism in the regulation of breathing in the rat, *Eur. J. Pharmacol.* **106**:59–67.

White, T. D., 1985, Release of ATP from central and peripheral nerve terminals, in: *Purines: Pharmacology and Physiological Roles* (T. W. Stone, ed.), Macmillan Co., New York, pp. 95–105.

Williams, M., 1984, Adenosine—A selective neuromodulator in the CNS, *Trends Neurosci.* **7**:164–168.

Wu, P. H., and Phillis, J. W., 1984, Uptake by central nervous tissues as a mechanism for the regulation of extracellular adenosine concentrations, *Neurochem. Int.* **6**:613–632.

Wu, P. H., Phillis, J. W., and Thierry, D. L., 1982, Adenosine receptor agonists inhibit K^+-evoked Ca^{2+} uptake by rat brain cortical synaptosomes, *J. Neurochem.* **39**:700–708.

Yarbrough, G. G., and McGuffin-Clineschmidt, J. C., 1981, *In vivo* behavioral assessment of central nervous system purinergic receptors, *Eur. J. Pharmacol.* **76**:137–144.

27

Adenosine: A Molecule for Synaptic Homeostasis?

Evolution of Current Concepts on the Physiological and Pathophysiological Roles of Adenosine in the Brain

George K. Kostopoulos

1. Introduction

Among the neurotransmitters and other neuroactive substances discussed in the previous chapters, adenosine is the endogenous *molecule* with the most commonly appreciated effects on the *mind*, as each cup of coffee may remind us. However, in contrast to the relatively well-established ideas about the transmitter amino acids, acetylcholine, and catecholamines, research on adenosine is currently faced with an increasing amount of data in need of an integrated functional scheme. Reflections on the way our ideas have evolved regarding several possible schemes will emphasize the mutual dependence between our understanding of synaptic transmission and the specific roles we often assign to endogenous neuroactive molecules.

In a new field such as the neurosciences, perhaps we can only speak of hypothetical functional schemes and not real paradigms having the universality demanded by a Kuhnian epistemological approach (Kuhn, 1970). However, allowing for this limitation in scale it seems (Swazey and Worden, 1975) that one could apply Kuhn's concepts of paradigm to neuroscience: normal research as puzzle solving for the articulation and reinforcement of the paradigm, followed by awareness of anomaly (discovery and crisis) and invention of a new paradigm to resolve the crisis.

Probably the most important "paradigm" in neuroscience, the localization of function in brain, was supported and extended by the electrographic recordings of Penfield and Jasper (1954) to include the brain malfunction known as epilepsy. On the other hand, Jasper's (1949) work proposing different brain circuits for the activation of specific and nonspecific cortical inputs led to a new "paradigm" that was further established in later work by himself and others. A third "paradigm" in neuroscience, that of synaptic transmission, has been worked out primarily from

George K. Kostopoulos • Department of Physiology, University of Patras Medical School, Patras 261 10, Greece.

experiments in the cholinergic neuromuscular junction. In the normal research, which followed successful resolution of the puzzles concerning several synapses in both the peripheral and central nervous system, the "paradigm" was articulated (criteria for transmitter identification) and established (see Werman, 1966; Phillis, 1970). In parallel experiments culminating after the mid-1970s, the process of discovery identified anomalies in the classical neurotransmitter paradigm. These novel facts forced a restructuring of our concepts. Research on adenosine has made important contributions to the evolution of these concepts, but on the other hand, acceptance of the importance of the role of adenosine as a neurotransmitter had to wait for the evolution of our experimental paradigm.

2. The Early Studies

The seminal paper of Drury and Szent-Györgyi (1929) showed that adenosine and ATP had important cardiovascular roles but it also alluded to possible central effects. This possibility was investigated again only after a quarter of a century. Feldberg and Sherwood (1954) and Buday *et al.* (1961) demonstrated a decrease in locomotor activity following injection of adenosine into the ventricles of cats and the injection of ATP directly into the cerebral ventricles of rats. At this time, and increasingly thereafter, the scientific community became aware of the many other roles of purines. The importance of ATP in intermediate metabolism was explained in detail. The two classic studies on physiological effects of adenosine with possible CNS involvement as well as a few more appearing in the early 1970s (Marley and Nistico, 1972; Haulica *et al.*, 1973; Maitre *et al.*, 1974) were motivated primarily by the fact that adenosine was the obvious metabolite of ATP and AMP (Mandel, 1971) and the suspicion that its levels might reflect the energy state of the brain. The demonstration of release of adenosine derivatives from brainslices by excitation (Pull and McIlwain, 1973) suggested that these substances were "neurohumoral agents in the brain." However, even though Sattin and Rall (1970) demonstrated a potent depressive effect of adenosine on adenyl cyclase, a property shared with catecholamines and other neurotransmitters, the observed sedative actions of adenosine were discussed by most people at the time in terms of an interference with the energy state of the brain rather than in terms of a role in the brain's synaptic transmission.

In contrast, a central transmitter role was suggested for ATP as early as 1954 by Holton and Holton. This suggestion was not pursued further until Burnstock and his associates (Burnstock *et al.*, 1963) first encountered some relaxing effects of nerve stimulation on smooth muscle in guinea pig taenia coli, which were not blocked by adrenergic or cholinergic antagonists. Subsequent work in the peripheral autonomic nervous system led to a proposal of purinergic nerves most likely utilizing ATP as a transmitter (see Burnstock, 1986). In the past the notion of ATP being a central transmitter, especially one released by the primary afferents in spinal cord (Holton, 1959), was disputed on the grounds that the excitatory effect observed by microiontophoretic application could be attributed to the calcium-chelating ability of ATP (see Krnjević, 1974).

Adenosine itself started to interest some laboratories as a candidate for a role in synaptic transmission only after the discovery of the potent depressant effects which this nucleoside had on single central neurons (Phillis *et al.*, 1974, 1979a,b; Phillis and Kostopoulos, 1975; Kostopoulos *et al.*, 1975; Kostopoulos and Phillis, 1977). The initial finding was rather accidental. In an effort to find controls for some effect of ATP, we tried ADP, AMP, and adenosine only to find them increasingly more potent as depressants of single cortical neurons. The persuasiveness of those papers in contrast to the biochemical ones (Sattin and Rall, 1970; Pull and McIlwain, 1973) is probably not unrelated to the fact that adenosine was applied microiontophoretically and that this technique was believed to be the best way to identify transmitters in the brain.

The optimistic title of a 1975 publication—"Adenosine as a neurotransmitter: Studies with potentiators and antagonists"—reflects the satisfaction of putting new pieces in a familiar puzzle. The latter was the "paradigm" of classical transmitter identification referred to in the introduction. Indeed, several accepted criteria for such an identification were met. Adenosine along with the enzymes which can produce and metabolize it was present in synapses. It was released in a Ca^{2+}-dependent manner and a powerful uptake system could help terminate its action (Kuroda and McIlwain, 1973; Sulakhe and Phillis, 1975). Methylxanthines antagonized both its electrophysiological (depression of neuronal activity) and biochemical (stimulation of adenyl cyclase) effects. The effects and their antagonism resulted from specific interaction with an extracellular receptor with stringent requirements for adenosine or a similar molecule as demonstrated by structure–activity relationships. The depressant effects were widespread in all regions of brain examined and were mimicked by adenosine uptake inhibition, suggesting a role for endogenous adenosine.

Awareness of alternative possible roles for endogenous adenosine came from reports of a presynaptic effect in the neuromuscular junction (Ginsborg and Hirst, 1972) but was more clearly established for brain tissue with intracellular recordings from cortical neurons *in situ* (Edstrom and Phillis, 1976; Phillis *et al.*, 1979a,b). The latter experiments showed that microiontophoretically applied adenosine hyperpolarizes the neurons without significantly affecting membrane resistance (Fig. 1). Evoked EPSPs had smaller sizes and rates of rise. Spontaneous EPSPs disappeared and the threshold for action potentials generated by direct depolarizing pulses was unchanged. These observations, soon confirmed and extended by others (Lekic, 1977; Scholfield, 1978), were best explained by an inhibition of excitatory transmitter release. Adenosine could therefore be considered as a neuromodulator rather than as a neurotransmitter.

Ten years later we still do not have strong evidence that adenosine is stored and released by any specific purinergic (central or peripheral) pathway. Thus, key steps in the proof that it is a primary transmitter are still lacking. However, recently many elegant experiments have described adenosine's involvement in synaptic transmission and established its importance in several aspects. A search of the pertinent literature reveals that after 1980 there has been an explosive increase in the number of laboratories actively involved in adenosine research; the early studies on adenosine had a strong but delayed impact. The fact that the early 1970s brought other perhaps more important subjects, such as the second messenger hypothesis (Bloom, 1975) and later the discovery of endogenous opioids (Kosterlitz, 1976), only explains part of this delay. Similarly, the confusing controversy between the claim that microiontophoresed cAMP works on adenosine receptors to produce a depression reversed by caffeine (Phillis and Kostopoulos, 1975) and the proposition that cAMP mimics noradrenaline as a second messenger potentiated by methylxanthines (Siggin *et al.*, 1969) was resolved quickly to the benefit of both the second messenger hypothesis and the adenosine story (see Phillis, 1977).

Thus, the main reason for the delayed impact may be that in 1976, to consider a neuroactive substance a "neuromodulator" was not very conducive to further research, as this term was the wastebasket for all endogenous neuroactive molecules which failed to meet the criteria for transmitter identification. As long as the "paradigm" of central synaptic transmission remained more or less constrained to substances that actually relayed the message across the synaptic junction, most scientists were involved in searching for the substance which carried this signal. The demonstration, however, in the mid and late 1970s of more than 50 neuropeptides which coresided with transmitters in specific terminals, and which were released to have several non-orthodox (indirect, long term) effects on the synapse, enriched the "paradigm" of synaptic transmission (Cuello, 1982; Schmitt, 1984). The focus changed to incorporate the many mechanisms by which the enormous plasticity of the synaptic response is achieved. Interest in adenosine was thereby rekindled.

A final conceptual and methodological reason for the flurry of activity on adenosine in the 1980s is that with the use of potent adenosine analogues two opposite effects on adenyl cyclase were discovered. The distinct pharmacological profile of the inhibition and the activation of

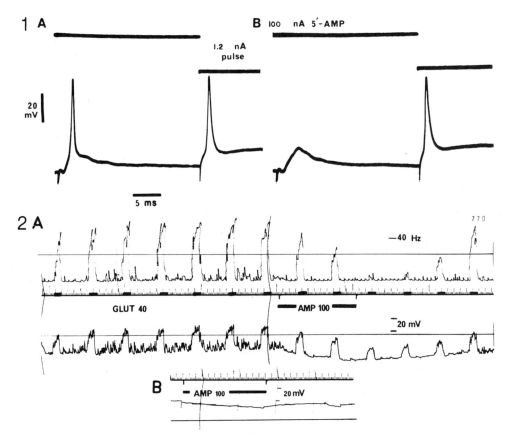

Figure 1. Effects of AMP on two rat cortical neurons recorded intracellularly *in vivo*, suggest activation of presynaptic adenosine receptors. (1) EPSPs and action potentials are successively evoked by epicortical stimulation and by an intracellular current pulse (A). Microiontophoretic application of 5′-AMP (100 nA) will raise the excitability threshold to epicortical stimulation without affecting that to the intracellular current pulse. The membrane potential of our other neuron (2) is resting at 65 mV (middle trace). Successive applications of glutamate will depolarize and induce bursts of action potentials, the frequency of which is counted on the upper trace. The application of 100-nA AMP hyperpolarizes this neuron by about 9 mV (after correction for electrode polarization shown in B). During and after AMP application, spontaneous depolarizing synaptic activity was almost eliminated and glutamate-evoked depolarizations were reduced in amplitude, becoming subthreshold for action potential generation. (From Phillis *et al.*, 1979a.)

adenyl cyclase led to the classification of adenosine receptors into two classes—A_1 and A_2, respectively (van Calker *et al.*, 1979; Londos *et al.*, 1980)—and provided a new framework within which to approach the problem. The availability of radiolabeled adenosine analogues further enabled the localization of adenosine receptors and a biochemical characterization of the effects of different experimental manipulations (see Daly, 1983).

3. Current Questions Related to Adenosine in the Brain

Several recent publications review the latest findings on adenosine (Phillis and Wu, 1981; Stone, 1981; Su, 1983; Williams, 1984; Dunwiddie, 1985; Snyder, 1985; Marangos and Boulenger, 1985) while proceedings from meetings dedicated to this subject have appeared recently at an increasing pace (Daly *et al.*, 1983; Berne *et al.*, 1983; Stone, 1985; Stefanovich *et al.*, 1986).

Therefore, this review will be limited to a discussion of the major issues concerning endogenous adenosine that are currently of interest. They fall into the four categories of what adenosine is doing, how, when, and where in the brain. The focus of the discussion is on those findings which triggered questions at either the behavioral or the cellular level. Although the "where" questions (Section 3.3) are currently considered the real essence of the identity problem of adenosine (specific neuromodulator or general regulator of synaptic homeostasis), the relatively neglected "when" questions (Section 3.4) may be the ones of greatest importance.

3.1. What Roles Does Endogenous Adenosine Play in the Brain?

3.1.1. Is Central Adenosine Tonically Controlling the Level of Arousal?

This question was raised by two lines of evidence: (1) the effects of adenosine's administration and, even more substantially, (2) the effects of drugs which are known to interfere with adenosine. Feldberg and Sherwood's (1954) basic claim that intracerebroventricularly applied adenosine induces sedation and probably sleep in cats has been repeatedly confirmed and amplified in many species (Buday *et al.*, 1961; Marley and Nistico, 1972; Haulica *et al.*, 1973; Vapaatalo *et al.*, 1975; Snyder *et al.*, 1981; Dunwiddie and Worth, 1982; Radulovacki *et al.*, 1984; Phillis *et al.*, 1986).

Phillis (this volume) summarizes the most recent findings on adenosine's inhibitory effects on locomotor activity as well as the evidence suggesting a hypnogenic role of adenosine. Brain adenosine receptors may be physiologically involved in a similar function since (1) antagonists of adenosine receptors such as the methylxanthines increase by themselves locomotor activity and (2) adenosine uptake inhibitors and adenosine deaminase inhibitors have sedative effects. Three lines of evidence have led to the proposal that the brain is continuously under a mild inhibitory purinergic tone: (1) adenosine analogues can decrease locomotor activity at brain concentrations (10 nM; Katims *et al.*, 1983) not significantly higher than that required for 50% occupation of adenosine receptors and the latter happens with the physiologically available adenosine (Williams, 1983), (2) adenosine depresses neuronal activity and caffeine antagonizes adenosine depression while being itself excitatory (Phillis and Kostopoulos, 1975; Greene *et al.*, 1985), and (3) caffeine's antagonism of adenosine receptors is observed in animals in doses (50–250 mg equivalent to 1–3 cups of coffee; Snyder, 1985) which in humans produce a feeling of awakening. Is this, however, a proof for adenosine involvement in control of arousal mechanisms? Since the exact nature of the latter is hardly understood, a conservative approach limiting adenosine involvement to the observed hypoactivity and certain changes in sleep pattern may be necessary. In some studies, adenosine analogues reduced locomotor activity without apparently affecting righting reflexes or causing sleep (Snyder *et al.*, 1981) while the electrographic (Radulovacki *et al.*, 1984) as well as biochemical data (Yanik *et al.*, 1985) point to an interference with REM rather than total sleep time. Stimulation of brain adenosine receptors may control the arousal state of the brain but alternatively they may interfere with the initiative or the competence for organizing movements. Experiments combining long-term polygraphic recordings and specific behavioral tests using a whole range of adenosine analogue doses and possibly human experimentation are needed. Particular attention should be given to the lowest part of the dose–effect relationship as some recent paradoxical but confirmed findings (Katims *et al.*, 1983; Coffin *et al.*, 1984) suggest that stimulation of some adenosine receptors at very low concentrations can actually increase locomotor activity. The question of adenosine involvement in regulation of the arousal level has tremendous importance not only for the understanding of the physiology and pathophysiology of sleep and its disorders but also for the toxicology of several important drugs which interfere with adenosine (Major *et al.*, 1981; Phillis and Wu, 1982) including, of course, coffee (Rall, 1985).

3.1.2. Does Adenosine Mediate Cerebral Blood Flow (CBF) Autoregulation?

This issue was raised after the demonstration of the remarkable vasodilatory effects of adenosine in a variety of other tissues and most notably the heart (for review, see Berne et al., 1983; Su, 1983). The potent effect of adenosine on cerebral vessels first demonstrated by Berne et al. (1974) and later more directly by Wahl and Kuschinsky (1976) had immediately recognizable pharmacological implications, extended lately even to brain tumor chemotherapy (Panther et al., 1985). Does, however, endogenous adenosine play any significant physiological role in cerebral blood flow autoregulation? Among the arguments favoring such a role are (Winn, 1985): (1) adenosine levels rise in the brain following small decreases in arterial blood pressure within the autoregulatory range or any other conditions which will decrease the supply or increase the consumption of energy by the brain; (2) the speed of this increase (5 sec after aortic transection) is comparable to that of CBF autoregulation; by comparison, changes in pH and other factors are much slower; (3) the released amounts are sufficient to dilate cerebral arteries and arterioles and thus increase CBF (threshold 10^{-8} M); (4) the dilatory effects of adenosine and those in response to hypoxia or hypotension are antagonized by methylxanthines and adenosine deaminase and potentiated by dipyridamole, an adenosine deaminase inhibitor. Applied by themselves, methylxanthines decrease and dipyridamole increases CBF. Adenosine is therefore recognized as a likely candidate chemical factor linking metabolism to CBF within the physiological autoregulatory range (Siesjo, 1984, Winn, 1985).

Nevertheless, there is no clear answer to the question of adenosine involvement in CBF autoregulation. We do not know whether adenosine itself or ATP (Forrester et al., 1979) is the actual endogenous ligand since the threshold for vessel dilation by the latter is much lower (10^{-11} M). Furthermore, we do not know the source of the endogenous vasodilatory purine, nor whether it is released from neurons, glia, or vascular elements. Most importantly, we need to learn the relationship between the vasoactive and the neuronal depressant roles of adenosine; this information should be particularly useful for understanding the role of purines in life-threatening situations. Comparison of experimentally derived thresholds for the respective effects of exogenous adenosine suggests that following a mild hypoxia, CBF regulation will be called into action first to increase the supply of energy while further increases in adenosine levels—if hypoxia persists—will suppress synaptic activity thus reducing the energy demand. However, it is not at all clear whether the two roles of adenosine—vascular and neuronal—are actually acting in concert toward a certain goal as this scheme suggests.

Both in situ and in isolated preparations (see Dunwiddie, 1985; Winn, 1985) adenosine starts to dilate cerebral vessels at physiological concentrations of 10^{-8} M but the respective dose–response curve does not plateau even at 10^{-3} M. This may be an even more important role of adenosine in pathophysiological regulation of CBF when, in emergency situations, adenosine levels may increase a hundred- to a thousandfold (see references in Snyder, 1985). It is entirely possible, however, that different mechanisms underlie the vasodilatory effects at the two ends of the adenosine concentration spectrum. Quantitative studies of adenosine levels at specific synaptic locations correlated with conditions of release and the state of CBF regulation are certainly needed. Finally, the possibility of an interdependence between adenosine effects on CBF and the sympathetic tone of cerebral vessels should be scrutinized.

3.1.3. Does Endogenous Adenosine Mediate Central Autonomic Control?

Adenosine can influence the CNS component of at least four autonomic regulatory systems: cardiovascular, respiratory, thermoregulatory, as well as the center regulating thirst and hunger (see Dunwiddie, 1985; Phillis, this volume). This has been shown by intracerebroventricular injections of adenosine analogues which produce hypotension and bradycardia, a decreased respiratory rate, hypothermia, and suppression of food and water intake.

The pharmacological significance of these central effects of adenosine cannot be over-emphasized. However, it would be important to learn whether they simply reflect the depression of command neurons at the respective vital CNS centers by the administered adenosine analogues, or alternatively whether they reflect a physiological and/or pathophysiological role of endogenous adenosine in regulating the excitability of these centers [e.g., during hypoxia and epilepsy when adenosine levels rise or even during parts of the wake–sleep cycle when the number of adenosine receptors is reportedly changing (Virus *et al.*, 1984)].

3.1.4. Does Adenosine Suppress Endogenous Pain?

An involvement of adenosine in brain mechanisms suppressing pain has been suggested on the grounds (1) of its possible involvement in the mechanism of action of endogenous opioids and (2) of the antinociceptive effects of adenosine analogues. Even before the acceptance of the importance of methylxanthine antagonism of adenosine receptors, caffeine and theophylline were shown to antagonize the analgesic action of morphine and endogenous opioids (see Phillis and Wu, 1981). When it was subsequently demonstrated that morphine increases the levels of extracellular adenosine (Fredholm and Vernet, 1978; Jiang *et al.*, 1980), this was suggested to be part of morphine's mechanism of action. On the other hand, adenosine and its nonmetabolized analogues have significant analgesic effects (Vapaatalo *et al.*, 1975; Yarbrough and McGuffin-Clineschmidt, 1981; Phillis, this volume), and potentiate those of morphine (Ahlijanian and Takemori, 1985) and norepinephrine (Acan *et al.*, 1985). Methylxanthines but not naloxone reverse these effects of adenosine.

One could at least partly explain the interaction between opioids and adenosine by the anxiolytic properties they supposedly share (Marangos and Boulenger, 1985). Even if we accept a role of endogenous adenosine in antinociceptive mechanisms, we would still need to know where this effect is expressed. Antinociceptive effects of adenosine analogues following intrathecal administration (Post, 1984; Hedner *et al.*, 1986) might act at the primary sensory level. Again human experimentation is probably needed to differentiate between true antinociception and alternative explanations of the animal experiments.

3.1.5. Neuronal Plasticity and Memory

The question of adenosine involvement in memory formation is intriguing although it actually rests on relatively little evidence. The demonstrated effects of ATP on operant behavior in rats (Coffin and Carney, 1983) and monkeys (Glowa and Spealman, 1984) and the well-known behavioral effects of caffeine (Rall, 1985) are not proven to be independent of their respective effects on vigilance. Although long-term potentiation is rather attenuated by adenosine (Dolphin, 1983), Kuroda (1983) suggested an involvement of adenosine in posttetanic potentiation and heterosynaptic facilitation, two phenomena presumed to be related to cellular processes of learning and memory. The proposed mechanism is similar to that proposed for other neurotransmitters and modulators which can increase presynaptic cAMP and thereby accumulate Ca^{2+} and facilitate subsequent transmitter release (Klein and Kandel, 1978). One might further speculate that adenosine would be unique among the other molecules because its presence and effects are widespread in the brain (Kostopoulos and Phillis, 1977) and its extracellular concentrations reflect the energy state of the local cell populations, increasing upon intense excitation of neighboring neurons.

3.1.6. Are There Any Brain Diseases Caused by an Inefficiency of the Adenosine System?

The demonstrated involvement of adenosine in central synaptic transmission and the other physiological functions mentioned have prompted speculation about its involvement in pathophysiological states.

a. Epilepsy. Any substance which can influence neuronal activity as potently as adenosine does, is expected to modulate the expression of epilepsy at the neuronal as well as the behavioral level. The strongest argument in favor of adenosine being involved in epilepsy is not its pharmacological effects but the biochemical evidence of its release in the brain at the onset of epileptic seizures.

The first studies on this subject (Maitre *et al.*, 1974) were not actually prompted by the knowledge of the ability of adenosine to depress neurons but from considerations related to a link between energy metabolism and epilepsy. This idea, introduced years ago by the Montreal group (Elliott and Penfield, 1948), led to important observations establishing that the enormous energy consumption during seizures is to some extent compensated by a brief functional hyperemia and increased glucose utilization immediately following seizures (Plum *et al.*, 1968; Meldrum and Nilsson, 1976).

The indirect suggestion from *in vitro* studies (Pull and McIlwain, 1973) that adenosine, a breakdown product of ATP, would increase during seizures, initially led to speculations on an epileptogenic role of adenosine (Walker *et al.*, 1973; Lewin, 1976), a view reinforced by the demonstration of epileptiform waves following epicortical adenosine applications. We also observed that epicortical application of adenosine could enhance some epileptic bursts in the cat (Fig. 2A) and the effect was mimicked by the adenosine uptake blocker papaverine (Fig. 2B). However, the effect (slow negative wave enhancement) is most easily explained by the specific depression of the upper layers of the cortex, and since it is also displayed by other depressant substances such as GABA (Iwama and Jasper, 1957; Gloor *et al.*, 1979), it cannot be attributed to a specific epileptogenic effect of adenosine. It may be relevant to note here that, during hypoglycemia characterized by a progressive increase in the amplitude of slow negative EEG waves, brain adenosine levels dramatically increase (Winn *et al.*, 1983). Because of its sedative actions, however, one cannot rule out the possibility that adenosine is involved in epileptogenesis to the extent that the level of arousal plays a determining role in many types of seizures (Sterman *et al.*, 1982).

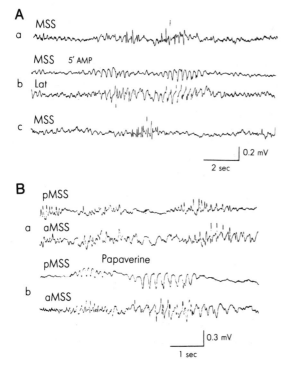

Figure 2. (A) Epicortical EEG from the medial suprasylvian gyrus (MSS) of a cat undergoing generalized epilepsy with spike and wave discharges. In (b) a piece of filter paper soaked in 10 mM 5′-AMP was placed on MSS but not on lateral gyros. The result is an elimination of negative (up-going) spikes and augmentation on negative slow waves. (B) Similar effects are produced by epicortical application of papaverine, an adenosine uptake inhibitor. pMSS and aMSS refer respectively to posterior and anterior MSS, (a) before and (b) after papaverine (10 mM) application. Data from Gloor *et al.* (1979). This effect was interpreted as being due to depression of upper cortical layers and is not consistent with an epileptogenic effect of epicortical adenosine (see text).

The dramatic increase in brain adenosine levels within seconds following the onset of seizures was finally demonstrated in animal models (Winn et al.,1978; Schrader et al., 1980). The two important effects of adenosine (regulation of CBF and neuronal depression) were by then established. Adenosine release during seizures was accordingly explained in teleological terms: adenosine raised CBF levels (1) producing the functional hyperemia necessary for compensating for the increased energy consumption during seizures and preventing cellular damage, and (2) depressing neurons to act as an "endogenous anticonvulsant" (Dragunow et al., 1985).

The pharmacological importance of the antiepileptic effects of adenosine cannot be over-emphasized. Work in the hippocampal slice (Dunwiddie, 1980; Haas and Jefferys, 1984; Lee et al., 1984; Schubert, this volume) shows that adenosine and its analogues can block epileptiform afterdischarges induced by penicillin, biculline, high K^+, or low Ca^{2+} at concentrations slightly lower than those necessary for blocking normal synaptic transmission. Activation of an adenosine receptor (possibly leading in some studies to an enhancement of g_K) is held responsible for this effect. Since slices can only have epileptiform spikes, not epilepsy, it was important to study these effects in vivo. The initial claim of Maitre et al. (1974) was confirmed in at least three more animal seizure models: pentylenetetrazol (Snyder et al., 1981; Dunwiddie and Worth, 1982), electroshock (Burley and Ferendelli, 1984), and amygdala-kindled seizures (Albertson et al., 1983; Barraco et al., 1984; Dragunow et al., 1985) were reduced by adenosine. Both in vitro and in vivo methylxanthines antagonized the antiepileptic effect of adenosine.

The argument was strengthened by two other pharmacological lines of evidence. First, drugs which enhance adenosine levels reduce epileptiform spikes in vitro and convulsions in vivo while adenosine deaminase and adenosine receptor antagonists promote them (see above references). Second, adenosine seems to be implicated in the action of important antiepileptic drugs (see next chapter). All the above electrophysiological evidence, however, hardly goes beyond the obvious ability of endogenous adenosine—a potent depressant—to stop the epileptic process. Does it play such a role? Can epilepsy, at least in part, be explained as a failure of adenosine depression? A controversy raised recently by the kindling experiments may help focus electrophysiological research into this direction. The controversy centers on whether or not exogenous adenosine increases the postkindling afterdischarge threshold in ways other than its suppression of discharge duration and spread (Dragunow et al., 1985). If endogenous adenosine is tonically suppressing neuronal activity and thus partially protecting brain tissue from seizures, an increase in threshold should be demonstrable. Alternatively, adenosine might be brought into play only after the onset of seizures, when it could suppress their duration and spread.

In conclusion, it seems that the right questions with regard to adenosine involvement in epilepsy have not been asked yet. It is unfortunate that Elliott and Penfield's (1948) specimens of human epileptic cortex are not available for analysis by today's biochemical techniques to see whether abnormalities of the adenosine system (receptors, metabolizing enzymes) could actually explain the hyperexcitability of their neurons. Experimental models with an adenosine system deficiency should be developed and studied. Repeated anoxic episodes for example might release enough adenosine to down-regulate its receptors (Lee and Tetzlaff, 1985) and thus lead to hyperexcitability. The perinatal literature certainly suggests a link between anoxia and seizure episodes (Volpe, 1981).

b. Stress and Anxiety Disorders. Indirect pharmacological and experimental pathophysio-logical evidence implicates an ineffectiveness of the central adenosine system in the development of stress-related diseases and anxiety disorders. Caffeine is now recognized as a specific aden-osine antagonist. The first suggestion that it might cause various anxiety disorders was made over a century ago (Legrand du Saulle, 1878) and is substantiated by strong clinical evidence today (see Marangos and Boulenger, 1985). Several anxiolytics including benzodiazepines increase extracellular concentrations of adenosine in the brain, thus facilitating the depressant effect of adenosine (Phillis and Wu, 1982). On the other hand, activation of central adenosine receptors can protect animals from developing stress-induced ulcers in some experimental paradigms

(Geiger and Glavin, 1985; but see Ushijima *et al.*, 1985) while chronic stress (and caffeine) increases central adenosine receptors (Boulenger *et al.*, 1986).

For the moment, however, there are only speculations on the role of endogenous adenosine in brain systems maintaining affective stability. Alternative interpretations of the above studies can be given because changes in arousal function, where adenosine is more likely to be involved, are a part of the CNS reaction to stress and anxiety states (Lader, 1983). It would be interesting in this respect as well as in relation to the analgesic effect of adenosine to design an experiment where rats could press a bar to receive an intracerebroventricular injection of an adenosine analogue or its antagonist.

c. Neurological Syndromes Associated with Deranged Metabolism of Adenosine. Numerous syndromes including "purine seizure disorders" are listed in a recent publication by Coleman *et al.* (1986). In some of them, adenosine levels are changed. It has been hypothesized that low levels of adenosine in the basal ganglia of patients with Lesch–Nyhan (1964) syndrome are due to a genetic deficiency in a purine salvage enzyme, and that this might lead to increased release of catecholamines and cause the involuntary movements which are one of the many neurological manifestations of this syndrome (Stone, 1981).

A substantial decrease in brain adenosine levels is predicted to be caused by a different metabolic error—homocystinemia. McIlwain (1985) proposed that the convulsive episodes and mental changes often observed in homocystinemia are mediated by the release from adenosine depression. Finally, adenosine deaminase deficiency, primarily a disease of the immune system (Seegmiller, 1979), may offer important neurological clues to the role of adenosine in the brain.

3.1.7. Are There Any Important Drug Effects Mediated through Endogenous Adenosine?

The suggestion that the most widely used drug, caffeine, produces central stimulation by removing a tonic inhibition of central neurons caused by endogenous adenosine was first proposed mainly on the basis of microiontophoretic experiments (Phillis and Kostopoulos, 1975). This idea, which found support in behavioral (Snyder *et al.*, 1981) and other experiments, is today rather universally accepted as a more likely mechanism than phosphodiesterase inhibition (Rall, 1985). It was observed some time ago that benzodiazepines block adenosine uptake (Mah and Daly, 1976). This has been verified electrophysiologically (Phillis, 1979), suggesting that benzodiazepines may act partly via such a mechanism. There is, however, still a need to identify other possible adenosine uptake blockers (Phillis, 1985).

The possible interactions of different drugs with purinergic systems have been recently reviewed (Dunwiddie, 1985; Phillis, 1985; Marangos and Boulenger, 1985). An oversimplification would divide most of these drugs into adenosine antagonists with central stimulant properties and adenosine uptake blockers with mostly sedative properties. Research with adenosine antagonists is relatively more advanced. Recently, several methylxanthine analogues have been developed with extremely high potency (Bruns *et al.*, 1983; Daly *et al.*, 1985) and several nonxanthine receptor antagonists have been discovered (Psychoyos *et al.*, 1982; Davies *et al.*, 1983). The discovery of specific antagonists for adenosine receptors in different tissues may be the key to understanding adenosine roles as well as to developing stronger, safer, and more selective antagonists to its actions.

The list of drugs which have been proposed to work at least in part by enhancing central adenosine levels include certain members of the benzodiazepines, the phenothiazines, and some tricyclic antidepressants (diphenylhydantoin and meprobamate) (Phillis and Wu, 1982; Phillis, 1985). Morphine raises adenosine levels but via an enhancement of release rather than from blockade of uptake (Phillis, 1985). Finally, some barbiturates have been shown to decrease binding to adenosine receptors (Lohse *et al.*, 1985) and the effects of ethanol have been linked to adenosine indirectly (Proctor and Dunwiddie, 1984); perhaps explaining why coffee is used as an antidote to alcohol intoxication. The number and importance of drugs which may interfere with adenosine in the brain make this a most exciting and promising field of research.

3.2. What Is the Mechanism of Adenosine Action?

Each fact about adenosine raises several related questions. The answers so far given to some of these questions are inadequate and often contradictory. The mechanism of adenosine action is being readdressed continuously in the context of new findings. Below are some of the issues which must be resolved before we can understand the mechanisms of adenosine action on the brain.

3.2.1. Which Is the Primary Molecule?

Adenosine receptors can be activated by a remarkable variety of endogenous substances besides adenosine. These include ATP, NAD, acetyl-CoA, and AMP and each gives similar electrophysiological results (Phillis *et al.*, 1979a,b; Snell *et al.*, 1985). Furthermore, adenosine levels at rest are probably enough to activate most if not all its receptors (Williams, 1983). Therefore, one may have to look for a molecule that will change this status quo either by antagonizing adenosine at its receptor, like an endogenous xanthine, or by decreasing extracellular levels of adenosine. McIlwain (1985) proposed that l-homocysteine may play such a role in homocysteinemia and it is certainly important to investigate further the actions of this molecule in physiological conditions. If adenosine receptors play a more specific role in signal transmission than simply lowering the level of excitability, then we should perhaps look for a natural adenosine antagonist which is released in temporal relation to synaptic transmission. A candidate receptor for this endogenous antiadenosine molecule may actually be the one proposed to mediate the locomotor stimulant effects of an extremely low dose of adenosine analogues revealed in the presence of subthreshold doses of caffeine (Snyder *et al.*, 1981, Phillis, this volume).

3.2.2. Which Are the Main Physiological Factors Controlling Extracellular Adenosine Levels?

Adenosine is unique in that all of its precursor substances have other important roles, from ATP which may be released as cotransmitter, to *S*-adenosylmethionine, a by-product of methylation processes reportedly linked to synaptic transmission (Hirata and Axelrod, 1980). Hence, adenosine levels may be linked to metabolism as well as to synaptic activity of neighboring neurons. Effects of adenosine on both Ca^{2+} and K^+ current as well as on their possible interactions have been described in different preparations. Which of these potential mechanisms, however, actually play physiologically important mechanisms controlling presynaptic transmitter release and postsynaptic excitability? These questions are addressed and analyzed in depth in other chapters of this book by Fredholm *et al.*, Haas and Greene, and Schubert.

3.2.3. Correlating Specific Adenosine Receptors to Specific Effects

Adenosine receptor subtypes (for review see Daly, 1983) have not been properly identified yet. The terms A1, A2, and P reflect only adenosine effects on adenyl cyclase (van Calker *et al.*, 1979; Londos *et al.*, 1980) among its many other different actions. Until it can be confirmed, probably by using selective antagonists, these three classes of receptors should be regarded only as a working hypothesis (Stone, 1985, Chapter 1). On the basis of studies of potency ratios, the adenosine receptor subtypes have been assigned tentative roles to explain some of the effects of peripherally or centrally administered adenosine. Since in most paradigms peripheral administration suggests the involvement of A1 receptors (L-PIA better than NECA) while in most experiments with intracerebroventricular injections the opposite is true, the suspicion is created that the experiments may have been influenced by technical factors such as the recently demonstrated difficulty of NECA to pass the blood–brain barrier (Bickford et al., 1985) and the different solubility properties of PIA and NECA (Dunwiddie, 1985).

3.2.4. What Is the Threshold Concentration for Each of the Demonstrated Effects of Adenosine?

Because adenosine levels may increase in response to a variety of stimuli and over a wide range, different properties of adenosine may be brought into action only at an appropriate concentration level. Knowing this level is necessary for any correlation between causes of adenosine release and the resulting action as well as for understanding the limits between physiological synaptic and/or vascular roles of adenosine and the respective pathophysiological ones. Helpful in this respect will be studies using drugs known to elevate levels of endogenous adenosine. Questions related to mechanisms of action may be resolved by functional studies at the cellular level in vivo now that some pathways selectively carrying adenosine receptors (see below) are being identified.

3.3. Possible Sites of Adenosine Actions

The lack of evidence for storage in vesicles and release from specific pathways in the brain contributes substantially to the belief that adenosine may not be a neurotransmitter or a neuromodulator in specific pathways but rather a ubiquitous regulatory substance maintaining an inhibitory tone on neurons. However, some recent evidence based on the presence of its receptors rather than on the release of adenosine from specific terminals suggests a differential distribution of adenosine in the brain. The question of whether adenosine is employed in signal transmission or modification in some pathways and not in others is obviously important for any attempt to understand its many different roles.

3.3.1. Regional Localization

The arguments for a rather ubiquitous role of adenosine in the brain come from biochemical and electrophysiological data. Regional differences in the ability of brain tissue to release adenosine are relatively small and differences in existing adenosine levels even smaller (Wojcik and Neff, 1982). The demonstrated link between metabolism and adenosine release (Barberis et al., 1985) probably explains these findings and strengthens the argument. In a comparative microiontophoretic study (Kostopoulos and Phillis, 1977), adenosine depression was demonstrated in every region of the brain studied. In vitro experiments (see references in Dunwiddie, 1985) also failed to find dramatic differences in the depressant effect of adenosine on evoked or spontaneous activity in different brain regions. Quite exceptionally in superior collicular slices, even high doses of adenosine (1 mM) failed to affect the postsynaptic response to optic tract stimulation (Okada and Saito, 1979). However, we have been able to show a depression of collicular neuron responses to photic stimulation in vivo (Fig. 3; data from Kostopoulos and Phillis, unpublished) by the microiontophoretic application of rather moderate doses of AMP. This is consistent with the observation that in situ adenosine may affect neuronal excitability indirectly by influencing the cells delivering at least some of the many different inputs. In this respect it is very interesting that in the cerebellum, superfused adenosine affected only the response to parallel fiber volleys and not that to climbing fiber volleys (Kocsis et al., 1984). This indicates that the climbing fiber terminals and the apical dendrites of Purkinje cells have relatively few adenosine receptors. However, postsynaptic receptors on Purkinje cell somata should probably exist too, as microion-

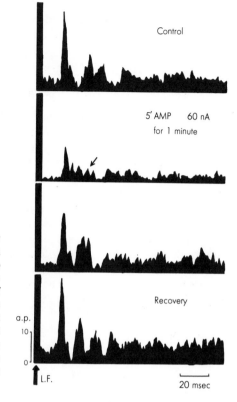

Figure 3. Poststimulus histograms (PSH) of extracellularly recorded activity of a superior colliculus neuron to light flash (L.F.) stimulation in anesthetized rat. The four PSH from top to bottom are taken successively every 1 min. 5′-AMP micro-iontophoresed with indicated dose during the entire period of the second PSH decreased both the background activity of the neuron and that evoked by light stimulation. Most readily, it apparently depressed a secondary excitatory effect (marked by arrow). Third and fourth PSH show partial and complete recovery. Sixty repetitions in each PSH. Similar effects were observed in all (five) neurons tested with light flash in this area.

tophoresis of adenosine close to the somata can depress nearly all spontaneous and glutamate-evoked activity (Kostopoulos *et al.*, 1975).

Experiments to localize pathways where adenosine is preferentially released or selectively effective have used several other techniques in addition to the above-mentioned ones. These include methods to localize adenosine-producing enzymes, adenosine deaminase-like immunoreactivity, adenosine uptake, and adenosine-sensitive adenyl cyclase. (1) While results on regional localization of 5′-nucleotidase are rather controversial (see Schubert *et al.*, 1979; Nagata *et al.*, 1984), the localization of the probably more important *S*-adenosyl homocysteine hydrolase has not been studied. (2) Adenosine deaminase-like immunoreactivity (Nagy *et al.*, 1984) produces a limited number of stained cells, mainly neurons in the basal hypothalamus projecting to various but not all brain regions. (3) Adenosine uptake sites labeled with [³H]nitroben-zylthioinosine (Nagy *et al.*, 1985; Bisserbe *et al.*, 1985; Davies and Hambley, 1986) overlap brain areas rich in adenosine deaminase (Nagy *et al.*, 1985); however, there is a poor correlation between adenosine uptake sites and areas rich in adenosine receptors (Marangos and Boulenger, 1985). (4) Regional localization of adenosine receptors and adenosine-sensitive adenyl cyclase (see Snyder, 1985; Reddington *et al.*, 1985; Marangos and Boulenger, 1985). The development of autoradiographic labeling techniques led to the first definite support for regional heterogeneity in brain adenosine systems. The molecular layer of cerebellar cortex and specific layers in the hippocampus and superior colliculus are particularly rich in adenosine receptors while other areas such as the hypothalamus appear virtually devoid of them (Lewis *et al.*, 1981; Goodman and Snyder, 1982). Furthermore, experimental lesions and the study of certain mouse mutants show that a large number of adenosine receptors are located on excitatory terminals; in the case of the parallel fibers in the cerebellum, the labeled terminals are believed to be glutamatergic (Goodman *et al.*, 1983; Wojcik and Neff, 1983b; Kocsis *et al.*, 1984). Corticothalamic and corticostriate axons are, however, not labeled. More recent autoradiographic experiments (Reddington *et al.*, 1985; Lee and Reddington, 1986) actually demonstrate differential localization of A1 and A2 receptors.

3.3.2. Cellular Localization of Adenosine

Indirect evidence of Wojcik and Neff (1983a) suggests that adenosine is released primarily from neurons rather than glial cells. The number of neurons releasing adenosine, however, appears to be much larger than the number of neurons stained for adenosine deaminase (Nagy *et al.*, 1984). The latter cells also stain for histidine decarboxylase and glutamate decarboxylase (Senba *et al.*, 1985). We really do not know if adenosine is released from any specific group of neurons. On the contrary, certain neurons which do not release adenosine may have adenosine receptors on their terminals, as do granule cells in the cerebellum (Goodman *et al.*, 1983; Wojcik and Neff, 1983b; Kocsis *et al.*, 1984). It appears from indirect evidence that adenosine receptors exist on noradrenergic terminals, since adenosine blocks noradrenaline release in the CNS (Fredholm and Hedquist, 1980). However, Murray and Cheney (1982) found no changes in hippocampal adenosine receptors following lesion of noradrenergic afferents to the hippocampus. The restriction to neurons may not be complete since adenosine may also affect glial cells (Bourke *et al.*, 1983) and cerebral vessels (see Section 3.1.2). These two effects, however, may come from a different pool.

3.3.3. Subcellular Localization

Using electron microscopy, adenosine-synthesizing enzymes (Kreutzberg and Hussain, 1984; Nagata *et al.*, 1984) have been localized in some synaptic regions. Adenosine release is more likely to take place from neuronal somata than from terminals (Wojcik and Neff, 1983a). Adenosine receptors are seen in both synaptic complexes and extrasynaptic sites (Tetzlaff *et al.*, 1987) while in hippocampal slices both microiontophoretic and autoradiographic experiments (see Reddington *et al.*, 1985) localize the receptors on the proximal part of apical dendrites of pyramidal cells. Finally, adenosine receptors appear to exist both on the outside of the neuronal membrane (A1 and A2) as well as on the inside (P receptors) (see Daly, 1983). In conclusion, it appears unlikely that a specific group of neurons exist which exclusively release adenosine. However, differential sensitivities and different effects may be achieved because of the heterogeneous localization of adenosine receptors.

3.4. When Does Adenosine Act?

Several questions have arisen which make a direct or indirect reference to the time dimension of adenosine effects; they deserve much more attention than they are currently receiving. There is no evidence to suggest that endogenous adenosine has any of the effects of either a fast or slow neurotransmitter as defined by Bloom (1984). Therefore, we are forced to the conclusion that adenosine may not be a transmitter. However, even as a neuromodulator (if adenosine is modulating the efficacy of single synaptic events following pre- or postsynaptic release), an action in the range of milliseconds should be demonstrable. Alternatively, the synaptic role of adenosine may be limited to a tonic inhibitory tone which slowly varies in response to metabolism-related changes in extracellular levels of adenosine over a time course of seconds.

On a longer time scale, we also know very little about the possible changes in the membrane response to adenosine after prolonged over- or underexposure to adenosine. It would be useful to know whether neurons and/or vessels grow tolerant after a prolonged hypoxia-induced rise in adenosine concentration. Of no less importance would be an understanding of the neuronal mechanisms underlying tolerance to caffeine. Evidence on down-regulation of adenosine receptors following exposure to adenosine analogues as well as up-regulation after chronic caffeine treatment (Marangos *et al.*, 1984; Porter *et al.*, 1985) has appeared. Circadian variations in the number of adenosine receptors have been described (Virus *et al.*, 1984). What is their importance in our daily-clock-related functions such as sleep and waking?

Turning to developmental issues, Marangos *et al.* (1982) and Geiger *et al.* (1984) have described the ontogenesis of adenosine receptors. It is a challenge to physiologists to correlate the time of development of adenosine receptors in different brain regions to the time of appearance of the several functional roles assigned to adenosine in the brain (see Section 3.1). Any information on the fate of adenosine receptors at the other end of the ontogenetic scale would be important for the pathophysiology of age-related brain disease.

4. Summary and Conclusion

A thematic listing of current questions on the role of endogenous adenosine in the brain has been presented after providing a historical framework of their development. Biochemical, electrophysiological, and behavioral experiments conducted in the early 1970s established that endogenous adenosine had a powerful influence on central synaptic transmission. However, the criteria identifying adenosine as a transmitter in specific pathways were not produced. Rather, strong evidence evolved for a presynaptic depressant action and therefore for a neuromodulatory role. Independently, evidence accumulated suggesting that adenosine is the metabolic link for CBF autoregulation. In the following years, interest in adenosine and appreciation of its role in the brain grew in parallel to conceptual developments which led to a broadening of the paradigm of synaptic transmission. One of the more important roles for endogenous adenosine may be related to its involvement in controlling arousal mechanisms. Less well established is adenosine's involvement in central autonomic and pain control, in the pathophysiology of several diseases, including epilepsy, and in the mechanism of action of several drugs of major clinical importance. Among the numerous questions related to the mechanisms of action of endogenous adenosine, understanding the conditions of its release and the locus and the temporal characteristic of its action are judged necessary for assigning to adenosine a particular role in synaptic transmission. The possible existence of an excitatory endogenous ligand to adenosine receptors is an important issue to resolve. Unique among other neuroactive substances, adenosine is released in response to energy shortages of brain cells resulting from reduced supply or increased neuronal activity. This provides a negative feedback action having an important role in pathological processes.

Understanding the role of endogenous adenosine in brain function may require further modification of the present conceptual paradigm of synaptic transmission. One useful modification may be to include the concept of *synaptic homeostasis* as an important function and to recognize that some neuroactive molecules may play a homeostatic role rather than a role in the transmission of specific signals. Adenosine may be part of such a synaptic homeostasis system controlling the level of excitability. In selective pathways with a high concentration of adenosine receptors, this may help a synaptic signal enjoy an appropriately set signal-to-noise ratio. In emergency situations, however, when the level of adenosine rises so as to influence most neurons, adenosine's depressive effects may have a protective role (from overexcitability in general to Ca^{2+} entry in particular). It would be important to understand the limits between a physiological modulatory and a pathophysiological protective role as well as the extent to which they might be connected to the CBF regulating role and possibly other actions of adenosine toward an integrated regulation of the brain's activity.

ACKNOWLEDGMENTS. At the time of this presentation, the author was a recipient of a grant from the Greek Ministry of Research and Technology. The skillful secretarial assistance of Miss G. Robillard is gratefully acknowledged.

References

Acan, S., Porter, N. M., and Proudfit, H. K., 1985, Potentiation of the antinociceptive effect of norepinephrine by the adenosine analog, 5'-N-ethylcarboxamide adenosine, *Soc. Neurosci. Abstr.* **41:**6.

Ahlijanian, M. K., and Takemori, A. E., 1985, Effects of (−)-N⁶-(R-phenyl-isopropyl)-adenosine (PIA) and caffeine on nociception and morphine-induced analgesia, tolerance and dependence in mice, *Eur. J. Pharmacol.* **112:**171–179.

Albertson, T. E., Stark, L. G., Joy, R. M., and Bowyer, J. F., 1983, Aminophylline and kindled seizures, *Exp. Neurol.* **81:**703–713.

Barberis, C., Leviel, V., and Daval, J. L., 1985, Metabolism and release of purines from nervous tissue, in: *Purines, Pharmacology and Physiological Roles* (T. W. Stone, ed.), Macmillan Co., New York, pp. 107–114.

Barraco, R. A., Swanson, T. H., Phillis, J. W., and Berman, R. F., 1984, Anticonvulsant effects of adenosine analogs on amygdaloid-kindled seizures in rats, *Neurosci. Lett.* **46:**317–322.

Bender, A. S., Wu, P. H., and Phillis, J. W., 1981, The rapid uptake and release of [³H] adenosine by rat cerebral cortical synaptosomes, *J. Neurochem.* **36:**651–660.

Berne, R. M., Rubio, R., and Curnish, R. R., 1974, Release of adenosine from ischemic brain: Effect on cerebral vascular resistance and incorporation into cerebral adenine nucleotides, *Circ. Res.* **35:**262–271.

Berne, R. M., Rall, T. W., and Rubio, R., 1983, *Regulatory Function of Adenosine,* Nijhoff, The Hague.

Bickford, P. C., Fredholm, B. B., Dunwiddie, T. V., and Freedman, R., 1985, Inhibition of Purkinje cell firing by systemic administration of phenylisopropyl adenosine: Effect of central noradrenaline depletion by DSP4, *Life Sci.* **37:**289–297.

Bisserbe, J. C., Patel, J., and Marangos, P. J., 1985, Autoradiographic localization of adenosine uptake sites in rat brain using [³H]nitrobenzylthioinosine, *J. Neurosci.* **5:**544–550.

Bloom, F. E., 1975, The role of cyclic nucleotides in central synaptic function, in: *Reviews of Physiology, Biochemistry and Pharmacology,* Vol. 74, (R. H. Adrian, E. Helmzeich, H. Holzec *et al.,* eds.) Springer-Verlag, Berlin, pp. 1–103.

Bloom, F. E., 1984, The functional significance of neurotransmitter diversity, *Am. J. Physiol.* C184–C194.

Boulenger, J. P., Marangos, P. J., Zander, K. J., and Hanson, J., 1986, Stress and caffeine: Effects on central adenosine receptors, *Clin. Neuropharmacol.* **9:**79–83.

Bourke, R. S., Kimelberg, H. K., Dazé, M. A., and Church, G., 1983, Swelling and ion uptake in cat cerebrocortical slices: Control by neurotransmitters and ion transport mechanisms, *Neurochem. Res.* **8:**5–24.

Bruns, R. F., Daly, J. W., and Snyder, S. H., 1983, Adenosine receptor binding: Structure–activity analysis generates extremely potent xanthine antagonists, *Proc. Natl. Acad. Sci. USA* **80:**2077–2080.

Buday, P. V., Carr, C. J., and Miya, T. S., 1961, A pharmacologic study of some nucleosides and nucleotides, *J. Pharm. Pharmacol.* **13:**290–299.

Burley, E. S., and Ferendelli, J. A., 1984, Regulatory effects of neurotransmitters on electroshock and pentylenetetrazol seizures, *Fed. Proc.* **43:**2521–2524.

Burnstock, G., 1986, The changing face of autonomic neurotransmission, *Acta Physiol. Scand.* **126:**67–91.

Burnstock, G., Campbell, G., Bennett, M., and Holman, M. E., 1963, Inhibition of the smooth muscle of the taenia coli, *Nature* **200:**581–582.

Coffin, V. L., and Carney, J. M., 1983, Behavioral pharmacology of adenosine analogs, in: *Physiology and Pharmacology of Adenosine Derivatives* (J. W. Daly, Y. Kuroda, J. W. Phillis, H. Shimizu, and M. Ui, eds.), Raven Press, New York, pp. 267–274.

Coffin, V. L., Taylor, J. A., Phillis, J. W., Altman, H. J., and Barraco, R. A., 1984, Behavioral interaction of adenosine and methylxanthines in central purinergic systems, *Neurosci. Lett.* **47:**91–98.

Coleman, M., Langrebe, M., and Landgrebe, A., 1986, Purine seizure disorders, *Epilepsia* **27:**263–269.

Cuello, A. C. (ed.), 1982, *Co-transmission,* Macmillan & Co., London.

Daly, J. W., 1983, Role of ATP and adenosine receptors in physiologic processes: Summary and prospective, in: *Physiology and Pharmacology of Adenosine Derivatives* (J. W. Daly, Y. Kuroda, J. W. Phillis, H. Shimizu, and M. Ui, eds.), Raven Press, New York, pp. 275–290.

Daly, J. W., Kuroda, Y., Phillis, J. W., Shimizu, H., and Ui, M. (eds.), 1983, *Physiology and Pharmacology of Adenosine Derivatives,* Raven Press, New York.

Daly, J. W., Padgett, W., Shamin, M. T., Butts-Lamb, P., and Waters, J., 1985, 1,3-Dialkyl-8-(p-sulfophenyl) xanthines: Potent water-soluble antagonists for A₁- and A₂-adenosine receptors, *J. Med. Chem.* **28:**487–492.

Davies, L. P., and Hambley, J. W., 1986, Regional distribution of adenosine uptake in guinea-pig brain slices and the effect of some inhibition: Evidence for nitrobenzylthioinosine-sensitive and insensitive sites? *Neurochem. Int.* **8:**103–108.

Davies, L. P., Brown, D. J., Chen Chow, S., and Johnston, G. A. R., 1983, Pyrazolo [3,4-d] pyrimidines, a new class of adenosine antagonists, *Neurosci. Lett.* **41:**189–193.

Dolphin, A. C., 1983, The adenosine agonist 2-chloroadenosine inhibits the induction of long term potentiation of the perforant path, *Neurosci. Lett.* **39:** 83–89.

Dragunow, M., Goddard, G. V., and Laverty, R., 1985, Is adenosine an endogenous anticonvulsant? *Epilepsia* **26:**480–487.

Drury, A. N., and Szent-Györgyi, A., 1929, The physiological activity of adenine compounds with especial reference to their action upon the mammalian heart, *J. Physiol. (London)* **68:**213–237.

Dunwiddie, T. V., 1980, Endogenously released adenosine regulates excitability in the in vitro hippocampus, *Epilepsia* **21:**541–548.

Dunwiddie, T. V., 1985, The physiological role of adenosine in the central nervous system, *Int. Rev. Neurobiol.* **27:**63–139.

Dunwiddie, T. V., and Worth, T., 1982, Sedative and anticonvulsant effects of adenosine analogs in mouse and rat, *J. Pharmacol. Exp. Ther.* **220:**70–76.

Edstrom, J. P., and Phillis, J. W., 1976, The effects of AMP on the potential of rat cerebral cortical neurons, *Can. J. Physiol. Pharmacol.* **54:**787–790.

Elliott, K. A. C., and Penfield, W., 1948, Respiration of glycolysis of focal epileptogenic human brain tissue, *J. Neurophysiol.* **11:**485–490.

Feldberg, W., and Sherwood, S. L., 1954, Injections of drugs into the lateral ventricle of the cat, *J. Physiol. (London)* **123:**148–167.

Forrester, T., Harper, A. M., MacKenzie, E. T., and Thompson, E. M., 1979, Effect of adenosine triphosphate and some derivatives on cerebral blood flow and metabolism, *J. Physiol. (London)* **296:**343–355.

Fredholm, B. B., and Hedquist, P., 1980, Modulation of neurotransmission by purine nucleotides and nucleosides, *Biochem. Pharmacol.* **29:**1635–1643.

Fredholm, B. B., and Vernet, L., 1978, Morphine increases depolarization induced purine release from hypothalamic synaptosomes, *Acta Physiol. Scand.* **104:**502–504.

Geiger, J. D., and Glavin, G. B., 1985, Adenosine receptor activation in brain reduces stress-induced ulcer formation, *Eur. J. Pharmacol.* **115:**185–190.

Geiger, J. D., Labella, F. S., and Nagy, J. J., 1984, Ontogenesis of adenosine receptors in the central nervous system of the rat, *Dev. Brain Res.* **13:**97–104.

Ginsborg, B. L., and Hirst, G. D. S., 1972, The effect of adenosine on the release of the transmitter from the phrenic nerve of the rat, *J. Physiol. (London)* **224:**629–645.

Gloor, P., Pellegrini, A., and Kostopoulos, G., 1979, Effects of changes in cortical excitability upon the epileptic bursts in generalized penicillin epilepsy of the cat, *Electroencephalogr. Clin. Neurophysiol.* **46:**274–289.

Glowa, G. R., and Spealman, R. D., 1984, Behavioral effect of caffeine, N^6-(L-phenyl-isopropyl) adenosine and their combination in the squirrel monkey, *J. Pharmacol. Exp. Ther.* **231:**665–670.

Goodman, R. R., and Snyder, S. H., 1982, Autoradiographic localization of adenosine receptors in rat brain using [^{3}H] cyclohexyladenosine, *J. Neurosci.* **2:**1230–1241.

Goodman, R. R., Kuhar, M. J., Hester, L., and Snyder, S. H., 1983, Adenosine receptors: Autoradiographic evidence for their location on axon termials of excitatory neurons, *Science* **220:**967–969.

Greene, R. W., Haas, H. L., and Hermann, A., 1985, Effects of caffeine on hippocampal pyramidal cells in vitro, *Br. J. Pharmacol.* **85:**163–169.

Haas, H. L., and Jefferys, J. G. R., 1984, Low-calcium field burst discharges of CA_1 pyramidal neurons in rat hippocampal slices, *J. Physiol. (London)* **354:**185–201.

Haulica, I., Ababei, L., Branisteanu, D., and Topoliceanu, F., 1973, Preliminary data on the possible hypnogenic role of adenosine, *J. Neurochem.* **21:**1019–1020.

Hedner, T., Fredholm, B. B., Hedner, J., Holmgren, M., Nordberg, G., and Sollevi, A., 1986, Intrathecally administered 2-dichloroadenosine produces spinal analgesia in the rat, *Pfluegers Arch.* **407:**543.

Hirata, F., and Axelrod, J., 1980, Phospholipid methylation and biological signal transmission, *Science* **209:**1082–1090.

Holton, F. A., and Holton, P., 1954, The capillary dilator substances in dry powders of spinal roots; a possible role of adenosine triphosphate in chemical transmission from nerve endings, *J. Physiol. (London)* **126:**124–140.

Holton, P., 1959, The liberation of adenosine triphosphate on antidromic stimulation of sensory nerves, *J. Physiol. (London)* **145:**494–504.

Iwama, K., and Jasper, H. H., 1957, The action of gamma aminobutyric acid upon cortical electrical activity in the cat, *J. Physiol. (London)* **138:**365–380.

Jasper, H. H., 1949, Diffuse projection systems: The integrative action of the thalamic reticular system, *Electroencephalogr. Clin. Neurophysiol.* **1:**405–420.

Jiang, Z. G., Chelack, B. J., and Phillis, J. W., 1980, Effects of morphine and caffeine on adenosine release from rat cerebral cortex: Is caffeine a morphine antagonist? *Can. J. Physiol. Pharmacol.* **58:**1513–1515.

Katims, J. J., Annau, J., and Snyder, S. H., 1983, Interactions in the behavioral effects of methylxanthines and adenosine derivatives, *J. Pharmacol. Exp. Ther.* **227:**167–173.

Klein, M., and Kandel, E. R., 1978, Presynaptic modulation of voltage-dependent Ca^{++} current: Mechanism for behavioral sensitization in *Aplysia californica, Proc. Natl. Acad. Sci. USA* **75:**3512–3516.

Kocsis, J. D., Eng. D. L., and Bhisitkul, R. B., 1984, Adenosine selectively blocks parallel-fiber-mediated synaptic potentials in rat cerebellar cortex, *Proc. Natl. Acad. Sci. USA* **81:**6531–6534.

Kosterlitz, H. W. (ed.), 1976, *Opiates and Endogenous Opioid Peptides,* North-Holland, Amsterdam.

Kostopoulos, G. K., and Phillis, J. W., 1977, Purinergic depression of neurons in different areas of the rat brain, *Exp. Neurol.* **55:**719–724.

Kostopoulos, G. K., Limacher, J. J., and Phillis, J. W., 1975, Action of various adenine derivatives on cerebellar Purkinje cells, *Brain Res.* **88:**162–165.

Kreutzberg, G. W., and Hussain, S. T., 1984, Cytochemical localization of 5′-nucleotidase activity, *Neuroscience* **11:**857–866.

Krnjević, K., 1974, Chemical nature of synaptic transmission in vertebrates, *Physiol. Rev.* **54:**418–540.

Kuhn, T. S., 1970, *The Structure of Scientific Revolutions,* 2nd ed., University of Chicago Press, Chicago.

Kuroda, Y., 1983, Neuronal plasticity and adenosine derivatives in mammalian brain, in: *Physiology and Pharmacology of Adenosine Derivatives* (J. W. Daly, Y. Kuroda, J. W. Phillis, H. Shimizu, and M. Ui, eds.), Raven Press, New York, pp. 245–256.

Kuroda, Y., and McIlwain, H., 1973, Subcellular localization of [^{14}C] adenine derivatives newly formed in cerebral tissues and the effects of electrical excitation, *J. Neurochem.* **21:**889–900.

Lader, M., 1983, Biological differentiation of anxiety, arousal and stress, in: *The Biology of Anxiety* (R. J. Mathew, ed.), Brunner/Mazel, New York, pp. 11–22.

Lee, K. S., and Reddington, M., 1986, 1,3-Dipropyl-8-cyclopentylxanthine (DPCPX) inhibition of [^{3}H] N-ethylcarboxamidoadenosine (NECA) binding allows the visualization of putative non-A$_1$ adenosine receptors, *Brain Res.* **368:**394–398.

Lee, K. S., and Tetzlaff, W., 1985, Rapid down regulation of hippocampal adenosine receptors following brief anoxia, *Soc. Neurosci. Abstr.* **15:**19.

Lee, K. S., Schubert, P., and Heineman, U., 1984, The anticonvulsive action of adenosine: A postsynaptic dendritic action by a possible endogenous anticonvulsant, *Brain Res.* **321:**160–164.

Legrand du Saulle, H., 1878, *Étude Clinique sur la Peur des Espaces (Agoraphobie des Allemands) Nevrose émotive,* Delahaye, Paris.

Lekic, D., 1977, Presynaptic depression of synaptic response of Renshaw cells by adenosine 5′monophosphate, *Can. J. Physiol. Pharmacol.* **55:**1391–1393.

Lesch, M., and Nyhan, W. L., 1964, A familial disorder of uric acid metabolism and CNS functions, *Am. J. Med.* **36:**561–570.

Lewin, E., 1976, Endogenously released adenine derivatives: A possible role in epileptogenesis, *Arch. Neurol.* **23:**393.

Lewis, E., Patel, J., Moon Edley, S., and Marangos, P. J., 1981, Autoradiographic visualization of rat brain adenosine receptors using N^6 cyclohexyl [^{3}H] adenosine, *Eur. J. Pharmacol.* **73:**109–110.

Lohse, M. S., Klotz, K. N., Jakobs, K. H., and Schwabe, U., 1985, Barbiturates are selective antagonists at A$_1$ adenosine receptors, *J. Neurochem.* **45:**1761–1770.

Londos, C., Cooper, D. M. F., and Wolff, J., 1980, Subclasses of external adenosine receptors, *Proc. Natl. Acad. Sci. USA* **77:**2551–2554.

McIlwain, H., 1985, The endogenously formed adenosine of the brain: Its status as a regulatory signal appraised in relation to actions of homocysteine, in: *Purines, Pharmacology and Physiological Roles* (T. W. Stone, ed.), Macmillan Co., New York, pp. 215–221.

Mah, H. D., and Daly, J. W., 1976, Adenosine-dependent formation of cyclic AMP in brain slices, *Pharmacol. Res. Commun.* **8:**65–79.

Maitre, M., Ciesielski, Z., Lehmann, A., Kempf, E., and Mandel, P., 1974, Protective effect of adenosine and nicotinamide against audiogenic seizure, *Biochem. Pharmacol.* **23:**2807–2816.

Major, P. P., Agarwal, R. P., and Kufe, D. W., 1981, Deoxycoformycin: Neurological toxicity, *Cancer Chemother. Pharmacol.* **5:**193–196.

Mandel, P., 1971, Free nucleotides, in: *Handbook of Neurochemistry,* Vol. 5 (A. Lajtha, ed.), Plenum Press, New York, pp. 249–282.

Marangos, P. J., and Boulenger, J. P., 1985, Basic and clinical aspects of adenosinergic neuromodulation, *Neurosci. Biobehav. Rev.* **9:**421–430.

Marangos, P. J., Patel, J., and Stivers, J., 1982, Ontogeny of adenosine binding sites in rat forebrain and cerebellum, *J. Neurochem.* **39:**267–270.

Marangos, P. J., Boulenger, J. P., and Patel, J., 1984, Effects of chronic caffeine on brain adenosine receptors: Anatomical and autogenic studies, *Life Sci.* **34:**899–907.

Marley, E., and Nistico, G., 1972, Effects of catecholamines and adenosine derivatives given into the brain of fowls, *Br. J. Pharmacol.* **36**:619–636.

Meldrum, B. S., and Nilsson, B., 1976, Cerebral blood flow and metabolic rate early and late in prolonged epileptic seizures induced in rat by bicuculline, *Brain* **99**:523–542.

Murray, T. F., and Cheney, D. L., 1982, Neuronal location of N^6-cyclohexyl [^{3}H] adenosine binding sites in rat and guinea-pig brain, *Neuropharmacology* **21**:575–580.

Nagata, H., Mimori, Y., Nakamura, S., and Kameyama, M., 1984, Regional and subcellular distribution in mammalian brain of enzymes producing adenosine, *J. Neurochem.* **42**:1001–1007.

Nagy, J. I., Labella, L. A., and Buss, M., 1984, Immunohistochemistry of adenosine deaminase: Implications for adenosine neurotransmission, *Science* **224**:166–168.

Nagy, J. I., Geiger, J. D., and Daddova, P. E., 1985, Adenosine uptake sites in rat brain: Identification using [^{3}H] nitrobenzylthioinosine and co-localization, *Neurosci. Lett.* **55**:47–53.

Okada, Y., and Saito, M., 1979, Inhibitory action of adenosine, 5-HT (serotonin) and GABA (γ-aminobutyric acid) on the postsynaptic potential (PSP) of slices from olfactory cortex and superior colliculus in correlation to the level of cyclic AMP, *Brain Res.* **160**:368–371.

Panther, L. A., Baumbach, G. L., Bigner, D. D., Piegors, D., Groothuis, D. R., and Heistad, D. D., 1985, Vasoactive drugs produce selective changes in flow to experimental brain tumors, *Ann. Neurol.* **18**:712–715.

Penfield, W. G., and Jasper, H. H. (eds.), 1954, *Epilepsy and the Functional Anatomy of the Human Brain*, Little, Brown, Boston.

Phillis, J. W., 1970, *The Pharmacology of Synapses*, Pergamon Press, Elmsford, N.Y.

Phillis, J. W., 1977, The role of cyclic nucleotides in the CNS, *Can. J. Neurol. Sci.* **4**:151–195.

Phillis, J. W., 1979, Diazepam potentiation of purinergic depression on central neurons, *Can. J. Physiol. Pharmacol.* **57**:432–435.

Phillis, J. W., 1985, The pharmacology of purines in the CNS: Interaction with psychoactive agents, in: *Purines, Pharmacology and Physiological Roles* (T. W. Stone, ed.), Macmillan Co., New York, pp. 45–55.

Phillis, J. W., and Kostopoulos, G. K., 1975, Adenosine as a putative transmitter in the cerebral cortex: Studies with potentiation and antagonists, *Life Sci.* **17**:1085–1094.

Phillis, J. W., and Wu, P. H., 1981, The role of adenosine and its nucleotides in central synaptic transmission, *Prog. Neurobiol.* **16**:187–239.

Phillis, J. W., and Wu, P. H., 1982, The effect of various centrally active drugs on adenosine uptake by the central nervous system, *Comp. Biochem. Physiol.* **72C**:179–187.

Phillis, J. W., Kostopoulos, G. K., and Limacher, J. J., 1974, Depression of corticospinal cells by various purines and pyrimidines, *Can. J. Physiol. Pharmacol.* **52**:1226–1229.

Phillis, J. W., Edstrom, J. P., Kostopoulos, G. K., and Kirkpatrick, J. R., 1979a, Effects of adenosine and adenine nucleotides on synaptic transmission in the cerebral cortex, *Can. J. Physiol. Pharmacol.* **57**:1289–1312.

Phillis, J. W., Kostopoulos, G. K., Edstrom, J. P., and Ellis, S. W., 1979b, Role of adenosine and adenine nucleotides in central nervous function, in: *Physiological and Regulatory Functions of Adenosine and Adenine Nucleotides* (H. P. Baer and G. T. Drummond, eds.), Raven Press, New York, pp. 343–359.

Phillis, J. W., Barraco, R. A., Delong, R. E., and Washington, D. O., 1986, Behavioral characteristics of centrally administered adenosine analogs, *Pharmacol. Biochem. Behav.* **24**:261–270.

Plum, F., Posner, J. B., and Troy, B., 1968, Cerebral metabolic and circulatory responses to induced convulsions in animals, *Arch. Neurol.* **18**:1–13.

Porter, N. M., Clark, F. M., Green, R. D., and Radulovacki, M., 1985, Effects of chronic intracerebroventricular infusion of adenosine agonists and deoxyformycin on brain adenosine and receptors and sleep in the rat, *Soc. Neurosci. Abstr.* **11**:576.

Post, C., 1984, Antinociceptive effects in mice after intrathecal injection of 5'-N-ethylcarboxamide adenosine, *Neurosci. Lett.* **51**:325–330.

Proctor, W. R., and Dunwiddie, T. V., 1984, Behavioral sensitivity to purinergic drugs parallels ethanol sensitivity in selectively bred mice, *Science* **224**:519–521.

Psychoyos, S., Ford, C. J., and Phillips, M. A., 1982, Inhibition by etazolate (SQ20009) and cartazolate (SQ65396) of adenosine-stimulated [^{3}H] cAMP formation in [2-^{3}H] adenosine prelabeled vesicles prepared from guinea pig cerebral cortex, *Biochem. Pharmacol.* **31**:1441–1442.

Pull, I., and McIlwain, H., 1973, Output of [^{14}C] adenine nucleotides and their derivatives from cerebral tissues, *Biochem. J.* **136**:893–901.

Radulovacki, M., Virus, R. M., Djuricic-Nedelson, M., and Green, R. D., 1984, Adenosine analogs and sleep in rats, *J. Pharmacol. Exp. Ther.* **228**:268–274.

Rall, T. W., 1985, Central nervous system stimulants: The methylxanthines, in: *The Pharmacological Basis of Therapeutics*, 7th ed. (A. G. Gilman, L. S. Goodman, T. W. Rall, and F. Murod, eds.), Macmillan Co., New York, pp. 589–603.

Reddington, M., Lee, K. S., Schubert, P., and Kreutzberg, G. W., 1985, Characterization of adenosine receptors in the hippocampus and other regions of rat brain, in: *Purines, Pharmacology and Physiological Roles* (T. W. Stone, ed.), Macmillan Co., New York, pp. 17–26.

Sattin, A., and Rall, T. W., 1970, The effect of adenosine and adenine nucleotides on the cyclic adenosine 3′,5′-phosphate content of guinea pig cerebral cortex slices, *Mol. Pharmacol.* **6:**13–23.

Schmitt, F. O., 1984, Molecular regulation of brain function: A new view, *Neuroscience* **13:**991–1001.

Scholfield, C. N., 1978, Depression of evoked potentials in brain slices by adenosine compounds, *Br. J. Pharmacol.* **63:**239–244.

Schrader, J., Wahl, M., Kuschinsky, W., and Kreutzberg, G. N., 1980, Increase of adenosine content in cerebral cortex of the cat during bicuculline-induced seizures, *Pfluegers Arch.* **387:**245–251.

Schubert, P., Komp, W., and Kreutzberg, G. W., 1979, Correlation of 5′nucleotidase activity and selective transneuronal transfer of adenosine in the hippocampus, *Brain Res.* **168:**419–424.

Seegmiller, J. E., 1979, Abnormalities of purine metabolism in human immunodeficiency diseases, in: *Physiological and Regulatory Functions of Adenosine and Adenine Nucleotides* (H. P. Baer and G. I. Drummond, eds.), Raven Press, New York, pp. 395–408.

Senba, E., Daddona, R. E., Watanabe, T., Wu, J. Y., and Nagy, J. I., 1985, Coexistence of adenosine deaminase, histidine decarboxylase, and glutamate decarboxylase in hypothalamic neurons in the rat, *J. Neurosci.* **5:**3393–3402.

Siesjo, B. K., 1984, Central circulation and metabolism, *J. Neurosurg.* **60:**883–908.

Siggins, G. R., Hoffer, B. J., and Bloom, F. E., 1969, Cyclic adenosine monophosphate: Possible mediator for norepinephrine effects on cerebellar Purkinje cells, *Science* **165:**1018–1020.

Snell, C. R., Richards, G. D., Candy, J. M., and Snell, P. H., 1985, Nicotinamide adenine dinucleotide as an endogenous modulator of synaptic activity, in: *Purines, Pharmacology and Physiological Roles* (T. W. Stone, ed.), Macmillan Co., New York, p. 272.

Snyder, S. H., 1985, Adenosine as a neuromodulator, *Annu. Rev. Neurosci.* **8:**103–124.

Snyder, S. H., Katims, J. J., Annau, Z., Bruns, R. F., and Daly, J. W., 1981, Adenosine receptors and behavioral actions of methylxanthines, *Proc. Natl. Acad. Sci. USA* **78:**3260–3264.

Stefanovich, J., Rudolphi, K., and Schubert, P., 1986, *Adenosine: Receptors and Modulation of Cell Function*, IRL Press, Oxford.

Sterman, M. B., Shouse, M. N., and Passouant, P., 1982, *Sleep and Epilepsy*, Academic Press, New York.

Stone, T. W., 1981, Physiological roles for adenosine and adenosine 5′-triphosphate in the nervous system, *Neuroscience* **6:**523–555.

Stone, T. W. (ed.), 1985, *Purines, Pharmacology and Physiological Roles*, Macmillan Co., New York.

Su, C., 1983, Purinergic neurotransmission and neuromodulation, *Annu. Rev. Pharmacol. Toxicol.* **23:**397–411.

Sulakhe, P. V., and Phillis, J. W., 1975, The release of [^{3}H] adenosine and its derivatives from cat sensorimotor cortex, *Life Sci.* **17:**551–556.

Swazey, J. P., and Worden, F. G., 1975, On the nature of research in neuroscience, in: *The Neurosciences: Paths of Discovery* (F. G. Worden, J. P. Swazey, and G. Adelman, eds.), MIT Press, Cambridge, Mass., pp. 569–587.

Tetzlaff, W., Schubert, P., and Kreutzberg, G. W., 1987, Synaptic and extrasynaptic localization of adenosine binding sites in the rat hippocampus, *Neuroscience* **21(3):**869–875.

Ushijima, I., Mizuki, Y., and Yamada, M., 1985, Development of stress-induced gastric lesions involves central adenosine A_1-receptor stimulation, *Brain Res.* **339:**351–355.

van Calker, D., Muller, M., and Hamprecht, B., 1979, Adenosine regulates via two different types of receptors the accumulation of cyclic AMP in cultured brain cells, *J. Neurochem.* **33:**999–1005.

Vapaatalo, H., Onken, D., Neuvonen, P., and Westerman, E., 1975, Stereospecificity in some central and circulatory effects of phenylisopropyl adenosine, *Arzneim. Forsch.* **25:**407–410.

Virus, R. M., Baglajewski, T., and Radulovacki, M., 1984, Circadian variation of [^{3}H] N^6-(L-phenylisopropyl) adenosine binding in rat brain, *Neurosci. Lett.* **46:**219–222.

Volpe, J. J. (ed.), 1981, *Neurology of the Newborn*, Saunders, Philadelphia.

Wahl, M., and Kuschinsky, W., 1976, The dilatory action of adenosine in pial arteries of cats and its inhibition by theophylline, *Pfluegers Arch.* **362:**55–59.

Walker, J. E., Lewin, E., and Moffitt, B. C., 1973, Production of epileptiform discharges by application of agents which increase cyclic AMP levels in rat cortex, in: *Epilepsy, Proceedings of the Hans Berger Centenary Symposium*, Churchill Livingstone, Edinburgh, pp. 30–36.

Werman, R., 1966, Criteria for identification of a central nervous system transmitter, *Comp. Biochem. Physiol.* **18:**745–766.

Williams, M., 1983, Mammalian central adenosine receptors, in: *Handbook of Neurochemistry*, Vol. 6 (A. Lajtha, ed.), Plenum Press, New York, pp. 1–26.

Williams, M., 1984, Adenosine—A selective neuromodulator in the mammalian CNS? *Trends Neurosci.* **7:**164–168.

Winn, H. R., 1985, Metabolic regulation of cerebral blood flow by adenosine, in: *Purines, Pharmacology and Physiological Roles* (T. W. Stone, ed.), Macmillan Co., New York, pp. 131–141.

Winn, H. R., Welsh, J. E., Rubio, R., and Berne, R. M., 1978, Brain adenosine levels during bicuculline seizures, *Physiologist* **21:**392–433.

Winn, H. R., Norii, S., Weaver, D. P., Reed, J. C., Ngai, A. C., and Berne, R. M., 1983, Changes in brain adenosine concentration during hypoglycemia and posthypoxic hyperemia, *J. Cereb. Blood Flow Metab.* **3**(Suppl. 1):449–450.

Wojcik, W. J., and Neff, N. H., 1982, Adenosine measurement by rapid HPLC-fluorometric method: Induced changes of adenosine content in regions of cat brain, *J. Neurochem.* **39:**280–282.

Wojcik, W. J., and Neff, N. H., 1983a, Location of adenosine release and adenosine A_2 receptors to rat striatal neurons, *Life Sci.* **33:**755–763.

Wojcik, W. J., and Neff, N. H., 1983b, A_1 receptors are associated with cerebellar granule cells, *J. Neurochem.* **41:**759–763.

Yanik, G., Porter, N. M., and Radulovacki, M., 1985, Effects of REM sleep deprivation on adenosine A_1 and A_2 receptors in rat brain region, *Neurosci. Abstr.* p. 576.

Yarbrough, G. G., and McGuffin-Clineschmidt, J. C., 1981, In vivo behavioral assessment of central nervous system purinergic receptors, *Eur. J. Pharmacol.* **76:**137–144.

28

Formation and Actions of Adenosine in the Rat Hippocampus, with Special Reference to the Interactions with Classical Transmitters

Bertil B. Fredholm, Marianne Dunér-Engström, Johan Fastbom, Bror Jonzon, Eva Lindgren, and Christer Nordstedt

1. Introduction

Adenosine and related compounds can probably play a transmitter or cotransmitter role at least in some tissues (e.g., Burnstock, 1985). However, this seems to be rare and the major functional role of adenosine not only in the periphery but also in the nervous system appears to be that of a modulator. Adenosine is released not only from nerve terminals but also from cell bodies and from glial cells or endothelial cells lining the cerebral blood vessels. Besides its role in blood-flow regulation, adenosine clearly plays a role in modulation of nervous activity, pre- and postjunctionally.

There are many possible interactions of the neuromodulator adenosine with classical transmitter substances, including: (1) the formation, or metabolism, of adenosine could be modified by a transmitter; (2) the release, or metabolism, of the transmitter may be modified by adenosine; and (3) the magnitude of the cellular response to the transmitter may be modified by adenosine. Over the past couple of years we have examined aspects of all three mechanisms, and in the present paper we will give a brief overview of this research. First, we will examine the mechanisms behind the release of adenosine and related compounds in the CNS. Thereafter, the effect of adenosine as an inhibitor of transmitter release will be considered, with a special emphasis on the mechanisms that underlie this prejunctional receptor action. After briefly discussing the effects of adenosine on cAMP generation in the CNS, we will consider some interactions between adenosine and classical transmitters at the receptor level.

2. Materials and Methods

Male Sprague–Dawley rats (ALAB strain) weighing 180–300 g were used. After decapitation, the hippocampus was dissected out and cut into 400-μm-thick slices using a McIlwain tissue

Bertil B. Fredholm, Marianne Dunér-Engström, Johan Fastbom, Bror Jonzon, Eva Lindgren, and Christer Nordstedt • Farmakologiska Institutionen, Karolinska Institutet, S-104 01 Stockholm, Sweden.

chopper. The slices were preincubated for at least 1 hr, first at room temperature and then at 37°C. Thereafter, the slices were loaded with [³H]adenine, [³H]noradrenaline, [³H]choline, [³H]seroto-nin, [³H]glutamate, or [¹⁴C][-GABA essentially as previously described (Fastbom and Fredholm, 1985; Jackisch et al., 1984; Jonzon and Fredholm, 1984). In the case of the labeled transmitter substances, the appropriate precautions against oxidation or metabolic degradation were taken.

Release of purines, labeled and unlabeled, was studied essentially as previously described (Fredholm et al., 1984a; Jonzon and Fredholm, 1985). The effect of various depolarizing stimuli including veratridine (50 μM), potassium, and electrical field stimulation was investigated. In addition, we studied the effect of gassing the slices with nitrogen instead of oxygen for 30 min. At the end of this anoxic period, the slices were taken out and homogenized. The content of unlabeled and labeled adenine nucleotides was determined in the slice using HPLC technique. The energy charge was calculated from the determined nucleotide levels. In addition, the amount of purines released from the slice into the medium was determined. In some instances the composition of the radioactivity released into the medium was determined by HPLC, followed by liquid scintillation counting.

Release of the transmitter substances was studied as previously described (Jonzon and Fredholm, 1984, 1985) using either electrical field stimulation or depolarization with potassium (25 to 50 mM) or veratridine (50 μM). The transmitter release was calcium-dependent and blocked by tetrodotoxin under the conditions used. Two to three stimulation periods were given and the drugs to be tested were administered during the second and/or third period. The results are expressed as $S_2(S_3)/S_1(S_2)$ ratios.

The effect of drugs on the accumulation of [³H]cAMP in the hippocampal slices was studied as previously described (Fredholm et al., 1982). In brief, the effect of different drugs on the accumulation of [³H]cAMP in [³H]-adenine-labeled slices was studied using incubation times of 15 to 90 min. The results are expressed as [³H]cAMP, separated by combined alumina and Dowex chromatography, in percent of the total radioactivity in the slice, which is mainly in the form of adenine nucleotides of which ATP dominates.

In some instances the slices were treated with N-ethylmaleimide (NEM; 50–100 μM) for 5 to 10 min to inactivate N-proteins as described elsewhere (Fredholm and Vernet, 1978).

The following chemicals were used: [2-³H]adenine (25 Ci/mmole), L-[7,8-³H]noradrenaline (44 Ci/mmole), [methyl-[³H]choline chloride (80 Ci/mmole), 5-hydroxy [side chain-1,2-³H]tryp-tamine creatinine sulfate (13 Ci/mmole), L-[G-³H]glutamic acid (39 Ci/mmole), (−)-N⁶-R-[G-³H]phenylisopropyladenosine (46 Ci/mmole), 4-amino-[U-¹⁴C]butyric acid (132 mCi/mmole) were all from the Radiochemical Centre, Amersham, U.K. NEM, 2-chlo-roadenosine, dithiotreitol (DTT), noradrenaline (NA), 12-O-tetradecanoyl-phorbol-13-acetate (TPA), and yohimbine were from Sigma, St. Louis. The two diastereoisomers of phe-nylisopropyladenosine were from Boehringer, Mannheim, West Germany. Pertussis toxin from List Biological Laboratories Inc., Campbell, California, was activated before use with DTT. Clonidine was a gift from Boehringer, Ingelheim, West Germany. Idazoxane ([2-(2-[1,4-ben-zodioxanyl])-2-imidazoline HCl]) was from Reckitt and Coleman, Pharmaceutical Division, Kingston-upon-Hull, U.K. 8-para-Sulfo-phenyltheophylline was from Research Biochemicals Inc., Wayland, Massachusetts. Morphine and naloxone were from ACO Läkemedel, Stockholm, Sweden.

3. Results and Discussion

3.1. Regulation of Adenosine Release

3.1.1. Mechanisms of Purine Release

Purines, particularly adenosine, inosine, and hypoxanthine, are released from brain slices following depolarization or hypoxia. There is also a substantial basal rate of purine release.

Finally, it has been repeatedly proposed that another purine, perhaps ATP, is released as a transmitter or cotransmitter.

Some of the major modes of purine release are diagrammatically shown in Fig. 1. In the upper panels are shown three modes of release from prejunctional elements (nerve endings). Adenosine may be formed secondarily to ATP, being released as a transmitter in its own right (A) or as a cotransmitter together with some other transmitter (B). The purine nucleotides could also be released from nerve endings (and from any other cell) secondarily to a change in the permeability characteristics of the cell membrane. Abood et al. (1962) presented evidence that depolarization of nerves may be associated with release of purine nucleotides. The mechanism was postulated to be an alteration of the membrane permeability. It should also be pointed out here that a very important situation in which adenine nucleotides are released from a preparation is where the cells are dying. In view of the extremely high intracellular content of adenine nucleotides, the presence of only one dying cell in a group of perhaps 10^5 to 10^6 cells could be quite easily detected. In our opinion there is little doubt that release of adenine nucleotides from dead or dying cells has been a major factor behind the repeatedly demonstrated release of adenine nucleotides in different in vitro preparations.

In the lower panels of Fig. 1 are shown three ways in which adenosine may be released from any cell, including postjunctional cellular elements. Panel D schematically illustrates how a lack of metabolizable substrate, e.g., glucose and oxygen, leads to a reduced rate of ATP synthesis and hence to a relative increase in ADP and AMP. Similarly, as shown in panel E, an increase in the work load—e.g., pumping out Na ions in the restitution phase following depolarization—could lead to an increase in the proportion of relatively energy-poor adenine nucleotides. For

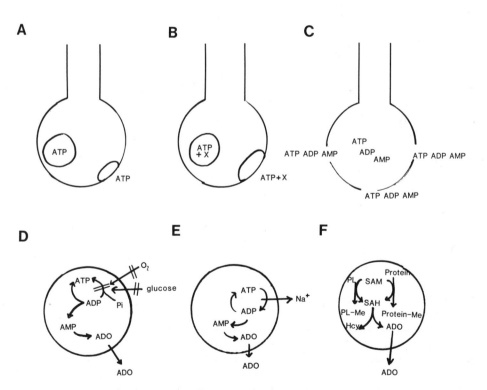

Figure 1. Schematic representation of different modes of purine release in nervous tissue. A–C represent three ways in which adenine nucleotides may be released from nerve endings. D–F are more general mechanisms that may be operative both pre- and postjunctionally. Mechanisms D–F have proved to be operative in both the peripheral and central nervous system. Mechanisms A–C are more speculative. For further details see text.

several reasons it would be disadvantageous if AMP was allowed to accumulate intracellularly. For example, the enzyme adenylate kinase would then tend to convert ATP to ADP. Therefore, there exists an efficient mechanism whereby AMP is eliminated, namely cytosolic 5'-nucleotidase. This enzyme rapidly converts the AMP to adenosine. Finally, and as outlined in panel F, adenosine may be formed intracellularly also under conditions when the energy metabolism is quite undisturbed. This is important because it explains why there may be a substantial adenosine formation even in metabolically intact tissues. The mechanism here is the enzyme hydrolysis of S-adenosylhomocysteine (SAH), which is formed from S-adenosylmethionine as a by-product of various cellular transmethylation reactions. The rapid removal of SAH, and the consequent formation of adenosine, is important since SAH is a potent inhibitor of various transmethylation reactions. Schrader et al. (1981) have convincingly shown that this mechanism is the most important for the formation of adenosine in the heart under basal conditions.

There is evidence that the basal concentration of adenosine in the extracellular fluid in the brain is around 0.5–1 μmole/liter (Zetterström et al., 1982). The adenosine concentration is enhanced by hypoxia, by sustained activity as during a seizure, and by hypotension (Zetterström et al., 1982; Winn et al., 1980). When we want to examine the mechanism by which adenosine is formed, an in vitro model is needed. We have used several such systems, but mainly the hippocampal slice preparation. In such slice preparations the adenosine level is similar to that found in vivo (see Fig. 3). Moreover, the concentration of adenosine in the slice is raised by procedures such as hypoxia, depolarization, or the addition of some neurotransmitters, i.e., by procedures similar to those found to be relevant in vivo.

3.1.2. Depolarization-Induced Release of Adenosine from Brain Slices Does Not Involve ATP Release and Is Probably Not Exocytotic

Depolarization of a brain-slice preparation (e.g., Fredholm and Vernet, 1978; Fredholm and Jonzon, 1981; Jonzon and Fredholm, 1985), of synaptosomes (Fredholm and Vernet, 1979), or of retina (Perez et al., 1986) by several different types of stimuli including high potassium, veratridine, and electrical pulses leads to an enhanced overflow of purines. The time course of this release as well as its calcium dependence are different from those of a more traditional neurotransmitter such as NA or GABA (see Jonzon and Fredholm, 1985). The potent inhibitor of ecto-5'-nucleotidase, α,β-methylene-adenosine diphosphate (AOPCP), had at most a modest effect on the efflux of purines or on the contents of adenine nucleotides in the efflux, which was small in the preparations studied. This suggests that at most a very small fraction of the radioactive adenosine released could be derived from adenine nucleotides released as transmitters or as cotransmitters. Quinacrine, which has been suggested to be a marker for "purinergic" nerves (see Burnstock, 1985), was not released in parallel with the purines (Fredholm and Jonzon, 1981). These findings indicate that ATP released from "purinergic" nerves or as cotransmitter is not a major source of purines released by nerve stimulation.

As shown in Fig. 2, dipyridamole, an inhibitor of purine nucleoside carrier-mediated transport (Plagemann and Wohlhueter, 1983), can be used as a tool to differentiate between different possible mechanisms of adenosine release. If the release is exocytotic (in the form of either an adenine nucleotide or adenosine itself), the overflow of transmitter should be enhanced by this transport inhibitor. This is very similar to the effect of cocaine on the overflow of a catecholamine from central and peripheral catecholaminergic neurons. By contrast, if adenosine is not released from a storage pool but as a consequence of increased intracellular formation, and if it escapes into the extracellular fluid at least partly via the carrier mechanism, then we should expect dipyridamole to actually inhibit the overflow of the purine. As seen in Fig. 2, the experimental results agree very well with the second prediction. This provides additional evidence that exocytotic release is not a major factor in the release of adenosine even by depolarizing stimuli. That exocytosis is not the major factor in releasing adenosine into the extracellular fluid during basal conditions and during hypoxia is obvious.

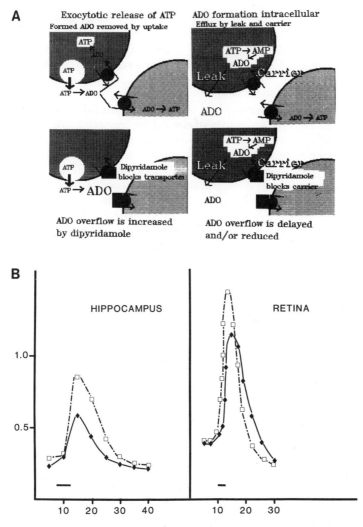

Figure 2. The effect of dipyridamole on the evoked release of radioactive purines after labeling of the purine pool by [³H]adenine. (A) Schematic representation of the mechanisms of action of dipyridamole in relation to purine release from nerve endings induced in either of two ways. The left-hand part shows the release of adenine nucleotides in a transmitter-like fashion (essentially as in Fig. 1A or B) or due to nonspecific increase in adenine nucleotide permeability. The right-hand part shows the release of purines according to a model more similar to panels D–F in Fig. 1. (B) The outcome of experiments with 10 μM dipyridamole in the hippocampus (left) or rabbit retina (right). The tissues were labeled and release induced by veratridine (500 μM) in the hippocampus or by potassium (43 mM) in the retina. □, control; ♦, the release in the presence of dipyridamole. Note that the outcome of the experiment is compatible with the model on the right, but not with the model on the left.

3.1.3. Modulation of Adenosine Formation by Transmitter Substances

Depolarizing stimuli can, however, cause an adenosine release that is dependent upon exocytosis. This relies on the fact that a classical transmitter, following its exocytotic release, may also cause the formation of adenosine by a receptor-mediated action. This is most clearly demonstrated in the PNS where adenosine release following stimulation of sympathetic nerves can be blocked by receptor antagonists (see Fredholm and Hedqvist, 1980). In the CNS, where many more transmitter systems are operating simultaneously, the results are less clear-cut. It is likely that the situation is similar to that in the PNS. In agreement with this view, depolarizing transmitter substances (including glutamate and aspartate) cause purine release and an increased formation of cAMP that can be blocked by adenosine receptor antagonists (Fredholm et al., 1982). Clearly, the possible role that excitatory neurotransmitters play in the release of adenosine in the brain requires more study.

Many years ago we found that morphine was able to stimulate the overflow of purines from veratridine-stimulated rat cortical slices (Fredholm and Vernet, 1978). We have recently shown that morphine also affected purine release following veratridine or potassium depolarization, and even hypoxia in the rat hippocampal slice preparation (Fredholm et al., 1987). The morphine-induced increase in purine release from hypoxic hippocampal slices was associated with an enhanced fall in the energy charge (Fredholm et al., 1987). It occurs at low concentrations and is blocked by naloxone, suggesting that it is receptor mediated. The receptor involved, however, is unknown, as is the mechanism by which morphine exerts this action. It is interesting to note that a possible role of endogenous opioids in the control of metabolic and neuronal damage in shock and trauma has been postulated based on the beneficial effects of naloxone (see Holaday, 1983). Our results are clearly compatible with the idea that endogenous opioids could enhance the loss of high-energy phosphates during metabolic injury, and prevention of this by naloxone may in some conditions be beneficial.

There is thus some evidence that the rate of formation of adenosine is regulated by classical transmitters. These transmitter substances may influence the rate of energy consumption or substrate delivery and in this way influence adenosine release. They could release purines secondarily to depolarization. They may also modulate the formation of adenosine in more subtle ways as there is some evidence that endorphins do. The rest of this chapter will be concerned with the role of adenosine as a modulator of transmitter release and/or transmitter actions.

3.2. Modulation by Adenosine of Transmitter Release

An inhibitory effect of adenosine on transmitter release was first demonstrated by Ginsborg and Hirst (1972), who used electrophysiological methods. About 10 years ago we and others demonstrated that adenosine inhibits transmitter release, as measured by the outflow of radioactive or endogenous transmitter (Hedqvist and Fredholm, 1976; Gustafsson et al., 1981; Vizi and Knoll, 1976). The early studies were carried out in the periphery, and since that time much evidence has accumulated showing that transmitter release is also modulated by adenosine in the CNS (see Fredholm and Hedqvist, 1980; Phillis and Wu, 1981). An inhibitory effect of adenosine and adenosine analogues on the evoked release of dopamine, NA, serotonin, acetylcholine, and excitatory amino acids has been repeatedly demonstrated in several brain regions. By contrast, it has proven difficult to convincingly demonstrate an effect of adenosine receptor active compounds on the release of the inhibitory neurotransmitter GABA (Limberger et al., 1986, and our own unpublished data). It has been argued that adenosine receptors are mainly localized to the nerve endings of excitatory neurons (Snyder, 1985). The magnitude of the prejunctional inhibitory effect of adenosine on the release of different transmitters agrees with this kind of distribution. A teleological argument for a preferential distribution of prejunctional adenosine receptors to excitatory nerve endings can perhaps be as follows: since adenosine is formed by excitatory stimulus control of the amount of excitatory transmitter released by adenosine, a meaningful feedback loop would be formed. By contrast, an inhibitory neurotransmitter may be expected to cause a smaller degree of metabolic derangement of the target cells and therefore to cause less adenosine formation.

The prejunctional inhibitory effects of adenosine are exerted over a range of concentrations that are quite similar to the levels that can be found in the CNS (Fig. 3). This supports the idea that the prejunctional effects are physiologically important. There is some evidence that transmitter

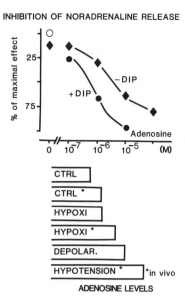

INHIBITION OF NORADRENALINE RELEASE

Figure 3. Concentration-dependent inhibition of [³H]-NA by adenosine in relation to the concentration of adenosine in brain under different conditions. The upper panel shows the concentration-dependent inhibition of NA release. ○, the transmitter release in the presence of 1 μM 8-phenyltheophylline. A maximal effect is taken to be that of 100 μM adenosine. Also shown are the dose–response curve for adenosine in the presence and in the absence of dipyridamole to block adenosine elimination via uptake. Data from Jonzon and Fredholm (1984). The lower panel shows the concentration of adenosine in brain as taken from several independent studies. The *in vitro* data are from rat hippocampal slices (Fredholm *et al.*, 1984a; Jonzon and Fredholm, 1985). The *in vivo* data are either from brain dialysis (control and hypoxia; Zetterström *et al.*, 1982) or from freeze blowing (hypotension; Winn *et al.*, 1980).

release is controlled already by the amounts of adenosine present under resting conditions. First, an inhibitory effect is seen already at about 0.1 μmole/liter, which is probably well below the basal adenosine concentration extracellularly. Second, xanthine derivatives have a slight, but definite effect on transmitter overflow. Finally, there is evidence that xanthines can influence transmitter turnover and even NA receptor functions, which is clearly compatible with such a physiological role of the purine (Fredholm *et al.*, 1984b).

In the first report on a prejunctional effect of adenosine, Ginsborg and Hirst (1972) did not describe a change in the efflux of radioactive transmitter, but rather a change in a postsynaptic response as determined by electrophysiology of a skeletal muscle preparation. In the CNS, electrophysiological methods have also been used to study the inhibitory effects of adenosine on transmitter release. The rat hippocampus has been commonly used for such studies, and there is good evidence that the adenosine-induced inhibition of field EPSPs recorded in the CA1 field after stimulation of the afferent input, is largely due to inhibition of transmitter release (whatever the transmitter may eventually prove to be) rather than an inhibition of the responses of the pyramidal cells to that transmitter (see Dunwiddie, 1985). Other chapters in this volume will cover these effects in more detail.

The prejunctional inhibitory effect of adenosine analogues on transmitter outflow as measured by radioactive transmitters or by electrophysiological techniques appears to be mediated via adenosine receptors that are similar to A1 receptors (e.g., Fredholm *et al.*, 1983; Dunwiddie and Fredholm, 1984; Dunwiddie, 1985). This is illustrated in Fig. 4, where the potency of some adenosine receptor active compounds as inhibitors of NA outflow or field EPSPs in the hippocampus is compared to their potency as displacers of R-PIA from A1 receptors or as stimulators via A2 receptors of cAMP accumulation. It is clearly seen that the response is correlated with A1-receptor potency, but not with A2-receptor potency.

The mechanism behind the prejunctional inhibitory effect is not known. The A1 receptors, which appear to mediate the prejunctional inhibitory effect, were originally defined on the basis of inhibitory effects on cAMP formation (van Calker *et al.*, 1979). Inhibition of cAMP formation is clearly an important mechanism behind the antilipolytic effect of A1-receptor stimulation in fat cells (cf. Fredholm, 1982). However, all A1-receptor effects may not be mediated via changes in

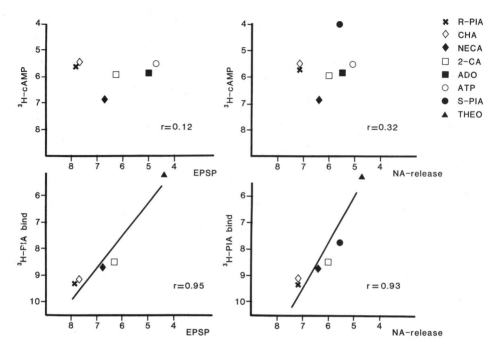

Figure 4. Relationship between the potency of several adenosine-receptor active compounds to raise the accumulation of [³H]cAMP in rat hippocampal slices (along ordinate on two upper graphs), to inhibit the binding of [³H]-R-PIA to membranes from rat cortex (along ordinate on two lower graphs), to inhibit field EPSPs (along abscissa of two left-hand graphs), and to inhibit the outflow of [³H]-NA by field stimulation from the rat or rabbit hippocampus (along abscissa of two right-hand graphs). No regression line was drawn for the data shown in the two upper panels since the slopes were not significantly different from 0. In the two lower panels the slopes were significant at the 0.015 and 0.007 level, respectively. Also shown are the correlations coefficient. Data from Dunwiddie and Fredholm (1984), Jackisch *et al.* (1985), Jonzon and Fredholm (1984), Ukena *et al.* (1984), and Fredholm *et al.* (1982).

cAMP. We have earlier argued that it is unlikely that the inhibitory effect of adenosine on NA release in the kidney is due to inhibition of adenylate cyclase (Fredholm *et al.*, 1983).

The inhibitory effect of A1-receptor stimulation on adenylate cyclase is mediated by the regulatory GTP-binding N_i (or G_i) protein. There is recent evidence that the N_i protein causes inhibition of adenylate cyclase by dissociating free $N_i\beta\tau$ subunits, which are indistinguishable from $N_s\beta\tau$ subunits and can therefore bind to $N_s\alpha$ subunit, which is thereby inactivated and can no longer cause any stimulation of the cyclase enzyme (Smigel *et al.*, 1985). The possibility clearly exists that the N_i protein may not also interact with other effector mechanisms. For example, it is possible that the α subunit may interact with some effector other than adenylate cyclase. Alternatively, the β,γ subunits may interact not only with the $N_s\alpha$ subunit thereby causing inhibition of adenylate cyclase but also with other as yet incompletely defined N proteins that could interact either with calcium channels or with phospholipase C.

In order to examine the possible involvement of an N protein in the prejunctional inhibitory effect of adenosine analogues, we examined the effects of NEM. NEM apparently does not bind directly to adenosine receptors, even though the binding of an agonist is markedly reduced, because the binding sites are shifted from a high- to a low-affinity configuration (Fredholm *et al.*, 1985; Ukena *et al.*, 1984). Adenylate cyclase is not substantially affected by NEM in doses that interact with N_i, and neither is the ability of adenosine analogues to activate the enzyme via the A2 receptor (Fredholm *et al.*, 1985; Ukena *et al.*, 1984; Yeung and Green, 1983). Therefore, it is of interest to note that NEM treatment markedly reduces the prejunctional inhibitory effect of R-PIA (Fig. 5).

Recently, Allgaier *et al.* (1985) reported that pertussis toxin (PTX) caused a significant inhibition of the prejunctional inhibitory effect of α2-adrenoceptor agonists on NA release in rabbit hippocampus. Dolphin and Prestwich (1985) reported similar findings regarding adenosine receptor-mediated control of glutamate release in cultured cells (but reported that PTX was not a useful tool in slices). PTX is quite selective in that ADP ribosylates mainly 39,000- and 41,000-dalton components, probably identical with the α subunits N_i and N_o proteins (and of transducin where this exists). While it is obviously much more selective than NEM, it has the drawback that if it is active at all with intact cells, PTX requires a long time to inactivate the N proteins. Such long incubation times could cause adaptive changes in other regulatory systems. Even though it is probably relatively less selective, NEM acts very rapidly (within a few minutes) to block N_i proteins. Together the findings with NEM and PTX strongly implicate an N protein different from N_s in the regulation of transmitter release.

As mentioned above, the N_i protein is generally coupled to adenylate cyclase. However, the results with forskolin (Fig. 5) do not indicate an important role in the regulation of transmitter release. Thus, we suggest that either the N protein involved in these prejunctional effects may not

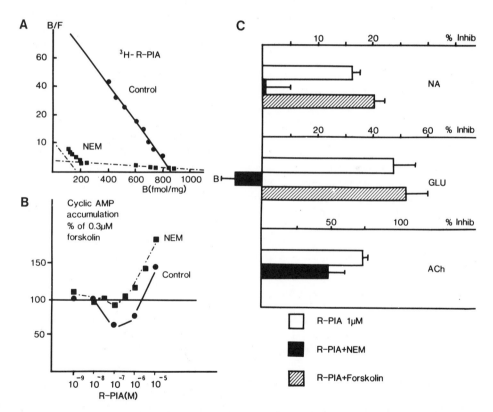

Figure 5. The effect of NEM treatment on the binding of [³H]-R-PIA to hippocampal membranes (panel a), the effect of R-PIA on forskolin-activated accumulation of [³H]cAMP (panel b), and the R-PIA (1 μM)-induced inhibition of the release of NA, glutamate, and acetylcholine. In all experiments, slices (or membranes in the binding experiments) were treated with 50–100 μM NEM for 10 min. [³H]-NA and [³H]-glutamate release was evoked by stimulation with 3 Hz at 10 V. [³H]-Acetylcholine release was evoked by stimulating with 0.2 Hz at 10 V. In all cases the release was calcium-dependent and tetrodotoxin-sensitive. (Results from Fredholm and Lindgren, 1987; Fredholm, Lindgren, and Lindström, 1985, and unpublished.)

be N_i, but perhaps the N_o that is quite ubiquitous in the CNS and is also a good substrate for PTX and apparently for NEM (unpublished). Alternatively, the N_i protein may be coupled to other effectors than adenylate cyclase. There are reports that the N_i protein may be involved in biological effects that are independent of adenylate cyclase (e.g., see Bokoch and Gilman, 1984).

3.3. Adenosine Regulation of cAMP

Sattin and Rall (1970) were the first to observe that adenosine stimulates the accumulation of cAMP in brain slices and that this action was antagonized by methylxanthines including theophylline and caffeine. Stimulation of cAMP accumulation by adenosine analogues has since been demonstrated in slices from several regions and many species (see Daly, 1977). On the other hand, it has proven quite difficult to demonstrate adenosine stimulation of adenylate cyclase activity, except in a few dopamine-rich regions. Instead, adenosine receptor-mediated inhibition of adenylate cyclase has been often and reproducibly found (Cooper et al., 1980; Yeung and Green, 1983). Thus, there is the interesting apparent paradox: a slice from a brain region such as the hippocampus responds with a rise in cAMP accumulation, whereas membranes prepared from the same region respond only with a decrease in cAMP accumulation.

The slices are composed of cells of many different types. There is some evidence that there may be differences in the sensitivity of cells of neuronal and glial origin to the actions of adenosine (Elfman et al., 1984). However, both types of cultured cells responded with an increase in cAMP content. The cAMP accumulation in slices is not dependent on prostaglandin synthesis or on release of other transmitters (unpublished data). Thus, we have no good explanation for the finding that cAMP levels rise in slices even though no stimulation can be found in most CNS membrane preparations. The possibility remains that the homogenization of the tissue and the preparation of membranes somehow disrupts the coupling of the A2 receptors responsible for cAMP accumulation and the N_s protein or the cyclase, whereas the association between the A1 receptor and N_i protein and the cyclase is more resistant to such disruption. The recent finding that the A1 receptor is very closely associated with the α subunit of the N_i protein (Stiles, 1985) is compatible with such an interpretation.

The question why we do not see inhibition of cAMP accumulation in brain slices recently received a tentative answer, when it was shown that such inhibition can indeed be observed provided that cAMP accumulation is stimulated by forskolin (Fredholm et al., 1983). This can be seen in Fig. 5 (lower left-hand side). Possibly the failure to observe an inhibitory effect of adenosine analogues under normal circumstances is due to the fact that the cyclase activity is basal and there is no activity to inhibit.

3.4. Interactions with Classical Neurotransmitters

It has been known for many years that adenosine can interact with drugs that stimulate cAMP formation, via an action on A1 receptors. For example, adenosine is a potent endogenous regulator of lipolysis in fat cells by virtue of its ability to antagonize primarily β-receptor-mediated lipolytic effects (e.g., Fredholm, 1982). The inhibitory effect of adenosine on the actions of β-adrenoceptor-stimulating substances in the heart is another example. It is possible that similar interactions occur in the CNS between adenosine A1 receptors and various cAMP-stimulating drugs. This possibility warrants a closer examination.

It has been repeatedly shown that some drugs that do not normally stimulate adenylate cyclase, such as NA interacting with $\alpha1$ adrenoceptors or histamine with H1 receptors, are able to do so if adenosine is simultaneously present (Daly, 1977). This interaction between adenosine and classical transmitters may be physiologically relevant. Hollingsworth and Daly (1985) recently reported that these drugs were able to stimulate the formation of inositol phosphates from [3H]inositol-labeled cerebral microsomes. We have recently confirmed the effect of NA in intact rat hippocampal slices. Presumably the accumulation of inositol phosphates is due to the break-down of phosphatidylinositol-1, 4-bisphosphate into $InsP_3$ and diacylglycerol (DAG), the $InsP_3$ being rapidly converted to the less phosphorylated inositol phosphate derivatives. The formed DAG could be expected to activate protein kinase C (Nishizuka, 1984). This enzyme is also potently activated by phorbol esters, and phorbol esters were found to mimic the effect of α1-receptor stimulation on cAMP accumulation in a cell-free preparation of guinea pig cortex (Hollingsworth et al., 1985).

We have recently shown that phorbol esters are potent stimulators of cAMP accumulation in brain slices (Fredholm et al., 1987). The effect of α1-adrenoceptor-stimulating drugs was shared by phorbol esters. In the synaptosomal preparation studied by Hollingsworth and co-workers, the phorbol esters had no effect by themselves (Hollingsworth et al., 1985). By contrast, in the brain slice the phorbol esters did have an effect. As seen in Fig. 6, the phorbolester phorbol 12,13-dibutyrate (PBB) stimulated basal cAMP accumulation by a mechanism that was blocked by the adenosine receptor antagonist 8-p-sulfophenyl theophylline. The adenosine uptake inhibitor di-pyridamole markedly enhanced the effect of the phorbol ester. There was also evidence for a synergism between exogenous adenosine and dipyridamole. These results suggest that phorbol esters can enhance the cAMP accumulation stimulated by endogenous and/or exogenous adenosine.

These results are compatible with the notion that drugs that activate α1 adrenoceptors can potentiate the effect of an adenylate cyclase-stimulating drug by enhancing the formation of DAG, which activates protein kinase C which in turn, by some as yet unknown mechanism, enhances cyclase activity. What this mechanism is we can only speculate about. It is possibly relevant that the phorbol ester is more efficient in stimulating adenosine-induced cAMP ac-cumulation than in enhancing the effect of forskolin (unpublished data). Moreover, the effect of high concentrations (> 3 μM) of forskolin is not really stimulated at all by PDBu. This could indicate that the phorbol ester, and by implication protein kinase C, does not act on the cyclase directly, but requires the activity of N (or G) proteins. It was recently shown by Jakobs and co-workers (Katada et al., 1985) that protein kinase C can phosphorylate and inactivate the N_i protein in blood platelets. A protein kinase C-mediated inhibition of the N_i protein in brain slices could be a mechanism by which to enhance the activity of adenylate cyclase-stimulating drugs

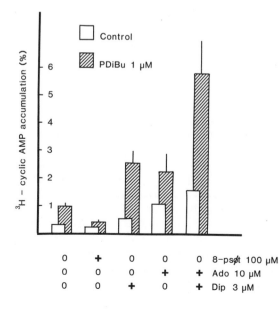

Figure 6. Interactions between phorbol di-butyrate and drugs that affect adenosine recep-tors on cAMP accumulation in the rat hippo-campus.

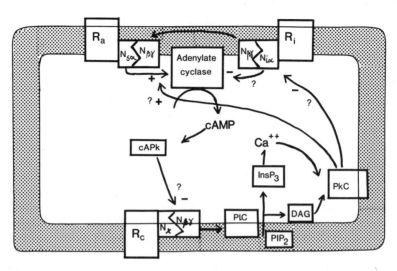

Figure 7. Schematic representation of some possible interactions between different types of receptor-active compounds. Drugs that bind to receptors that stimulate (R_s) or inhibit (R_i) adenylate cyclase via intermediary N proteins will alter the levels of cAMP and thereby the activity of cAMP-dependent protein kinase (cAPk). This kinase is postulated to be able to regulate by phosphorylation the cascade of events between receptor (R_c) and phospholipase C (PlC). Conversely, drugs that affect this pathway are supposed to alter the activity of the calcium- and phospholipid-sensitive protein kinase (PkC), which is postulated to be able to regulate, perhaps at the N protein level, the activation of adenylate cyclase.

such as adenosine or NECA. Indeed, we find that the ability of R-PIA to decrease cAMP accumulation (see Fig. 5) is blocked by PBB. However, we found (Nordstedt and Fredholm, 1987) that PBB is able to enhance the stimulatory effect of NECA also in NEM-treated hippocampal slices where the N_i protein is largely inactivated, although the effect may be smaller. Thus, it seems unlikely that an action on N_i is the only mechanism behind this intriguing potentiation. Some of the different types of interaction are indicated in Fig. 7. Obviously there exists a rich supply of possible sites of interaction that deserve study.

4. Conclusions

Adenosine is present in the CNS in concentrations that are sufficient to produce clear-cut effects. Therefore, we have to seriously consider adenosine as one among the many factors that influence central nervous activity. Clearly, adenosine is different from many of the classical transmitters. Among the classical transmitters we may differentiate between "fast" and "slow" chemical signals (Iversen, 1984). The fast signals, exemplified mainly by excitatory and inhibitory amino acids, provide the basis for quick information transfer at well-defined and anatomically distinct synapses. This forms what has been called a "hard-wired" nervous system. Superimposed on this we have a "soft-wired" nervous system. This uses other types of signals including monoamines and peptides. These signals operate over a longer time scale and mainly act by setting the stage for the fast chemical signals. The major factor that determines whether a neuron will respond to these neuromodulatory neurotransmitters is if it is in possession of the relevant receptor. This is then a chemically coded signaling system that is also characterized by important interactions between different transmitters. The large number of different peptide and monoamine signals as well as the existence of several types of receptors for each of them, combined with the possibilities for interactions at receptor or postreceptor levels (e.g., as in Fig. 7), provide a basis for a specificity in this chemically coded neurotransmission system. The interactions between different signals also provide a basis for a kind of memory—and this is the closest we will come in this chapter to the title of the present symposium.

Adenosine must be seen as a representative of still another type of chemical signal. The amount of adenosine in a given CNS region is not determined by its release from nerve endings following exocytosis. Instead, the amount of adenosine is controlled by local metabolic factors, including the rate of substrate delivery and the relative magnitude of the work carried out. For example, an intense excitation of a given neuronal structure will increase the local adenosine level.

Adenosine could play a role in the regulation of blood flow in the CNS and possibly also in the utilization of substrate. In addition, it could interact with classical transmitters in several different ways. For example, adenosine is a powerful inhibitor of the release of several (but probably not all) transmitters. This effect appears to be exerted via adenosine receptors of the A1 subtype and is apparently mediated via an N protein, but not N_s. The involvement of cAMP in these prejunctional effects of adenosine is uncertain and further studies are required to elucidate the mechanism of action. Adenosine may also influence the actions of other transmitter substances at the effector cell level. There are probably a large number of such interactions which we have only begun to explore. Considering the widespread occurrence of adenosine, it seems likely that these interactions at the receptor, transducer, or effector level between adenosine and classical transmitters may prove to be very significant physiologically.

ACKNOWLEDGMENTS. These studies were supported by the Swedish Medical Research Council (Project No. 2553), by Ostermans Foundation, by Stiftelsen Gamla Tjänarinnor, King Gustaf V 80-years fund, and by the Karolinska Institutet.

References

Abood, L. G., Koketsu, K., and Miyamoto, S., 1962, Outflux of various phosphates during membrane depolarization of excitable tissues, *Am. J. Physiol.* **202**:469–474.

Allgaier, C., Feuerstein, T. J., Jackish, R., and Hertting, G., 1985, Islet-activating protein (pertussis toxin) diminishes α_2-adrenoceptor mediated effects on noradrenaline release, *Naunyn-Schmiedebergs Arch. Pharmacol.* **331**:235–239.

Bokoch, G. M., and Gilman, A. G., 1984, Inhibition of receptor-mediated release of arachidonic acid by pertussis toxin, *Cell* **39**:301–308.

Burnstock, G., 1985, Purinergic transmitters and receptors: New directions, in: *Adenosine: Receptors and Modulation of Cell Function* (V. Stefanovich, K. Rudolphi, and P. Schubert, eds.), IRL Press, Oxford, pp. 3–14.

Cooper, D. M. F., Londos, C., and Rodbell, M., 1980, Adenosine receptor-mediated inhibition of rat cerebral cortical adenylate cyclase by a GTP-dependent process, *Mol. Pharmacol.* **18**:598–601.

Daly, J. W., 1977, *Cyclic Nucleotides in the Nervous System*, Plenum Press, New York.

Dolphin, A. C., and Prestwich, S. A., 1985, Pertussis toxin reverses adenosine inhibition of neuronal glutamate release, *Nature* **316**:148–150.

Dunwiddie, T. V., 1985, The physiological role of adenosine in the central nervous system, *Int. Rev. Neurobiol.* **27**:63–139.

Dunwiddie, T. V., and Fredholm, B. B., 1984, Adenosine receptors mediating inhibitory electrophysiological responses in rat hippocampus are different from receptors mediating cyclic AMP accumulation, *Naunyn-Schmiedebergs Arch. Pharmacol.* **326**:294–301.

Elfman, L., Lindgren, E., Walum, E., and Fredholm, B. B., 1984, Adenosine analogues stimulate cyclic AMP accumulation in cultured neuroblastoma and glioma cell lines, *Acta Pharmacol. Toxicol.* **55**:297–302.

Fastbom, J., and Fredholm, B. B., 1985, Inhibition of [³H]-glutamate release from rat hippocampal slices by L-phenylisopropyladenosine, *Acta Physiol. Scand.* **125**:121–123.

Fredholm, B. B., 1982, Adenosine receptors, *Med. Biol.* **60**:289–293.

Fredholm, B. B., and Hedqvist, P., 1980, Modulation of neurotransmission by purine nucleotides and nucleosides, *Biochem. Pharmacol.* **29**:1635–1643.

Fredholm, B. B., and Jonzon, B., 1981, Quinacrine and release of purines from the rat hypothalamus, *Med. Biol.* **59**:262–267.

Fredholm, B. B., and Lindgren, E., 1987, Effects of N-ethylmaleimide and forskolin on noradrenaline release from rat hippocampal slices: Evidence that prejunctional adenosine and α-receptors are linked to N-proteins, but not to adenylate cyclase, *Acta Physiol. Scand.* **130**:95–105.

Fredholm, B. B., and Vernet, L., 1978, Morphine increases depolarization induced purine release from rat cortical slices, *Acta Physiol. Scand.* **104**:502–504.

Fredholm, B. B., and Vernet, L., 1979, Release of [³H]-nucleosides from [³H]-adenine labelled hypothalamic synaptosomes, *Acta Physiol. Scand.* **106**:97–107.

Fredholm, B. B., Jonzon, B., Lindgren, E., and Lindström, K., 1982, Adenosine receptors mediating cyclic AMP production in the rat hippocampus, *J. Neurochem.* **39**:165–175.

Fredholm, B. B., Jonzon, B., and Lindström, K., 1983, Adenosine receptor mediated increases and decreases in cyclic AMP in hippocampal slices treated with forskolin, *Acta Physiol. Scand.* **117**:461–463.

Fredholm, B. B., Dunwiddie, T. V., Bergman, B., and Lindström, K., 1984a, Levels of adenosine and adenine nucleotides in slices of rat hippocampus, *Brain Res.* **295**:127–136.

Fredholm, B. B., Jonzon, B., and Lindgren, E., 1984b, Changes in beta-receptor number and noradrenaline release following long term treatment with theophylline or L-phenylisopropyl adenosine, *Acta Physiol. Scand.* **122**:55–59.

Fredholm, B. B., Lindgren, E., and Lindström, K., 1985, Treatment with N-ethylmaleimide selectively reduced receptor-mediated decreases in cyclic AMP accumulation in rat hippocampal slices, *Br. J. Pharmacol.* **86**:509–513.

Fredholm, B. B., Dunér-Engström, M., Fastbom, J., Jonzon, B., Lindgren, E., Nordstedt, C., van der Ploeg, I., and Pedata, F., 1987, Interactions of the neuromodulator adenosine with classical transmitters, in: *Topics and Perspectives in Adenosine Research* (E. Gertach and B.S. Becker, eds.), Berlin, Springer-Verlag, pp. 509–520.

Ginsborg, B. L., and Hirst, G. D. S., 1972, The effect of adenosine on the release of the transmitter from the phrenic nerve of the rat, *J. Physiol. (London)* **224**:629–645.

Gustafsson, L., Fredholm, B. B., and Hedqvist, P., 1981, Theophylline interferes with the modulatory role of endogenous adenosine on cholinergic neurotransmission in guinea pig ileum, *Acta Physiol. Scand.* **111**:269–280.

Hedqvist, P., and Fredholm, B. B., 1976, Effects of adenosine on adrenergic neurotransmission: Prejunctional inhibition and postjunctional enhancement, *Naunyn-Schmiedebergs Arch. Pharmacol.* **293**:217–223.

Holaday, J. W., 1983, Cardiovascular consequences of endogenous opiate antagonism, *Biochem. Pharmacol.* **32**:573–585.

Hollingsworth, E. B., and Daly, J. W., 1985, Accumulation of inositol phosphates and cyclic AMP in guinea-pig cerebral cortical preparations: Effects of norepinephrine, histamine, carbamylcholine and 2-chloroadenosine, *Biochim. Biophys. Acta* **847**:207–216.

Hollingsworth, E. B., Sears, E. B., and Daly, V. W., 1985, An activator of protein kinase C (phorbol-12-myristate-13-acetate) augments 2-chloroadenosine-elicited accumulation of cyclic AMP in guinea pig cerebral cortical particulate preparations, *FEBS Lett.* **184**:339–342.

Iversen, L. L., 1984, The Ferrier Lecture 1983: Amino acids and peptides: Fast and slow chemical signals in the nervous system? *Proc. R. Soc. London Ser. B* **221**:246–260.

Jackisch, R., Strittmatter, H., Fehr, R., and Hertting, G., 1984, Endogenous adenosine as a modulator of hippocampal acetylcholine release, *Naunyn-Schmiedebergs Arch. Pharmacol.* **327**:319–325.

Jackisch, R., Fehr, R., and Hertting, G., 1985, Adenosine: An endogenous modulator of hippocampal noradrenaline release, *Neuropharmacology* **24**:499–507.

Jonzon, B., and Fredholm, B. B., 1984, Adenosine receptor-mediated inhibition of noradrenaline release from slices of the rat hippocampus, *Life Sci.* **35**:1971–1979.

Jonzon, B., and Fredholm, B. B., 1985, Release of purines, noradrenaline, and GABA from rat hippocampal slices by field stimulation, *J. Neurochem.* **44**:217–224.

Katada, T., Gilman, A. G., Watanabe, Y., Bauer, S., and Jakobs, K. H., 1985, Protein kinase C phosphorylates the inhibitory guanine-nucleotide-binding regulatory component and apparently suppresses its function in hormonal inhibition of adenylate cyclase, *Eur. J. Biochem.* **151**:431–437.

Limberger, N., Späth, L., and Starke, K., 1986, A search for receptors modulating the release of γ-[³H]aminobutyric acid in rabbit caudate nucleus slices, *J. Neurochem.* **46**:1109–1117.

Nishizuka, Y., 1984, The role of protein kinase C in cell surface signal transduction and tumour promotion, *Nature* **308**:693–698.

Nordstedt, C., and Fredholm, B. B., 1987, Phorbol-12,13-dibutyrate enhances the cyclic AMP accumulation in rat hippocampal slices induced by adenosine analogues, *Naunyn-Schmiedebergs Arch. Pharmacol.* **335**:136–142.

Perez, M. T. R., Ehinger, B. E., Lindström, K., and Fredholm, B. B., 1986, Release of endogenous and radioactive purines from the rabbit retina, *Brain Res.* **398:**106–112.

Phillis, J. W., and Wu, P. H., 1981, The role of adenosine and its nucleotides in central synaptic transmission, *Prog. Neurobiol.* **16:**187–239.

Plagemann, P. G. W., and Wohlhueter, R. M., 1983, Nucleoside transport in mammalian cells and interaction with intracellular metabolism, in: *Regulatory Function of Adenosine* (R.M. Berne, T.W. Rall, and R. Rubio, eds.), Nijhoff, The Hague, pp. 179–201.

Sattin, A., and Rall, T. W., 1970, Cyclic AMP content of guinea pig cerebral cortex slices, *Mol. Pharmacol.* **6:**13–23.

Schrader, J., Schütz, W., and Barbenheuer, H., 1981, Role of S-adenosyl homocysteine hydrolase in adenosine metabolism in mammalian heart, *Biochem. J.* **196:**65–70.

Smigel, M. D., Ferguson, K. M., and Gilman, A. G., 1985, Control of adenylate cyclase by G proteins, *Adv. Cyclic Nucleotide Res.* **19:**103–111.

Snyder, S. H., 1985, Adenosine as a neuromodulator, *Annu. Rev. Neurosci.* **8:**103–124.

Stiles, G. L., 1985, The A1 adenosine receptor, *J. Biol. Chem.* **260:**6728–6732.

Ukena, D., Poeschla, E., Huttemann, E., and Schwabe, U., 1984, Effects of N-ethylmaleimide on adenosine receptors of rat fat cells and human platelets, *Naunyn-Schmiedebergs Arch. Pharmacol.* **327:**247–253.

van Calker, D., Muller, M., and Hamprecht, B., 1979, Adenosine regulates via two different types of receptors the accumulation of cyclic AMP in cultured brain cells, *J. Neurochem.* **33:**999–1005.

Vizi, E. S., and Knoll, J., 1976, The inhibitory effect of adenosine and related nucleotides on the release of acetylcholine, *Neuroscience* **1:**391–398.

Winn, H. R., Welsh, J. E., Rubio, R., and Berne, R. M., 1980, Brain adenosine production in rat during sustained alteration in systemic blood pressure, *Am. J. Physiol.* **239:**H636–H641.

Yeung, S. M., and Green, R. D., 1983, Agonist and antagonist affinities for inhibitory adenosine receptors are reciprocally affected by 5′-guanylylimidodiphosphate or N-ethylmaleimide, *J. Biol. Chem.* **258:**2334–2339.

Zetterström, T., Vernet, L., Ungerstedt, U., Tossman, U., Jonzon, B., and Fredholm, B. B., 1982, Purine levels in the intact rat brain: Studies with an implanted perfused hollow fibre, *Neurosci. Lett.* **29:**111–115.

29

Mediation of Nonclassical Postsynaptic Responses by Cyclic Nucleotides

Benjamin Libet

Like Herbert Jasper, whom I have had the privilege of knowing as a stimulating colleague and friend for more than 35 years, I have approached the issue of brain function along more than one experimental strategy. One involved direct studies of human cerebral processes in relation to conscious, subjective experience (e.g., Libet, 1973, 1982, 1985a). The other has been at the synaptic transmitter level, as it relates to slow functions of the brain. This stemmed from early work with Ralph Gerard on slow or "steady" potentials in brain (e.g., Gerard and Libet, 1940; Libet and Gerard, 1941) in which we had discovered modes of cerebral neuronal interaction that seemed to require mechanisms different from those available in fast axonal and synaptic transmissions. That expectation attracted me to investigate the slow potentials observed by Rose Eccles in sympathetic ganglia (Eccles, 1952), and that led to discoveries and analyses of a whole new class of slow synaptic mechanisms by myself and then many others. The characteristics of these slow synaptic actions greatly expanded the availability of processes that could help to mediate the slower and many of the higher functions of the brain (e.g., Libet, 1978, 1986).

1. Classical and Nonclassical Synaptic Actions

Classical synaptic functions of neurotransmitters are those involved in eliciting the (fast) EPSPs and IPSPs. These PSPs have synaptic delays in fractions of a millisecond and durations in tens of milliseconds; they produce direct and additive changes in postsynaptic level of excitation leading to firing; they are generated by increases in specific ionic conductances, induced by the respective transmitter–receptor interactions; their synaptic junctions are morphologically highly organized with pre- and postsynaptic elements closely apposed though separated by a structured cleft of 200 Å (e.g., Eccles, 1964). Nonclassical transmitter functions may be categorized into two groups: (1) production of slow PSPs and (2) neuromodulatory actions that affect the efficacy of synaptic functions.

Benjamin Libet • Department of Physiology, School of Medicine, University of California, San Francisco, California 94143.

1.1. Slow PSPs

Mammalian sympathetic ganglia exhibit two cholinergic, muscarinically mediated slow PSPs, the s-IPSP and s-EPSP, and a noncholinergic ss-EPSP (see Fig. 1) (Libet, 1970, 1979a; Ashe and Libet, 1981a). The muscarinic step for the mammalian s-IPSP is postulated to occur at dopamine (DA)-containing interneurons (the SIF cells), and the DA released thereby would be the direct inhibitory transmitter (Eccles and Libet, 1961; Libet, 1970; Libet and Tosaka, 1970). Although this view is further supported by several lines of evidence (Libet and Owman, 1974; Dun and Karczmar, 1978; Ashe and Libet, 1982), the possibility of an additional s-IPSP component mediated by a direct muscarinic action on the principal neurons is not excluded (see Cole and Shinnick-Gallagher, 1984; Libet, 1985b). The noncholinergic ss-EPSP is probably mediated by an as yet inadequately identified peptide [possibly substance P or vasoactive intestinal peptide (VIP); e.g., Konishi *et al.*, 1979; Dun and Karczmar, 1979; Katayama and North, 1978; Kawatani *et al.*, 1985). In frog ganglia, the peptide LH-RF has in fact been identified as the transmitter for the similar noncholinergic ss-EPSP there; see Jan and Jan (1982).] The mammalian sympathetic ganglion thus contains analyzable models for the postsynaptic actions of ACh, both nicotinic and muscarinic, of a catecholamine (DA), and of one or more neuropeptides. Additionally, DA serves also as a postsynaptic neuromodulator, enhancing the responses to ACh (see below).

s-IPSP, s-EPSP, and ss-EPSP have synaptic delays of 10s, 100s, and 1000s of milliseconds, respectively; durations are from seconds up to 30 min; responses to repetitive inputs integrate over seconds to minutes; electrogenic mechanisms include novel ones, with no change in membrane conductance (Kobayashi and Libet, 1968; Hashiguchi *et al.*, 1978, 1982), or a decrease (Kobayashi and Libet, 1968, 1970; Weight and Votava, 1970; Brown and Adams, 1980; Constanti and Brown, 1981), or a small increase in membrane conductance (Nishi, 1979; Cole and Shinnick-Gallagher, 1984; Brown and Selyanko, 1985; Mochida and Kobayashi, 1986); this

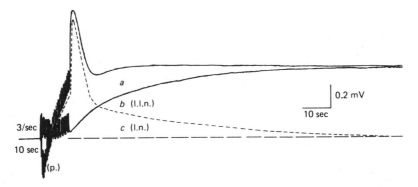

Figure 1. Various postsynaptic potentials of rabbit superior cervical ganglion, elicited by supramaximal stimulation of preganglionic (cervical sympathetic) nerve at 3 per sec for 10 sec and recorded extracellularly. D-Tubocurarine is present to prevent firing by the nicotinic fast EPSPs; the depressed f-EPSPs appear spike-like in this slow-speed tracing. In tracing b, taken after also adding the potent muscarinic antagonist QNB (quinuclidinyl benzilate hydrochloride at 0.05 μM), only the nicotinic f-EPSPs (during the 10-sec stimulus train) and the noncholinergic ss-EPSP ("l.l.n.," late–late surface negative component) are visible; the ss-EPSP continued beyond the tracing shown, declining slowly over 20 min. In tracing a, taken before adding QNB, the s-IPSP ("p.," surface positive) and the s-EPSP ("l.n.," late negative), each of which involves a muscarinic step, are seen superimposed on the nicotinic f-EPSPs and the noncholinergic ss-EPSP that remained in tracing b. Tracing c shows a subtraction of tracing b from a; it shows the presumed contributions of s-IPSP and s-EPSP ("l.n.") to the tracing in a. The muscarinic s-EPSP peaks at about 15 sec from start of the preganglionic train and persists for 1–2 min. The noncholinergic ss-EPSP begins after a delay of some seconds, peaks at about 1.5 min, and persists for 20 min (or 30 min after a stimulus train at 10–20 per sec). (From Ahse and Libet, 1981a.)

contrasts with the large increases in membrane conductance characteristic of fast PSPs. Transmitter delivery is often by way of more diffuse, longer distances from release sites to postsynaptic receptors; such morphological arrangements have been termed "loose synaptic" (Libet, 1965, 1979a,b, 1980, 1986) or "nonsynaptic" (e.g., Descarries *et al.*, 1977; Dismukes, 1979) or "parasynaptic" (Schmitt, 1984). (For reviews of all these features, see Libet, 1970, 1979a, 1986.)

1.2. Neuromodulatory Actions

Neuromodulatory actions may be distinctively defined as those in which a neurotransmitter alters synaptic efficacy of the neural inputs by means other than itself eliciting an EPSP or IPSP, whether these be fast or slow (Libet, 1979b, 1986; Schmitt, 1984). Known modes of modulation are growing in number, including various forms of control of presynaptic function, but they will not be reviewed here. In mammalian sympathetic ganglia a modulatory action was discovered (Libet and Tosaka, 1970) that is especially interesting for issues of long-lasting postsynaptic interactions among different inputs in brain. In this, DA (whether applied exogenously or released intraganglionically by orthodromic neural input) can induce a long-term enhancement (LTE) of the slow PSPs (or of the equivalent responses to test applications of ACh or its muscarinic agonists, methacholine or bethanechol; see Fig. 2). (1) The enhancement lasts for more than 3 hr after DA is gone. (2) It is mediated by a specific DA receptor, the so-called D_1 type coupled to adenylate cyclase (Ashe and Libet, 1981b; Mochida *et al.*, 1981, 1987; Libet and Mochida, 1987); by contrast, the inhibitory action of DA is mediated by an α_2 (adrenergic) receptor (Brown

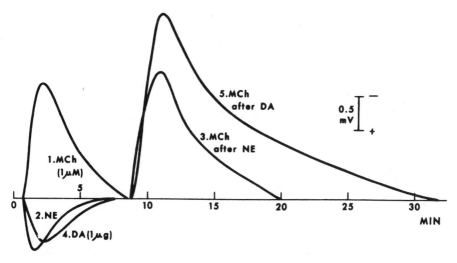

Figure 2. Modulatory enhancement of slow muscarinic depolarizations by DA. Surface-recorded responses of rabbit SCG (22°C) in a sucrose-gap chamber. The ganglion was pretreated with the potent muscarinic agonist bethanechol (BCh) to deplete intraganglionic DA; this procedure eliminates the initial hyperpolarizing component normally seen in the responses to methacholine (MCh) (see Libet and Owman, 1974). The first test shown is the response to a single-bolus injection of 1 μM MCh (approximately 200 μg) into the ganglionic superfusate. Test 2 is the response to 1 μg NE. Test 3 is a repeat of MCh, as in test 1, done shortly after the hyperpolarizing response to NE finished. Test 4 shows the response to 1 μg DA injected after the conclusion of MCh response 3. Test 5 is a repeat of MCh, as in test 1, shortly after the hyperpolarizing response to DA finished. The substantial increase in amplitude and duration of the MCh response seen in test 5 after DA, but not in test 3 after NE, can be seen in succeeding tests with MCh, repeated for some hours, even though no further DA is applied. (From Libet, 1979a, based on experiments reported in Libet and Tosaka, 1970.)

and Caulfield, 1979; Ashe and Libet, 1982). (3) The LTE can be elicited heterosynaptically (Mochida and Libet, 1985); i.e., orthodromic conditioning impulses, e.g., 10/sec for 120 sec, in one preganglionic bundle can induce LTE of test s-EPSP responses to brief trains of impulses in another bundle. This feature introduced a modulatory interaction among inputs from different sources, in which one neurotransmitter (DA) induces a persisting conditioning of the postsynaptic mechanism mediating PSP responses to another neurotransmitter (ACh here). Such heterosynaptic interaction distinguishes this LTE from the so-called long-term potentiation (LTP) described in the hippocampus (e.g., Bliss, 1979) and also in sympathetic ganglia (Brown and McAfee, 1982).

2. cGMP as Intracellular Messenger for s-EPSP

For the membrane changes mediating muscarinic s-EPSP in mammalian sympathetic ganglia, we found either no changes in conductance or, at more depolarized levels of resting membrane potential (V_m), decreases in conductance (Kobayashi and Libet, 1968, 1970; Hashiguchi et al., 1978). [In frog sympathetic neurons, no s-EPSP is exhibited by intact cells (Libet et al., 1968), but depolarized cells do exhibit an s-EPSP correlated with a decrease in conductance (Kobayashi and Libet, 1968, 1970; Brown and Adams, 1980; cf. Weight and Votava, 1970).] The decreases in conductance were subsequently explained as a muscarinic closure of "M" channels, a new class of voltage-sensitive K^+ channels which are otherwise opened relatively slowly by depolarizations to V_m between -60 and -20 mV (Brown and Adams, 1980; Constanti and Brown, 1981; Hashiguchi et al., 1982); muscarinic action blocks this outward M current, resulting in a decrease in conductance and a slow further depolarizing change. In s-EPSP responses of mammalian ganglion cells at normal resting V_m of about -70 mV, an M component of s-EPSP depolarization is absent, since the M channels are already closed without a muscarinic action (Hashiguchi et al., 1982). More recently, an additional component of inward current due to voltage-independent increases in conductance (perhaps of Cl^- ion) has also been attributed to the muscarinic action (Brown and Selyanko, 1985; Mochida and Kobayashi, 1986). The significance of such a component remains to be established but it appears likely to be a main source of the later "secondary" phase of the mammalian s-EPSP (Mochida and Libet, 1987); the latter phase appears as a 1- to 2-min-long "tail" of depolarization following the initial larger phase of about 10–20 sec in duration, as in Fig. 1, tracing c.

The predominant contribution to muscarinic slow depolarization appears to come from an electrogenic mechanism associated with no detectable change in conductance, within intact mammalian ganglia in neurons with resting V_m at -70 mV, or at all V_m values negative to -60 mV (Hashiguchi et al., 1978, 1982) (see Fig. 3). cGMP meets the criteria for designation as an intracellular mediator of this component of muscarinic depolarization: (1) Muscarinic agents activate guanylate cyclase, inducing an increase in neuronal cGMP in mammalian sympathetic ganglia (Kebabian et al., 1975; Volle et al., 1982). It should be noted that Volle et al. reported that the increase in cGMP, induced in rat SCG by stimulation of preganglionic nerve, could not be blocked by 10 μM atropine. One may suggest that Volle et al. uncovered an additional non-muscarinic activating mechanism which provides cGMP for a function other than slow muscarinic depolarization. (2) Dibutyryl-cGMP applied exogenously can mimic the muscarinic action in question. cGMP produces a slow depolarization in rabbit SCG (McAfee and Greengard, 1972; Hashiguchi et al., 1978, 1982). But, more importantly, the depolarization induced by cGMP at concentrations of 100 μM or less, occurs with no change in membrane conductance (Hashiguchi et al., 1978, 1982; Fig. 3). This mechanism is voltage-independent and matches the characteristics of the depolarization by muscarine when obtained at resting V_m values more negative than about -55 mV (Hashiguchi et al., 1978, 1982). Higher concentrations of cGMP can elicit a further depolarizing component that is associated with an increase in membrane conductance (Hashiguchi et al., 1978). The depolarizing effect of higher concentrations could represent a

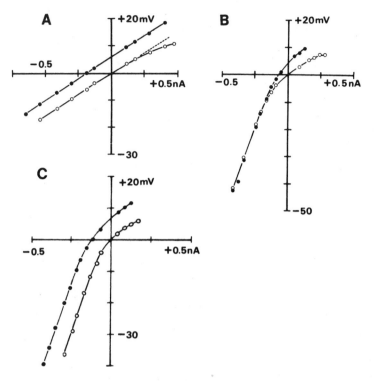

Figure 3. Changes in membrane conductance with depolarizations by muscarine or by cGMP, as seen in voltage–current (V–I) curves. V–I points were obtained with the current-clamp method, using 1-sec pulses of constant current. For each cell, V–I curves with no agent (○) and with agent present (●) are shown. (A) (±)-Muscarine-Cl (10 μM), and (C) dibutyryl-cGMP (100 μM), both in rabbit SCG cells; (B) muscarine (10 μM) in a frog sympathetic ganglion cell. Resting membrane potentials (V_m) before application of the chemical agent, plotted as zero voltages at the origin, were -61.5 mV in A, -51 mV in B, and -51 mV in C. Note that a muscarinic depolarization accompanied by an *increased* membrane resistance (increased slope of V–I), i.e., one due to block of "M" channels, occurs only at depolarized V_m values (less negative than about -60 mV) in both A and B. However, in A, the rabbit cell exhibits a large depolarization (upward displacement of V–I line) at all V_m values with no change in resistance (slope), i.e., one *not* due to M channel blockade. Frog cells (B) show no muscarinic depolarization at all V_m values negative to -60 mV, i.e., they only have a muscarinic M component of slow depolarization. The cGMP depolarizing shift in a rabbit cell (C) occurs with no change in resistance at all V_m values, i.e., cGMP mimics only the main component of muscarinic depolarization in the mammalian neuron (in A), but not the ability of muscarine to block M channels. (From Hashiguchi *et al.*, 1978, 1982.)

different, nonspecific action by cGMP which can be exerted even on peripheral nerve (McAfee and Greengard, 1972) and it is also seen with the other cyclic nucleotide, cAMP (Gallagher and Shinnick-Gallagher, 1977). (3) Specific pharmacological antagonists of cGMP have not been tested. Inhibitors of phosphodiesterases should enhance a cGMP-mediated muscarinic depolarization; however, they would also protect cAMP which, as seen below, exerts a potent modulatory effect on muscarinic depolarizing responses and that would confound the interpretation relative to cGMP (see Libet, 1979c).

cGMP and Muscarinic Responses in the CNS

In most spinal motoneurons tested, Krnjević *et al.* (1976) found that cGMP applied intracellularly produced an increase in membrane conductance (fall in resistance) and, most commonly, some depolarization (with a smaller number exhibiting a consistent hyperpolarization). This did not match the action of ACh, which produced a decrease in conductance; since ACh also had this effect when applied intracellularly, there is a question of how this ACh effect is related to any physiological one that would be mediated via extracellular attachment to the muscarinic receptor. The increase in conductance with cGMP (Krnjević *et al.*, 1976) is also at variance with a decrease, reported for intracellular application in some cerebral neurons (Woody *et al.*, 1978), and with no change, found for depolarizations by minimal extracellular applications to mammalian sympathetic neurons (Hashiguchi *et al.*, 1978, 1982). Perhaps intracellular injections can engage processes that reflect the potentially multiple roles of cGMP as a cell messenger. Extracellular applications within the CNS can also produce effects not limited to the presumed target cell, a problem that is not a serious one in the case of the relatively homogeneous population of neurons in sympathetic ganglia.

3. Role of cAMP In the Postsynaptic Actions of DA

3.1. DA Activation of Adenylate Cyclase

Following on our evidence that DA appeared to be a synaptic transmitter in mammalian sympathetic ganglia (Libet and Tosaka, 1970; Libet, 1970), DA was shown to stimulate adenylate cyclase and raise the cAMP content of bovine SCG when chopped into small bits of tissue (Kebabian and Greengard, 1971). Although stimulation of preganglionic nerve also raises cAMP in rabbit and rat SCG (Aleman *et al.*, 1974; Kalix *et al.*, 1974; Volle *et al.*, 1982), DA applied exogenously in the bathing medium of whole SCGs of rabbit and rat was reported to produce only small (Kalix *et al.*, 1974) or insignificant increases in cAMP (Lindl and Cramer, 1975; Quenzer *et al.*, 1979) although more substantial increases have also been reported (Wamsley *et al.*, 1980).

COMT Barriers

The reports of ineffectiveness of DA activation of adenylate cyclase in whole ganglia are now explicable in terms of intraganglionic catechol-*o*-methyl transferase (COMT), which could limit the ability of DA to reach the appropriate postsynaptic receptors within the ganglion. Although exogenous DA has been found to induce LTE of slow depolarizing responses of surface-recorded neurons to an exogenous muscarinic agonist (Libet and Tosaka, 1970; Libet *et al.*, 1975), exogenous DA was relatively ineffective for inducing enhancement of the s-EPSP recorded as an extracellular response of the whole rabbit SCG unless COMT was blocked by the inhibitor U-0521 (3′,4′-dihydroxy-2-methylproPriophenone) (see Fig. 4) (Ashe and Libet, 1981b). Similarly, in the presence of U-0521, DA does consistently induce a substantial increase (> 50%) in the cAMP content of the intact rabbit SCG (Mochida *et al.*, 1981, 1987). It should be noted that the β adrenergic agonist, isoproterenol, can also induce a substantial rise in ganglionic cAMP (Lindl and Cramer, 1975; Volle *et al.*, 1982; Mochida *et al.*, 1987). Which receptors may be involved in synaptically significant activations of adenylate cyclase will be discussed below.

Suitable conditioning stimulation of preganglionic nerve can induce an apparently DA-mediated enhancement of s-EPSP responses even in the absence of a COMT inhibitor (Libet and Mochida, 1987); this suggests that synaptically released DA can, at the presumably high local concentrations achieved, reach postsynaptic sites adequately. Stimulation of preganglionic nerve can also deplete the DA content of intraganglionic interneurons, the small intensely fluorescent (SIF) cells in rabbit SCG (Libet and Owman, 1974); this is taken to signify that an orthodromic, muscarinically mediated release of DA from these cells occurs. One may therefore assume that DA released synaptically by orthodromic, preganglionic input can induce a postsynaptic increase in ganglionic cAMP. This would not exclude additional mechanisms from contributing to the

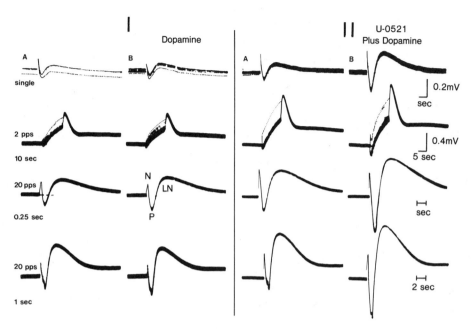

Figure 4. Enhancement of slow PSPs by DA; effect of a COMT inhibitor. Pair of rabbit SCGs, I and II, curarized (D-tubocurarine, 50 μM) to abolish firing of ganglion cells by f-EPSP. (Dihydroergotamine, 45 μM, was present in both ganglia.) Responses were recorded with surface electrodes, one on ganglion and the other on postganglionic nerve. Preganglionic nerve was stimulated supramaximally, as indicated at left for each horizontal row. For each ganglion, column A gives test responses *before* and column B test responses approximately 45 min *after* the exposure to and washout of DA (and of U-0521). For ganglion II, U-0521 (0.3 mM) was added to bathing medium 30 min before the addition of DA (50 μM); after an additional 30 min with both agents they were washed out. Components labeled N (surface negative), P (positive), and LN (late negative) indicate net recordable f-EPSP, s-IPSP, and s-EPSP, respectively. Voltage calibration in second row of column II applies to rows 2–4. (From Ashe and Libet, 1981b.)

orthodromically induced increase in cAMP, e.g., in glia cells or in presynaptic terminals (Volle *et al.*, 1982).

COMT may thus play a role less potent but analogous to that of cholinesterase in ACh transmission (Ashe and Libet, 1981b). The access of exogenous ACh to its receptors is clearly limited by cholinesterase; an anticholinesterase drug is often required in order to obtain a response. Postsynaptic responses to endogenous, synaptically released ACh obviously are producible in spite of cholinesterase, but the latter presumably does limit the spread of such ACh to more distant sites. COMT may act in a qualitatively similar manner, not only in ganglia but perhaps also in brain, although its potency in such a function is probably well below that of the powerful cholinesterase enzymes. It should be noted that our findings, on the kind and significance of the effects of COMT inhibition, are in good general accord with the earlier report by Belfrage *et al.* (1977). These authors found that COMT blockade was much more influential for peripheral vasodilator responses to exogenous noradrenaline than to nerve stimulation; this would be analogous to our similar distinction between the effects of exogenous versus neurally released (endogenous) DA, for inducing either LTE (of s-EPSP responses) or an increase in cAMP. The proposal by Belfrage *et al.* (1977) that COMT is of physiological importance mainly at receptor sites not in close contact with peripheral sympathetic effector nerve endings, would also have a bearing on our synaptically mediated actions by DA; as indicated above, the inhibitory and modulatory actions of DA are apparently mediated mostly via "loose" or "nonsynaptic" morphological arrangements between release sites and postsynaptic receptors.

3.2. cAMP Does Not Mediate s-IPSP

It was initially proposed (McAfee and Greengard, 1972; Greengard, 1976) that the cAMP produced in response to DA is the intracellular mediator of the hyperpolarizing inhibitory (s-IPSP) action of DA, one of the two synaptic actions we had established (Libet and Tosaka, 1970; Libet, 1970; Libet and Owman, 1974). The electrophysiological and pharmacological evidence on which that proposal was based turned out to be interpretable in a different manner, and further evidence argued against an inhibitory role for cAMP in sympathetic ganglia (reviewed by Libet, 1979c). It should be noted that a separate proposal for cAMP as mediator of noradrenergic inhibition of Purkinje cells in the cerebellum has been developed with several lines of supporting evidence (Bloom, 1979) although even that proposal has been subjected to serious questioning (e.g., Phillis, 1977; reviewed in Drummond, 1983).

3.3. cAMP Appears to Mediate the Modulatory Action of DA

Exogenous bath application of dibutyryl-cAMP at 100 µM for 5 min can induce the same kind of LTE of slow muscarinic depolarizations that had been found to be induced by a brief exposure to DA (see Fig. 5) (Libet, 1979c; Libet *et al.*, 1975; Mochida *et al.*, 1981, 1987). An intracellular injection of cAMP also induced a similar LTE of s-EPSP responses (Kobayashi *et al.*, 1978). The similarity of these postsynaptic actions by DA and cAMP extends to the ability of cGMP to block the LTE induced either by DA or by applied cAMP; both LTEs are antagonized by cGMP in the same time-dependent manner (see below).

3.3.1. D_1 Receptor as Mediator Both of LTE and cAMP Increases

The receptors in brain that are relatively specific for DA, as distinguished from the α and β adrenergic receptors, are largely classifiable into those which are coupled to and activate adeny-

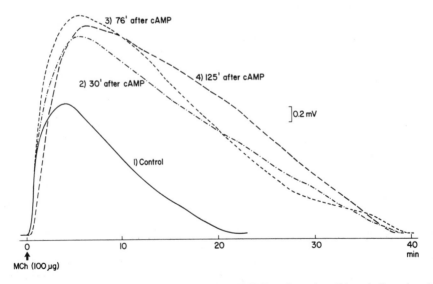

Figure 5. Modulation of slow muscarinic depolarizations by cAMP. Experimental conditions similar to those in Fig. 2. After "control" depolarizing response (1) to a test dose of MCh, the ganglion was superfused for 8 min with Ringer containing dibutyryl-cAMP (1 mM) (instead of being briefly exposed to DA or NE, as in Fig. 2). Subsequent test responses to MCh were made at 30, 76, and 125 min after ending the exposure to cAMP (shown in tracings 2–4, respectively). (From data reported in Libet, 1984, based on data reported in Libet *et al.*, 1975.)

late cyclase (D_1) and those which do not (D_2) (Kebabian and Calne, 1979; Kebabian *et al.*, 1986; Seeman, 1980). Pharmacological antagonists against DA may act against both types of receptors, but often with relative selectivity—especially SCH-23390 and flupenthixol on D_1, and sulpiride and domperidone on D_2. That DA induces LTE of slow muscarinic PSPs via a D_1 receptor was indicated by (1) the ability of DA to activate adenylate cyclase in ganglionic preparations (see Section 3.1); (2) the depression of DA-induced LTE (of s-EPSP) by the DA antagonists (+)-butaclamol or spiroperidol but not by the more selective D_2 antagonists sulpiride or metoclopramide (Ashe and Libet, 1981b); and (3) also not by the adrenergic antagonist dihydroergotamine (Ashe and Libet, 1981b). It should be noted that the other, hyperpolarizing action of DA is achieved via an adrenergic receptor (Libet and Tosaka, 1970) or, more precisely, an α_2 receptor (Brown and Caulfield, 1979).

It has now been demonstrated in the same sympathetic ganglion, the rabbit SCG (Mochida *et al.*, 1981, 1987), that DA and its analogue ADTN can each induce both (1) LTE of slow depolarizing responses to a muscarinic agonist and (2) a substantial increase in cAMP (Figs. 6 and 7). Conversely, antagonists of DA-induced LTE also depressed DA-induced increases in cAMP; these antagonists included those relatively specific against D_1 receptors, SCH-23390 and flupenthixol (see Iorio *et al.*, 1983; Hyttel, 1983; Seeman, 1980), as well as less specific ones, haloperidol and butaclamol (see Fig. 7). The relatively specific D_2 antagonists sulpiride and domperidone (see Seeman, 1980) affected neither of the two DA actions. Further, α_2 agonists (methylnorepinephrine and clonidine) produced no LTE, although they do produce a hyperpolarizing response, while the general α antagonist dihydroergotamine did not affect either of the DA actions listed as (1) and (2).

3.3.2. Adrenergic β Actions

The β antagonist propranolol did depress the DA-induced increase in cAMP to about the same degree as did the specific DA antagonists (like butaclamol), i.e., by about 50%. Application of butaclamol and propranolol together completely suppressed the increase in cAMP by DA (see Fig. 7). This suggests that DA can activate adenylate cyclase independently at both D_1 and β receptors. The β agonist isoproterenol could induce both a substantial LTE (of muscarinic depolarizations) and an increase in cAMP. Yet, the β antagonist propranolol had no effect on the LTE induced by DA or by isoproterenol. Putting all this together would indicate that not all receptor-coupled increases in intracellular cAMP are effective in producing the LTE modulatory change in muscarinic responses; cAMP produced at D_1 receptors is effective while that produced at β-adrenergic receptors may not be (Mochida *et al.*, 1987).

Perhaps β-induced increased in cAMP occur at different sites, e.g., in glia cells (Kalix *et al.*, 1974), or they may subserve other neuronal functions (Quenzer *et al.*, 1979; Dun *et al.*, 1984).

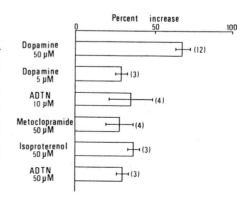

Figure 6. Induction of rise in cAMP content by treatment with DA and some other agents. Increase in one of the paired ganglia in response to an agent was compared with the cAMP levels in the contralateral ganglion without any treatment (baseline value) and expressed as the percentage increase over it. Each bar represents the mean percentage difference ± S.E.M. for the pairs of ganglia tested (numbers in parentheses) for each agent. COMT inhibitor U-0521 was present during the treatment with DA (5 and 50 μM) and ADTN (10 μM) but not for metoclopramide, isoproterenol, and ADTN 50 μM. (From Mochida *et al.*, 1987.)

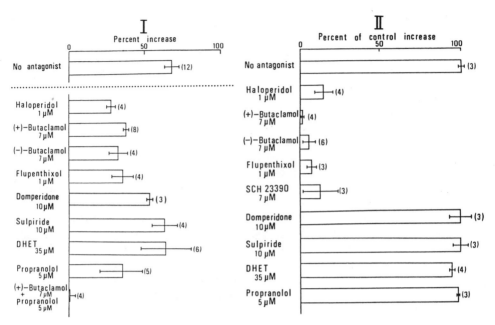

Figure 7. Effects of various antagonists on (column I) DA-induced increase in cAMP content, and on (column II) DA-induced LTE of muscarinic slow depolarizing responses.

Column I: In each experiment, one ganglion of a pair (rabbit SCGs) was treated with DA (50 μM in the presence of U-0521), the other ganglion was untreated. Horizontal bars indicate the percent increase in cAMP in DA-treated over that in the paired untreated ganglion, when no antagonist was present (topmost bar) and when an antagonist was present throughout (as in each lower bar). Each bar gives the mean percentage increase ± S.E.M. for the indicated number of paired ganglia tested for each antagonist. Note that (1) agents capable of D_1 antagonism (haloperidol, (+)-butaclamol, flupenthixol; see Seeman, 1980) produced substantial depression (about −50% ±) of the DA action; (2) (−)-butaclamol was equally effective, unlike the findings in cerebral striatal tissue; (3) the relatively selective D_2 antagonists (domperidone and sulpiride) and the α adrenergic antagonist [dihydroergotamine (DHET)] were rather ineffective. (4) The β adrenergic antagonist (propranolol) was about as effective as the D_1 antagonists, but (5) combined presence of butaclamol and propranolol produced an additive effect and completely suppressed the DA-induced increase in cAMP. (The incomplete blockade by D_1 or β antagonists, respectively, and the complete blockade by their combination, indicates DA is stimulating adenylate cyclase via actions separately at both D_1- and β-type receptors in this tissue.)

Column II: In each experiment, paired ganglia were tested at 30-min intervals (in a sucrose-gap chamber, as in Libet and Tosaka, 1970; Libet et al., 1975) with brief exposures to the muscarinic agonist acetyl-β-methacholine (MCh). After the initial two tests with MCh, all ganglia were exposed briefly to DA (15 μM); amplitudes of MCh slow depolarizations after DA were greater than in the tests before DA. For MCh tests at 60 min after DA, the mean increase, in three experiments (six ganglia) with no antagonist present (topmost horizontal bar), was about +68%. This was taken to be the "control" increase for comparison with experiments with an antagonist present. In the latter cases, one ganglion of the pair had an antagonist present throughout, starting 1 hr before the first tests with MCh. Each bar shows the fraction of DA enhancement still remaining in the presence of an antagonist, expressed as a percentage of the DA enhancement (increase in MCh response) in the paired ganglion with no antagonist present; each bar gives the mean value (± S.E.M.) of such percentile fractions, for the experiments (number indicated) with each antagonist. Note that D_1 antagonists (including the highly selective one, SCH-23390; see Iorio et al., 1983) strongly depress the DA-induced LTE; the D_2, α, and β antagonists have no significant effects. (Especially noteworthy is the lack of effect by propranolol on DA LTE, contrasting with its effect on DA-induced cAMP in column I.) (From Mochida et al., 1987.)

Indeed, Madison and Nicoll (1986) found that a norepinephrine β action, perhaps via cAMP, depresses the afterhyperpolarization and thus facilitates repetitive firing in hippocampal neurons.

4. cGMP as an Antagonist of cAMP

In the process of investigating whether DA modulatory enhancement would be demonstrable for depolarizing responses to cGMP, as the putative mediator of slow muscarinic depolarizations, surprising additional features of cGMP actions were discovered (Libet *et al.*, 1975): (1) Application of cGMP after a brief exposure of the ganglion to DA (or to cAMP) could antagonize or block the development of the modulatory LTE change (in muscarinic PSPs) that otherwise followed such treatment by either DA or cAMP. (2) But, additionally, this antagonist property of cGMP was time-dependent. It was only effective if cGMP was applied during the initial 5 to 10 min after the exposure to DA (or to cAMP); if cGMP was applied later than that, the enhancement of later muscarinic tests appears as usual for some hours (see Fig. 8). (3) Furthermore, a later exposure to DA (or cAMP), one not followed by cGMP, could still induce an LTE of subsequent muscarinic tests; i.e., cGMP did not destroy the production and storage process, but only antagonized the process while it (cGMP) was present. Clearly, cGMP did not affect the slow muscarinic depolarizing response itself; nor did it antagonize the expression of the neuronal change responsible for the enhanced muscarinic responses. Rather, cGMP apparently antagonized the *process of producing* the persisting modulatory change. In this, cGMP may be directly antagonizing the action of cAMP, the putative mediator of this production process.

4.1. Storage of a Neuronal Memory Trace and Its "Disruptability"

The foregoing findings provide features that are remarkably appropriate to the production and storage of an intermediate-term neuronal memory trace (Libet *et al.*, 1975; Libet, 1984). The time-dependence of the antagonistic action by cGMP indicates there is a qualitative distinction between a more durable form of the neuronal change, that expresses the DA-induced LTE, and the production or "storage" process by which that durable change is laid down in the cell. It is only the storage "consolidation" process that can be affected or antagonized by cGMP, during the initial 5 to 10 min following exposure to DA (or to cAMP). (A schema of the postulated intracellular processes is given in Fig. 9.) Such a pattern is highly reminiscent of the psychological–behavioral time factors in learning and memory; for these it is well known that there is an early period of some minutes after a learning experience during which the "consolidation" of the memory trace is more easily "disruptable" by other neural inputs, even though there is little effect on memory traces already stored at earlier times (e.g., Gerard, 1955; McGaugh, 1966; McGaugh and Gold, 1976).

The DA-modulating action thus provides a model in which development and storage of a memory trace and its retention as a durable change for at least many hours, are all accomplished within a single neuron. cAMP is the intracellular mediator of this DA action, suggesting the possibility that production of a phosphoprotein via a cAMP-dependent protein kinase may be a part of the durable neuronal alteration (e.g., Greengard, 1976; Rodknight, 1982). The postsynaptic location of such a memory trace, and the ability to induce such an LTE heterosynaptically (Mochida and Libet, 1985), provides the opportunity for "learning interactions" among different neural inputs that converge on the same neuron; in the present, specific case, the memory trace is initiated by a brief (dopaminergic) input in one synaptic line, while the "readout" of the memory consists simply in the enhanced ability of the postsynaptic unit to produce its specific response to another (cholinergic) input. This arrangement provides for a "learned" change in the response to one input as a result of an "experience" previously carried in by way of another input.

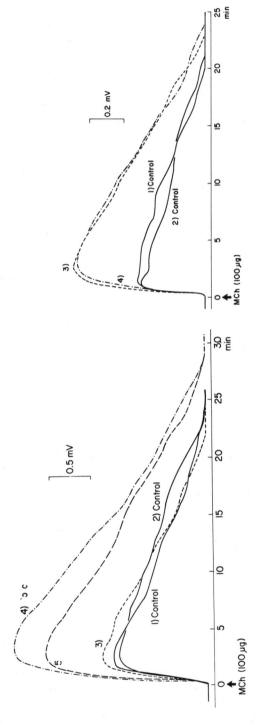

Figure 8. Time-dependent effect of cGMP, in antagonizing LTE, induced by DA. Experimental conditions similar to those in Fig. 2. After initial two control responses to MCh (1 and 2), each of the paired ganglia was exposed to a single dose of DA injected into the superfusing fluid. In the left ganglion, superfusion with dibutyryl-cGMP (50 μM) was begun 4 min after DA and maintained for 8 min (i.e., until 12 min after DA). Test 3, with MCh applied 35 min after DA (23 min after end of cGMP), shows no enhancement. A second exposure to DA followed test 3, but no cGMP was applied after this DA. MCh tests 4 and 5 followed the second DA by 35 and 85 min, respectively, and do show LTE; this demonstrates (1) that this ganglion was in fact capable of developing the LTE response to DA and (2) that cGMP antagonized only that LTE induced by a preceding DA action. In the right ganglion, similar superfusion with cGMP was delayed until 30 min after the first dose of DA. MCh test 3, applied 60 min after the DA (22 min after the end of cGMP), shows the usual good enhancement. A second exposure to DA followed test 3. MCh test 4, applied 60 min after the second DA, shows no further change; this demonstrates that the first DA had already elicited a maximal LTE in spite of its being followed by the cGMP that started 30 min after the DA. (From Libet *et al.*, 1975.)

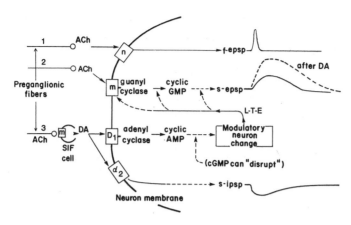

Figure 9. Schema summarizing slow postsynaptic responses to ACh and DA, and the roles therein of cAMP and cGMP, in the principal neuron ("ganglion cell") of rabbit SCG. ACh released by preganglionic axons acts at nicotinic receptors (n) to elicit f-EPSP (by increasing ionic conductance for Na^+ and K^+); at muscarinic receptor (m), to stimulate guanylate cyclase and lead to an s-EPSP (with no change in membrane conductance); at muscarinic receptor (m) on the SIF cell, which then releases DA. DA acts at α_2 receptors to elicit an s-IPSP (not mediated by cAMP; see Libet, 1979c). [An additional component of s-IPSP mediated by a direct muscarinic action of ACh on the ganglion cell is not excluded (see Cole and Shinnick-Gallagher, 1984; Libet, 1985).]

DA also acts at D_1-type receptors, separate and distinct from the α_2 receptors, to stimulate adenylate cyclase; the resultant cAMP induces LTE of the s-EPSP response to ACh (as shown by the dashed s-EPSP tracing). cGMP can antagonize ("disrupt") the storage process for producing the more enduring form of the modulatory change responsible for the LTE. Possible alternative sites at which the modulatory change is operative are indicated by the dashed arrow to points in the sequence that leads to the s-EPSP response. (From Libet, 1984, as modified from Libet *et al.*, 1975.)

4.2. Interactions between cAMP and cGMP

The kinds of interactions displayed in these neural actions are noteworthy. The interactions do not follow the simple, proposed rule "that cAMP and cGMP act in a dualistic ('yin–yang') opposing fashion" (Goldberg *et al.*, 1975; Stone *et al.*, 1975; Kebabian *et al.*, 1975). cAMP, as mediator of the DA-induced LTE, acts to synergize rather than to oppose the s-EPSP response that is apparently mediated by cGMP. However, cGMP does have the additional capability of antagonizing or opposing this modulatory action of cAMP. It seems likely that this antagonistic action of cGMP may become physiologically significant only when cGMP levels in the cell achieve sufficiently high and sustained values; under those conditions the cAMP-mediated enhancement of the cGMP-mediated s-EPSP would be suppressed in a kind of negative feedback manner (Libet, 1979c, 1984). Obviously, the present model does not exhaust the possibilities for the roles and interactions of cAMP and cGMP in neurons and other cells generally.

5. Possible Significance for Cerebral Functions

Many functions of the brain are (1) relatively slow and (2) broadly distributed. Among such are the slow electrophysiological manifestations, including slow EEG waves with periodicities in seconds; and slow components of event-related potentials (ERP), including the P_{300} component, readiness (Bereitschafts) potentials, CNVs, and other steady potential shifts lasting seconds and even minutes. Such slow potentials appear related to processes of cognition, states of attention and expectancy, decision, preparation to act, and so forth (e.g., Callaway *et al.*, 1978).

The neuronal sources of such slow potentials and even their long latencies may now be explained in terms of slow PSPs at single synapses, like those observed in sympathetic neurons; it is no longer necessary to invoke complex networks involving the brief neuronal actions of classical fast PSPs (see Libet, 1978).

The even slower, enduring, and broadly distributed cerebral processes involved in altered states of motivation, vigilance, learning and memory, and so forth may also become more tractable at neuronal levels, in terms of nonclassical synaptic actions some of which involve cyclic nucleotide mediation. The slow EPSPs, both cholinergic and peptidergic, provide for interactions of convergent inputs at a single neuron for periods of 1 to 30 min after a given input; this makes it unnecessary to postulate that reverberating circuits, based on brief synaptic actions, must underlie processes like short-term memory (see Libet, 1984). Neuromodulatory actions can form models for more enduring contingent actions. The DA–LTE model for formation of a memory trace was already discussed above. One may note that the function of D_1 receptors in the brain (those coupled to activation of adenylate cyclase) still remains to be characterized (e.g., Snyder, 1984; Krieger, 1983); the ganglionic role of D_1 receptors, in inducing LTE of muscarinic responses, is one that merits cerebral investigation. Also, muscarinic action in the brain has been reported capable of stimulating guanylate cyclase, increasing the cGMP levels for example in rat hippocampus (Black et al., 1979), as in mammalian sympathetic ganglia (see above). How this mode of muscarinic action contributes to the physiological muscarinic ACh actions in the brain is yet to be clearly established (Krnjević et al., 1976; Woody et al., 1978; Woody, and Gruen, this volume). Perhaps there is more than one membrane mechanism for generating slow muscarinic depolarizing responses, as is now evident in ganglia (Brown and Selyanko, 1985; Mochida and Kobayashi, 1986). These is a large additional repertoire of modulatory synaptic actions becoming available (e.g., see other chapters in this volume), acting at both pre- and postsynaptic sites.

The morphological substrates in the brain for such slow and broadly distributed processes have been appearing. The monoamine projections from the brain stem innervate wide regions of the brain. Their synaptic relationships to the receptors involved are often not closely organized (e.g., Descarries et al., 1977; Reader et al., 1979, this volume) and have been termed nonsynaptic, loose synaptic (Libet, 1965, 1979b), or parasynaptic (Schmitt, 1984). The small number of dopaminergic SIF cell-interneurons in rabbit SCG similarly give rise to a profuse network of beaded fibers which surround all principal neurons (Libet and Owman, 1974) but make appositions largely by less specialized contacts, with pre- to postdistances greater than the classical 200 Å (see Dail and Evan, 1978). The ACh-receptor system in the brain is predominantly muscarinic in nature and also widely distributed (Dykes et al., this volume; Mesulam, this volume). The extraordinary number of different neurally identified peptides in the brain (see elsewhere in this volume; also Hökfelt et al., 1980; Krieger, 1983) offers many speculative possibilities, although specific synaptic functions have mostly not been defined for these potentially potent substances.

In short, nonclassical synaptic functions, including those shown to involve mediation by cyclic nucleotides, may provide mechanisms relevant to the more interesting and unique features of brain function, while classical synaptic functions are more suitable to functions that require relatively fast and discretely localized messages.

ACKNOWLEDGMENT. The work on synaptic processes in sympathetic ganglia was supported by USPHS Grant NS-00884.

References

Aleman, V., Bayon, A., and Molina, J., 1974, Functional changes of synapses, Adv. Behav. Biol. **10:**115–124.
Ashe, J. H., and Libet, B., 1981a, Orthodromic production of noncholinergic slow depolarizing response in superior cervical ganglion of rabbit, J. Physiol. (London) **320:**333–346.
Ashe, J. H., and Libet, B., 1981b, Modulation of slow postsynaptic potentials by dopamine, in rabbit sympathetic ganglion, Brain Res. **217:**93–106.

Ashe, J. H., and Libet, B., 1982, Pharmacological properties and monoaminergic mediation of the slow IPSP, in mammalian sympathetic ganglion, *Brain Res.* **242**:345–349.

Belfrage, E., Fredholm, B. B., and Rosell, S., 1977, Effect of catechol-O-methyl-transferase (COMT) inhibition on the vascular and metabolic responses to noradrenaline, isoprenaline and sympathetic nerve stimulation in canine subcutaneous adipose tissue, *Naunyn-Schmiedebergs Arch. Pharmacol.* **300**:11–17.

Black, A. C., Sandquist, D., West, J. R., Wamsley, J. K., and Williams, T. H., 1979, Muscarinic cholinergic stimulation increases cyclic GMP levels in rat hippocampus, *J. Neurochem.* **33**:1165–1168.

Bliss, T. V. P., 1979, Synaptic plasticity in the hippocampus, *Trends Neurosci.* **2**:42–45.

Bloom, F. E., 1979, Cyclic nucleotides in central synaptic function, *Fed. Proc.* **38**:2203–2207.

Brown, D. A., and Adams, P. R., 1980, Muscarinic suppression of a novel voltage-sensitive K^+ current in a vertebrate neurone, *Nature* **283**:673–676.

Brown, D. A., and Caulfield, M. P., 1979, Hyperpolarizing "α_2" adrenoreceptors in rat sympathetic ganglia, *Br. J. Pharmacol.* **65**:435–445.

Brown, D. A., and Selyanko, A. A., 1985, Membrane currents underlying the cholinergic slow excitatory postsynaptic potential in the rat sympathetic ganglion, *J. Physiol. (London)* **365**:365–387.

Brown, T. H., and McAfee, D. A., 1982, Long-term synaptic potentiation in the superior cervical ganglion, *Science* **215**:1411–1413.

Callaway, E., Tueting, P., and Koslow, S. H. (eds.), 1978, *Event-Related Brain Potentials in Man*, Academic Press, New York.

Cole, A. E., and Shinnick-Gallagher, P., 1984, Muscarinic inhibitory transmission in mammalian sympathetic ganglia mediated by increased potassium conductance, *Nature* **307**:270–271.

Constanti, A., and Brown, D. A., 1981, M-current in voltage-clamped mammalian sympathetic neurones, *Neurosci. Lett.* **24**:289–294.

Dail, W. G., and Evan, A. P., 1978, Ultrastructure of adrenergic terminals and SIF cells in the superior cervical ganglion of the rabbit, *Brain Res.* **148**:469–477.

Descarries, L., Watkins, K. C., and Lapierre, Y., 1977, Noradrenergic axon terminals in the cerebral cortex of rat. III. Topometric ultrastructural analysis, *Brain Res.* **133**:197–222.

Dismukes, R. K., 1979, New concepts of molecular communication among neurons, *Behav. Brain Sci.* **2**:409–448.

Drummond, G. I., 1983, Cyclic nucleotides in the nervous system, *Adv. Cyclic Nucleotide Res.* **15**:373–494.

Dun, N. J., and Karczmar, A. G., 1978, Involvement of the interneuron in the generation of the slow inhibitory postsynaptic potential in mammalian sympathetic ganglia, *Proc. Natl. Acad. Sci. USA* **75**:4029–4032.

Dun, N. J., and Karczmar, A. G., 1979, Actions of substance P on sympathetic neurons, *Neuropharmacology* **18**:215–218.

Dun, N. J., Jiang, Z. G., and Mo, N., 1984, Long-term facilitation of peptidergic transmission by catecholamines in guinea-pig inferior mesenteric ganglia, *J. Physiol. (London)* **357**:37–50.

Eccles, J. C., 1964, *The Physiology of Synapses*, Springer, Berlin.

Eccles, R. M., 1952, Responses of isolated curarized sympathetic ganglia, *J. Physiol. (London)* **117**:196–217.

Eccles, R. M., and Libet, B., 1961, Origin and blockade of the synaptic responses of curarized sympathetic ganglia, *J. Physiol. (London)* **157**:484–503.

Gallagher, J. P., and Shinnick-Gallagher, P., 1977, Cyclic nucleotides injected intracellularly into rat superior cervical ganglion cells, *Science* **198**:851–852.

Gerard, R. W., 1955, The academic lecture: The biological roots of psychiatry, *Am. J. Psychiatry* **112**:81–90.

Gerard, R. W., and Libet, B., 1940, The control of normal and "convulsive" brain potentials, *Am. J. Psychiatry* **96**:1125–1151.

Goldberg, N. D., Haddox, M. K., Nicol, S. E., Glass, D. B., Sanford, C. H., Kuehl, F. A., Jr., and Estensen, R., 1975, Biologic regulation through opposing influences of cyclic GMP and cyclic AMP: The Yin-Yang hypothesis, *Adv. Cyclic Nucleotide Res.* **5**:307–330.

Greengard, P., 1976, Possible role for cyclic nucleotides and phosphorylated membrane proteins in postsynaptic actions of neurotransmitters, *Nature* **260**:101–108.

Hashiguchi, T., Ushiyama, N., Kobayashi, H., and Libet, B., 1978, Does cyclic GMP mediate the slow excitatory postsynaptic potential: Comparison of changes in membrane potential and conductance, *Nature* **271**:267–268.

Hashiguchi, T., Kobayashi, H., Tosaka, T., and Libet, B., 1982, Two muscarinic depolarizing mechanisms in mammalian sympathetic neurons, *Brain Res.* **242**:378–383.

Hökfelt, T., Johansson, O., Ljungdahl, A., Lundberg, J. M., and Schultzberg, M., 1980, Peptidergic neurones, *Nature* **284**:515–521.

Hyttel, J., 1983, SCH-23390—The first selective dopamine D-1 antagonist, *Eur. J. Pharmacol.* **91**:153–154.

Iorio, L. C., Barnett, A., Heitz, F. H., Houser, V. P., and Korduba, C. A., 1983, SCH-23390, a potent benzazepine antipsychotic with unique interactions on dopamine system, *J. Pharmacol. Exp. Ther.* **226**:462–468.

Jan, L. Y., and Jan, Y. N., 1982, Peptidergic transmission in sympathetic ganglia of the frog, *J. Physiol. (London)* **327:**219–246.

Kalix, P., McAfee, D. A., Schorderet, M., and Greengard, P., 1974, Pharmacological analysis of synaptically mediated increase in cyclic adenosine monophosphate in rabbit superior cervical ganglion, *J. Pharmacol. Exp. Ther.* **188:**676–687.

Katayama, Y., and North, R. A., 1978, Does substance P mediate slow synaptic excitation within the myenteric plexus? *Nature* **274:**387–388.

Kawatani, M., Rutigliano, M., and De Groat, W. C., 1985, Depolarization and muscarinic excitation induced in a sympathetic ganglion by vasoactive intestinal polypeptide, *Science* **229:**879–881.

Kebabian, J. W., and Calne, D. B., 1979, Multiple receptors for dopamine, *Nature* **277:**93–96.

Kebabian, J. W., and Greengard, P., 1971, Dopamine-sensitive adenyl cyclase: Possible role in synaptic transmission, *Science* **174:**1346–1349.

Kebabian, J. W., Steiner, A. L., and Greengard, P., 1975, Muscarinic cholinergic regulation of cyclic guanosine 3',5'-monophosphate in autonomic ganglia: Possible role in synaptic transmission, *J. Pharmacol. Exp. Ther.* **193:**474–488.

Kebabian, J. W., Agui, T., van Oene, J. C., Shigematsu, K., and Saavedra, J. M., 1986, The D1 dopamine receptor: New perspectives, *Trends Pharmacol. Sci.* **7:**96–99.

Kobayashi, H., and Libet, B., 1968, Generation of slow postsynaptic potentials without increases in ionic conductance, *Proc. Natl. Acad. Sci. USA* **60:**1304–1311.

Kobayashi, H., and Libet, B., 1970, Actions of noradrenaline and acetylcholine on sympathetic ganglion cells, *J. Physiol. (London)* **208:**353–372.

Kobayashi, H., Hashiguchi, T., and Ushiyama, N. S., 1978, Postsynaptic modulation of excitatory process in sympathetic ganglia by cyclic AMP, *Nature* **271:**268–270.

Konishi, S., Tsunoo, A., and Otsuka, M., 1979, Substance P and noncholinergic excitatory synaptic transmission in guinea pig sympathetic ganglia, *Proc. Jpn. Acad. Ser. B* **55:**525–530.

Krieger, D. T., 1983, Brain peptides: What, where, and why? *Science* **222:**975–985.

Krnjević, K., Puil, E., and Werman, R., 1976, Is cyclic guanosine monophosphate the internal "second messenger" for cholinergic actions on central neurons? *Can. J. Physiol. Pharmacol.* **54:**172–176.

Libet, B., 1965, Slow synaptic responses in autonomic ganglia, in: *Studies in Physiology* (D. R. Curtis and A. K. McIntyre, eds.), Springer-Verlag, Berlin, pp. 160–165.

Libet, B., 1970, Generation of slow inhibitory and excitatory postsynaptic potentials, *Fed. Proc.* **29:**1945–1956.

Libet, B., 1973, Electrical stimulation of cortex in human subjects and conscious sensory aspects, in: *Handbook of Sensory Physiology,* Vol. II (A. Iggo, ed.), Springer-Verlag, Berlin, pp. 743–790.

Libet, B., 1978, Slow postsynaptic responses in sympathetic ganglion cells, as models for the slow potential changes in the brain, in: *Multidisciplinary Perspectives in Event-Related Brain Potential Research* (D. Otto, ed.), Superintendent of Documents, Washington, D.C., pp. 12–18.

Libet, B., 1979a, Slow synaptic actions in ganglionic functions, in: *Integrative Functions of the Autonomic Nervous System* (C. M. Brooks, K. Koizumi, and A. Sato, eds.), Tokyo University Press and Elsevier/North-Holland, Amsterdam, pp. 197–222.

Libet, B., 1979b, Neuronal communication and synaptic modulation: Experimental evidence vs. conceptual categories. Commentary, pp. 431–433 to R. K. Dismukes, "New concepts of molecular communication among neurons," *Behav. Brain Sci.* **2:**409–448.

Libet, B., 1979c, Which postsynaptic action of dopamine is mediated by cyclic AMP? *Life Sci.* **24:**1043–1058.

Libet, B., 1980, Functional roles of SIF cells in slow synaptic actions, *Adv. Biochem. Psychopharmacol.* **25:**111–118.

Libet, B., 1982, Brain stimulation in the study of neuronal functions for conscious sensory experiences, *Hum. Neurobiol.* **1**(4):235–242.

Libet, B., 1984, Heterosynaptic interaction at a sympathetic neurone as a model for induction and storage of a postsynaptic memory, in: *Neurobiology of Learning and Memory* (G. Lynch, J. L. McGaugh, and N. M. Weinberger, eds.), Guilford Press, New York, pp. 405–430.

Libet, B., 1985a, Unconscious cerebral initiative and the role of conscious will in voluntary action, *Behav. Brain Sci.* **8:**529–566.

Libet, B., 1985b, Mediation of slow-inhibitory postsynaptic potentials, *Nature* **313:**161–162.

Libet, B., 1986, Non-classical synaptic functions of transmitters, *Fed. Proc.* **45:**2678–2686.

Libet, B., and Gerard, R. W., 1941, Steady potential fields and neurone activity, *J. Neurophysiol.* **4:**438–455.

Libet, B., and Mochida, S., 1987, Long-term-enhancement (LTE) of postsynaptic potentials, following neural conditioning, in mammalian sympathetic ganglia, *Brain Res.* (submitted).

Mochida, S., and Libet, B., 1987, A later secondary component of the muscarinic slow-excitatory postsynaptic potential, in mammalian sympathetic ganglia, *J. Autonomic Nerv. Sys.,* (submitted).

Libet, B., and Owman, C., 1974, Concomitant changes in formaldehyde-induced fluorescence of dopamine inter-neurones and in slow inhibitory postsynaptic potentials of rabbit superior cervical ganglion, induced by stimulation of preganglionic nerve or by a muscarinic agent, *J. Physiol. (London)* **237:**635–662.

Libet, B., and Tosaka, T., 1970, Dopamine as a synaptic transmitter and modulator in sympathetic ganglia: A different mode of synaptic action, *Proc. Natl. Acad. Sci. USA* **67:**667–673.

Libet, B., Chichibu, S., and Tosaka, T., 1968, Slow synaptic responses and excitability in sympathetic ganglia of the bullfrog, *J. Neurophysiol.* **31:**383–395.

Libet, B., Kobayashi, H., and Tanaka, T., 1975, Synaptic coupling into the production and storage of a neuronal memory trace, *Nature* **258:**155–157.

Lindl, T., and Cramer, H., 1975, Evidence against dopamine as a mediator of the rise of cyclic AMP in the superior cervical ganglion of the rat, *Biochem. Biophys. Res. Commun.* **65:**731–739.

McAfee, D. A., and Greengard, P., 1972, Adenosine 3′,5′-monophosphate: Electrophysiological evidence for a role in synaptic transmission, *Science* **178:**310–312.

McGaugh, J. L., 1966, Time-dependent processes in memory storage, *Science* **153:**1351–1358.

McGaugh, J. L., and Gold, P., 1976, Modulation of memory by electrical stimulation of the brain, in: *Neural Mechanisms of Learning and Memory* (M. R. Rosenzweig and E. L. Bennett, eds.), MIT Press, Cambridge, Mass.

Madison, D. V., and Nicoll, R. A., 1986, Actions of noradrenaline recorded intracellularly in rat hippocampal CA1 pyramidal neurons, *J. Physiol. (London)* **372:**221–244.

Mochida, S., and Kobayashi, H., 1986, Three types of muscarinic conductance changes in sympathetic neurons discriminately evoked by the different concentrations of acetylcholine, *Brain Res.* **383:**299–304.

Mochida, S., and Libet, B., 1985, Synaptic long-term-enhancement (LTE) induced by a heterosynaptic neural input, *Brain Res.* **329:**360–363.

Mochida, S., Kobayashi, H., Tosaka, T., Ito, J., and Libet, B., 1981, Specific dopamine receptor mediates the production of cyclic AMP in the rabbit sympathetic ganglia and thereby modulates the muscarinic postsynaptic responses, *Adv. Cyclic Nucleotide Res.* **14:**685.

Mochida, S., Kobayashi, H., and Libet, B., 1987, Stimulation of adenylate cyclase in relation to dopamine-induced long-term-enhancement (LTE) of muscarinic depolarization, in rabbit SCG, *J. Neurosci.* **7:**311–318.

Nishi, S., 1979, The catecholamine-mediated inhibition in ganglionic transmission, in: *Integrative Functions of the Autonomic Nervous System* (C. M. Brooks, K. Koizumi, and A. Sato, eds.), Tokyo University Press and Elsevier/North-Holland, Amsterdam, pp. 223–233.

Phillis, J. W., 1977, The role of cyclic nucleotides in the CNS, *Can. J. Neurol. Sci.* **4:**151–195.

Quenzer, L., Yahn, D., Alkadhi, K., and Volle, R. L., 1979, Transmission blockade and stimulation of ganglionic adenylate cyclase by catecholamines, *J. Pharmacol. Exp. Ther.* **208:**31–36.

Reader, T. A., Ferron, A., Descarries, L., and Jasper, H. H., 1979, Modulatory role for biogenic amines in the cerebral cortex: Microiontophoretic studies, *Brain Res.* **160:**217–229.

Rodknight, R., 1982, Aspects of protein phosphorylation in the nervous system with particular reference to synaptic transmission, *Prog. Brain Res.* **56:**1–25.

Schmitt, F. O., 1984, Molecular regulators of brain function: A new view, *Neuroscience* **13:**991–1001.

Seeman, P., 1980, Brain dopamine receptors, *Pharmacol. Rev.* **32:**229–313.

Snyder, S. H., 1984, Drug and neurotransmitter receptors in the brain, *Science* **224:**22–31.

Stone, T. W., Taylor, D. A., and Bloom, F. E., 1975, Cyclic AMP and cyclic GMP may mediate opposite neuronal responses in the rat cerebral cortex, *Science* **187:**845–847.

Volle, R. L., Quenzer, L. F., and Patterson, B. A., 1982, The regulation of cyclic nucleotides in a sympathetic ganglion, *J. Autonom. Nerv. Syst.* **6:**65–72.

Wamsley, J. K., Black, A. C., Jr., West, J. R., and Williams, T. H., 1980, Cyclic AMP synthesis in guinea pig superior cervical ganglia: response to pharmacological and preganglionic physiological stimulation, *Brain Res.* **182:**415–421.

Weight, F. F., and Votava, J., 1970, Slow synaptic excitation in sympathetic ganglion cells: Evidence for synaptic inactivation of potassium conductance, *Science* **170:**755–758.

Woody, C. D., Swartz, B. E., and Gruen, E., 1978, Effects of acetylcholine and cyclic GMP on input resistance of cortical neurons in awake cats, *Brain Res.* **158:**373–395.

30

Modulation of Synaptically Evoked Neuronal Calcium Fluxes by Adenosine

Peter Schubert

1. Introduction

The functioning of the brain is characterized by a surprisingly high degree of flexibility. This phenomenon, which is usually described as neuronal plasticity, has not only been observed during development and repair, but also seems to be an essential criterion of signal processing. The flow of activity generated in a neuronal circuit as the result of transmitter action can be modified by neuromodulators which interfere with synaptic transmission and change the pattern of evoked neuronal firing.

Neuromodulation by adenosine has been studied intensely in recent years; it has been found to differ in several respects from the action of a classical transmitter. Whereas the latter is released from a defined source, i.e., the axon terminal, release of adenosine is less well specified and occurs from axon terminals as well as from postsynaptic neurons (Schubert and Kreutzberg, 1975). Moreover, adenosine is released from glial cells as well as from neurons (Lewin and Bleck, 1979). The most common physiological trigger by which a transmitter is released is by the arrival of action potentials to the axon terminal. Some adenosine is also released in an activity-dependent manner from central axon terminals (Schubert *et al.*, 1976), presumably as ATP together with the transmitter. A rapid extracellular formation of adenosine is guaranteed by a cascade of ectoenzymes; large amounts of the AMP-splitting enzyme 5-nucleotidase are present in the glial cell membranes which encapsulate synaptic complexes (Kreutzberg *et al.*, 1978). However, in addition to nerve cell activity, changes in cell metabolism influence the release of adenosine from intracellular compartments. During ischemia, for example, the release of adenosine from both nerve and glial cells can be dramatically increased (e.g., see Berne *et al.*, 1974) by a pathologically increased breakdown of intracellular ATP. It is interesting to note that it is the metabolic breakdown product which acts as "emergency signal" and modifies nerve cell activity.

Thus, adenosine seems to function as a neuromodulator under physiological as well as pathological conditions. However, depending on whether the extracellular concentration is in the physiologically low or pathologically high range, different effects of adenosine can be dis-

Peter Schubert • Department of Neuromorphology, Max Planck Institute for Psychiatry, 8033 Martinsried, West Germany.

tinguished (see below). This raises the question of how adenosine action is determined. Unlike a transmitter for which the site of action is controlled by a defined site of release, adenosine will be distributed rather diffusely in the extracellular space after being released from nerve endings, neurons, and glial cells. In this respect, adenosine resembles more a hormone for which the site and mode of action are determined by the presence of specific receptors.

There is evidence for the existence of several adenosine receptors; receptors of the A1 and A2 types can be distinguished by pharmacological criteria (Bruns *et al.*, 1980; Van Calker *et al.*, 1979). They were originally classified according to the observed effect on cAMP synthesis, i.e., a low-affinity A2 receptor responsible for the adenosine-induced increase of cAMP in brain tissue, and a high-affinity A1 receptor which leads to an inhibition of adenylate cyclase. This does not necessarily mean that all the adenosine effects observed are linked to a primary influence on cAMP synthesis. Further investigations favored the presence of one or more subtypes of adenosine receptors which may be responsible for the variety of effects observed (Londos *et al.*, 1980).

The well-known depression of synaptic transmission has been shown to be mediated by the A1 receptor (Reddington *et al.*, 1982; Dunwiddie and Fredholm, 1984). Binding sites for A1 receptor agonists were found to be associated with synaptic complexes as recently demonstrated in the hippocampus by electron microscopic autoradiography (Tetzlaff *et al.*, 1987). In addition, significant numbers of A1 binding sites were found at extrasynaptic sites associated with the dendritic membrane of hippocampal pyramidal neurons suggesting that adenosine not only modulates synaptic transmission but is also able to influence the membrane properties of the target neuron. This latter effect could change the way in which a neuron responds to a given input. The following sections explore this effect, examining in particular the stimulus-evoked calcium fluxes which are modified by adenosine.

2. Methodological Considerations

The experiments were performed *in vitro* on rat hippocampal slices. Combined ion-sensitive and recording electrodes were prepared as previously described (Heinemann *et al.*, 1977). These were used to measure stimulus-evoked changes in the extracellular concentration of free calcium ions, $[Ca^{2+}]_o$, while recording nerve cell activity. There is evidence from previous studies that the decreases in $[Ca^{2+}]_o$ measured in response to orthodromic synaptic activation or to direct antidromic stimulation of neurons provide a reliable measure of the activity-dependent influx of Ca^{2+} ions (Heinemann and Jones, 1987; Konnerth and Heinemann, 1983; Schubert *et al.*, 1986). To differentiate between stimulus-evoked Ca^{2+} fluxes at synaptic sites and postsynaptic Ca^{2+} influx into the somas of the activated neurons, experiments were performed with two ion-sensitive electrodes. One was located in the stratum radiatum of the CA1 area where the stimulated commissural and Schaffer collateral fibers terminated on the dendrites of the CA1 neurons. The second electrode was located in the soma layer of the pyramidal neurons to measure the Ca^{2+} fluxes into the nerve cell bodies elicited by synaptic stimulation or by direct antidromic activation (Fig. 1).

To differentiate further between pre- and postsynaptic Ca^{2+} fluxes, some experiments were performed under conditions such that synaptic transmission was blocked. This was achieved by lowering the Ca^{2+} concentration in the superfused medium from 2.4 to 0.2 mM free Ca^{2+}. In 0.2 mM Ca^{2+}, orthodromic stimulation of the radiatum fibers by a train of 200 stimuli at 20 Hz generated presynaptic fiber potentials, but no postsynaptic potentials (Fig. 1). Under these conditions the synaptic Ca^{2+} signal is thought to reflect predominantly the action potential-induced presynaptic Ca^{2+} entry into the axon terminals. The CA1 neurons were still excitable by antidromic stimulation. A stimulus train applied to the alvear fibers generated antidromic population spikes which were followed by afterpotentials. The latter is a characteristic finding in low-Ca^{2+}

Figure 1. Experiments were performed on a 400-μm rat hippocampal slice preparation. They were started in continuously superfused normal medium containing (in mM): $CaCl_2$, 2.2; $MgSO_4$, 2.4; KCl, 3.3; NaCl, 124; $NaHCO_3$, 25.7; KH_2PO_4, 1.25; glucose, 10. Upon orthodromic stimulation of the afferent fibers in the stratum radiatum (by Sr in s.rad), evoked responses were recorded extracellularly in the CA1 pyramidal neurons, i.e., an EPSP in the synaptic area and a population spike in the soma layer (ORTHO left). Antidromic stimulation of the pyramidal neurons (by Sa in s.pyr) elicited an antidromic population spike (ANTI left). In low-Ca^{2+} medium (0.2 mM Ca^{2+} and 3.0 mM Mg^{2+}), presynaptic fiber volleys were elicited upon orthodromic synaptic stimulation, but no postsynaptic potentials (ORTHO middle showing the superimposed oscillographic recordings generated by a train of 200 stimuli at 20 Hz). Antidromic stimulation generated afterpotentials during the first stimuli of the train (ANTI middle).

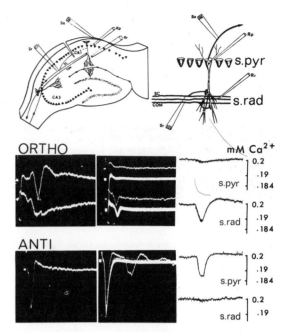

Two ion-sensitive/recording electrodes were used. These were located in s.pyr and s.rad,

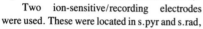

allowing simultaneous and independent measurements of stimulus-evoked decreases of $[Ca^{2+}]_o$ occurring in the synaptic area (s.rad) and in the soma cell layer (s.pyr). To ensure that no synaptic Ca^{2+} fluxes contributed to the soma signal, afferent radiatum fibers were transected. In spite of the short distance between the two electrodes, measurements did not interfere. Upon orthodromic stimulation (ORTHO right) a large decrease of $[Ca^{2+}]_o$ could be recorded in s.rad which was not reflected by a concomitant decrease of $[Ca^{2+}]_0$ in s.pyr. Antidromic stimulation (ANTI right) produced a large signal in s.pyr, but not in s.rad. (From Schubert and Kreutzberg, 1987.)

medium indicating a pathologically increased excitability of the CA1 neurons under these conditions (e.g., see Taylor and Dudek, 1982).

Measuring the local stimulus-evoked decreases in $[Ca^{2+}]_o$ simultaneously in the synaptic area (stratum radiatum) and in the CA1 soma cell layer (stratum pyramidale) revealed that the measurements made by the one electrode did not interfere with those made by the other. Orthodromic synaptic stimulation resulted in a marked decrease of $[Ca^{2+}]_o$ in the stratum radiatum and only a slight deflection in the stratum pyramidale. On the other hand, a marked decrease of $[Ca^{2+}]_o$ was seen in the stratum pyramidale upon antidromic stimulation of the CA1 neurons which was not accompanied by a significant change of $[Ca^{2+}]_o$ in the stratum radiatum. This demonstrates that the technique can be used to differentiate between neuronal Ca^{2+} fluxes occurring at the synaptic sites and those Ca^{2+} fluxes which were evoked in response to synaptic activation in the soma of the target neurons.

The sensitivity of this method is illustrated in Fig. 2. If a hippocampal slice is superfused with low-Ca^{2+} medium containing the potassium channel blocker 4-aminopyridine (4-AP), an increase of the stimulus-evoked neuronal Ca^{2+} fluxes is observed. 4-AP has been reported to interfere in particular with those potassium channels which control the spike duration in hippocampal radiatum fibers (Haas *et al.*, 1983). Therefore, the increase of the synaptic Ca^{2+} signal in the presence of 50 μM 4-AP presumably reflects an increase of the presynaptic Ca^{2+} influx resulting from the blockade of these 4-AP-sensitive K^+ channels and from a consecutive prolongation of the spike duration (Schubert and Heinemann, 1987). Also, 4-AP has recently been reported to effectively enhance synaptic transmission and to overcome the blockade in low-Ca^{2+} medium (Riker *et al.*, 1985). The partial restoration of synaptic transmission by 4-AP is clearly

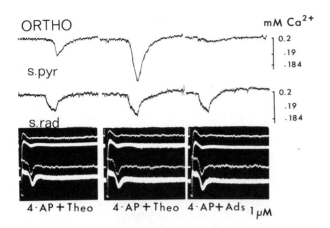

Figure 2. The local decreases of $[Ca^{2+}]_0$ elicited in 0.2 mM Ca^{2+} medium by orthodromic synaptic stimulation were simultaneously measured by two electrodes in the synaptic area (s.rad) and in the (clearly postsynaptic) soma layer of the CA1 neurons (s.pyr). In the presence of 50 μM theophylline (Theo) to antagonize a possible adenosine action, infusion of 50 μM 4-AP increased the synaptic Ca^{2+} signal (left and middle). This increase was accompanied by a steadily growing Ca^{2+} signal in the soma layer indicating a marked postsynaptic Ca^{2+} influx (which was not reflected by a significant generation of evoked potentials; see superimposed extracellular recordings below). However, in the presence of only 1 μM adenosine, the decrease of $[Ca^{2+}]_0$ measured in the soma layer was almost abolished (right). (From Schubert and Kreutzberg, 1987.)

demonstrated by the continuously growing Ca^{2+} signal measured in the soma layer during wash-in of 4-AP-containing medium (Fig. 2). An interesting observation was that the postsynaptic somatic Ca^{2+}-influx was already markedly increased before significant numbers of extracellularly recorded evoked potentials were generated. The somatic Ca^{2+} signal may be therefore used as a more sensitive indicator for the presence of synaptic transmission and its amplitude as a measure of the strength of the evoked postsynaptic activation.

3. Control of Synaptic Transmission and Postsynaptic Ca²⁺-Influx by Physiological Adenosine Concentrations

Modulation of signal processing by adenosine has been usually studied at high extracellular concentrations in the order of 20–40 μM, levels which are reached in the brain only under pathological conditions. Less is known about the physiological modulation by adenosine exerted at concentrations of about 1μM, which are reported to be present in the normally functioning brain (Zetterstroem *et al.*, 1984). Since the physiological function is difficult to extrapolate from the available information on the "high-dosage" adenosine actions (see also below), we investigated the effect of removing the action of endogenous adenosine. This can be done by performing experiments in the presence of an adenosine receptor-blocker, like theophylline (Theo), or by an enzymatic breakdown with adenosine deaminase (ADA). Specifically, we measured in the presence and absence of theophylline or ADA the stimulus-evoked synaptic and somatic calcium fluxes, which, as described above, provide a sensitive measure for detecting changes in the efficiency of synaptic transmission.

If tested in 0.2 mM Ca^{2+} medium, theophylline or ADA alone did not significantly change synaptic Ca^{2+} influx. However, in conjunction with 4-aminopyridine (4-AP), the above described increase in the synaptic calcium signal accompanied by a dramatic enlargement of the evoked Ca^{2+} influx into the soma region was observed, indicating the partial recovery of synaptic transmission (Fig. 2). Such a recovery upon combined treatment with Theo or ADA and 4-AP often revealed signs of frequency potentiation, i.e., the generation of evoked potentials later during the stimulus train (Schubert and Heinemann, 1987; see also Fig. 4). This points to a presynaptic site of action. After washing out theophylline and in the presence of a baseline concentration of 1 μM adenosine, the somatic Ca^{2+}-influx was almost completely depressed although 4-AP remained present (Fig. 2).

A partial recovery of synaptic transmission by ADA or theophylline was seen also in the absence of 4-AP, when an increased presynaptic Ca^{2+} influx was obtained by increasing the Ca^{2+} concentration in the superfused medium. In these experiments, performed in 0.6 mM Ca^{2+}, a marked synaptic Ca^{2+} signal was accompanied by only a small Ca^{2+} influx into the postsynaptic nerve cell bodies, if 1 μM adenosine was present (Fig. 3). In contrast, the somatic Ca^{2+} influx elicited by direct antidromic activation of the pyramidal neurons was about the same regardless of whether adenosine was present or not (Fig. 3 bottom). This rules out the possibility that the depression of synaptically evoked somatic Ca^{2+}-influx results from an adenosine-induced overall change of the neuronal membrane properties.

In conclusion, these findings reveal a powerful control of the efficiency of synaptic transmission by physiological adenosine concentrations. Although this effect, exerted by these low adenosine concentrations, is apparently not achieved by a primary depression of presynaptic Ca^{2+} influx, it seems to be highly dependent on the intracellular calcium level reached in the axon terminal upon activation. This is indicated by the observed potentiation of the theophylline- or ADA-effect by 4-AP, which is thought to act by increasing presynaptic Ca^{2+} influx (see above). The most likely explanation for this powerful adenosine effect on synaptic transmission is that this nucleoside acts by decreasing the sensitivity of transmitter release to calcium thus changing the stimulus/secretion coupling.

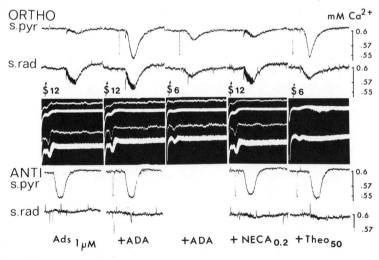

Figure 3. Technical details similar to those described in Figs. 1 and 2. In 0.6 mM Ca^{2+} medium, removal of the baseline adenosine concentration (1 μM) by adenosine deaminase (ADA) led to an increase of the orthodromic Ca^{2+} signal in the synaptic area (s.rad), which was accompanied by a large increase of the postsynaptic Ca^{2+} influx reflected by the Ca^{2+} signal in s.pyr. Even when the synaptic Ca^{2+} signal was considerably reduced by lowering the stimulus strength from 12 V to 6 V, an enlarged postsynaptic Ca^{2+} signal was seen. It was depressed by 0.2 μM NECA; the further addition of 50 μM theophylline considerably increased the Ca^{2+} signal in s.pyr which, in this case, went along with the generation of some extracellularly recorded evoked responses. There are only minor changes of the somatic Ca^{2+} signals generated by direct antidromic stimulation (ANTI, below). (From Schubert and Kreutzberg, 1987.)

4. Modulation of the Presynaptic Ca^{2+} Influx by Increased Adenosine Concentrations

In the absence of detectable synaptic transmission, the stimulus-evoked decrease of $[Ca^{2+}]_0$ elicited in 0.2 mM Ca^{2+} by orthodromic stimulation of the afferent fibers is attributed largely to a presynaptic Ca^{2+} entry into the axon terminals of the activated fibers. This conclusion is supported by studies revealing that intracellularly recorded evoked postsynaptic potentials were abolished at these low Ca^{2+} concentrations (Andersen et al., 1980; Heinemann et al., 1977; Konnerth and Heinemann, 1983). Therefore a modulation of presynaptic Ca^{2+} fluxes should be reflected by measurable changes of the orthodromic Ca^{2+} signal.

The enzymatic removal of the 1 μM baseline concentration of adenosine by ADA had almost no effect; but further addition of 20–40 μM adenosine resulted in a significant depression of the orthodromic Ca^{2+} signal (Schubert et al., 1986). When testing the enantiomers of PIA, a marked depression was obtained with low concentrations of L-PIA (0.02 μM) whereas 100-fold greater concentrations of D-PIA were ineffective. This stereospecificity points to an A1 receptor-mediated effect. The data suggest that higher concentrations of adenosine are able to depress the action potential-induced entry of Ca^{2+} into the axon terminals.

4.1. Effect of a K^+ Channel Blocker

It may well be that adenosine reduces the action potential-induced presynaptic Ca^{2+} entry by increasing primarily the membrane potassium conductance, thus shortening the action potential-induced depolarization of the presynaptic membrane. An effect of adenosine on the extracellularly recorded presynaptic fiber volley has been observed in the early experiments when testing the effect of adenosine on evoked potentials (Schubert and Mitzdorf, 1979). In order to test this possibility, experiments were performed in the presence of K^+ channel blockers (Schubert et al., 1986). As outlined above, those potassium channels which control the repolarization of the action potentials generated in hippocampal radiatum fibers are particularly sensitive to 4-AP (Haas et al., 1983). Accordingly, addition of 4-AP to the superfused medium considerably increased the orthodromic Ca^{2+} signal which, in the absence of adenosine, was often accompanied by the reappearance of extracellularly recorded postsynaptic potentials (Fig. 4). Adenosine at 1 μM effectively blocked the postsynaptic Ca^{2+} influx, but the synaptic Ca^{2+} signal was not, or only slightly, reduced (see above, Fig. 2). However, if higher adenosine concentrations (in the range of 20–60 μM) or equivalent concentrations of L-PIA (p.02–0.1 μM) were added to the 4-AP-containing medium, an almost complete depression of the orthodromic Ca^{2+} signal was still seen (Fig. 4). This means that a depression of the presynaptic Ca^{2+} influx can be obtained by greater adenosine concentrations even when the potassium channels thought to control the spike duration are not functioning.

4.2. Effect of an Organic Ca^{2+} Channel Blocker

The presynaptic Ca^{2+} influx seems to be more sensitive to adenosine modulation than the voltage-dependent Ca^{2+} influx elicited by direct antidromic stimulation. Whereas 20 μM adenosine depressed the orthodromic Ca^{2+} signal by about 25%, the antidromic Ca^{2+} signal was reduced by only 7% (Schubert et al., 1986).

Such a differential sensitivity of pre- and postsynaptic Ca^{2+} fluxes has been described also for "nonphysiological" Ca^{2+} blockers. Thus, verapamil was found to depress preferentially the postsynaptic Ca^{2+} entry, whereas the presynaptic Ca^{2+} fluxes measured in low-Ca^{2+} medium were almost unaffected (Heinemann and Jones, 1987). This differential effect of verapamil on pre- and postsynaptic Ca^{2+} fluxes was used as a further criterion to characterize those Ca^{2+} fluxes modulated by adenosine. Addition of 50 μM verapamil to the superfused medium led to a

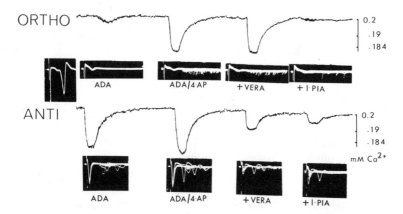

Figure 4. Stimulus-evoked decreases in $[Ca^{2+}]_0$ elicited by orthodromic (ORTHO) and antidromic (ANTI) stimulation trains. Black inserts show the superimposed oscillographic recordings. Addition of 50 μM 4-aminopyridine (4-AP) to the adenosine-free, 0.2 mM Ca^{2+} medium [containing adenosine deaminase (ADA)] led to a considerable increase of the orthodromic Ca^{2+} signal and a partial recovery of synaptic transmission. Whereas the orthodromic Ca^{2+} signal is not affected by the further addition of 50 μM verapamil, it is completely depressed by 0.02 μM L-PIA. The highly verapamil-sensitive antidromic Ca^{2+} signal is less affected by L-PIA. (From Schubert and Kreutzberg, 1987.)

pronounced depression of the antidromic Ca^{2+} signal, leaving the orthodromic Ca^{2+} signal relatively unaffected. Adenosine and its analogues depressed particularly these verapamil-insensitive Ca^{2+} currents (Fig. 4). One may speculate that the Ca^{2+} fluxes which are preferentially modulated by higher adenosine concentrations are the transient (low threshold) Ca^{2+} currents which, in contrast to the persistent (high threshold) Ca^{2+} currents, were reported not to be blocked by organic Ca^{2+} blockers (Boll and Lux, 1985; Carbone and Lux, 1984).

4.3. Evaluation of Reported Data

It may be that the inconsistency of data reported so far on the effects of adenosine on neuronal Ca^{2+} fluxes is related to the fact that to study the different Ca^{2+} currents, different experimental conditions are required, and that in addition adenosine modulates these Ca^{2+} currents in a differential manner. Thus, Ca^{2+} uptake into brain synaptosomes elicited by increasing K^+ concentration has been reported either to be depressed (Ribeiro *et al.*, 1979; Wu *et al.*, 1982) or not to be affected by adenosine (Barr *et al.*, 1985). Directly measured Ba^{2+} currents in dorsal root ganglion cells, thought to be a model to study presynaptic Ca^{2+} fluxes, were found to be depressed by chloroadenosine (Dolphin *et al.*, 1986), whereas Ca^{2+} currents in guinea pig hippocampal neurons were not affected (Halliwell and Scholfield, 1984). A depression of Ca^{2+} spikes was observed in ganglionic (Henon and McAffee, 1979) and rat hippocampal neurons (Proctor and Dunwiddie, 1983); recent voltage clamp studies on cultured sensory neurons showed a depression of Ca^{2+} currents accompanied by an increase of the membrane resistance (MacDonald *et al.*, 1986). The authors concluded that this reflects a direct effect of adenosine on Ca^{2+} currents not mediated by a primary effect on the membrane potassium conductance. Our finding that the depression of the orthodromic Ca^{2+} signal in low-Ca^{2+} medium is also seen in the presence of effective doses of the potassium channel blocker 4-AP as well as of TEA is consistent with such a direct action.

However, the possibility remains that adenosine also controls neuronal Ca^{2+} influx indirectly by modulating primarily membrane potassium currents (e.g., see Trussel and Meyer, 1985). Most likely, the early adenosine-induced membrane hyperpolarization, which occurs in conjunction with a decrease of the membrane resistance (Segal, 1982; Siggins and Schubert, 1981), reflects an increase of the membrane potassium conductance. This effect was found to be rather insensitive to K^+ channel blockers (Segal, 1982).

5. Differential Dependence of the Adenosine-Mediated Modulation on Mg^{2+} Ions

In normal Ca^{2+} medium (containing 2.0 mM Ca^{2+} and 2.4 mM Mg^{2+}), synaptic transmission and the evoked postsynaptic potentials were depressed in a concentration-dependent manner by adenosine. This depression coincides with a diminution of the stimulus-evoked decrease of $[Ca^{2+}]_o$ in the synaptic area and also in the postsynaptic somal layer (Fig. 5). The synaptic Ca^{2+} signal reflecting presynaptic and postsynaptic Ca^{2+} influx, was markedly depressed when the adenosine concentration was raised to 20 μM.

This effect was not seen when the medium lacked Mg^{2+} (Fig. 5, top). The stimulus-evoked Ca^{2+} influx measured in the synaptic area was considerably increased in Mg^{2+}-free medium and this increase was largely antagonized by the NMDA receptor antagonist 2-amino-5-phosphonovaleric acid (APV). This indicates that the enlarged synaptic Ca^{2+} signal elicited in Mg^{2+}-free medium includes a synaptically evoked postsynaptic Ca^{2+} influx which is mediated by the

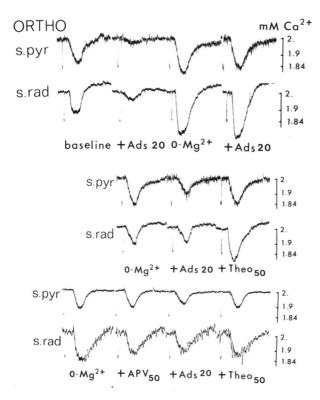

Figure 5. Experiments were performed in "normal" 2.0 mM Ca^{2+} medium (i.e., in the presence of synaptic transmission). The decreases in $[Ca^{2+}]_0$ elicited in the synaptic area (s.rad) upon orthodromic stimulation of the stratum radiatum fibers should reflect both presynaptic and evoked postsynaptic Ca^{2+} entry. (Top) Addition of 20 μM adenosine to the "normal" medium containing 2.4 mM Mg^{2+} and a baseline concentration of 1 μM adenosine resulted in a marked depression of the synaptic Ca^{2+} signal. This signal was markedly increased in a medium lacking Mg^{2+} and remained almost unaffected by the addition of 20 μM adenosine. (Middle) In an analogous experiment, the addition of 20 μM adenosine to Mg^{2+}-free medium containing the 1 μM baseline concentration of adenosine was rather ineffective. But antagonism of the 1 μM adenosine action by 50 μM theophylline (Theo) resulted in a marked increase of the synaptic Ca^{2+} signal. (Bottom) The increase of the synaptic response observed in Mg^{2+}-free medium was sensitive to the NMDA-receptor antagonist APV. Addition of 50 μM APV considerably decreased the synaptic Ca^{2+} signal. But in the presence of APV, the further addition of theophylline was ineffective and the observed synaptic Ca^{2+} signal was about the same as in APV alone. (From Schubert and Kreutzberg, 1987.)

Mg^{2+}-sensitive NMDA receptors. The enlarged synaptic signal remains almost unaffected by the addition of 20 μM or even higher concentrations of adenosine. This could mean that an adenosine effect is masked by such enlarged Ca^{2+} signals. Another possibility is that the "high threshold" adenosine action on the synaptic Ca^{2+} influx which includes a depression of the presynaptic Ca^{2+} influx, is Mg^{2+}-sensitive and no longer operative in low Mg^{2+} (Schubert, in preparation).

This explanation would be in agreement with recent pharmacological data demonstrating that Mg^{2+} ions control the functioning of A1 receptors (Reddington et al., 1986). In particular, the affinity and number of detectable receptor sites were found to increase at increasing Mg^{2+} concentrations. However, there was one subtype of A1 receptors which seemed to be Mg^{2+}-insensitive. For the latter, an interesting functional parallel was found when testing the Mg^{2+}-dependency of the "low-threshold" adenosine modulation of the postsynaptic Ca^{2+} influx. Thus, the enlarged Ca^{2+} signal which was recorded in Mg^{2+}-free medium and which remained rather unaffected by 20 μM adenosine, increased considerably when the action of the 1 μM baseline adenosine concentration was antagonized by theophylline (Fig. 5, middle). However, theophylline was ineffective when tested in the presence of APV (Fig. 5, bottom). This means that there is an APV-sensitive synaptic Ca^{2+} influx that is mediated by NMDA-receptors and is apparently controlled by the physiologically available adenosine concentrations.

6. Conclusions

Adenosine controls the efficiency of synaptic transmission and the evoked Ca^{2+} influx into the postsynaptic neurons in the concentration range present physiologically. The data suggest a presynaptic effect on transmitter release resulting from a change of the stimulus/secretion coupling. The finding that adenosine also has some influence on the amount of NMDA receptor-mediated postsynaptic Ca^{2+} entry may be of functional significance under those particular physiological and/or pathological conditions when these receptors are brought into play. This Mg^{2+}-insensitive adenosine action may be little reflected in a change of the evoked electrical potentials, but involved in the regulation of calcium-dependent metabolic processes in the target neuron.

The "high threshold" depression of the presynaptic Ca^{2+} fluxes is presumably more important under (pathological) conditions when the extracellular adenosine concentration is increased. By this action, transmitter release and synaptic transmission will be depressed, reducing the afferent activation of a neuron. Together with the previously reported antagonistic effect of adenosine on the generation of repetitive nerve cell firing (Schubert and Lee, 1986) and its effect on NMDA receptor-mediated events, a depression of presynaptic Ca^{2+} influx may contribute to counteraction of abnormal nerve cell activity.

ACKNOWLEDGMENTS. I thank Dr. Georg Kreutzberg for his continuous support of these studies. I am also indebted to Regina Kolb and Maria Koebet who cooperated in performing the experiments.

References

Andersen, P., Dingledine, R., Gjerstad, L., Langmoen, I. A., and Mosfeldt Laursen, A., 1980, Two different responses of hippocampal pyramidal cells to application of gamma-aminobutyric acid, J. Physiol. (London) 305:279–296.

Barr, E., Daniell, L. C., and Leslie, S. W., 1985, Synaptosomal calcium uptake unaltered by adenosine and 2-chloroadenosine, Biochem. Pharmacol. 34:713–715.

Berne, R. M., Rubio, R., and Curnish, R. R., 1974, Release of adenosine from ischaemic brain, Circ. Res. 35:262–272.

Boll, W., and Lux, H. D., 1985, Action of organic antagonists on neuronal calcium currents, *Neurosci. Lett.* **56:**336–339.

Bruns, R., Daly, J., and Synder, S., 1980, Adenosine receptors in brain membranes: Binding of N_6-cyclohexyl (^{3}H)adenosine and 1,3-diethyl-8-(^{3}H)phenylxanthine, *Proc. Natl. Acad. Sci. USA* **77:**5547–5551.

Carbone, E., and Lux, H. D., 1984, A voltage-activated, fully inactivating Ca channel in vertebrate sensory neurones, *Nature* **310:**501–505.

Dolphin, A. C., Forda, S. R., and Scott, R. H., 1986, The adenosine analogue 2-chloroadenosine inhibits Ba currents in dorsal root ganglion neurones in culture, *J. Physiol. (London)* **373:**47–61.

Dunwiddie, T., and Fredholm, B., 1984, Adenosine receptors mediating inhibitory electrophysiological responses in rat hippocampus differ from receptors mediating cyclic AMP accumulation, *Naunyn-Schmiedeberg Arch. Pharmacol.* **326:**294–301.

Haas, H. L., Wieser, H. G., and Yasargil, M. G., 1983, 4-Aminopyridine and fiber potentials in rat and human hippocampal slices, *Experientia* **39:**114–115.

Halliwell, J. V., and Scholfield, C. N., 1984, Somatically recorded Ca currents in guinea pig hippocampal and olfactory cortex neurones are resistant to adenosine action, *Neurosci. Lett.* **50:**13–18.

Heinemann, U., and Jones, P., 1987, Reduction of stimulus-evoked post-, but not presynaptic calcium influx in rat hippocampus by organic calcium antagonists, *Br. J. Pharmacol.* **87:**5P.

Heinemann, U., Lux, H. D., and Gutnick, M. J., 1977, Extracellular free calcium and potassium during paroxysmal activity in cerebral cortex of the cat, *Exp. Brain Res.* **27:**237–243.

Henon, B. K., and McAffee, D. A., 1979, Cyclic AMP and other adenine nucleotides inhibit Ca-dependent potentials in sympathetic postganglionic neurons, *Soc. Neurosci. Abstr.* **5:**559.

Konnerth, A., and Heinemann, U., 1983, Effects of GABA on presumed presynaptic Ca entry in hippocampal slices, *Brain Res.* **270:**185–189.

Kreutzberg, G. W., Barron, K., and Schubert, P., 1978, Cytochemical localization of 5′-nucleotidase in glial plasma membranes, *Brain Res.* **158:**247–257.

Lewin, E., and Bleck, V., 1979, Uptake and release of adenosine by cultured astrocytoma cells, *J. Neurochem.* **33:**365–367.

Londos, C., Cooper, D. M. F., and Wolff, J., 1980, Subclasses of external adenosine receptors, *Proc. Natl. Acad. Sci. USA* **77:**2551–2554.

MacDonald, R. L., Skerritt, J. H., and Werz, M. A., 1986, Adenosine agonists reduce voltage-dependent calcium conductance of mouse sensory neurones in cell culture, *J. Physiol. (London)* **370:**75–90.

Proctor, W. R., and Dunwiddie, T. V., 1983, Adenosine inhibits calcium spikes in hippocampal pyramidal neurons in vitro, *Neurosci. Lett.* **35:**197–201.

Reddington, M., Lee, K. S., and Schubert, P., 1982, An A_1-adenosine receptor, characterized by ^{3}H-cyclohexyladenosine binding, mediates the depression of evoked potentials in a rat hippocampal slice preparation, *Neurosci. Lett.* **28:**275–279.

Reddington, M., Alexander, S. P., Erfurth, A., and Lee, K., 1986, Biochemical and autoradiographic approaches to the characterization of adenosine receptors in brain, in: *Topics and Perspectives in Adenosine Research* (E. Gerlach and B. Becker, eds.), Springer-Verlag, Berlin, pp. 49–58.

Ribeiro, J. A., Sa-Almeida, A. M., and Namorado, J. M., 1979, Adenosine and adenosine triphosphate decrease 45 Ca uptake by synaptosomes stimulated by potassium, *Biochem. Pharmacol.* **28:**1297–1300.

Riker, W. K., Matsumoto, M., and Takashima, K., 1985, Synaptic facilitation by 3-aminopyridine and its antagonism by verapamil and diltiazem, *J. Pharmacol. Exp. Ther.* **235:**431–435.

Segal, M., 1982, Intracellular analysis of a postsynaptic action of adenosine in the rat hippocampus, *Eur. J. Pharmacol.* **79:**193–199.

Siggins, G. R., and Schubert, P., 1981, Adenosine depression of hippocampal neurons in vitro: An intracellular study of dose-dependent actions on synaptic and membrane potentials, *Neurosci. Lett.* **23:**55–60.

Schubert, P., Heinemann, U., 1987, Adenosine antagonists combined with 4-aminopyridine can recover synaptic transmission in low Ca media, (submitted).

Schubert, P., and Kreutzberg, G. W., 1987, Pre- versus postsynaptic effects of adenosine on neuronal calcium fluxes, in: *Topics and Perspectives in Adenosine Research* (E. Gerlach and B. Becker, eds.), Springer Verlag, Berlin, pp. 521–532.

Schubert, P., and Kreutzberg, G. W., 1975, Dendritic and axonal transport of nucleoside derivatives in single motoneurons and release from dendrites, *Brain Res.* **90:**319–323.

Schubert, P., and Lee, K. S., 1986, Non-synaptic modulation of repetitive firing by adenosine is antagonized by 4-aminopyridine in a rat hippocampal slice, *Neurosci. Lett.* **67:**334–338.

Schubert, P., and Mitzdorf, U., 1979, Analysis and quantitative evaluation of the depressive effect of adenosine on evoked potentials in hippocampal slices, *Brain Res.* **172:**186–190.

Schubert, P., Heinemann, and Kolb, R., 1986, Differential effect of adenosine on pre- and postsynaptic calcium fluxes, *Brain Res.* **376:**382–386.

Schubert, P., Lee, K., West, M., Deadwhyler, S., and Lynch, G., 1976, Stimulation dependent release of 3H-adenosine derivatives from central axon terminals to target neurones, *Nature* **260**:541–542.

Taylor, C. P., and Dudek, F. E., 1982, Synchronous neural afterdischarges in rat hippocampal slices without active chemical synapses, *Science* **218**:810–812.

Tetzlaff, W., Schubert, P., and Kreutzberg, G. W., 1987, Synaptic and extrasynaptic localization of adenosine binding sites in the rat hippocampus, *Neuroscience* **21**:869–875.

Trussel, L. O., and Meyer, B. J., 1985, Adenosine-activated potassium conductance in cultured striatal neurons, *Proc. Natl. Acad. Sci. USA* **82**:4857–4861.

Van Calker, D., Mueller, M., and Hamprecht, B., 1979, Adenosine regulates via two different types of receptors the accumulation of cyclic AMP in cultured brain cells, *J. Neurochem.* **33**:999–1000.

Wu, P. H., Phillis, J. W., and Thierry, D. L., 1982, Adenosine receptor agonists inhibit K-evoked Ca uptake by rat brain cortical synaptosomes, *J. Neurochem.* **39**:700–708.

Zetterstrom, T., Vernet, L., Ungerstedt, U., Tossmann, U., Jonzon, B., and Fredholm, B. B., 1984, Purine levels in the intact rat brain: Studies with an implanted perfused hollow fibre, *Neurosci. Lett.* **29**:111–115.

31

Electrophysiological Analysis of Effects of Exogenous and Endogenous Adenosine in Hippocampal Slices

H. L. Haas and R. W. Greene

1. Introduction

Little doubt remains that adenosine serves a modulatory role in the nervous system (Sattin and Rall, 1970; Shimizu and Daly, 1970; Fredholm and Hedqvist, 1980; Phillis and Wu, 1981; Stone, 1981; Daly *et al.*, 1984; Dunwiddie, 1985). While electrophysiologically active concentrations of adenosine have been found in the extracellular fluid, the source and control of the levels of this active adenosine are unclear. There are indications that adenosine is released (or coreleased) from synaptic endings, fulfilling a typical transmitter role (Burnstock, 1975, 1981; Nagy *et al.*, 1986). A synaptic hyperpolarization in autonomic neurons has been identified as an adenosine-mediated potential (Akasu *et al.*, 1984). Regardless of the magnitude of adenosine's role in the CNS as a classical transmitter, the ubiquitous but uneven occurrence of adenosine in the CNS and its marked inhibitory actions on nervous activity (Kostopoulos and Phillis, 1977) implicate it as a major neuromodulator, which could provide the negative feedback link between the metabolic state and the electrophysiological activity of nerve cells (Pull and McIlwain, 1973).

Brain slice preparations have permitted major advances in our understanding of the actions of adenosine at the cellular and subcellular levels (Kuroda *et al.*, 1976; Scholfield, 1978; Schubert and Mitzdorf, 1979; Okada and Ozawa, 1980; Dunwiddie and Hoffer, 1980). In the hippocampus, adenosine reduces the efficacy of synaptic transmission by acting on presynaptic sites, decreasing transmitter release, and on postsynaptic sites by altering the cellular response to the transmitter. The mechanism for the postsynaptic action is an increase in membrane potential and in potassium conductance (Okada and Ozawa, 1980; Segal, 1982; Siggins and Schubert, 1981).

We have investigated these actions in detail and have shown that adenosine increases a calcium-dependent and a nonvoltage-, noncalcium-dependent potassium current in hippocampal pyramidal cells. In this chapter we summarize our own published contribution to the analysis of

H. L. Haas • Department of Physiology, Johannes Gutenberg-University, D65 Mainz, Federal Republic of Germany. *R. W. Greene* • Harvard Medical School, V.A. Medical Center, Brockton, Massachusetts 02401.

adenosine action in the hippocampus (Hood *et al.*, 1983; Haas *et al.*, 1984; Haas and Greene, 1984; Greene and Haas, 1985, 1987) and in addition provide some recent unpublished material.

2. Methods

All the experiments described below were conducted on hippocampal slices from rats (some guinea pigs and mice) *in vitro,* kept completely submerged in a modified Ringer solution at 30–34°C in a perfusion chamber (Haas *et al.*, 1979; Greene and Haas, 1985). Extra- and intracellular recording (current and single electrode voltage clamp) and stimulation of fiber tracts were performed under direct observation through a stereomicroscope.

3. Action of Exogenous Adenosine

3.1. Presynaptic Actions

A postsynaptic action on distal dendritic sites is very difficult to differentiate from a presynaptic action on nerve terminals. These presynaptic sites are not amenable to direct electrophysiological analysis but indirect methods allow an estimation of transmitter release. Although hippocampal circuitry is more complex than a simple excitatory junction, paired pulse facilitation occurs in much the same way as has been described at the neuromuscular junction (Katz and Miledi, 1968; Rahaminoff, 1968; Andersen, 1960; Dunwiddie and Lynch, 1978; Buckle and Haas, 1982). Facilitation of a test response by a preceding conditioning response is believed to depend on residual calcium in nerve terminals. Under conditions of high transmitter release a depression of the test response occurs, presumably due to exhaustion of the immediately releasable transmitter (Betz, 1970; McNaughton *et al.*, 1981). A reduction in the paired pulse facilitation would indicate an increase in release while an enhancement would suggest less transmitter depletion and thus decreased release. This indirect approach has been used to ascribe a presynaptic action to 4-aminopyridine (Buckle and Haas, 1982) which blocks a transient potassium current (Gustafsson *et al.*, 1982) and increases transmitter release. Adenosine had an

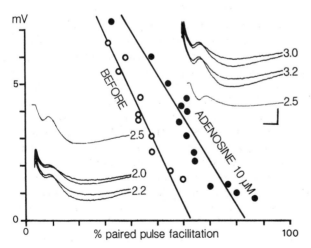

Figure 1. Facilitation is increased by adenosine. EPSPs were evoked in stratum radiatum at 60-msec intervals. Facilitation of the test response (abscissa) is plotted against the amplitude of the conditioning response (ordinate). As facilitation depends on the response amplitude, it is necessary to compare responses at several stimulation intensities before and during adenosine action. Therefore, facilitation is shown here as a function of the conditioning response. Inserts show field EPSPs with an initial afferent fiber volley. At 2.5 V stimulation intensity averaged single pulse responses are shown before (left), and during (right), adenosine 10 μM. Furthermore, oscilloscope tracings of superimposed conditioning and test responses at 2.0 and 2.2 V stimulation before and at 3.0 and 3.2 V during adenosine action are illustrated. The conditioning responses for these two groups are similar but the test responses during adenosine are larger. Calibration 2 mV, 1 msec.

opposite effect on the paired pulse paradigm: it increased synaptic facilitation. This effect was enhanced in media containing higher calcium concentrations when release is high (Dunwiddie and Haas, 1985). These findings were explained by a presynaptic action of adenosine on nerve terminals, resulting in reduced transmitter release. Although the following paragraphs show that adenosine has marked postsynaptic actions, it seems likely that a presynaptic action contributes to its depressant effects in the CNS, perhaps mediated by a mechanism similar to that observed postsynaptically.

3.2. Membrane Potential and Conductance

Adenosine hyperpolarized all CA1 pyramidal neurons when added at 20 μM or higher concentration to the perfusate (Fig. 2). This increase in membrane potential was accompanied by an increase in potassium conductance (gK). The effect was independent of chloride equilibrium potential but followed the Nernst relationship for changes in the extracellular potassium concentration (Fig. 3). It was not secondary to an inflow of Ca^{2+} ions as it occurred with sufficient cadmium in the medium to block Ca^{2+} currents, Ca^{2+}-activated potassium currents, and synaptic activity. The adenosine effect is not due to an increase of Ca^{2+} concentration from intracellular sources because buffering intracellular Ca^{2+} to very low levels with injected EGTA did not prevent it.

Furthermore, blockers of several voltage-dependent potassium currents, including tetraethylammonium (TEA), 4-aminopyridine, and barium, left the hyperpolarization by adenosine virtually unaltered. Forskolin, which blocks the Ca^{2+}-activated gK through maximal stimulation of cAMP, had no antagonistic effect on this adenosine action (Fig. 2B). Only intra- and extracellular cesium, a nonselective blocker of potassium currents, antagonized hyperpolarization and conductance increase evoked by adenosine. Adenosine did not alter any of the known voltage-dependent potassium currents such as the delayed outward rectifier, I_K, the transient rectifier, I_A, the

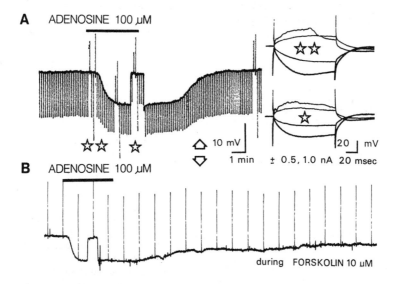

Figure 2. Hyperpolarization of CA1 pyramidal cells by adenosine. (A) In the presence of TTX. Short voltage excursions are from current injection which is illustrated at an expanded time base on the right: oscilloscope tracings of four superimposed sweeps, ±0.5 and 1.0 nA, before (two stars) and during (one star, manual voltage clamp) adenosine action, taken at the original resting potential. (B) In the presence of TTX and forskolin which has removed the Ca^{2+}-dependent potassium conductance. Upstrokes are calcium spikes without afterhyperpolarization.

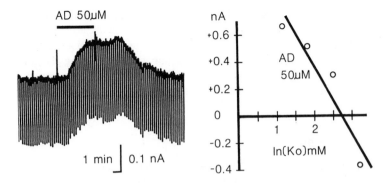

Figure 3. Adenosine induces potassium current. (Left) Single electrode voltage clamp (SEVC) record at -70 mV and 3 mM extracellular potassium. This response varied with the extracellular potassium as predicted by the Nernst equation for a change in potassium permeability, shown in the diagram on the right. The response was reversed (the current induced by adenosine became inward) at 24 mM extracellular potassium.

acetylcholine-sensitive rectifier, I_M, or the anomalous inward rectifier, I_Q. However, the Ca^{2+}-dependent potassium currents were increased in addition to the activation of a non-Ca^{2+} and nonvoltage-sensitive gK.

In order to learn more about the molecular mechanism of the adenosine action, we have treated hippocampal slices with N-ethylmaleimide (NEM), which interacts with the GTP-dependent inhibitory protein N_i, and adenosine-induced cAMP decrease (Fredholm *et al.*, 1985). With 100 μM NEM we found no difference in the capacity of adenosine to evoke hyperpolarizations (three cells) or reductions in synaptic potentials (two experiments). The sensitivity of these effects to pertussis toxin, which reverses the adenosine-induced inhibition of glutamate release (Dolphin and Prestwich, 1985), remains to be tested.

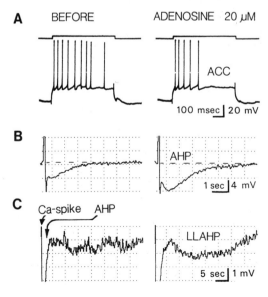

Figure 4. Adenosine increases accommodation of firing and afterhyperpolarizations. (A) The response of a CA1 pyramidal cell to depolarizing current injection ($+0.4$ nA for 600 msec, upper trace is current), before and during adenosine 20 μM. (B) Amplitude and time course of afterhyperpolarizations following a burst of action potentials are enhanced by adenosine. (C) The AHP following a Ca^{2+} spike in a TTX-poisoned preparation is enhanced. A much longer-lasting low-amplitude AHP (LLAHP) is also increased.

3.3. Calcium-Activated Potassium Current

This current is composed of at least two components, a transient voltage-dependent (Brown and Griffith, 1983) and a long-lasting nonvoltage-dependent current I_{kAHP} (Lancaster and Adams, 1986). Both components were increased by adenosine added to the bath at low concentrations (5–20 μM). In conventional voltage recordings this effect was manifested by an increase in adaptation of action potential frequency as well as an increase and prolongation of the long-lasting afterhyperpolarization (AHP) following action potentials (Fig. 4). With higher concentrations, a reduction of the AHP was usually observed presumably due to a shunting effect of the non-Ca^{2+}-, nonvoltage-sensitive potassium conductance. Thus, at least two different gK's were enhanced by adenosine, one Ca^{2+} dependent and one independent of Ca^{2+} and voltage. In some cells a further, much longer-lasting AHP was also enhanced by adenosine (LLAHP in Fig. 4C). The increase in an outward tail current without alteration of the preceding inward (Ca^{2+}) current is illustrated in Fig. 5. The effects on gK and on gK(Ca) were probably A_1 effects as they were seen also with cyclohexyladenosine and phenylisopropyladenosine, while NECA was much weaker in this respect.

As the effects on gK(Ca) occurred with relatively low concentrations of adenosine, it may be functionally more important than the general reduction in excitability produced by higher concentrations. This provides a means for the extracellular adenosine concentration to regulate the responsiveness to longer-duration excitatory signals without having much effect on basal activity. Thus, when there is an accumulation of adenosine after increased nervous activity, the nervous system is protected from exaggerated excitation, such as epileptic discharges.

The most likely manner by which adenosine interferes with gK(Ca) is through an alteration of intracellular Ca^{2+} regulation. More specifically, the increase in the AHP duration is best explained by increased Ca^{2+} concentration near the membrane following inflow during the action potential. This could be achieved by reduction of the Ca^{2+} uptake into intracellular stores, perhaps a reduction in Ca^{2+} affinity of the Ca^{2+}-binding proteins resulting from cAMP-dependent phosphorylation: histamine, noradrenaline, and cAMP reduce accommodation of firing, amplitude, and time course of the long-lasting AHP [gK(Ca)] on the same cell population

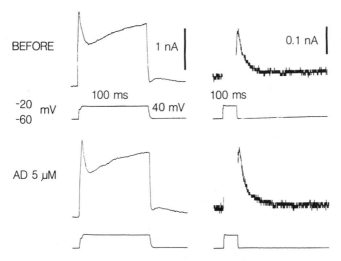

Figure 5. Adenosine increases the delayed outward currents without altering the slow inward currents. Single electrode voltage clamp records before (upper row) and during (lower row) adenosine exposure. Records in the left column are identical to those on the right except for a slower time course and greater current amplification on the right.

(Madison and Nicoll, 1982; Haas and Konnerth, 1983; Haas and Greene, 1984). These amines enhance intracellular cAMP and the evidence for mediation of this effect through cAMP is good (Madison and Nicoll, 1986; Haas, 1984). In contrast, adenosine, acting on the A_1 receptor, inhibits adenylate cyclase (Fredholm *et al.*, 1985) and increases all the above-mentioned electrophysiological parameters [gK(Ca)].

3.4. Calcium Currents

Available evidence from the peripheral nervous system suggests a direct interference of adenosine with Ca^{2+} currents (Henon and McAfee, 1983; Dolphin *et al.*, 1986; MacDonald *et al.*, 1986). This possibility seems to receive support from the observation that Ca^{2+} spikes were reduced in tetrodotoxin (TTX)-poisoned hippocampal slices (Proctor and Dunwiddie, 1983; Haas and Greene, 1984; Greene and Haas, 1985; but see Halliwell and Scholfield, 1984). Figure 6 shows clear evidence that inward currents were generated and affected at distant (dendritic) sites and could not be properly clamped. A closer analysis of adenosine's action on Ca^{2+} spikes and Ca^{2+} currents under conditions where outward currents were maximally blocked led us to the

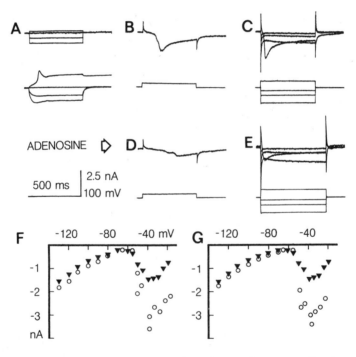

Figure 6. At high concentrations, adenosine reduces slow inward currents but does not affect Q current. A consists of records made during sample and hold current clamp mode of a cesium-loaded cell with Ba^{2+} (2 mM) and Mg^{2+} (10 mM) in the perfusion media. Note the new stable membrane potential of +5 mV which was returned to −55 mV with a 5-sec hyperpolarizing current pulse (not illustrated). The same switching frequency was used as for the voltage clamp records from this neuron shown in B–E. The holding potential was −55 mV for all. D and E were recorded during exposure to adenosine (50 μM). B and D illustrate multiphasic kinetics of inward currents especially obvious near threshold and indicative of escape from membrane potential control at electrotonically distant sites. F and G are graphs of the peak inward currents of this neuron (ordinate) with respect to the command membrane potential (abscissa, holding potential equals −55 mV). F shows values obtained before (○) and during (▼) exposure to adenosine (50 μM). G is the same except the circles represent values obtained on recovery from exposure to adenosine.

conclusion that the primary action occurred on potassium currents and the reduction in Ca^{2+} spikes and Ca^{2+} currents is secondary and due to shunting by adenosine-evoked gK's at sites electronically distant from the recording electrode. This interpretation received strong support by a patch-clamp analysis on cultured striatal neurons (Trussell and Jackson, 1985). This mechanism could also explain the presynaptic reduction of release. However, a direct effect on Ca^{2+} currents as occurs undoubtedly in presynaptic endings on dorsal root ganglion cells (Dolphin et al., 1986; MacDonald et al., 1986) cannot be excluded.

3.5. Action on Epileptiform Activity

Burst discharges or lasting depolarizations like the paroxysmal depolarization shift (PDS) are modulated by $gK(Ca)$ (Hotson and Prince, 1980; Alger and Nicoll, 1980; Schwartzkroin and Stafstrom, 1980; Hablitz, 1981; Haas, 1984). The described actions of adenosine are perfectly suited to attenuate such firing or depolarizations. Anticonvulsant effects of adenosine have been reported by several authors working on different in vivo models (Maitre et al., 1974; Weir et al., 1984; Dunwiddie, 1985; Ault and Wang, 1986; Dragunow, 1986). As exaggerated activity is correlated with significant release of adenosine, this compound may be an endogenous antiepileptic, which reduces epileptic discharges and could contribute to the long-lasting depression after a seizure. Adenosine-like binding has been found with the antiepileptic carbamazepine (Skerritt et al., 1982). Electrophysiological analysis in our laboratory, however, revealed different mechanisms of action for carbamazepine and adenosine (Hood et al., 1983).

Antagonism of extracellularly recorded epileptiform discharges by adenosine is found in hippocampal slices exposed to low Ca^{2+} and high Mg^{2+} (Hood et al., 1983; Haas et al., 1984; Haas and Jefferys, 1984; Lee et al., 1984; Schubert, this volume) or to penicillin (Dunwiddie et al., 1981). Adenosine blocks evoked (Fig. 7A) and spontaneous (Fig. 7B) field bursts (or spreading excitation) in Ca^{2+}-deficient medium. These results can only be explained by an action of adenosine independent of Ca^{2+} inflow.

4. Endogenous Adenosine Action

Adenosine levels in brain tissue are normally about 1 μM with relatively little variation between different brain regions (see Dunwiddie, 1985) but may increase by at least two orders of magnitude in hyperactive tissue. An enhanced topological resolution might reveal much larger

Figure 7. Adenosine blocks epileptiform activity in low Ca^{2+} (0.2 mM)/high Mg^{2+} (4 mM) medium. (A) Averaged records on the right show the multiple discharge of pyramids following alveus stimulation (antidromic activation) before and during adenosine. The trace on the left displays the size of the second population spike (star) through a sample and hold amplifier. Note the larger antidromic spike during adenosine (lower left, cells are hyperpolarized) and the rebound increase in the second population spike after washout. (B) Adenosine blocks spontaneous field bursts, registered here through a ratemeter counting a single unit and, during the bursts, the synchronized population spikes (upstrokes). CPS, counts per second.

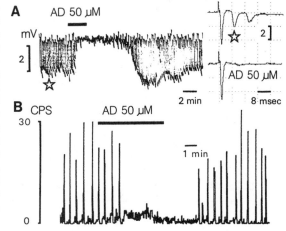

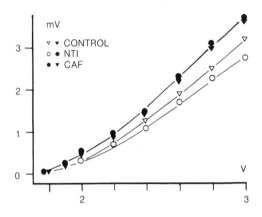

Figure 8. Interference of an adenosine uptake blocker (nitrobenzylthioinosine, NTI) with the action of caffeine. In the presence of NTI, caffeine enhances EPSPs more than under control conditions. A range of stimuli (1.8–3 V, abscissa) are plotted versus extracellular EPSP amplitude (mV, ordinate). NTI decreased the EPSP (O); caffeine increased the potentials to the same level in control and during NTI.

variations even under normal conditions. Although the concept of purinergic tonus is not new, we have provided good, new evidence for endogenous adenosine action in the hippocampus using several approaches: Caffeine and theophylline not only antagonized the actions of adenosine on hippocampal neurons but produced the opposite effect, a blockade of a nonvoltage-, non-Ca^{2+}-dependent potassium current and the long-lasting Ca^{2+}-dependent potassium current (Greene *et al.*, 1985). A depolarization and a blockade of accommodation of firing and the long-lasting AHP were observed with 100 μM caffeine. Caffeine increased EPSPs (measured extra- and intracellularly) and population spikes. The efficacy of caffeine was increased in the presence of exogenous adenosine, consistent with the action of a competitive inhibitor. Although other effects of caffeine such as a reduction of action potential amplitude and a reduction of the depolarizing plateau following slow spikes in the presence of barium and TTX (probably a persistent Ca^{2+}/Ba^{2+} current) were also observed, these occurred usually with higher concentrations and prolonged applications. The adenosine uptake blocker nitrobenzylthioinosine (NTI) produced a hyperpolarization and activation of potassium currents similar to those seen with adenosine (Fig. 8; see also Motley and Collins, 1983; Sebastiao and Ribeiro, 1985; Sanderson and Scholfield, 1986). The efficacy of caffeine in increasing synaptic potentials was significantly enhanced in the presence of NTI. Furthermore, the catabolic enzyme adenosine deaminase (ADA) had effects like caffeine, opposite to adenosine (Fig. 9), notably, also during perfusion with low $Ca^{2+}/high$ Mg^{2+} medium, when the Ca^{2+}-dependent synaptic source of adenosine would be eliminated. In the presence of ADA, the effect of caffeine was greatly reduced, presumably due to the reduction

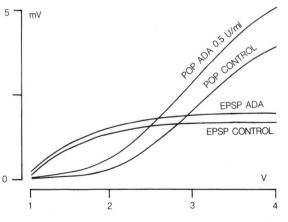

Figure 9. Adenosine deaminase (ADA) has actions opposite to those of adenosine, indicating a tonic inhibitory action of the latter. EPSPs and population spikes were recorded from strata radiatum and pyramidale in response to stratum radiatum stimulation. Potentials were measured (in mV, ordinate) for 15 different stimulation intensities (abscissa) and lines drawn through these points. The points are not retained in the figure for clarity.

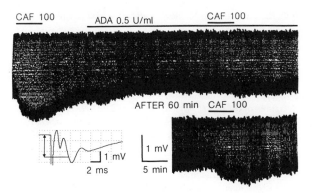

Figure 10. The excitatory action of caffeine is blocked in the presence of adenosine deaminase (ADA). Amplitude of EPSP, measured at a fixed time interval (as indicated in the insert, lower left hand), is continuously displayed through a sample and hold amplifier. Caffeine (CAF 100 μM) and ADA (0.5 U/ml) are present in the perfusion fluid during the time indicated by bars above the trace.

of electrophysiologically active adenosine (Fig. 10). Taken together, these results strongly suggest that many neurons are under a tonic endogenous inhibitory influence by adenosine. The excitation and, perhaps more importantly, the potentiation of excitatory signals by caffeine are a consequence of the antagonistic effects on adenosine present in electrophysiologically active concentrations in brain tissue.

5. Summary and Conclusion

Both pre- and postsynaptic actions are likely to contribute to the central effects of adenosine. In the hippocampus, an indirect quantal analysis suggests a reduction of transmitter release (Dunwiddie and Haas, 1985). The mechanism of the postsynaptic action is an increase in at least two potassium conductances, one Ca^{2+} dependent and one independent of Ca^{2+} and voltage (Haas and Greene, 1984; Haas et al., 1984; Greene and Haas, 1985). All these actions seem to occur through A_1 receptors at physiological concentrations and provide a powerful modulation of neuronal excitability, possibly as part of a feedback system linking neuronal activity to the available energy. The energy-rich ATP allows excitation (Akasu et al., 1983; Jahr and Jessell, 1983), while adenosine released by strong and, in particular, exaggerated activity is inhibitory and protects neurons from overexcitation. Experiments interfering with endogenous adenosine through antagonism, uptake block, or enzymatic breakdown strongly support a physiological role for adenosine (Greene et al., 1985; Haas et al., 1987). The molecular mechanisms have not yet been fully revealed but a mediation through the GTP-dependent inhibitory protein, which is blocked by pertussis toxin, is an attractive possibility (Dolphin and Prestwich, 1985). A direct coupling of this protein to a potassium channel might be responsible for the increase in a gK insensitive to Ca^{2+} and voltage while the effect on gK(Ca) could be mediated through decreased cAMP and intracellular Ca^{2+} binding (see Silinsky, 1984).

References

Akasu, T., Hirai, K., and Koketsu, K., 1983, Modulatory actions of ATP on membrane potentials of bullfrog sympathetic ganglion cells, *Brain Res.* **258:**313–317.

Akasu, T., Shinnick-Gallagher, P., and Gallagher, J. P., 1984, Adenosine mediates a slow hyperpolarizing synaptic potential in autonomic neurones, *Nature* **311:**26–65.

Alger, B. E., and Nicoll, R. A., 1980, Epileptiform burst afterhyperpolarization: A calcium-dependent potassium potential in hippocampal CA1 pyramidal cells, *Science* **210:**1122–1124.

Andersen, P., 1960, Interhippocampal impulses. II. Apical dendritic activation of CA1 neurons, *Acta Physiol. Scand.* **48:**178–208.

Ault, B., and Wang, C. M., 1986, Adenosine inhibits epileptiform activity arising in hippocampal area CA3, *Br. J. Pharmacol.* **87**:695–703.

Betz, W. J., 1970, Depression of transmitter release at the neuromuscular junction of the frog, *J. Physiol. (London)* **206**:629–644.

Brown, D. A., and Griffith, W. H., 1983, Calcium-activated outward current in voltage-clamped hippocampal neurones of the guinea-pig, *J. Physiol. (London)* **337**:287–301.

Buckle, P. J., and Haas, H. L., 1982, Enhancement of synaptic transmission by 4-aminopyridine in hippocampal slices of the rat, *J. Physiol. (London)* **326**:109–122.

Burnstock, G., 1975, Purinergic transmission, in: *Handbook of Psychopharmacology*, Vol. 5 (L. L. Iversen, S. D. Iversen, and S. H. Snyder, eds.), Raven Press, New York, pp. 131–194.

Burnstock, G., 1981, Neurotransmitter and trophic factors in the autonomic nervous system, *J. Physiol. (London)* **313**:1–35.

Daly, J. W., Butts-Lamb, P., and Padgett, W., 1984, Subclasses of adenosine receptors in the cortical nervous system: interaction with caffeine and related methylxanthines, *Cell. Mol. Neurobiol.* **3**:69–80.

Dolphin, A. C., and Prestwich, S. A., 1985, Pertussis toxin reverses adenosine inhibition of neuronal glutamate release, *Nature* **316**:148–150.

Dolphin, A. C., Forda, S. R., and Scott, R. H., 1986, Calcium-dependent currents in cultured rat dorsal root ganglion neurones are inhibited by an adenosine analogue, *J. Physiol. (London)* **373**:47–61.

Dragunow, M., 1986, Adenosine: The brain's natural anticonvulsant? *Trends Pharmacol. Sci.* **7**:128–130.

Dunwiddie, T. V., 1985, The physiological role of adenosine in the central nervous system, *Int. Rev. Neurobiol.* **27**:63–139.

Dunwiddie, T. V., and Haas, H. L., 1985, Adenosine increases synaptic facilitation in the in vitro rat hippocampus: Evidence for a presynaptic site of action, *J. Physiol. (London)* **369**:365–377.

Dunwiddie, T. V., and Hoffer, B. T., 1980, Adenine nucleotides and synaptic transmission in the in vitro hippocampus, *Br. J. Pharmacol.* **69**:59–68.

Dunwiddie, T. V., and Lynch, G. S., 1978, Long-term potentiation and depression of synaptic responses in the rat hippocampus: Localization and frequency dependency, *J. Physiol. (London)* **276**:353–367.

Dunwiddie, T. V., Hoffer, B. T., and Fredholm, B. B., 1981, Alkylxanthines elevate hippocampal excitability: Evidence for a role of endogenous adenosine, *Naunyn-Schmeidebergs Arch. Pharmacol.* **316**:326–330.

Fredholm, B. B., and Hedqvist, P., 1980, Modulation of neurotransmission by purine nucleotides and nucleosides, *Biochem. Pharmacol.* **29**:1635–1643.

Fredholm, B. B., Lindgren, E., and Lindström, K., 1985, Treatment with N-ethylmaleimide selectivity reduces adenosine receptor-mediated decreases in cyclic AMP accumulation in rat hippocampal slices, *Br. J. Pharmacol.* **86**:509–513.

Greene, R. W., and Haas, H. L., 1985, Adenosine actions on CA1 pyramidal neurones in rat hippocampal slices, *J. Physiol. (London)* **366**:110–127.

Greene, R. W., and Haas, H. L., 1987, Adenosine increases outward and decreases inward currents in hippocampal pyramidal cells of the rat in vitro, *Pfluegers Arch.* **408**:R87,339.

Greene, R. W., Haas, H. L., and Hermann, A., 1985, Effects of caffeine on hippocampal pyramidal cells in vitro, *Br. J. Pharmacol.* **85**:163–169.

Gustafsson, B., Galvan, M., Grafe, P., and Wigstroem, H., 1982, A transient outward current in a mammalian central neurone blocked by 4-aminopyridine, *Nature* **199**:252–254.

Haas, H. L., 1984, Histamine potentiates neuronal excitation by blocking a calcium-dependent potassium conductance, *Agents Actions* **16**:3–4.

Haas, H. L., and Greene, R. W., 1984, Adenosine enhances afterhyperpolarization and accommodation in hippocampal pyramidal cells, *Pfluegers Arch.* **402**:244–247.

Haas, H. L., and Jefferys, J. G. R., 1984, Low-calcium field burst discharges of CA1 pyramidal neurones in rat hippocampal slices, *J. Physiol. (London)* **354**:185–201.

Haas, H. L., and Konnerth, A., 1983, Histamine and noradrenaline decrease calcium-activated potassium conductance in hippocampal pyramidal cells, *Nature* **302**:432–434.

Haas, H. L., Schaerer, B., and Vosmansky, M. T., 1979, A simple perfusion chamber for the study of nervous tissue slices in vitro, *J. Neurosci. Methods* **1**:323–325.

Haas, H. L., Greene, R. W., and Heimrich, B., 1987, Endogenous adenosine actions on CA1 pyramidal cells in hippocampal slices of the rat, *Pfluegers Arch.* **408**:R87,340.

Haas, H. L., Jefferys, J. G. R., Slater, N. T., and Carpenter, D. O., 1984, Modulation of low calcium induced field bursts in the hippocampus by monoamines and cholinomimetics, *Pfluegers Arch.* **400**:28–33.

Hablitz, J. J., 1981, Altered burst responses in hippocampal Ca3 neurons injected with EGTA, *Exp. Brain Res.* **42**:483–485.

Halliwell, J. V., and Scholfield, C. N., 1984, Somatically recorded Ca-currents in guinea-pig hippocampal and olfactory cortex neurones are resistant to adenosine action, *Neurosci. Lett.* **50**:13–18.

Henon, B. K., and McAfee, D. A., 1983, The ionic basis of adenosine receptor actions on post-ganglionic neurones in the rat, *J. Physiol. (London)* **336**:607–620.

Hood, T. W., Siegfried, J., and Haas, H. L., 1983, Analysis of carbamazepine actions in hippocampal slices of the rat, *Cell. Mol. Neurobiol.* **3**:213–222.

Hotson, J. R., and Prince, D. A., 1980, A calcium-activated hyperpolarization follows repetitive firing in hippocampal neurones, *J. Neurophysiol.* **43**:409–419.

Jahr, C. E., and Jessell, T. M., 1983, ATP excites a subpopulation of rat dorsal horn neurones, *Nature* **304**:730–733.

Katz, B., and Miledi, R., 1968, The role of calcium in neuromuscular facilitation, *J. Physiol. (London)* **195**:481–492.

Kostopoulos, G. K., and Phillis, J. W., 1977, Purinergic depression of neurons in different areas of the rat brain, *Exp. Neurol.* **55**:719–724.

Kuroda, Y., Saito, M., and Kobayashi, K., 1976, Concomitant changes in cyclic AMP level and postsynaptic potentials of olfactory cortex induced by adenosine derivatives, *Brain Res.* **109**:196–201.

Lancaster, B., and Adams, P. R., 1986, Calcium-dependent current generating the afterhyperpolarization of hippocampal neurons, *J. Neurophysiol.* **55**:1268–1283.

Lee, K. S., Schubert, P., and Heinemann, U., 1984, The anticonvulsive action of adenosine: A postsynaptic, dendritic action by a possible endogenous anticonvulsant, *Brain Res.* **321**:160–164.

MacDonald, R. L., Skerritt, J. H., and Werz, M. A., 1986, Adenosine agonists reduce voltage-dependent calcium conductance of mouse sensory neurones in cell culture, *J. Physiol. (London)* **370**:75–90.

McNaughton, B. L., Barnes, C. A., and Andersen, P., 1981, Synaptic efficacy and epsp summation in granule cells of rat fascia dentata studied in vitro, *J. Neurophysiol.* **46**:952–966.

Madison, D. V., and Nicoll, R. A., 1982, Noradrenaline blocks accommodation of pyramidal cell discharge in the hippocampus, *Nature* **299**:636–638.

Madison, D. V., and Nicoll, R. A., 1986, Cyclic adenosine 3′,5′-monophosphate mediates beta-receptor actions of noradrenaline in rat hippocampal pyramidal cells, *J. Physiol. (London)* **372**:245–259.

Maitre, M., Ciesielski, L., Lehmann, A., Kempf, E., and Mandel, P., 1974, Protective effect of adenosine and nicotinamide against audiogenic seizures, *Biochem. Pharmacol.* **23**:2807.

Motley, S. J., and Collins, G. G. S., 1983, Endogenous adenosine inhibits excitatory transmission in the rat olfactory cortex slice, *Neuropharmacology* **22**:1081–1086.

Nagy, J. I., Buss, M., and Daddona, P. E., 1986, On the innervation of trigeminal mesencephalic primary afferent neurons by adenosine deaminase-containing projections from the hypothalamus in the rat, *Neuroscience* **17**:141–156.

Okada, Y., and Ozawa, S., 1980, Inhibitory action of adenosine on synaptic transmission in the hippocampus of the guinea pig in vitro, *Eur. J. Pharmacol.* **68**:483–492.

Phillis, J. W., and Wu, P. H., 1981, The role of adenosine and its nucleotides in central synaptic transmission, *Prog. Neurobiol.* **16**:187–239.

Proctor, W. R., and Dunwiddie, T. V., 1983, Adenosine inhibits calcium spikes in hippocampal pyramidal neurones in vitro, *Neurosci. Lett.* **35**:197–201.

Pull, I., and McIlwain, H., 1972, Output of 14C adenine derivatives on electrical excitation of tissues from the brain: Calcium ion sensitivity and an accompanying reuptake process, *Biochem. J.* **127**:91.

Rahaminoff, R., 1968, A dual action of calcium ions on neuromuscular facilitation, *J. Physiol.* **195**:471–480.

Sanderson, G., and Scholfield, C. N., 1986, Effects of adenosine uptake blockers and adenosine on evoked potentials of guinea-pig olfactory cortex, *Pfluegers Arch.* **406**:25–30.

Sattin, A., and Rall, T. W., 1970, The effect of adenosine and adenine nucleotides on the cyclic adenosine 3′-5′-monophosphate content of guinea-pig cerebral cortex slices, *Mol. Pharmacol.* **6**:13–23.

Scholfield, C. N., 1978, Depression of evoked potentials in brain slices by adenosine compounds, *Br. J. Pharmacol.* **63**:239–244.

Schubert, P., and Mitzdorf, U., 1979, Analysis and quantitative evaluation of the depressive effect of adenosine on evoked potentials in hippocampal slices, *Brain Res.* **172**:186–190.

Schwartzkroin, P. A., and Stafstrom, C. E., 1980, Effects of EGTA on the calcium-activated afterhyperpolarization in hippocampal CA3 pyramidal cells, *Science* **210**:1125–1126.

Sebastiao, A. M., and Ribeiro, J. A., 1985, Enhancement of transmission at the frog neuromuscular junction by adenosine deaminase: Evidence for an inhibitory role of endogenous adenosine on neuromuscular transmission, *Neurosci. Lett.* **62**:267–270.

Segal, M., 1982, Intracellular analysis of a post-synaptic action of adenosine in the rat hippocampus, *Eur. J. Pharmacol.* **79**:193–199.

Shimizu, H., and Daly, J., 1970, Formation of adenosine 3′,5′-monophosphate from adenosine in brain slice, *Biochim. Biophys. Acta* **222**:465–473.

Siggins, G. R., and Schubert, P., 1981, Adenosine depression of hippocampal neurons in vitro: An intracellular study of dose-dependent actions on synaptic and membrane potentials, *Neurosci. Lett.* **23**:55–60.

Silinsky, E. M., 1984, On the mechanism by which adenosine receptor activation inhibits the release of acetylcholine from motor nerve endings, *J. Physiol. (London)* **346**:243–256.

Skerritt, J. H., Davies, L. P., and Johnston, G. A. R., 1982, A purinergic component in the anticonvulsant action of carbamazepine? *Eur. J. Pharmacol.* **82**:195–197.

Stone, T. W., 1981, Physiological roles for adenosine and adenosine 5′-triphosphate in the nervous system, *Neuroscience* **6**:523–555.

Trussell, L. O., and Jackson, M. B., 1985, Adenosine-activated potassium conductance in cultured striatal neurons, *Proc. Natl. Acad. Sci. USA* **82**:4857–4861.

Weir, R. L., Padgett, W., Daly, J. W., and Anderson, S. M., 1984, Interaction of anticonvulsant drugs with adenosine receptors in the central nervous system, *Epilepsia* **25**:492–498.

32

Electrophysiology of a Peptidergic Neuron
The Hypothalamic Magnocellular Neurosecretory Cell

Leo P. Renaud

1. Introduction

The "peptide-synthesizing" or "peptidergic" neurons have recently become the object of intense interest in neurobiology (for reviews see Krieger, 1983; Beal and Martin, 1986). While neurophysiological research has usually been directed toward an understanding of the long- and short-term synaptic or receptor actions of neuropeptides, comparatively little attention has been directed toward the electrophysiology of the peptide-secreting neurons themselves. In part, this reflects the apparent lack of unique electrophysiological signals comparable to immunocytochemical staining that would serve to identify the peptidergic nature of any specified neuron under examination. Since peptides are quite possibly present in *all* neurons, other criteria (e.g., uniformity of immunocytochemical identity in a specific location) may prove more fruitful. One of the more obvious instances of the above is the collection of magnocellular neurosecretory cells (MNCs) in the mammalian hypothalamic supraoptic (SON) and paraventricular (PVN) nuclei, and accessory magnocellular cell groups. These "classic" neurosecretory neurons have long been viewed as "peptidergic" neurons by Bargmann (1949), Scharrer and Scharrer (1975), Sachs (1970), and others. Immunocytochemical studies have clearly revealed that these neurons synthesize either oxytocin or vasopressin (Swaab *et al.*, 1975; Vandesande and Dierickx, 1975). Their axons project almost exclusively into the neurohypophysis, where vasopressin and oxytocin are released in proportion to their levels of excitability. This chapter will review selected aspects of the neurophysiology of this class of peptidergic neurons based on observations acquired during *in vivo* and *in vitro* experiments in the rat.

2. Identification of MNCs in Vivo

2.1. Antidromic Identification

In the course of *in vivo* extracellular recordings from SON and PVN neurons in anesthetized preparations, MNCs can be readily identified on the basis of their antidromic activation following

Leo P. Renaud • Neurosciences Unit, Montreal General Hospital and McGill University, Montreal, Quebec H3G 1A4, Canada.

the delivery of an electrical stimulus sufficient to activate their axon terminals in the neurohypophysis (Yagi *et al.,* 1964; for review see Renaud *et al.,* 1979). Criteria for identity include constant-latency all-or-none response at threshold, constant-latency following of two or more stimuli presented at high frequency, and evidence of collision cancellation between spontaneously occurring and antidromically activated spikes within a critical interval (one latency period) of the stimulus. Further differentiation as to whether the observed activity arises from either an oxytocin- or a vasopressin-secreting neuron can be achieved on the basis of pattern of firing and sensitivity to specific sensory stimuli.

2.2. Oxytocin-Secreting MNCs

Bursting activity patterns are a feature of both types of neurosecretory neurons, but the pattern and stimulus for their generation are uniquely different for oxytocin- as compared with vasopressin-secreting MNCs. Recordings from MNCs in lactating rats with suckling pups have revealed a stereotyped behavior among a population of SON and PVN neurons which are otherwise silent or (more frequently) display an irregular continuous firing pattern. The suckling stimulus appears to promote the intermittent (every few minutes) occurrence of an abrupt high-frequency (up to 60–80 Hz) discharge lasting for 2–4 sec followed by a 10- to 30-sec depression in their excitability (Lincoln and Wakerley, 1974). This event is synchronized not only between adjacent "oxytocin-secreting" cells, but also between such cells in different nuclei (Belin and Moos, 1986). Within 10–12 sec of this neuronal burst, oxytocin released by the impulses reaching the neural lobe axon terminals has had time to circulate and cause a contraction of the myoepithelial tissues in the mammary glands whereupon intramammary pressure is increased and milk is ejected. In the rat, this bursting behavior from putative oxytocin-secreting MNCs is not confined to the milk ejection reflex. During the late phase of gestation, certain MNCs appear to have an increased level of spontaneous activity (Negoro *et al.,* 1973; Boer and Nolten, 1978). High-frequency bursting is present during the expulsive phase of parturition and precedes strong uterine contractions (Summerlee, 1983).

The specific afferent pathways that convey the suckling stimulus to the hypothalamus remain poorly defined (reviewed in Poulain and Wakerley, 1982). There is substantial convergence of sensory inputs from the nipple to neurons at the spinal segmental level (Poulain and Wakerley, 1986). Ascending sensory information courses through the midbrain tegmentum (Dubois-Dauphin *et al.,* 1985). Although there is no clear evidence that catecholamine afferents to SON and PVN are involved, this neuronal reflex can be facilitated by catecholamines (Moos and Richard, 1982) and by oxytocin itself (Freund-Mercier and Richard, 1984). The latter observation has led to the proposal that during parturition and lactation (and possibly at other times) oxytocin may be released both into the neurohypophysis and from synaptic sites in brain (Theodosis, 1985). Moreover, oxytocin may favor the development of a special form of neuronal plasticity that favors interaction of oxytocin cells during lactation (Theodosis *et al.,* 1986a) and chronic dehydration (Perlmutter *et al.,* 1985).

On the basis of immunocytochemical data, there is little difference between the numbers of MNCs with oxytocin-like immunoreactivity in male and female brains. Aside from oxytocin's influence on smooth muscle tissue at parturition and during lactation in the female, there is little known concerning other more general functions for plasma oxytocin that would encompass both males and females. Little is known of stimuli that selectively activate oxytocin-secreting neurons in both sexes. However, in the rat, there are features that permit their differentiation from vasopressin-secreting cells on electrophysiological grounds. First, oxytocin-secreting MNCs appear to be unresponsive to a rise in mean arterial pressure sufficient to activate peripheral baroreceptors (Fig. 1). Second, in the rat, a majority of these neurons which show continuous irregular firing patterns and no response to transient elevation of arterial pressure demonstrate a 50–200% increase in firing within seconds of the administration of cholecystokinin octapeptide

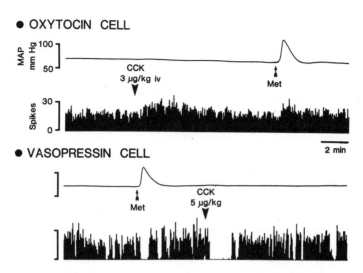

Figure 1. Mean arterial pressure (MAP) traces (above) and ratemeter records (below) from two different SON neurons in a Nembutal-anesthetized male rat. Oxytocin-secreting MNCs are distinguished by their lack of response when an intravenous α agonist (metaraminol, arrow) is used to raise MAP sufficient to activate peripheral baroreceptors. Note also that this cell's firing is *increased* following an intravenous injection of CCK-8. Vasopressin-secreting MNCs are often phasically active and their firing is transiently depressed during drug-induced increases in MAP. Note that this cell's firing is *decreased* after CCK-8 injection.

(CCK-8) by intravenous or intraperitoneal injection (Tang *et al.*, 1986; Fig. 1). This neuronal activity and associated hormone release in the neurohypophysis would explain the dramatic elevation in plasma oxytocin levels reported to follow CCK injections (Verbalis *et al.*, 1986). Since food ingestion also elevates plasma oxytocin, although to a lesser degree than CCK, and aversive agents (e.g., lithium chloride, copper sulfate, apomorphine, and hypertonic saline), Verbalis *et al.*, (1986) have postulated that a vagally mediated central nausea pathway, with activation of hypothalamic oxytocin-secreting neurons, is largely responsible for CCK-induced satiety. We have recently reported (Tang *et al.*, 1986) that gastric distension selectively enhances the firing of oxytocin-secreting neurons in SON, an observation that may have a bearing on their involvement in a vagally mediated central satiety mechanism in the rat. At the moment, there is little further information on this specific stimulus for oxytocin neurons, and whether it is unique to this species.

2.3. Vasopressin-Secreting Neurons

In their pioneering studies, Lincoln and Wakerley (1974) noted that "phasic" discharges could be recorded from a separate population of neurohypophysial-projecting neurons whose activity was not synchronized to milk ejection. It is now apparent that the firing patterns of such neurons may alternate between continuous and phasic activity in response to situations favorable to vasopressin release, e.g., hyperosmolar or hypovolemic states (Poulain *et al.*, 1977). Moreover, these cells are uniquely responsive to cardiovascular input such that their firing can be transiently *enhanced* by stimulation of carotid chemoreceptors or alternatively *depressed* by abrupt drug-induced elevations of mean arterial pressure sufficient to activate peripheral baroreceptors (Kannan and Yagi, 1978; Harris, 1979; Fig. 1). The latter feature has been of particular assistance in the differentiation between putative vasopressin- and oxytocin-secreting neurons during experiments designed to examine the functional nature of selected afferent pathways to neurosecretory neurons.

The critical issue as to whether those MNCs that display phasic discharges are in fact the same cells that synthesize and release vasopressin cannot be adequately tested *in vivo* owing to the instability of intracellular recordings in this brain region. However, the matter has been addressed using brain slice preparations where a majority of phasically firing neurons also display vasopressin-like immunoreactivity (Yamashita *et al.*, 1983; Cobbett *et al.*, 1986).

3. Possibilities for Synaptic Modulation

Physiological stimuli known to alter the release of vasopressin and/or oxytocin from the neurohypophysis include plasma hyperosmolality, hypovolemia, chemoreceptor and baroreceptor activation, suckling, emesis, pain, and emotionality. However, as earlier mentioned in reference to milk ejection, the identity and functional organization of the specific afferent pathways whereby any one of these stimuli engaged MNCs remain poorly defined. This is partly due to inherent difficulties in the morphological and functional analysis of complex polysynaptic pathways from a peripheral receptor to a centrally located perikaryon. Of added concern is the question of distinguishing between input pathways that are modulatory in nature rather than intrinsic to the reflex (Lebrun *et al.*, 1983).

A major contribution in defining the structural framework for the conduction of information to MNCs has ensued from recent progress with anterograde and retrograde tracers (e.g., Miselis, 1981; Iijima and Ogawa, 1981; Silverman *et al.*, 1981; Sawchenko and Swanson, 1983; Tribollet *et al.*, 1985). These studies have been successful in identifying groups of neurons that, when stimulated, will alter the excitability of MNCs synaptically. Of the various known afferents to SON and PVN, those that arise in the amygdala, septum, diagonal band, subfornical organ, and brain-stem A1 and A2 cell groups have been subjected to detailed electrophysiological analysis and will be reviewed here briefly. Supplementary information derived from studies of the sensitivity of MNCs to direct application of neurotransmitters or neuromodulators has, in specific instances, been integrated into the analysis of specific afferent pathways. The following section provides a brief overview of this information.

3.1. Catecholamines

3.1.1. Noradrenaline (NA)

The dense catecholamine innervation of MNCs reported in several earlier studies (e.g., Fuxe, 1965) is due primarily to NA-containing terminals. Retrograde and anterograde tracer studies have identified the A1 neurons of the caudal ventrolateral medulla (CVLM) as a principal source (Sawchenko and Swanson, 1981) with a lesser contribution from the A2 noradrenergic cells in the dorsomedial medulla (Raby and Renaud, 1987). Electrical stimulation in the CVLM evokes a selective facilitation of vasopressin-secreting MNCs in SON and PVN (Day and Renaud, 1984; Day *et al.*, 1984). In contrast, stimulation of the dorsomedial medulla A2 neurons facilitates the firing of a population of both vasopressin- and oxytocin-secreting MNCs (Day *et al.*, 1984; Raby and Renaud, 1987). Latencies of response (~ 40 msec) agree with the slow conduction velocities recorded from monoaminergic fibers, and the loss of response following depletion of terminal catecholamines after 6-hydroxydopamine pretreatment indicates that the A1- and A2-evoked excitations are the result of the monosynaptic release of NA on MNCs. Confirmation of the excitatory nature of NA on MNCs has been obtained both *in vivo* (Day *et al.*, 1985b) and *in vitro* (Armstrong *et al.*, 1986; Inenaga *et al.*, 1986; Randle *et al.*, 1986a,b). These studies indicate that the activation of an adrenergic receptor of the α_1 type causes a slow membrane depolarization and promotes bursting activity, most likely through alteration of a membrane potassium conductance. Moreover, this action culminates in the release of both vasopressin and oxytocin from the neurohypophysis (Randle *et al.*, 1986c).

The above represents a dramatic departure from the impressions obtained through iontophoretic (Barker *et al.*, 1971a; Arnauld *et al.*, 1983) and functional (Armstrong *et al.*, 1982; Blessing *et al.*, 1982) studies which inferred that noradrenergic pathways exert a tonic inhibitory influence on the excitability of vasopressin-secreting neurons. However, iontophoretic studies have indicated that the NA-induced depressions were mediated through a β adrenoreceptor mechanism (Barker *et al.*, 1971a). That this action does occur at concentrations of the drug that are possibly much higher than the physiological range can be confirmed using voltametric (Armstrong-James and Fox, 1983) and pressure ejection methods (Day *et al.*, 1985b). The massive increase in plasma vasopressin after electrolytic lesions in the CVLM (Blessing *et al.*, 1982) may be partly due to the stimulatory action of the iron deposited by stainless steel electrodes; lesions in CVLM made with platinum electrodes produce little change in plasma vasopressin levels (P. Korner, personal communication).

3.1.2. Dopamine

Recent ultrastructural studies utilizing an antiserum against glutaraldehyde-conjugated dopamine (Buijs *et al.*, 1984; Lindvall *et al.*, 1984) leave little doubt as to the presence of a substantial dopaminergic innervation of MNCs, possibly from cells located in the ventral tegmental area. While data from earlier iontophoretic studies (Moss *et al.*, 1972b) gave equivocal results, more recent experiments generally indicate an excitatory action of dopamine on both oxytocin- and vasopressin-secreting MNCs when tested not only *in vivo* (e.g., Moos and Richard, 1982) but also *in vitro* (e.g., Bridges *et al.*, 1976; Mason, 1983).

3.1.3. Histamine

Centrally injected histamine has been noted to enhance the release of vasopressin from the neurohypophysis (Roberts and Calcutt, 1983; Bhargava *et al.*, 1983). Axon terminals with histamine-like immunoreactivity can be visualized among MNCs and may arise from neurons in the posterior hypothalamus (e.g., Watanabe *et al.*, 1984). Although some have reported little or no effect (Barker *et al.*, 1971a; Sakai *et al.*, 1974), others have observed that histamine has excitatory actions on SON neurons *in vivo* (Haas *et al.*, 1975) and *in vitro* (Armstrong and Sladek, 1985), presumably mediated through an H_1-type receptor.

3.1.4. Serotonin

Double label studies have recently revealed that SON and PVN neurons receive a distinct input from brain-stem serotoninergic cells (Sawchenko *et al.*, 1983). Although the innervation is sparse as compared to the noradrenergic innervation, it has a preferential distribution for those portions of SON and PVN where oxytocin-secreting MNCs are concentrated. Earlier iontophoretic studies suggest a depressant action on MNCs (Barker *et al.*, 1971a; Moss *et al.*, 1972b). In view of the distribution of serotonin fibers mentioned above, it is of interest to note that serotonin appears to depress milk ejections in the anesthetized rat, although opposite effects are noted in the conscious animal (Moos and Richard, 1983).

3.2. Limbic

Connections from the amygdala and septum to SON and PVN (Zaborszky *et al.*, 1975; Sawchenko and Swanson, 1983; Oldfield *et al.*, 1985) likely contribute to the anatomical basis for any alterations in posterior pituitary hormone release accompanying stressful and emotional stimuli (e.g., Cross, 1955; Keil and Severs, 1977).

3.2.1. Amygdala

Electrophysiological studies suggest that projections from the amygdala to SON and PVN follow the ventral amygdalofugal pathway and are most often inhibitory to both vasopressin- (Fig. 2) and oxytocin-secreting cells (Negoro et al., 1973; Pittman et al., 1981; Thomson, 1982; Hamamura et al., 1982; Ferreyra et al., 1983). Responses may depend upon stimulus frequency, species, and sites within the amygdala (Tomas, 1975; Hayward et al., 1977).

3.2.2. Lateral Septum

Ipsilateral stimulation in this location has a predominantly depressant influence on the excitability of both vasopressin- (Fig. 2) and oxytocin-secreting MNCs in SON (Poulain et al., 1980; Cirino and Renaud, 1985). Since stimulation in the amygdala and lateral septum evokes similar patterns of response from approximately 30% of MNCs (see Fig. 2A), there would seem to be some convergence of input. Whether these inputs share a common mechanism (e.g., transmitter and/or interneuron) is not known. In any event, the ability to demonstrate that stimulation in these limbic areas is capable of attenuating ongoing *phasic* activity (from putative vasopressin-secreting cells) depends on several factors, including the intensity of the stimulus, its duration, and (especially) its temporal relationship to the onset of a burst (Fig. 2). With oxytocin-secreting MNCs, which lack phasic variations in excitability, stimulus intensity and frequency appear to be the most relevant variables (Cirino and Renaud, 1985).

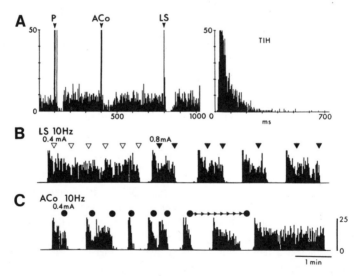

Figure 2. Spike train data from a phasic (vasopressin-secreting) SON MNC reveals the depressant effects of stimulation in the cortical nucleus of amygdala (ACo) and the lateral septum (LS). (A) Peristimulus histogram during sequential single shock stimuli applied to the posterior pituitary (P, to monitor the antidromic response), ACo, and LS reveals a brief depression in excitability. On the right, a time interval histogram during 1000 spontaneous spikes. (B) Repeated applications of brief 20-pulse trains of 10-Hz stimulation in LS (symbols) given at two different intensities (0.4 and 0.8 mA) reveal that the higher intensity is more effective in arresting ongoing phasic discharges. (C) Similar to B, but with ACo stimulation revealing that a silent period may also be initiated by this input, although not necessarily sustained when the stimulus is prolonged (horizontal arrowheads). (From Cirino and Renaud, 1985.)

The septum has been identified with a variety of roles including control of salt and water balance, regulation of blood pressure and milk ejection (Mogenson, 1976; Harris, 1978; Lebrun *et al.*, 1983). With respect to the latter, the observation that septal stimulation at 10 Hz, but not at 1 Hz, can modulate (delay) the frequency of milk ejections (Lebrun *et al.*, 1983) correlates reasonably well with the extracellular single-cell data (Poulain *et al.*, 1980; Cirino and Renaud, 1985). Information on vasopressin is scant at present.

3.3. Amino Acids

3.3.1. Aspartate and Glutamate

Iontophoretic data indicate that a majority of vasopressin- and oxytocin-secreting MNCs are briskly responsive to both L-aspartate and L-glutamate (Arnauld *et al.*, 1983). MNCs may demonstrate depolarizing block to excessive quantities of these agents, but their continuous application in low concentration *in vitro* or *in vivo* may reveal either continuous or phasic activity in otherwise quiescent cells (Haller and Wakerley, 1980; Arnauld *et al.*, 1983).

3.3.2. GABA: In Vivo Observations

GABA has a potent depressant action on the excitability of most MNCs and this action is readily reversible by the GABA$_A$ receptor antagonist bicuculline (Nicoll and Barker, 1971a; Moss *et al.*, 1972b; Bioulac *et al.*, 1978; Arnauld *et al.*, 1983). An abundance of synaptic terminals with GABA-like immunoreactivity have recently been visualized in SON at the ultrastructural level (van den Pol, 1985; Theodosis *et al.*, 1986b), thus confirming earlier light microscopic (Perez de la Mora *et al.*, 1981; Tappaz *et al.*, 1983) and biochemical (Tappaz *et al.*, 1977) evidence of GABA's prominence in the regulation of MNC excitability.

3.3.3. GABAergic Inputs: In Vivo Studies

Several inhibitory inputs to MNCs can be observed with *in vivo* recordings (e.g., septum, amygdala, subfornical organ) but only that evoked by stimulation in the ventral portion of the vertical limb of the diagonal band of Broca (DBB) has been characterized as GABA-mediated. Interestingly, this depressant action is selectively directed toward vasopressin-secreting neurons. Bicuculline also selectively blocks the depression in excitability of vasopressin-secreting neurons consequent to peripheral baroreceptor activation (Jhamandas and Renaud, 1986a). The simultaneous observation of a reciprocal activity pattern among a population of DBB neurons that project to SON (Jhamandas and Renaud, 1986b) suggests their participation either as inhibitory neurons or as interneurons in the baroreflex inhibitory pathway to vasopressin-secreting neurons. However, this is only a portion of the neural network since lesions in ascending catecholamine pathways at the level of the locus coeruleus or ventrolateral medulla also block baroreceptor input to SON (Banks and Harris, 1984).

3.3.4. GABAergic Inputs: In Vitro Observations

A more detailed intracellular characterization of the inhibitory input to SON MNCs from DBB has now been achieved *in vitro* using a perfused explant of rat hypothalamus (Randle *et al.*, 1986d). In this preparation, recordings obtained with potassium acetate-filled micropipettes reveal frequent spontaneous IPSPs. In addition, DBB stimulation evokes a prominent compound IPSP of 60- to 100-msec duration (Fig. 3C). The mean evoked IPSP time constant of decay (average of 37.0 msec; $N = 16$ cells) is approximately 2.5 times the cell time constant. Conductance increases

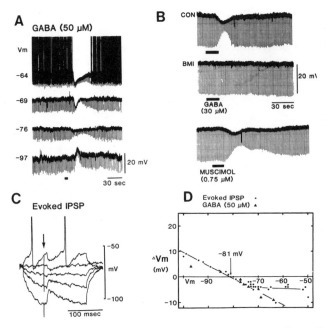

Figure 3. Composite diagram of *in vitro* observations in SON that illustrate the similarity in membrane response of MNCs to exogenously applied GABA and the IPSP evoked by diagonal band stimulation. (A) Addition of GABA (50 μM) to the perfusion media causes an abrupt cessation in firing at resting membrane potential levels (top trace) accompanied by a membrane hyperpolarization and prominent increase in membrane conductance. Subsequent additions of GABA while the membrane potential (V_m) was maintained at the levels indicated on the left by intracellular current injection reveal the approximate GABA reversal potential. (B) Membrane hyperpolarization and conductance increase induced by addition of GABA (30 μM, top panel) are blocked by the GABA$_A$ receptor antagonist bicuculline (BMI, 100 μM, middle panel) and mimicked by the GABA$_A$ receptor agonist muscimol. (C) IPSP evoked by stimulation of the diagonal band (arrow) is reversed as V_m is adjusted to more hyperpolarized levels by an intracellular current pulse. (D) Amplitude of the voltage response to GABA and the IPSP are plotted as a function of the membrane potential. Note the similar reversal potential (~ -81 mV). (From Randle and Renaud, 1987.)

up to 22.0 nS at the peak of the IPSP reflect enhanced membrane permeability to chloride ions. In control media, IPSPs reverse at approximately -80 mV (Fig. 3D). The IPSP reversal potential can be shifted to more depolarized levels by intracellular injection of chloride ions or by reduction in the extracellular chloride concentration. Both spontaneous and evoked IPSPs are blocked by addition of bicuculline (10–100 μM) to the bath media whereas their durations can be prolonged in the presence of pentobarbital.

3.3.5. GABA Action: Intracellular Observations

The preceding features are strongly suggestive of a GABA-mediated postsynaptic inhibition. Indeed, the addition of GABA (30–50 μM) to the media depresses spontaneous activity of all SON neurons recorded *in vitro* (Randle *et al.*, 1986a; Randle and Renaud, 1987). Cells usually display an associated membrane hyperpolarization which reverses at membrane potentials similar to that for evoked IPSPs (Randle and Renaud, 1987; Fig. 3A,D). The additional features of sensitivity of GABA's actions to transmembrane chloride ionic gradient, reversible blockade in the presence of bicuculline, and mimicry by the potent GABA agonist muscimol (Fig. 3B) are characteristics of GABA$_A$ receptor activation. The slope of the log–log plots of drug-induced currents as a function of drug concentration is approximately 1.7 for both GABA and muscimol, indicating that two molecules combine to activate the ionophore which, in this case, is specific for chloride ions. It is presumably the consequence of this receptor–ionophore interaction that underlies the depression in vasopressin-secreting MNC excitability consequent both to DBB stimulation and (*in vivo*) to peripheral baroreceptor activation.

3.4. Acetylcholine

The antidiuretic action of acetylcholine initially reported by Pickford is due to stimulation of nicotinic cholinergic receptors and subsequent release of vasopressin. Iontophoretic application of acetylcholine to MNCs reveals an excitatory nicotinic action (Dreifuss and Kelly, 1972a) and depressant muscarinic effect (Barker *et al.*, 1971a). Further study suggests that these are preferentially distributed to vasopressin- and oxytocin-secreting MNCs, respectively (Bioulac *et al.*, 1978; Arnauld *et al.*, 1983). In SON, Hatton *et al.* (1983) proposed that the nicotinic cholinergic input to phasic MNCs may arise from lateral hypothalamic neurons located near the nucleus. On a functional note, nicotinic cholinergic receptors facilitate the release of vasopressin from hypothalamic explants (Sladek and Joynt, 1979). Conversely, nicotinic antagonists administered systemically block the excitation of both oxytocin and vasopressin neurons resulting from hemorrhage, and the excitation of oxytocin neurons by suckling (Clarke *et al.*, 1978; Bisset and Chowdrey, 1981; Clarke and Merrick, 1985).

3.5. Angiotensin II and the Subfornical Organ

3.5.1. Action of Angiotensin II on MNCs

The presence of receptors for angiotensin II on MNCs is proposed in part by the observation that iontophoretic application of angiotensin II produces an increase in their excitability (Nicoll and Barker, 1971b). Intracerebroventricular angiotensin II also promotes activation of MNCs (Akaishi *et al.*, 1980), although this route of administration may be indirect through involvement of angiotensin II receptors located in the walls of the rostral third ventricle. Increases in both vasopressin and oxytocin levels in plasma suggest a nonselective action of this peptide on MNCs. Intravenous angiotensin II increases the excitability of both vasopressin- and oxytocin-secreting MNCs (Fig. 4B). This is clearly an indirect effect mediated through angiotensin II-sensitive neurons in a circumventricular structure, the subfornical organ (SFO), since the response is abolished by SFO lesions (Ferguson and Renaud, 1986).

3.5.2. SFO Influence on MNCs

The SFO is one of two forebrain circumventricular structures [the other is the organum vasculosum of the lamina terminalis (OVLT)] whose neurons project directly to SON and PVN (Miselis, 1981; Silverman *et al.*, 1981; Sawchenko and Swanson, 1983; Tribollet *et al.*, 1985). SFO has a role in the maintenance of body fluid balance, certain autonomic (e.g., blood pressure) functions, and the regulation of anterior and posterior pituitary hormone release. While the neural circuitry pertaining to these roles is reviewed elsewhere (Renaud *et al.*, 1985; Gutman *et al.*, 1986), that to MNCs deserves special mention. Electrical stimulation in SFO exerts a unique prolonged increase in the excitability of a majority of MNCs in SON and PVN and involves both vasopressin- and oxytocin-secreting neurons (Sgro *et al.*, 1984; Ferguson *et al.*, 1984; see Fig. 4A). Recent studies in unanesthetized rats indicate that this stimulation produces a prominent rise in both vasopressin and oxytocin in the plasma (Ferguson and Kasting, 1986).

3.5.3. Central Angiotensin Pathways

Angiotensin II-like immunoreactivity has recently been reported by Lind *et al.*, (1985) in neural circuitry that is both afferent and efferent to SFO. The possibility that angiotensin may have a transmitter role at one or more of these sites finds support in the observations by Tanaka *et al.* (1986a,b) that saralasin, an angiotensin antagonist, can selectively block both synaptic excitation and neuronal firing induced by microiontophoretically applied angiotensin II in median

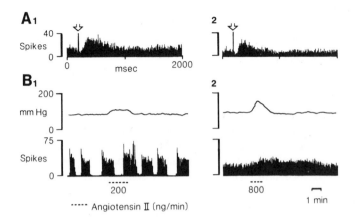

Figure 4. Spike train data from a vasopressin-secreting (1) and an oxytocin-secreting (2) MNC in PVN. (A) Peristimulus histograms reveal that both neurons display a prolonged increase in excitability after a single electrical stimulus in the subfornical organ (arrow). (B) During intravenous infusion of angiotensin II (horizontal dashed line) there is an increase in mean arterial pressure (top traces) and action potential frequency (lower ratemeter traces). Note the phasic discharge from the vasopressin cell and the continuous discharge from the oxytocin cell. (From Ferguson and Renaud, 1986.)

preoptic nucleus and lateral hypothalamus. The demonstrated sensitivity of neurosecretory neurons to locally applied angiotensin II and reduction in their level of spontaneous activity by saralasin (Jhamandas and Renaud, unpublished data) would be in keeping with the notion that angiotensin II also maintains a tonic facilitatory drive on neurosecretory cells and may possibly act as a peptidergic neurotransmitter to MNCs.

3.6. Other Peptides

3.6.1. Vasopressin and Oxytocin

As mentioned in Section 4.3.3 (see also Buijs and Heerikhuize, 1982), neurohypophyseal peptides may be involved in synaptic transmission at several CNS sites. Within SON and PVN, the possibility of a synaptic role for these peptides is further strengthened by the detection of synaptic profiles with oxytocin-like immunoreactivity (Theodosis, 1985). Moreover, evidence for peptide receptors on MNCs is based on earlier *in vivo* studies where iontophoretically applied vasopressin depressed (Nicoll and Barker, 1971a) and oxytocin excited MNCs (Moss *et al.*, 1972a). Recent *in vitro* observations suggest a predominantly excitatory action on unidentified PVN neurons following bath application (Abe *et al.*, 1983; Inenaga and Yamashita, 1986).

3.6.2. Neuropeptide Y (NPY)

The presence of a pancreatic polypeptide-like agent termed NPY coexisting with NA in A1 neurons as well as in axon terminals in SON and PVN (Hunt *et al.*, 1981; Jacobowitz and Olschowska, 1982; Everitt *et al.*, 1984) prompted an *in vivo* study to compare its actions with that of NA (Day *et al.*, 1985a). Although NPY and the structurally similar avian pancreatic polypeptide (APP) were found to mimic the actions of NA, and may therefore participate in the excitation of vasopressin-secreting MNCs following electrical stimulation in the A1 region, the effective concentrations of NPY and APP were comparatively high and appeared to interfere with, rather than potentiate, the actions of NA.

3.6.3. CCK-8

CCK-8 is reported to coexist with oxytocin in MNCs in SON and PVN (Vanderhaegen *et al.*, 1980). The function of CCK-8 in these neurons, and its actions on MNC excitability remain uncertain. However, it is indeed curious that peripheral (intravenous or intraperitoneal) injections of CCK-8 in the rat are followed by an abrupt and selective increase in firing of oxytocin-secreting MNCs (Tang *et al.*, 1986; see Fig. 1A) and a subsequent increase in the levels of circulating oxytocin (Verbalis *et al.*, 1986). This effect is vagally mediated, rather than a direct effect of CCK on the neurons themselves. An equally interesting, but not clearly related, finding is the similar selective response of oxytocin-secreting MNCs to gastric distension (Tang *et al.*, 1986).

3.6.4. Opioid Peptides

In the rat, reports of opioid peptides localized within MNCs or their axon terminals include dynorphin (Watson *et al.*, 1982), α-neoendorphin (Millan *et al.*, 1983), and leucine enkephalin (Martin and Voigt, 1981) in vasopressin-secreting cells, and methionine enkephalin in oxytocin-secreting cells (Martin *et al.*, 1983). There are substantial functional data indicating a role for these peptides in modulating vasopressin and especially oxytocin secretion, most often to depress release (e.g., Clarke *et al.*, 1979; Summy-Long *et al.*, 1984; Bicknell *et al.*, 1985).

The depressant action of opiates and opioid peptides at the cellular level also supports the notion of a selective action on oxytocin-secreting MNCs. Phasically active (vasopressin-secreting) neurons recorded *in vitro* (Wakerley *et al.*, 1983) and *in vivo* (Arnauld *et al.*, 1983) are only weakly inhibited. In contrast, the inhibitory action of opioids on oxytocin secretion appears due to reduction in the release of hormone from axon terminals in the neural lobe by interfering with the stimulus–secretion coupling mechanism (Clarke *et al.*, 1979; Bicknell and Leng, 1982).

4. Intrinsic Properties of MNCs

4.1. Osmosensitivity

Elevation of plasma osmotic pressure potently stimulates both oxytocin- and vasopressin-secreting MNCs *in vivo* (Brimble and Dyball, 1977) and consequent hormone release (e.g., Cheng and North, 1986). The mechanisms whereby this is achieved remain unclear. On the one hand, osmoreceptors appear to be located in several sites, including the hepatic portal vasculature and circumventricular organs (reviewed in Sladek and Armstrong, 1985). Verney's (1947) studies focused attention on the hypothalamic supraoptic nucleus where *in vivo* (Leng, 1980) and *in vitro* data (Mason, 1980; Abe and Ogata, 1982; Bourque and Renaud, 1984) support the notion of an intrinsic osmosensitivity of MNCs. With intracellular recordings, an increase of 8 mosm will produce membrane depolarization (Mason, 1980) and this depolarization may possibly involve change in a membrane potassium conductance (Abe and Ogata, 1982). However, comparatively large changes in osmotic pressure are required to induce brisk neuronal firing *in vitro*, especially under conditions of synaptic isolation (Bourque and Renaud, 1984). This lack of sensitivity contrasts sharply with the exquisite *in vivo* sensitivity of the system. Evidently multiple osmoreceptor elements, notably those in the anterior ventral third ventricle (AV3V), participate in the normal response to an osmotic challenge (Leng *et al.*, 1982, 1985). Thus, the intrinsic osmotic depolarization would likely interact with other intrinsic voltage-sensitive conductances (see Section 4.3) and these in turn would be augmented or modulated by incoming synaptic information of local or peripheral origin which utilize perhaps a variety of transmitters (e.g., acetylcholine, NA) and peptides (e.g., angiotensin). The ensuing changes in level and patterns of firing (e.g., change from slow irregular to phasic activity) would therefore be conducive to more efficient and maximal hormone release in the neural lobe (see Dutton and Dyball, 1979; Bicknell and Leng, 1981; Cazalis *et al.*, 1985).

4.2. Passive and Steady-State Properties of MNCs

Intracellular lucifer yellow injections and whole cell reconstructions of SON neurons reveal round or oval-shaped somata of 10–40 μm with a simple dendritic tree (two or three main branches) that usually remains confined to the nuclear boundaries but can extend into the ventral glial lamina (Randle *et al.*, 1986e). A single axon, originating from the soma or a dendrite, possesses irregularities (collaterals?) as it courses dorsomedial to the nucleus; these may be part of the morphological basis for "recurrent" events in this area after stimulation of the neural lobe (Leng, 1982; Mason *et al.*, 1984; see Section 4.3.3). In slice preparations, homotypic dye coupling (see Cobbett *et al.*, 1985) is regularly observed and its frequency can be correlated with certain variables (e.g., level of hydration) (Cobbett and Hatton, 1984). It is uncertain whether the gap junctions observed between MNCs (Andrew *et al.*, 1981) represent the molecular substrate for the dye coupling. The latter is seldom noted in perfused explant preparations (Randle *et al.*, 1986e).

Compared with other central neurons, MNCs possess high input resistances (50–350 MΩ) and relatively long cell time constants (~ 14 msec). The current–voltage relationship is linear between −60 and −80 mV (i.e., near the resting membrane potential; −60 to −70 mV). At more positive (depolarized) potentials there is strong outward rectification which is partially removed by calcium channel blockers (e.g., cobalt); at more negative potentials, the current–voltage relationship rectifies inwardly (Mason, 1983; Bourque and Renaud, 1985a). The combination of these passive properties and uncomplicated morphology predicts efficient electrotonic responses to synaptic currents of either direction. The long cell time constant favors summation of synaptic and spike afterpotentials.

4.3. Activity-Dependent Conductances

4.3.1. Spike Broadening

Intracellular recordings *in vitro* reveal that action potentials in MNCs are composed of a low-threshold tetrodotoxin-sensitive sodium conductance and a high-threshold tetrodotoxin-resistant calcium current (Bourque and Renaud, 1985a; Fig. 5A). Action potentials are broadened due to a prominent shoulder on the repolarization phase of the spike. That this is a contribution of the calcium conductance is verified by its loss in medium containing cobalt or lacking calcium (Bourque and Renaud, 1985b; Fig. 5C). Action potential duration in MNCs may broaden by 150% in proportion to firing frequency (Bourque and Renaud, 1985b; Andrew and Dudek, 1985). However, spike broadening is most obvious when a silent period precedes a spontaneous or current-evoked burst (Fig. 5B). Typically such bursts begin with several spikes with very short interspike intervals wherein broadening proceeds rapidly and then gradually achieves a stable state after 15–20 events. Recovery of the short spike duration occurs after a silent interval is initiated, and proceeds exponentially with a time constant approximating 5 sec. Therefore, spike duration is both time- and frequency-dependent. The actual mechanism for spike broadening is unclear but may reflect a frequency-dependent inactivation of a potassium conductance (Bourque *et al.*, 1986a).

A close correlation exists between the changes in spike duration due to firing frequency and pattern on the one hand, and the frequency- and pattern-dependent release of hormone in the isolated neurohypophysis (Dreifuss *et al.*, 1981; Dutton and Dyball, 1979; Bicknell and Leng, 1981; Cazalis *et al.*, 1985). Action potentials from neural lobe axon terminals also reflect sodium and calcium currents (Salzberg *et al.*, 1983). Any relationship between axon terminal spike

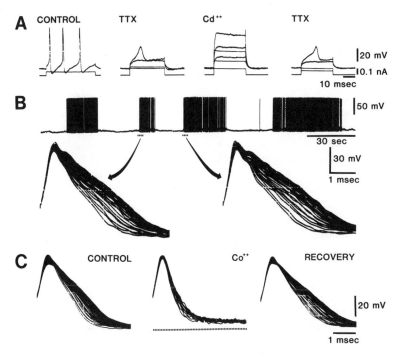

Figure 5. Intracellular recordings obtained from SON neurons in perfused hypothalamic explants. (A) Intracellular current pulses (lower traces) evoke action potentials (upper traces) with a prominent HAP (control); perfusion with 10 μM tetrodotoxin (TTX) blocks the sodium current and reveals a high-threshold cadmium-sensitive calcium spike. (B) Top trace is a record of spontaneous phasic firing, while the lower traces demonstrate a progressive broadening of action potentials occurring at the onset of the two middle bursts (dotted lines). (C) Action potential broadening during current-induced spike trains in normal media (control) is reversibly abolished by the addition of a calcium channel blocker (Co^{2+}, 2 mM) to the medium. In the presence of Co^{2+}, note the absence of both a shoulder on the repolarizing phase of the spike and a significant spike AHP, indicating their dependence on calcium influx. (From Bourque and Renaud, 1985a,b.)

broadening in this species and the known enhancement of hormone release by pattern and frequency of stimulation remains unclear. Should there be a correlation between spike durations in axon terminals and enhanced calcium inflow, this mechanism might underlie the efficiency of spike frequency and patterning in terms of hormone release.

4.3.2. Hyperpolarizing Afterpotential (HAP) and Afterhyperpolarization (AHP)

Single action potentials in MNCs are followed by an HAP (Andrew and Dudek, 1984a; Bourque *et al.*, 1985; see Fig. 5A). The HAP decays with a mean time constant of 17.5 msec, clearly exceeding the cell time constant of 9.5 msec, indicating a brief persistence of the ionic conductance underlying the HAP. These HAPs are intrinsic to MNCs, and persist during synaptic blockade with elevated magnesium. Their resistance to intracellular chloride iontophoresis, sensitivity to calcium channel blockers, and reversibility at the potassium equilibrium potential are features of a calcium-activated potassium conductance. HAP potentiation contributes to spike frequency adaptation during depolarizing current pulses. This potentiation also contributes to the appearance of a postburst AHP. This mechanism, rather than a recurrent synaptic mechanism, may account for the prolonged postburst silence observed from oxytocin-secreting cells *in vivo* during the milk ejection reflex (see Section 2.2). It is not yet clear whether a calcium-dependent potassium conductance also contributes to the termination of phasic bursts in vasopressin-secreting MNCs.

4.3.3. Nonsynaptic Depolarizing Potentials (NSDPs)

Intracellular recordings with potassium acetate-filled electrodes have revealed the presence of intrinsic, nonspike and nonsynaptic depolarizing membrane voltage fluctuations lasting 20–125 msec with a mean rise time of approximately 20 msec, a decay time of 16 msec, and often maintaining a constant peak amplitude for their duration (Bourque *et al.*, 1986b). These NSDPs are voltage-dependent and are detected only at membrane potentials within 5–7 mV of spike threshold. Their appearance is prompted by any membrane-depolarizing event (e.g., osmotic depolarization, depolarizing afterpotentials, drug-induced depolarizations, EPSPs) that causes membrane voltage to move into their range of activation. Since their voltage levels cross threshold for spike initiation, these events contribute to action potential generation in MNCs. Their lack of sensitivity to tetrodotoxin but clear reduction in size in the presence of cobalt or manganese suggests an underlying calcium conductance.

4.3.4. Depolarizing Afterpotentials (DAPs) and Phasic Bursting

The ability of a certain proportion of MNCs to adopt a phasic bursting pattern—a property of the vasopressin-secreting cell (Section 2.3) during activation—has been further examined *in vitro* with intracellular recordings. The mechanism for phasic bursting is intrinsic to MNCs (Hatton, 1982; Andrew and Dudek, 1983, 1984b) and is not driven by synaptic input, although the onset of an individual burst is likely to depend on the occurrence of a depolarizing synaptic or nonsynaptic event sufficient to trigger an action potential. The HAP is followed by a late DAP (Fig. 6A). Summation of DAPs from several rapidly occurring spikes establishes a plateau potential (Fig. 6B,C) that will then sustain regenerative activity for variable periods of time (Andrew and Dudek, 1984b).

Recent studies with voltage clamp (Bourque, 1986) reveal that the plateau-forming mechanism has a marked voltage-dependence and depends on calcium influx, while a calcium-dependent inactivation of a calcium conductance is thought to bring about the termination of the burst (Bourque *et al.*, 1986a). Although the steady-state current–voltage relationship is linear at resting potential, voltage-current analysis reveals that a narrow region of negative resistance between -65 and -60 mV is imparted by activation of the current underlying the DAP (Bourque, 1986). The regenerative inward current will further depolarize the cell toward threshold. This process may be enhanced by osmotically induced depolarization, also by synaptic release of NA which

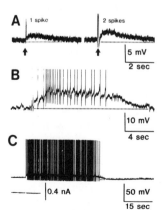

A   1 spike   2 spikes

|5 mV
2 sec

B

|10 mV
4 sec

C

── |0.4 nA |50 mV
15 sec

Figure 6. Intracellular voltage traces from SON MNC in perfused hypothalamic explants. (A) Intracellular depolarizing current pulses (arrow) evoke one or two spikes and a late DAP of long duration. (B) A spontaneous burst reveals initial summation of DAPs and a brief plateau that sustains firing for several seconds. Typically there is a gradual reduction in spike frequency and arrest of firing after which the plateau collapses. (C) Current-induced burst reveals the underlying plateau, eventual arrest of firing, and membrane repolarization. (From Bourque, 1984.)

can be seen to increase DAPs and to promote bursting activity through activation of an α_1 adrenergic receptor. Conversely, any hyperpolarizing (e.g., GABAergic) synaptic event will tend to remove the neuron from this zone of activation and initiate a silent period.

4.3.5. Recurrent Inhibition

The widespread yet specific distribution of neurohypophysial (and other) peptides in the CNS has clearly fostered the notion that they may participate in synaptic transmission (Buijs and Heerikhuize, 1982). Observation of a silent period following antidromic activation of MNCs prompted the suggestion that this might be due to an action of vasopressin and/or oxytocin released from recurrent axon collaterals (Nicoll and Barker, 1971a; Dreifuss and Kelly, 1972b). While the notion of a peptide mediating a recurrent synaptic inhibitory event was novel and received support from iontophoretic data indicating a depressant action of vasopressin on MNC excitability (Nicoll and Barker, 1971a), evidence for similar postantidromic silent periods in the vasopressin-deficient Brattleboro rat (Dreifuss et al., 1974; Dyball, 1974) and its resistance to several transmitter antagonists (Nicoll and Barker, 1971a) raised doubts as to the validity of this hypothesis. A synaptic mechanism is nonetheless favored by several items. Foremost is that the silent interval can clearly be observed in some MNCs at stimulus intensities that are subthreshold for antidromic activation (see Barker et al., 1971b; Dreifuss and Kelly, 1972b; Akaishi and Ellendorff, 1983). Moreover, anatomical and electrical evidence for axon collaterals of MNCs in SON has recently been reported (Mason et al., 1984). Whether the altered pattern observed in Brattleboro rats actually reflects involvement of vasopressin or neurophysin (Leng and Wiersma, 1981) remains uncertain. On the other hand, the intrinsic potassium conductances underlying the prominent HAPs and AHPs in MNCs (Andrew and Dudek, 1984a; Bourque et al., 1985) are clearly major factors in the early reductions in excitability at stimulus intensities above threshold for antidromic invasion.

5. Concluding Comments

Much can be gleaned from recent electrophysiological analysis of MNCs. The potential for combining observations obtained in vivo with the details of intracellular events provides a refreshing approach from which to advance our understanding of the complexity of intrinsic and synaptic mechanisms in operation to regulate their excitability. Among the known central peptidergic neurons in mammals, MNCs are perhaps the best characterized in terms of their neurophysiology, and the information obtained from them should prove beneficial to our understanding of the function of other less accessible peptidergic systems.

ACKNOWLEDGMENTS. The author is grateful to Gwen Peard for typing the manuscript, to the Canadian MRC and Quebec Heart Foundation for financial assistance, and to Charles Bourque, Trevor Day, Alastair Ferguson, Jack Jhamandas, and John Randle for their major contributions to this research program.

References

Abe, H., and Ogata, N., 1982, Ionic mechanisms for the osmotically-induced depolarization in neurons of the guinea-pig supraoptic nucleus in vitro, J. Physiol. (London) 327:157–171.

Abe, H., Inoue, M., Matsuo, T., and Ogata, N., 1983, The effects of vasopressin on electrical activity in the guinea-pig supraoptic nucleus in vitro, J. Physiol. (London) 337:665–685.

Akaishi, T., and Ellendorff, F., 1983, Electrical properties of paraventricular neurosecretory neurons with and without recurrent inhibition, Brain Res. 262:151–154.

Akaishi, T., Negoro, H., and Kobayasi, S., 1980, Responses of paraventricular and supraoptic units to angiotensin II, Sar[1]~Ile[8]-angiotensin II and hypertonic NaCl administered into the cerebral ventricle, *Brain Res.* **188**:499–511.

Andrew, R. D., and Dudek, F. E., 1983, Burst discharge in mammalian neuroendocrine cells involves an intrinsic regenerative mechanism, *Science* **221**:1050–1052.

Andrew, R. D., and Dudek, F. E., 1984a, Intrinsic inhibition in magnocellular neuroendocrine cells of rat hypothalamus, *J. Physiol. (London)* **353**:171–185.

Andrew, R. D., and Dudek, F. E., 1984b, Analysis of intracellular recorded phasic bursting by mammalian neuroendocrine cells, *J. Neurophysiol.* **51**:552–566.

Andrew, R. D., and Dudek, F. E., 1985, Spike broadening in magnocellular neuroendocrine cells of rat hypothalamic slices, *Brain Res.* **334**:176–179.

Andrew, R. D., MacVicar, B. A., Dudek, F. E., and Hatton, G. I., 1981, Dye transfer through gap junctions between neuroendocrine cells of rat hypothalamus, *Science* **211**:1187–1189.

Armstrong, W. E., and Sladek, C. D., 1985, Evidence for excitatory actions of histamine on supraoptic neurons in vitro: Mediation by an H_1-type receptor, *Neuroscience* **16**:307–322.

Armstrong, W. E., Sladek, C. D., and Sladek, J. R., Jr., 1982, Characterization of noradrenergic control of vasopressin release by the organ-cultured rat hypothalamo-neurohypophyseal system, *Endocrinology* **111**:273–279.

Armstrong, W. E., Gallagher, M. J., and Sladek, C. D., 1986, Noradrenergic stimulation of supraoptic neuronal activity and vasopressin release in vitro: Mediation by an α_1-receptor, *Brain Res.* **365**:192–197.

Armstrong-James, M., and Fox, K., 1983, Effects of iontophoresed noradrenaline on the spontaneous activity of neurons in rat primary somatosensory cortex, *J. Physiol. (London)* **335**:427–447.

Arnauld, E., Cirino, M., Layton, B. S., and Renaud, L. P., 1983, Contrasting actions of amino acids, acetylcholine, noradrenaline and leucine enkephalin on the excitability of supraoptic vasopressin-secreting neurons, *Neuroendocrinology* **36**:187–196.

Banks, D., and Harris, M. C., 1984, Lesions of the locus coeruleus abolish baroreceptor-induced depression of supraoptic neurones in the rat, *J. Physiol. (London)* **355**:383–398.

Bargmann, W., 1949, Über die neurosekretorische verknöpfung von hypothalamus und neurohypophyse, *Z. Zellforsch. Mikrosk. Anat.* **34**:610–634.

Barker, J. L., Crayton, J. W., and Nicoll, R. A., 1971a, Noradrenaline and acetylcholine response of supraoptic neurosecretory cells, *J. Physiol. (London)* **218**:19–32.

Barker, J., Crayton, J. W., and Nicoll, R. A., 1971b, Antidromic and orthodromic responses of paraventricular and supraoptic neurosecretory cells, *Brain Res.* **33**:353–366.

Beal, M. F., and Martin, J. B., 1986, Neuropeptides and neurological disease, *Ann. Neurol.* **20**:547–565.

Belin, V., and Moos, F., 1986, Paired recordings from supraoptic and paraventricular oxytocin cells in suckled rats: Recruitment and synchronization, *J. Physiol. (London)* **377**:369–390.

Bhargava, K. P., Kulshrestha, V. K., Santhakumari, G., and Stivastava, H. P., 1983, Mechanism of histamine-induced antidiuretic response, *Br. J. Pharmacol.* **47**:700–706.

Bicknell, R. J., and Leng, G., 1981, Relative efficiency of neural firing patterns for vasopressin release in vitro, *Neuroendocrinology* **33**:295–299.

Bicknell, R. J., and Leng, G., 1982, Endogenous opiates regulate oxytocin but not vasopressin secretion from the neurohypophysis, *Nature* **298**:161–162.

Bicknell, R. J., Chapman, C., and Leng, G., 1985, Effects of opioid agonists and antagonists on oxytocin and vasopressin release in vitro, *Neuroendocrinology* **41**:142–148.

Bioulac, B., Gaffori, O., Harris, M., and Vincent, J.-D., 1978, Effects of acetylcholine, sodium glutamate and GABA on the discharge of supraoptic neurons in the rat, *Brain Res.* **154**:159–162.

Bisset, G. W., and Chowdrey, H. S., 1981, A central cholinergic link in the neural control of the release of vasopressin, *Br. J. Pharmacol.* **74**:239.

Blessing, W. W., Sved, A. F., and Reis, D. J., 1982, Destruction of noradrenergic neurons in rabbit brainstem elevates plasma vasopressin, causing hypertension, *Science* **217**:661–663.

Boer, K., and Nolten, J. W. L., 1978, Hypothalamic paraventricular unit activity during labor in the rat, *J. Endocrinol.* **76**:155–163.

Bourque, C. W., 1984, Membrane properties of supraoptic nucleus neurons in vitro, Ph.D. thesis, McGill University, Montreal.

Bourque, C. W., 1986, Calcium-dependent spike after-currents induce burst firing in magnocellular neurosecretory cells, *Neurosci. Lett.* **70**:204–209.

Bourque, C. W., and Renaud, L. P., 1984, Activity patterns and osmosensitivity of rat supraoptic neurones in perfused hypothalamic explants, *J. Physiol. (London)* **349**:631–642.

Bourque, C. W., and Renaud, L. P., 1985a, Calcium-dependent action potentials in rat supraoptic neurosecretory neurones recorded in-vitro, *J. Physiol. (London)* **363:**419–428.

Bourque, C. W., and Renaud, L. P., 1985b, Activity-dependence of action potential duration in rat supraoptic neurosecretory neurones recorded in-vitro, *J. Physiol. (London)* **363:**429–439.

Bourque, C. W., Randle, J. C. R., and Renaud, L. P., 1985, A calcium-dependent potassium conductance in rat supraoptic neurosecretory cells, *J. Neurophysiol.* **54:**1375–1382.

Bourque, C. W., Brown, D. A., and Renaud, L. P., 1986a, Barium ions induce prolonged plateau depolarizations in neurosecretory neurones of the adult rat supraoptic nucleus, *J. Physiol. (London)* **375:**573–586.

Bourque, C. W., Randle, J. C. R., and Renaud, L. P., 1986b, Non-synaptic depolarizing potentials in rat supraoptic neurones recorded in vitro, *J. Physiol. (London)* **376:**493–505.

Bridges, T. E., Hillhouse, E. W., and Jones, M. T., 1976, The effect of dopamine on neurohypophysial hormone release in vivo and from the rat neural lobe and hypothalamus in vitro, *J. Physiol. (London)* **260:**647–666.

Brimble, M. J., and Dyball, R. E. J., 1977, Characterization of the responses of oxytocin- and vasopressin-secreting neurones in the supraoptic nucleus to osmotic stimulation, *J. Physiol. (London)* **271:**253–271.

Buijs, R. M., and Heerikhuize, J. J. V., 1982, Vasopressin and oxytocin release in the brain—a synaptic event, *Brain Res.* **252:**71–76.

Buijs, R., Geffard, M., Pool, C. W., and Hoorneman, E. M. D., 1984, The dopaminergic innervation of the supraoptic and paraventricular nucleus: A light and electron microscopical study, *Brain Res.* **323:**65–72.

Cazalis, M., Dayanithi, G., and Nordmann, J. J., 1985, The role of patterned burst and interburst interval on the excitation-coupling mechanism in the isolated rat neural lobe, *J. Physiol. (London)* **369:**45–60.

Cheng, S. W. T., and North, W. G., 1986, Responsiveness of oxytocin-producing neurons to acute salt loading in rats: Comparisons with vasopressin-producing neurons, *Neuroendocrinology* **42:**174–180.

Cirino, M., and Renaud, L. P., 1985, Influence of lateral septum and amygdala stimulation on the excitability of hypothalamic supraoptic neurons: An electrophysiological study in the rat, *Brain Res.* **326:**357–361.

Clarke, G., and Merrick, L. P., 1985, Electrophysiological studies of the magnocellular neurons, in: *Neurobiology of Vasopressin* (D. Ganten and D. Pfaff, eds.), Springer-Verlag, Berlin, pp. 17–59.

Clarke, G., Fall, C. H. D., Lincoln, D. W., and Merrick, L. P., 1978, Effects of cholinoceptor antagonists on the suckling-induced and experimentally evoked release of oxytocin, *Br. J. Pharmacol.* **63:**519–527.

Clarke, G., Wood, P., Merrick, L., and Lincoln, D. W., 1979, Opiate inhibition of peptide release from the neurohumoral terminals of hypothalamic neurones, *Nature* **282:**746–748.

Cobbett, P., and Hatton, G. I., 1984, Dye coupling in hypothalamic slices: Dependence on in vivo hydration state and osmolality of incubation medium, *J. Neurosci.* **4:**3034–3038.

Cobbett, P., Smithson, K. G., and Hatton, G. I., 1985, Dye-coupled magnocellular peptidergic neurons of the rat paraventricular nucleus show homotypic immunoreactivity, *Neuroscience* **16:**885–895.

Cobbett, P., Smithson, K. G., and Hatton, G. I., 1986, Immonoreactivity to vasopressin- but not oxytocin-associated neurophysin antiserum in phasic neurons of rat hypothalamic paraventricular nucleus, *Brain Res.* **362:**7–16.

Cross, B. A., 1955, Neurohormonal mechanisms in emotional inhibition of milk ejection, *J. Endocrinol.* **12:**29–37.

Day, T. A., and Renaud, L. P., 1984, Electrophysiological evidence that noradrenergic afferents selectively facilitate the activity of supraoptic vasopressin neurons, *Brain Res.* **303:**233–240.

Day, T. A., Ferguson, A. V., and Renaud, L. P., 1984, Facilitatory influence of noradrenergic afferents on the excitability of rat paraventricular nucleus neurosecretory cells, *J. Physiol. (London)* **355:**237–250.

Day, T. A., Jhamandas, J. H., and Renaud, L. P., 1985a, Comparison between the actions of avian pancreatic polypeptide, neuropeptide Y and norepinephrine on the excitability of rat supraoptic vasopressin neurons, *Neurosci. Lett.* **62:**181–185.

Day, T. A., Randle, J. C. R., and Renaud, L. P., 1985b, Opposing alpha- and beta-adrenergic mechanisms mediate actions of noradrenaline on supraoptic vasopressin neurones, *Brain Res.* **358:**171–179.

Dreifuss, J. J., and Kelly, J. S., 1972a, The activity of identified supraoptic neurones and their response to acetylcholine applied by iontophoresis, *J. Physiol. (London)* **220:**105–118.

Dreifuss, J. J., and Kelly, J. S., 1972b, Recurrent inhibition of antidromically identified rat supraoptic neurones, *J. Physiol. (London)* **220:**87–103.

Dreifuss, J. J., Nordmann, J. J., and Vincent, J. D., 1974, Recurrent inhibition of supraoptic neurosecretory cells in homozygous Brattleboro rats, *J. Physiol. (London)* **237:**25–27P.

Dreifuss, J. J., Tribollet, E., and Muhlethaler, M., 1981, Temporal patterns of neural activity and their relation to the secretion of posterior pituitary hormones, *Biol. Reprod.* **24:**51–72.

Dubois-Dauphin, M., Armstrong, W. E., Tribollet, E., and Dreifuss, J. J., 1985, Somatosensory systems and the milk-ejection reflex in the rat. I. Lesions of the mesencephalic tegmentum disrupt the reflex and damage mesencephalic somatosensory connections, *Neuroscience* **15:**1111–1130.

Dutton, A., and Dyball, R. E. J., 1979, Phasic firing enhances vasopressin release from the rat neurohypophysis, *J. Physiol. (London)* **290:**433–440.

Dyball, R. E. J., 1974, Single unit activity in the hypothalamo-neurohypophyseal system of Brattleboro rats, *J. Endocrinol.* **60:**135–143.

Everitt, B. J., Hökfelt, T., Terenius, L., Tatemoto, K., Mutt, V., and Goldstein, M., 1984, Differential coexistence of neuropeptide Y (NPY)-like immunoreactivity with catecholamines in the central nervous system of the rat, *Neuroscience* **11:**443–462.

Ferguson, A. V., and Kasting, N. W., 1986, Electrical stimulation in the subfornical organ increases plasma concentrations of oxytocin and vasopressin in the conscious rat, *Soc. Neurosci. Abstr.* **12:**445.

Ferguson, A. V., and Renaud, L. P., 1986, Systemic angiotensin acts at subfornical organ to facilitate activity of neurohypophysial neurons, *Am. J. Physiol.* **251:**R712–R717.

Ferguson, A. V., Day, T. A., and Renaud, L. P., 1984, Subfornical organ afferents influence the excitability of neurohypophysial and tuberoinfundibular paraventricular nucleus neurons in the rat, *Neuroendocrinology* **39:**423–428.

Ferreyra, H., Kannan, H., and Koizumi, K., 1983, Influences of the limbic system on hypothalamo-neurohypophysial system, *Brain Res.* **264:**31–45.

Freund-Mercier, M.-J., and Richard, P., 1984, Electrophysiological evidence for facilitatory control of oxytocin neurones by oxytocin during suckling in the rat, *J. Physiol. (London)* **352:**447–466.

Fuxe, K., 1965, Evidence for the existence of monoamine neurons in the central nervous system. IV. The distribution of monoamine nerve terminals in the central nervous system, *Acta Physiol. Scand.* **247:**37–85.

Gutman, M. B., Ciriello, J., and Mogenson, G. J., 1986, Electrophysiological identification of forebrain connections of the subfornical organ, *Brain Res.* **382:**119–128.

Haas, H. L., Wolf, P., and Nussbaumer, J.-C., 1975, Histamine: Action on supraoptic and other hypothalamic neurones of the cat, *Brain Res.* **88:**166–170.

Haller, E. W., and Wakerley, J. B., 1980, Electrophysiological studies of paraventricular and supraoptic neurones recorded in vitro from slices of rat hypothalamus, *J. Physiol. (London)* **302:**347–362.

Hamamura, M., Shibuki, K., and Yagi, K., 1982, Amygdalar inputs to ADH-secreting supraoptic neurones in rats, *Exp. Brain Res.* **48:**420–428.

Harris, M. C., 1978, The concept of the neuroendocrine reflex, in: *Cell Biology of Hypothalamic Neurosecretion* (J.D. Vincent and J.C. Kordon, eds.), CNRS, Paris, pp. 47–61.

Harris, M. C., 1979, Effects of chemoreceptor and baroreceptor stimulation on the discharge of hypothalamic supraoptic neurones in rats, *J. Endocrinol.* **82:**115–125.

Hatton, G. I., Ho, Y. W., and Mason, W. T., 1983, Synaptic activation of phasic bursting in rat supraoptic nucleus neurones recorded in hypothalamic slices, *J. Physiol. (London)* **345:**297–317.

Hayward, J. N., Murgas, K., Pavasuthipaisit, K., Perez-Lopez, F. R., and Sofroniew, M. V., 1977, Temporal patterns of vasopressin release following electrical stimulation of the amygdala and the neuroendocrine pathway in the monkey, *Neuroendocrinology* **23:**61–75.

Hunt, S. P., Emson, P. C., Gilbert, R., Goldstein, M., and Kimmel, J. R., 1981, Presence of avian pancreatic polypeptide-like immunoreactivity in catecholamine- and methionine enkephalin-containing neurons within the central nervous system, *Neurosci. Lett.* **21:**125–130.

Iijima, K., and Ogawa, T., 1981, An HRP study on the distribution of all nuclei innervating the supraoptic nucleus in the rat brain, *Acta Histochem.* **69:**274–295.

Inenaga, K., and Yamashita, H., 1986, Excitation of neurones in the rat paraventricular nucleus in vitro by vasopressin and oxytocin, *J. Physiol. (London)* **370:**165–180.

Inenaga, K., Dyball, R. E. J., Okuya, S., and Yamashita, H., 1986, Characterization of hypothalamic noradrenaline receptors in the supraoptic nucleus and periventricular region of the paraventricular nucleus of mice in vitro, *Brain Res.* **369:**37–47.

Jacobowitz, D. M., and Olschowska, J. A., 1982, Coexistence of bovine pancreatic polypeptide-like immunoreactivity and catecholamines in neurons of the ventral aminergic pathway of the rat brain, *Brain Res. Bull.* **9:**391–406.

Jhamandas, J. H., and Renaud, L. P., 1986a, A γ-aminobutyric acid-mediated baroreceptor input to supraoptic vasopressin neurones in the rat, *J. Physiol. (London)* **381:**595–606.

Jhamandas, J. H., and Renaud, L. P., 1986b, Diagonal band neurons may mediate arterial baroreceptor input to hypothalamic vasopressin-secreting neurons, *Neurosci. Lett.* **65:**214–218.

Kannan, H., and Yagi, K., 1978, Supraoptic neurosecretory neurones: Evidence for the existence of converging inputs from carotid baroreceptors and osmoreceptors, *Brain Res.* **145:**385–390.

Keil, L. C., and Severs, W. B., 1977, Reduction in plasma vasopressin levels of dehydrated rats following acute stress, *Endocrinology* **100:**30–38.

Krieger, D. T., 1983, Brain peptides: What, where and why? *Science* **222:**975–985.

Lebrun, C. J., Poulain, D. A., and Theodosis, D. T., 1983, The role of the septum in the control of the milk ejection reflex in the rat: Effects of lesions and electrical stimulation, *J. Physiol. (London)* **339:**17–31.

Leng, G., 1980, Rat supraoptic neurones: The effects of locally applied hypertonic saline, *J. Physiol. (London)* **304:**405–414.

Leng, G., 1982, Lateral hypothalamic neurones: Osmosensitivity and the influence of activating magnocellular neurosecretory neurones, *J. Physiol. (London)* **326:**35–48.

Leng, G., and Wiersma, J. H., 1981, Effects of neural stalk stimulation on phasic discharge of supraoptic neurones in Brattleboro rats devoid of vasopressin, *J. Endocrinol.* **90:**211–220.

Leng, G., Mason, W. T., and Dyer, R. G., 1982, The supraoptic nucleus as an osmoreceptor, *Neuroendocrinology* **34:**75–82.

Leng, G., Dyball, R. E. J., and Mason, W. T., 1985, Electrophysiology of osmoreceptors, in: *Vasopressin* (R. W. Schrier, ed.), Raven Press, New York, pp. 333–342.

Lincoln, D. W., and Wakerley, J. B., 1974. Electrophysiological evidence for the activation of supraoptic neurones during the release of oxytocin, *J. Physiol. (London)* **242:**533–554.

Lind, R. W., Swanson, L. W., and Ganten, D., 1985, Organization of angiotensin II immunoreactive cells and fibers in the rat central nervous system: An immunohistochemical study, *Neuroendocrinology* **40:**2–24.

Lindvall, O., Björklund, A., and Skagerberg, G., 1984, Selective histochemical demonstration of dopamine terminal systems in rat di- and telencephalon: New evidence for dopaminergic innervation of hypothalamic neurosecretory nuclei, *Brain Res.* **306:**19–30.

Martin, R., and Voigt, K. H., 1981, Enkephalins co-exist with oxytocin and vasopressin in nerve terminals of rat neurohypophysis, *Nature* **289:**502–504.

Martin, R., Geis, R., Holl, R., Schafer, M., and Voigt, K. H., 1983, Coexistence of unrelated peptides in oxytocin and vasopressin terminals of rat neurohypophysis: Immunoreactive methionine[5]enkephalin-, leucine[5]-enkephalin-, and cholecystokinin-like substances, *Neuroscience* **8:**213–227.

Mason, W. T., 1980, Supraoptic neurones of rat hypothalamus are osmosensitive, *Nature* **287:**154–157.

Mason, W. T., 1983, Excitation by dopamine of putative oxytocinergic neurones in the rat supraoptic nucleus in vitro: Evidence for two classes of continuously firing neurones, *Brain Res.* **267:**113–121.

Mason, W. T., Ho, Y. W., and Hatton, G. I., 1984, Axon collaterals of supraoptic neurones: Anatomical and electrophysiological evidence for their existence in the lateral hypothalamus, *Neuroscience* **11:**169–182.

Millan, M. J., Millan, M. H., and Herz, A., 1983, Contribution of the supraoptic nucleus to brain and pituitary pools of immunoreactive vasopressin and particular opioid peptides, and the interrelationships between these, in the rat, *Neuroendocrinology* **36:**310–319.

Miselis, R., 1981, The efferent projections of the subfornical organ of the rat: A circumventricular organ with a neural network subserving water balance, *Brain Res.* **230:**1–12.

Mogenson, G. J., 1976, Septal hypothalamic relationships, in: *The Septal Nuclei* (J.F. DeFrance, ed.), Plenum Press, New York, pp. 149–184.

Moos, F., and Richard, P., 1982, Excitatory effect of dopamine on oxytocin and vasopressin reflex releases in the rat, *Brain Res.* **241:**249–260.

Moos, F., and Richard, P., 1983, Serotonergic control of oxytocin release during suckling in the rat: Opposite effects in conscious and anesthetized rats, *Neuroendocrinology* **36:**300–306.

Moss, R. L., Dyball, R. E. J., and Cross, B. A., 1972a, Excitation of antidromically identified neurosecretory cells of the paraventricular nucleus by oxytocin applied iontophoretically, *Exp. Neurol.* **34:**95–102.

Moss, R. L., Urban, I., and Cross, B. A., 1972b, Microiontophoresis of cholinergic and aminergic drugs on paraventricular neurons, *Am. J. Physiol.* **233:**310–318.

Negoro, H., Visessuwan, S., and Holland, R. C., 1973, Inhibition and excitation of units in paraventricular nucleus after stimulation of the septum, amygdala and neurohypophysis, *Brain Res.* **57:**479–483.

Nicoll, R. A., and Barker, J. L., 1971a, The pharmacology of recurrent inhibition in the supraoptic neurosecretory system, *Brain Res.* **15:**501–511.

Nicoll, R. A., and Barker, J. L., 1971b, Excitation of supraoptic neurosecretory cells by angiotensin II, *Nature New Biol.* **233:**172–174.

Oldfield, B. J., Hou-Yu, A., and Silverman, A. J., 1985, A combined electron microscopic HRP and immunocytochemical study of the limbic projections to rat hypothalamic nuclei containing vasopressin and oxytocin neurons, *J. Comp. Neurol.* **231:**221–231.

Perez de la Mora, M., Possani, L. D., Tapia, R., Teran, L., Palacios, R., Fuxe, K., Hökfelt, T., and Ljungdahl, A., 1981, Demonstration of central γ-aminobutyric-containing nerve terminals by means of antibodies against glutamate decarboxylase, *Neuroscience* **6:**875–895.

Perlmutter, L. S., Tweedle, C. D., and Hatton, G. I., 1985, Neuronal/glial plasticity in the supraoptic dendritic zone in response to acute and chronic dehydration, *Brain Res.* **361:**225–232.

Pittman, Q. J., Blume, H. W., and Renaud, L. P., 1981, Connections of the hypothalamic paraventricular nucleus with the neurohypophysis, median eminence, amygdala, lateral septum and midbrain periaqueductal gray: An electrophysiological study in the rat, *Brain Res.* **215**:15–28.

Poulain, D. A., and Wakerley, J. B., 1982, Electrophysiology of hypothalamic magnocellular neurones secreting oxytocin and vasopressin, *Neuroscience* **7**:773–808.

Poulain, D. A., and Wakerley, J. B., 1986, Afferent projections from the mammary glands to the spinal cord in the lactating rat. II. Electrophysiological responses of spinal neurons during stimulation of the nipples, including suckling, *Neuroscience* **19**:511–521.

Poulain, D. A., Wakerley, J. B., and Dyball, R. E. J., 1977, Electrophysiological differentiation of oxytocin- and vasopressin-secreting neurones, *Proc. R. Soc. London Ser. B* **196**:367–384.

Poulain, D. A., Ellendorff, F., and Vincent, J. D., 1980, Septal connections with identified oxytocin and vasopressin neurones in the supraoptic nucleus of the rat: An electrophysiological investigation, *Neuroscience* **5**:379–387.

Raby, W., and Renaud, L. P., 1987, Characterization of a norepinephrine pathway from dorsomedial medulla (A2) to hypothalamic supraoptic nucleus in the rat, *Can. J. Physiol. Pharmacol.* **65**:Axxviii.

Randle, J. C. R., and Renaud, L. P., 1987, Actions of gamma-aminobutyric acid in rat supraoptic nucleus neurosecretory neurones in vitro, *J. Physiol. (London)* **387**:629–647.

Randle, J. C. R., Day, T. A., Jhamandas, J. H., Bourque, C. W., and Renaud, L. P., 1986a, Neuropharmacology of supraoptic nucleus neurons: Noradrenergic and GABAergic receptors, *Fed. Proc.* **45**:2312–2317.

Randle, J. C. R., Bourque, C. W., and Renaud, L. P., 1986b, α_1 adrenergic receptor activation depolarizes rat supraoptic neurosecretory neurons in vitro, *Am. J. Physiol.* **251**:R569–R574.

Randle, J. C. R., Mazurek, M., Kneifel, D., Dufresne, J., and Renaud, L. P., 1986c, α_1 adrenergic receptor activation releases vasopressin and oxytocin from perfused hypothalamic explants, *Neurosci. Lett.* **65**:219–223.

Randle, J. C. R., Bourque, C. W., and Renaud, L. P., 1986d, Characterization of spontaneous and evoked inhibitory postsynaptic potentials in rat supraoptic neurosecretory in vitro, *J. Neurophysiol.* **56**:1703–1717.

Randle, J. C. R., Bourque, C. W., and Renaud, L. P., 1986e, Serial reconstruction of lucifer yellow-labeled supraoptic nucleus neurons in perfused rat hypothalamic explants, *Neuroscience* **17**:453–467.

Renaud, L. P., Pittman, Q. J., and Blume, H. W., 1979, Neurophysiology of hypothalamic peptidergic neurons. in: *Central Regulation of the Endocrine System* (K. Fuxe, T. Hökfelt, and R. Luft, eds.), Plenum Press, New York, pp. 119–136.

Renaud, L. P., Ferguson, A. V., Day, T. A., Bourque, C. W., and Sgro, S., 1985, Electrophysiology of the subfornical organ and its hypothalamic connections—An in-vivo study in the rat, *Brain Res. Bull.* **15**:83–86.

Roberts, F., and Calcutt, C. R., 1983, Histamine and the hypothalamus, *Neuroscience* **9**:721–739.

Sachs, H., 1970, Neurosecretion, in: *Handbook of Neurochemistry,* Vol. 4 (A. Lajtha, ed.), Plenum Press, New York, pp. 373–428.

Sakai, K. K., Marks, B. H., George, J. M., and Koestner, A., 1974, The isolated organ-cultured supraoptic nucleus as a neuropharmacological test system, *J. Pharmacol. Exp. Ther.* **190**:482–491.

Salzberg, B. M., Obaid, A. L., Senseman, D. M., and Gainer, H., 1983, Optical recording of action potentials from vertebrate nerve terminals using potentiometric probes provides evidence for sodium and calcium components, *Nature* **306**:36–40.

Sawchenko, P. E., and Swanson, L. W., 1981, Central noradrenergic pathways for the integration of hypothalamic neuroendocrine and autonomic responses, *Science* **214**:685–687.

Sawchenko, P. E., and Swanson, L. W., 1983, The organization and biochemical specificity of afferent projections to the paraventricular and supraoptic nuclei, *Prog. Brain Res.* **60**:19–29.

Sawchenko, P. E., Swanson, L. W., Steinbusch, H. W. M., and Verhofstad, N. A. J., 1983, The distribution and cells of origin of serotonergic inputs to the paraventricular and supraoptic nuclei of the rat, *Brain Res.* **277**:355–360.

Scharrer, E., and Scharrer, B., 1975, Neurosecretion, *Physiol. Rev.* **25**:171–181.

Sgro, S., Ferguson, A. V., and Renaud, L. P., 1984, Subfornical organ–supraoptic nucleus connections: An electrophysiological study in the rat, *Brain Res.* **303**:7–13.

Silverman, A. J., Hoffman, D. L., and Zimmerman, E. A., 1981, The descending afferent connections of the paraventricular nucleus of the hypothalamus (PVN), *Brain Res. Bull.* **6**:47–61.

Sladek, C. D., and Armstrong, W. E., 1985, Osmotic control of vasopressin release, *Trends Neurosci.* **8**:166–168.

Sladek, C. D., and Joynt, R. J., 1979, Characterization of cholinergic control of vasopressin release by the organ-cultured rat hypothalamo-neurohypophyseal system, *Endocrinology* **104**:659–663.

Summerlee, A. J. S., 1983, Hypothalamic neurone activity: Hormone release and behaviour in freely moving rats, *Q.J. Exp. Physiol.* **68**:505–515.

Summy-Long, J. Y., Miller, D. S., Rosella-Dampman, L. M., Hartman, R. D., and Emmert, S. E., 1984, A functional role for opioid peptides in the differential secretion of vasopressin and oxytocin, *Brain Res.* **309**:362–366.

Swaab, D. F., Pool, C. W., and Nijveldt, F., 1975, Immunofluorescence of vasopressin and oxytocin in the rat hypothalamo-neurohypophyseal system, *J. Neural Transm.* **36**:195–215.

Tanaka, J., Kaba, H., Saito, H., and Seto, K., 1986a, Subfornical organ efferents influence the activity of median preoptic neurons projecting to the hypothalamic paraventricular nucleus in the rat, *Exp. Neurol.* **93**:647–651.

Tanaka, J., Kaba, H., Saito, H., and Seto, K., 1986b, Lateral hypothalamic area stimulation excites neurons in the region of the subfornical organ with efferent projections to the hypothalamic paraventricular nucleus in the rat, *Brain Res.* **379**:200–203.

Tang, M., McCann, M. J., Verbalis, J. G., Stricker, E. M., and Renaud, L. P., 1986, Selective excitation of rat supraoptic nucleus oxytocin-secreting neurons after systemic administration of cholecystokinin (CCK-8) and gastric distention, *Soc. Neurosci. Abstr.* **12**:447,

Tappaz, M. L., Brownstein, M. J., and Kopin, I. J., 1977, Glutamate decarboxylase (GAD) and γ-aminobutyric acid (GABA) in discrete nuclei of hypothalamus and substantia nigra, *Brain Res.* **125**:109–121.

Tappaz, M. L., Wassef, M., Oertel, W. H., Paut, L., and Pujol, J. F., 1983, Light- and electron-microscopic immunocytochemistry of glutamic acid decarboxylase (GAD) in the basal hypothalamus: Morphological evidence for neuroendocrine gamma-aminobutyrate (GABA), *Neuroscience* **9**:271–287.

Theodosis, D. T., 1985, Oxytocin-immunoreactive terminals synapse on oxytocin neurones in the supraoptic nucleus, *Nature* **313**:682–685.

Theodosis, D. T., Montagnese, C., Rodriguez, F., Vincent, J. D., and Poulain, D. A., 1986a, Oxytocin induces morphological plasticity in the adult hypothalamo-neurohypophysial system, *Nature* **322**:738–741.

Theodosis, D. T., Paut, L., and Tappaz, M. L., 1986b, Immunocytochemical analysis of the GABAergic innervation of oxytocin- and vasopressin-secreting neurons in the rat supraoptic nucleus, *Neuroscience* **19**:207–222.

Thomson, A. M., 1982, Responses of supraoptic neurones to electrical stimulation of the medial amygdaloid nucleus, *Neuroscience* **7**:2197–2205.

Tomas, T., 1975, ADH release from cut pituitary stalk and intact pituitary gland during amygdala stimulation at various frequencies in rats, *Neuroendocrinology* **17**:139–146.

Tribollet, E., Armstrong, W. E., Dubois-Dauphin, M., and Dreifuss, J. J., 1985, Extrahypothalamic afferent inputs to the supraoptic nucleus area of the rat as determined by retrograde and anterograde tracing techniques, *Neuroscience* **15**:135–138.

van den Pol, A., 1985, Dual ultrastructural localization of two neurotransmitter-related antigens: Colloidal gold-labeled neurophysin-immunoreactive supraoptic neurons receive peroxidase-labeled glutamate decarboxylase- or gold-labeled GABA-immunoreactive synapses, *J. Neurosci.* **5**:2940–2954.

Vanderhaegen, J. J., Lotstra, F., DeMey, J., and Gilles, C., 1980, Immunohistochemical localization of cholecystokinin- and gastrinlike peptides in the brain and hypophysis of the rat, *Proc. Natl. Acad. Sci. USA* **77**:1190–1194.

Vandesande, F., and Dierickx, K., 1975, Identification of the vasopressin producing and of the oxytocin producing neurons in the hypothalamic neurosecretory system of the rat, *Cell Tissue Res.* **164**:153–162.

Verbalis, J. G., McCann, M. J., McHale, C. M., and Stricker, E. M., 1986, Oxytocin secretion in response to cholecystokinin and food: Differentiation of nausea from satiety, *Science* **232**:1417–1419.

Verney, E. G., 1947, The antidiuretic hormone and the factors which determine its release, *Proc. R. Soc. London* **135**:25–106.

Wakerley, J. B., Noble, R., and Clarke, G., 1983, Effects of morphine and D-Ala, D-Leu enkephalin on the electrical activity of supraoptic neurosecretory cells in vitro, *Neuroscience* **10**:73–81.

Watanabe, T., Taguchi, Y., Shiosaka, S., Tanaka, J., Kubota, H., Terano, Y., Tohyama, M., and Wada, H., 1984, Distribution of the histaminergic neuron system in the central nervous system of rats: A fluorescent immunohistochemical analysis with histidine decarboxylase as a marker, *Brain Res.* **295**:13–25.

Watson, S. J., Akil, H., Fischli, W., Goldstein, A., Zimmerman, E., Nilaver, G., and van Wimersma Greidanus, T. B., 1982, Dynorphin and vasopressin: Common localisation in magnocellular neurons, *Science* **216**:85–87.

Yagi, K., Azuma, T., and Matsuda, K., 1964, Neurosecretory cell: Capable of conducting impulse in rats, *Science* **154**:778–779.

Yamashita, H., Inenaga, K., Kawata, M., and Sano, Y., 1983, Phasically firing neurons in the supraoptic nucleus of the rat hypothalamus: Immunocytochemical and electrophysiological studies, *Neurosci. Lett.* **37**:87–92.

Zaborszky, L., Leranth, C., Makara, G. B., and Palkovits, M., 1975, Quantitative studies on the supraoptic nucleus in the rat. II. Afferent fiber connections, *Exp. Brain Res.* **22**:525–540.

33

Neuronal and Endocrine Peptides
Diversity and Gene Expression

M. Chrétien, R. A. Sikstrom, C. Lazure, and N. G. Seidah

1. Introduction

How can we attempt to deal with the complexity of the central nervous system, let alone begin to understand how it functions? The numbers are baffling! The circuitry of this intricate network, comprising billions of cells with more than a thousand times that number of interconnections, suggests a vastly more involved system than any currently known communication structure. Add to this that nerve cells can convey information by synaptic transmission as well as by the secretion of hormone messengers as do other endocrine cells. Add to this the possibility that some of these messengers may act in dual roles as neurotransmitters or neuromodulators. Yet much has already been learned by focusing our consideration of the brain and its workings on specific anatomical regions or at the level of the cell. Even amid the complexity, the use of molecular probes has helped to describe more fully how the living nervous system may operate at the cellular level. Many of the known biologically active agents or hormones are protein in nature and in our study of them to the present we have gained a foothold in the understanding of many types of cells including those in the nervous system. A general observation might be that any expression of biological diversity is a form of flexibility which may lend itself to survival.

2. Biosynthesis

Among the known proteins, we see a great range of diversity in size and character representing, one surmises, many different functional adaptations to the needs and demands of the moment. How does this come to be? Let us examine some specific examples from neuronal and endocrine systems. Having developed the necessary techniques over the past four decades, life scientists were able to deal with macromolecules like proteins and nucleic acids and to examine their exact nature. The information obtained gives us hints on their biosynthesis as specific

M. Chrétien and R. A. Sikstrom • Laboratory of Molecular Neuroendocrinology, Clinical Research Institute of Montreal, Montreal, Quebec, H2W 1R7, Canada. *C. Lazure and N. G. Seidah* • Laboratory of Biochemical Neuroendocrinology, Clinical Research Institute of Montreal, Montreal, Quebec H2W 1R7, Canada.

molecules. The information defining each protein is passed from one generation of cells to the next through the genetic code. The code is transcribed in the form of messenger ribonucleic acid (mRNA) which can subsequently be translated into protein according to the classic dogma

Specific gene DNA → mRNA → protein

Without dealing with the immense amount of information now known about the process of protein biosynthesis, it is sufficient to say that protein must be produced for soluble and membrane-bound environments and for intracellular as well as extracellular destinations. In doing so, proteins are often synthesized as precursors. The structure of the precursor forms of the well-known peptides PTH, insulin, and β-endorphin are shown in Figs. 1 and 2.

Since most known polypeptide hormones are constructed as prohormones, it is now accepted that biologically active neuropeptides will also exhibit this characteristic and hence will require various modifications to liberate the active molecules.

3. Diversity of Hormonal Agents and Biological Regulation

By extending its ability to create a diverse array of peptide hormone products each with the potential to influence target organs, the cell has increased its chances to control and adapt. This molecular diversity can be expressed at the protein precursor processing level, in the synthesis of mRNA or in the complex process of selecting genetic elements of information to be transcribed. By focusing now at each of these steps in turn we shall attempt to illustrate how variability or potential change can provide a means of evolving or adapting at the molecular level by leading to an increase in the number of overall possibilities.

3.1. Processing of Precursors

Processing is generally understood to include any transformation which may occur during the total course of biosynthesis until the final mature and active hormone is produced. As such, the various modifications which take place during the maturation of a peptide may be in different cell locations or organelles. Clearly a key modification involved in the conversion of a prohormone to its active component is the cleaving of the peptide chain at the appropriate site(s). But the proteolytic cleavages are usually not the only events necessary to obtain a bioactive peptide from a precursor; specific amino acid residue modifications are also involved. The cell may greatly enhance its choice of final products by operating through a precursor which, although synthesized as a single polypeptide, contains many different potential hormones joined together or even many similar peptides in the form of repeating units.

3.1.1. Proteolysis

Proopiomelanocortin (POMC), a precursor polyprotein originally isolated from the pituitary, is an example of a proform which contains several active hormones including adrenocorticotropin (ACTH), β- and γ-lipotropic hormones (β-LPH, γ-LPH), α- and β-melanocyte-stimulating hormones (α-MSH, β-MSH) and β-endorphin (β-END) within its sequence as illustrated in Fig. 2. Although most studies on biological activities have been focused on ACTH, MSHs, and β-END, the possibility that other segments of POMC may come to show activity cannot be excluded. This means that from one precursor, many potentially active individual peptides can be produced (see below). In the structure of proenkephalin (Fig. 3), we can see a precursor consisting mainly of identical repeating units of Met-enkephalin (ME).

In the structures illustrated above, the ultimate mature peptides are flanked by specific

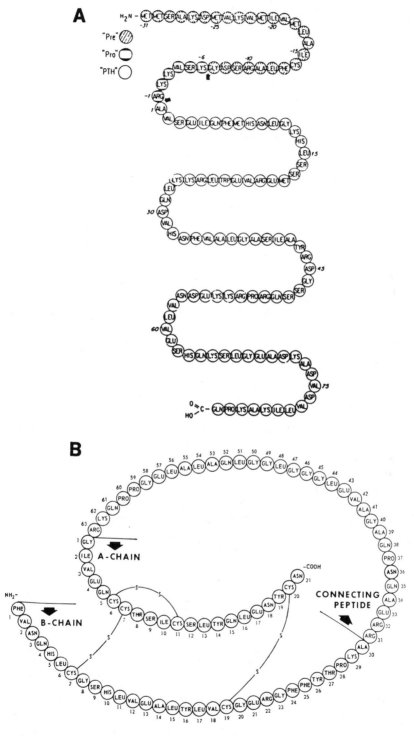

Figure 1. (A) The primary structure of prepro-PTH. Residues in open circles show the mature hormone which is liberated by peptide cleavage after the Lys-Arg site of the prosequence. (Adapted from Rosenblatt, 1982.) (B) The amino acid sequence of porcine proinsulin shows the proposed cleavage site at Arg_{31}-Arg_{32} and Lys_{62}-Arg_{63} which on proteolysis leaves the A and B chains joined by two disulfide bridges in active insulin.

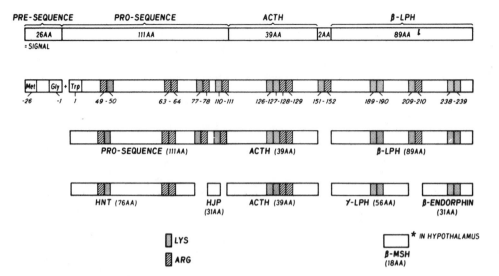

Figure 2. Schematic representation of the structure of human preproopiomelanocortin. Lysine residues are shown with dotted shading and arginine residues with cross-hatching. The locations of pairs of basic amino acid residues are shown to indicate sites where cleavage can give rise to ACTH, β- and γ-LPH, β-MSH, and β-END.

sequences of amino acids as first noted in the β- and γ-LPH model in 1967 (Chrétien and Li, 1967), which frequently seem to mark the sites to be cleaved during processing by a specific maturation enzyme. The cleavage sites, which represent an additional point of control, are often found to be pairs of basic amino acid residues, preferentially -Lys-Arg-, and first found in β-LPH (Chrétien and Li, 1967) and insulin (Chance *et al.*, 1968). The characteristics of processing have been described in recent reviews (Lazure *et al.*, 1983; Loh and Gainer, 1983; Steiner *et al.*, 1984). Among the precursor processing sequence sites known, most tend to be pairs of basic amino acid residues but a few hormones such as somatostatin, cholecystokinin, EGF, NGF, and other growth factors appear to be liberated through enzymatic cleavage at other recognition sites, often a single Arg residue (Douglas *et al.*, 1984; Schwartz, 1986).

An estimate of the amplification possible through a biosynthetic precursor containing multi-

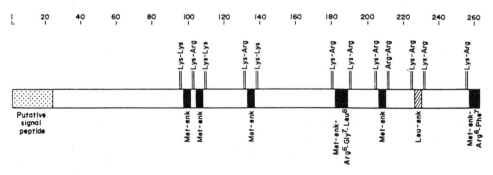

Figure 3. Structure of the enkephalin precursor. Potential Lys-Arg cleavage sites are shown. Four copies of Met-enkephalin and one of Leu-enkephalin are illustrated. (Adapted from Noda *et al.*, 1982.)

ple units can be seen in the following quantitation. The number of potential peptide products which can be derived on processing from a precursor can be expressed by the series

$$\sum_{i=1}^{n} i + 1 = (1 + 1) + (2 + 1) + (3 + 1) + \ldots + (n + 1)$$

where n represents the number of cleavage sites. In the molecule of POMC shown above which has 9 sites of paired basic amino acid residues, this leads to a possibility of 54 products theoretically available from the precursor while the enkephalin A precursor with 12 sites gives a possibility of 90 different products for each precursor, some of which will be the same due to the presence of identical repeating units.

3.1.2. Other Protein Modifications

From an original precursor, specific proteolytic cleavage is but one way of refining or augmenting the means of cell expression. Ample evidence now exists of several other non-proteolytic modifications by which a given polypeptide can be tailored to its specific goal. Although the functional role of most modifications is not yet well understood, the nature and the extent of one of them can be shown by a well-studied example on peptide acetylation of POMC-related products.

β-END, originally identified as the C-terminus of β-LPH (Fig. 2), is a 31-residue peptide biosynthesized in POMC and found to be a potent opiate. Several investigations have found that pituitary tissue also contains a 1 to 26 (β-END$_{1-26}$) and a 1 to 27 (β-END$_{1-27}$) residue form of this peptide. In addition, a β-END$_{1-31}$ form has been isolated from bovine intermediate lobe and in the hypothalamus which is acetylated on the N-terminal amino group resulting in an almost complete loss of opiate activity. The acetylated forms of β-END$_{1-27}$ and β-END$_{1-26}$ have also been well identified.

Another example of this modification is ACTH$_{1-14}$ (called α-MSH$_{1-14}$) and also found as α-MSH$_{1-13}$ (amidated C-terminal) both of which can be acetylated once on the amino group or once on the hydroxyl group of the N-terminal serine, or both creating thereby a possibility of eight different compounds.

Other processing modifications so far encountered are amidation, usually occurring at a terminal glycine residue, glycosylation, which is a realm of complexity in itself, phosphorylation on Tyr, Ser, or Thr, and sulfation.

3.1.3. Tissue-Specific Processing

In the rat the POMC precursor is synthesized in both the anterior and the intermediate lobes of the pituitary as well as other sites such as the hypothalamus. POMC is usually expressed from only a single gene. Yet, differences in the nature and/or extent of enzymatic processing of POMC in the anterior and the intermediate lobe tissues result in the production and secretion of different sets of end-product peptides. In the anterior lobe, intact N-terminal$_{1-74}$, ACTH$_{1-39}$, and β-LPH are the major POMC derivatives while in the intermediate lobe, further cleavage yields N-terminal$_{1-49}$ plus Lys-γ_3-MSH, α-MSH plus CLIP, and β-END as major products. Further processing of α-MSH- and β-END-related peptides via acetylation (as described above) also appears to be specific to intermediate lobe cells as well as the hypothalamus. As reported recently, the pattern of POMC processing in brain appears to be distinct from that in either the anterior or the intermediate pituitary lobe (Liotta *et al.*, 1984). In the light of studies showing that α-N-acetylation inactivates the opioid properties of β-END$_{1-31}$ and potentiates the behavioral effects of ACTH$_{1-13}$ NH$_2$ (MSH), the selective production of the acetylated peptides could represent another mechanism for additional regulation of the biological actions of neuronal POMC derivatives.

Also processed differently in the pituitary lobes is progastrin (Rehfeld, 1981; Udenfriend and Kilpatrick, 1983). In a manner comparable to POMC, the gastrin precursor undergoes more extensive processing in the neurointermediate lobe than the end products found in the anterior lobe.

Another family of opiate peptides, the enkephalins, are also generated biosynthetically as a precursor and are found in adrenal medulla and brain tissue (Douglas *et al.*, 1984). However, recent studies reveal that the processing of proenkephalin in the two tissues occurs very differently. In brain, cleavage appears to commence from the N-terminus producing free synenkephalin and enkephalin, while in adrenal one tends to find larger peptides suggesting less thorough processing (Liston *et al.*, 1983, 1984).

Prodynorphin, a precursor which has repeating copies of Leu-enkephalin and other peptides, is also processed with marked variation in several different regions of the brain (Zamir *et al.*, 1984).

3.1.4. Releasing Factors

The hypothalamic factors are other important brain peptides which act to mediate pituitary secretion. These peptides are synthesized in the hypothalamus and are secreted into the portal blood system to act upon various cells of the pituitary to rapidly increase the release of active pituitary hormones into the peripheral circulation. In short, the hypothalamic releasing factors can regulate peptide secretion of the pituitary. Specifically, TRH releases TSH and prolactin, GRF releases GH, LH-RH releases LH and FSH, while CRF releases POMC-related peptides. The releasing factors so far known appear to be biosynthesized similarly to the peptide hormones and other neuropeptides, i.e., as a precursor form subsequently processed to active components by similar proteolytic cleavages and other modifications (Douglas *et al.*, 1984). Recent cloning of the DNA sequence representing LH-RH has revealed a prospective new peptide identified as the long-sought-after prolactin-inhibiting factor (Nikolics *et al.*, 1985), and similar findings in this direction are likely to occur in the future.

3.2. Expression of Diversity at the Level of Transcription

As our abilities to analyze and manipulate genomic and cDNA structures increase, we can learn more about the ways in which the cell is able to provide multiple products at the level of mRNA. The following examples will give a view of the intricate means available.

3.2.1. Expression of Calcitonin and the Calcitonin Gene-Related Peptide

Calcitonin is biosynthesized in the thyroid. Its system of cellular expression and synthesis was examined in a medullary threshold carcinoma (MTC) which was able to spontaneously reduce its production of calcitonin (Douglas *et al.*, 1984). An examination of the mRNAs produced by the MTC (which was carried out by hybridizations with cloned cDNA probes) showed that the change was caused by transcription of the calcitonin gene to produce a series of new structurally related mRNAs. When one of the related mRNAs was cloned and sequenced, it was found to give rise by translation to peptides with sequence both in common and at variance with those found previously and hence one new peptide was designated as the calcitonin gene-related peptide (CGRP). In MTC cells one or the other mRNA is transcribed by splicing DNA genomic elements to give a specific mRNA depending upon the cellular environment (as shown in Fig. 4). The structure of the calcitonin gene has two exons (C_1 and C_2) which code for a sequence common to both calcitonin and CGRP, and their precursors. Therefore, based upon the structure

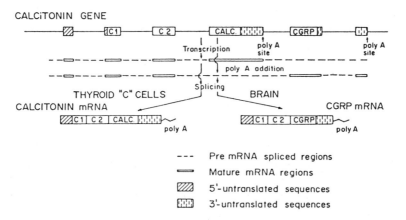

Figure 4. Scheme of the mRNA processing for calcitonin and CGRP peptide. C_1 and C_2 represent common domains present in both calcitonin mRNA and CGRP mRNA. Translated regions are denoted as open boxes and 5'- and 3'-untranslated sequences are shaded. (Adapted from Amara *et al.*, 1982.)

of the gene and its mRNA products, a model describing mRNA processing has been proposed (Amara *et al.*, 1982; Evans *et al.*, 1982), and is summarized in Fig. 4. In the thyroid, the calcitonin-specific exon is spliced onto the common region exons to generate preprocalcitonin, while in the hypothalamus CGRP-specific exons are spliced onto the same common region exons to generate prepro-CGRP.

Thus, we have an example in which transcriptional events regulate the expression of the rat calcitonin/CGRP gene so that two distinct species of mRNA (coding for functionally distinct bioactive peptides) can be generated from a single gene. Calcitonin has been studied as a thyroid hormone for some time but recent reports describe CGRP as having potent action as a vasodilator (Brain *et al.*, 1985). Also known is an additional function associated with a variant form of CGRP, called β-CGRP and differing by one amino acid, which is found in several regions of the brain and may come to have a functional importance distinct from both calcitonin and CGRP (Amara *et al.*, 1985). This illustrates a unique mechanism which tends to create flexibility and serves to increase the diversity of bioactive neuroendocrine peptides encoded by pluripotent genes.

3.2.2. Substance P Gene Tissue-Specific Splicing

Substance P is a well-known neuropeptide which acts as a neurotransmitter or neuromodulator in primary sensory neurons and in certain regions of the brain. Recently, however, the primary structure of two types of bovine brain substance P precursors revealed the existence of two related products, termed substance P and substance K, derived via alternative RNA splicing from a single gene (Nawa *et al.*, 1984). In a manner similar to that of the calcitonin/CGRP system, tissue-specific RNA splicing generates two distinct mRNAs encoding substance P alone or substance P as well as substance K. The latter is also known as neurokinin α, a peptide isolated from porcine spinal cord which has been shown to be active as a gut-contracting agent. In some tests, chemically synthesized substance K possesses biological activity greater than that of substance P, and this suggests that it may also have a different physiological role. Also suggesting dissimilar cellular roles are data showing that substance P and substance K are found in very different proportions in a series of CNS regions and in peripheral tissues, and that there are different receptors specific for substance P and substance K (Nawa *et al.*, 1984). mRNA splicing thus represents another interesting model not only to explore mechanisms responsible for tissue-specific regulation in the expression of the eukaryotic gene, but also to understand the molecular basis for the generation of the diversity of neuropeptides in the neuroendocrine system. Let us now briefly consider another system effective at expressing diversity of genetic information.

3.3. Multiplicity via Selection of Gene Elements

When many complex organisms are in contact with a foreign body, they recognize it as an invader and act in such a way as to remove or destroy it. Our immune system acts to produce a great variety of antibodies. There are millions of different chemical structures—protein, carbohydrate, and so on—that an organism has never been exposed to, but which it is able to recognize in a specific manner. Remarkably, the immune system can distinguish between different antigens, being any substance capable of eliciting an immune response, that are very similar to each other— such as between two proteins that differ in only a single amino acid or between two optical isomers. How does the immune system carry out this task with such a high degree of diversity and specificity? This is a question which has intrigued scientists for many years and has, as a result, been much studied and even continues to be the subject of intensive research. The number of lymphocytes in the body is about 2×10^{12} and a mouse can produce between 10^6 and 10^9 antibody molecules of different specificity. What genetic procedures lead to such diversity? Briefly, when a B cell is creating a particular antibody in response to the exposure of a foreign substance, it can draw upon a vast library of genetic sequence information expressing many antigenic characteristics. A typical antibody molecule is composed of two identical large or heavy (H) chains and two identical light (L) chains. Sequence studies have now established that both L and H chains consist of a constant (C) or unchanging sequence region and a variable (V) region which is different and unique for each type of antibody. Does this mean that the millions of protein antibodies require an equally large number of genes? As it turns out, the requirement is fulfilled by a unique genetic mechanism which selects from separate pools containing relatively few genes to ultimately produce a unique antibody protein. In each pool, separate gene segments that code for different parts of the variable regions of L and H chains can be brought together by site-specific combination events during B-cell differentiation. One simple but important mechanism that greatly increases antibody diversity is the combining of different L and H chains that occurs when an immunoglobulin molecule is assembled. In the mouse genome, there are close to 1000 genes encoding V_L regions and around 10,000 genes encoding V_H regions. Therefore, genetic combination could lead to $1000 \times 10,000$ different ways to construct an mRNA coding for one of 10^7 different antigen binding sites since the variable regions of both the L and H chains contribute to an antibody's binding site. Somatic mutations have recently been shown to occur in and around V region genes and probably increase the number of different antibodies by an additional factor of at least 10 to 100 (Tonegawa *et al.*, 1981). Hence, from relatively small numbers of genes, vast numbers of specific antibody molecules are synthesized. Thus, we see the immense potential for creating a vast array of diverse products by means of genetic selection from a given set of DNA information. What would we expect if the mechanisms described above were allowed to operate in the brain?

4. Neural Tissues and Diversity

As indicated in the opening paragraph, the brain is a complex biological system. The nature of brain and its relative sophistication can be indicated more clearly by the following specific points of comparison.

1. More structural genes are present in brain. It has been stated that as many or possibly more structural genes are required for the formation and function of brain as are necessary for all other tissues and organs combined (Chaudhari and Hahn, 1983).

2. Greater diversity of mRNA species is evident in CNS cells. A more diverse population of mRNA molecules is consistent with the extensive cellular heterogeneity and microdifferentiation of the various cell types found in brain. An estimate of as many as 500 different cell types present in brain has been made (Grouse et al., 1978).

3. The complexity of brain RNA sequences is considerably greater than that of other tissues or organs. This remarkable property of mammalian brain has been established recently as measured largely through the techniques of RNA–DNA hybridization (Kaplan and Finch, 1982). Studies on tumor cells of neural origin and nuclear RNA prepared from the neuronal fraction indicate that neurons contain RNA of higher complexity than do other types of mammalian cells (Ozawa et al., 1980). Hybridization studies have been carried out on RNA both of nuclear origin and from polysomes with even the latter showing complexity in whole brain equivalent to about 150,000 different sequences (Van Ness et al., 1979).

Given the above points of distinction, let us now consider that in many brain regions one or more would code for a precursor such as POMC (Fig. 2). It has been shown by immunohistochemical mapping of brain tissue that POMC is present in several defined brain regions (Khachaturian et al., 1985). It is conceivable that each of these separate neuronal sites may express a different form of biological activity through each POMC peptide produced on their respective target cells. In addition, as described above, the cleavage of POMC can give rise to 54 different potential peptides. Therefore, we can see that a single mRNA for POMC can be magnified in effect by 54× the number of sites where it is actively synthesized. This example illustrates a phenomenon which may be expressed by many other precursor mRNAs as yet unknown. Although we do not know enough about the cell biology and the diversity of brain to make calculations, as shown above, for the numbers of producible immunoglobulins, it is not inappropriate to anticipate an adaptability in brain much greater than that described for lymphoid cells.

Certainly, current facts make it tempting to suggest that many of the above-described mechanisms, as well as those we are as yet unaware of, may be operative in brain, all tending toward the amplification of neuropeptide end-products. Thus, it is easy to imagine how brain cells, beginning with a genetic repertoire of greater substance and more complexity, might be able to express a diversity and subtlety beyond anything so far encountered in biology.

ACKNOWLEDGMENTS. This work was supported by the Medical Research Council of Canada, the National Institutes of Health, and the J. A. De Sève Foundation.

References

Amara, S. G., Jonas, V., Rosenfeld, M. G., Ong, E. S., and Evans, R. M., 1982, Alternate RNA processing in calcitonin gene expression generates mRNAs encoding different polypeptide products, Nature 298:240–244.

Amara, S. G., Arriza, J. L., Leff, S. E., Swanson, L. W., Evans, R. M., and Rosenfeld, M. G., 1985, Expression in brain of a messenger RNA encoding a novel neuropeptide homologous to calcitonin gene-related peptide, Science 229:1094–1097.

Brain, S. D., Williams, T. J., Tippins, J. R., Morris, H. R., and MacIntyre, I., 1985, Calcitonin gene-related peptide is a potent vasodilator, Nature 313:54–56.

Chance, R. E., Ellis, R. M., and Bromer, W. W., 1968, Porcine proinsulin: Characterization and amino acid sequence, Science 161:165–167.

Chaudhari, N., and Hahn, W. E., 1983, Genetic expression in the developing brain, Science 220:924–928.

Chrétien, M., and Li, C. H., 1967, Isolation, purification and characterization of γ-lipotropic hormone from sheep pituitary glands, Can. J. Biochem. 45:1163–1174.

Douglas, J., Civelli, O., and Herbert, E., 1984, Polyprotein gene expression: Generation of diversity of neuroendocrine peptides, Annu. Rev. Biochem. 53:665–715.

Evans, R. M., Amara, S. G., and Rosenfeld, M. G., 1982, RNA processing regulation of neuroendocrine gene expression, DNA 1:323–328.

Grouse, L. D., Schrier, B. K., Bennett, E. L., Rosenzweig, M. R., and Nelson, P. G., 1978, Sequence diversity studies on rat brain RNA: Effects of environmental complexity on rat brain RNA diversity, *J. Neurochem.* **30:**191–203.

Kaplan, B. B., and Finch, C. E., 1982, The sequence complexity of brain ribonucleic acids, in: *Molecular Approaches to Neurobiology* (I. R. Brown, ed.), Academic Press, New York, pp. 71–98.

Khachaturian, H., Lewis, M. E., Schafer, M. K., and Watson, S. J., 1985, Anatomy of the CNS opioid systems, *Trends Neurosci.* **8:**111–119.

Lazure, C., Seidah, N. G., Pélaprat, D., and Chrétien, M., 1983, Proteases and post-translational processing of prohormones: A review, *Can. J. Biochem. Cell Biol.* **61:**501–515.

Liotta, A. S., Advis, J. P., Krause, J. E., McKelvy, J. F., and Krieger, D. T., 1984, Demonstration of *in vivo* synthesis of pro-opiomelanocortin-, β-endorphin-, and α-melanotropin-like species in the adult rat brain, *J. Neurosci.* **4:**956–965.

Liston, D., Vanderhaeghen, J., and Rossier, J., 1983, Presence in brain of synenkephalin, a proenkephalin-immunoreactive protein which does not contain enkephalin, *Nature* **302:**62–65.

Liston, D., Patey, G., Rossier, J., Verbanck, P., and Vanderhaeghen, J., 1984, Processing of proenkephalin is tissue-specific, *Science* **225:**734–737.

Loh, Y. P., and Gainer, H., 1983, Biosynthesis and processing of neuropeptides, in: *Brain Peptides* (D. T. Krieger, M. J. Brownstein, and J. B. Martin, eds.), Wiley, New York, pp. 80–116.

Nawa, H., Kotani, H., and Nakanishi, S., 1984, Tissue-specific generation of two preprotachykinin mRNA from one gene by alternate RNA splicing, *Nature* **312:**729–734.

Nikolics, K., Mason, A. J., Szönyi, E., Ramachandran, J., and Seeburg, P. H., 1985, A prolactin-inhibiting factor within the precursor for human gonadotropin-releasing hormone, *Nature* **316:**511–517.

Noda, M., Furutani, Y., Takahashi, H., Toyosato, M., Hirose, T., Inayoma, S., Nakanishi, S., and Numa, S., 1982, Cloning and sequence analysis of cDNA for bovine adrenal preproenkephalin, *Nature* **295:**202–205.

Ozawa, H., Kushiya, E., and Takahashi, Y., 1980, Complexity of RNA from neuronal and glial nuclei, *Neurosci. Lett.* **18:**191–196.

Rehfeld, J. F., 1981, Four basic characteristics of the gastrin–cholecystokinin system, *Am. J. Physiol.* **240:**G255–G266.

Rosenblatt, M., 1982, Pre-proparathyroid hormone: Intracellular transport and processing, *Miner. Electrolyte Metab.* **8:**118–129.

Schwartz, T. W., 1986, The processing of peptide precursors, *FEBS Lett.* **200:**1–10.

Steiner, D. F., Chan, S. J., Docherty, K., Emdin, S. O., Dodson, G. G., and Falkmer, S., 1984, Evolution of polypeptide hormones and their precursor processing mechanisms, in: *Evolution and Tumour Pathology of the Neuroendocrine System* (S. Falkmer, R. Hakanson, and F. Sundler, eds.), Elsevier, Amsterdam, pp. 203–223.

Tonegawa, S., Sakano, H., Maki, R., Traunecker, A., Heinrich, G., Roeder, W., and Kurosawa, Y., 1981, Somatic reorganization of immunoglobulin genes during lymphocyte differentiation, *Cold Spring Harbor Symp. Quant. Biol.* **45:**839–858.

Udenfriend, S., and Kilpatrick, D. L., 1983, Biochemistry of the enkephalins and enkephalin-containing peptides, *Arch. Biochem. Biophys.* **221:**309–323.

Van Ness, J., Maxwell, I. H., and Hahn, W. E., 1979, Complex population of nonpolyadenylated messenger RNA in mouse brain, *Cell* **18:**1341–1349.

Zamir, N., Weber, E., Palkovits, M., and Brownstein, M., 1984, Differential processing of prodynorphin and proenkephalin in specific regions of the rat brain, *Proc. Natl. Acad. Sci. USA* **81:**6886–6889.

34

Mechanisms of Neuropeptide Precursor Processing

Implications for Neuropharmacology

Harold Gainer

1. Introduction

In the past decade, more than 50 peptides have been identified in the nervous system as potential neurotransmitters and neuromodulators. These peptides produce distinct physiological and pharmacological effects on specific neurons, and are specifically localized and synthesized in the nervous system. Thus, in contrast to previous decades, when the neuropharmacologist needed to contend with only a few neurotransmitter candidates and receptor subtypes in the nervous system, the present situation abounds with an apparent "embarrassment of riches." This diversity of potential intercellular peptidic messengers in the nervous system promises to become even more complex in the future for two reasons. First, new biologically active peptides will undoubtedly be discovered, and second, the biosynthetic mechanism for the generation of peptides is itself a potential generator of diversity. The generation of biologically active peptides involves the posttranslational processing of protein precursors (Douglass *et al.*, 1984; Loh *et al.*, 1984), which, in addition to containing the peptide sequence(s) of interest, also contain other (unpredictable) peptide sequences. Since the proteolytic cleavage processes are usually located in the secretory vesicles (Gainer *et al.*, 1985), all these peptides will be cosecreted by exocytosis in response to a nerve impulse. While one of these secreted peptides may be the principal messenger at one site in the nervous system, any of the others could be the primary messenger at another site. In addition, variations in the posttranslational modifications of identical peptide precursors in different cells can lead to entirely different peptide products, with potentially different biological consequences (as for the case of proopiomelanocortin, see Chrétien *et al.*, this volume).

Although many cells and tissues synthesize peptides as intercellular messengers, the neuron is unique since in this cell type the sites of transcription, translation, and packaging of peptides into secretory vesicles (in the perikaryon) are separated by great distances (by the axon) from the

Harold Gainer • Laboratory of Neurochemistry and Neuroimmunology, National Institute of Child Health and Human Development, National Institutes of Health, Bethesda, Maryland 20892. *Present address:* Laboratory of Neurochemistry, National Institute of Neurological and Communication Disorders and Stroke, National Institutes of Health, Bethesda, Maryland 20892.

site of secretion (the nerve terminal). Because of this, certain mechanisms common to conventional neurotransmitter-secreting terminals, such as neurotransmitter reuptake and local recycling of vesicle membranes in the nerve terminal, are not functional in peptidergic nerve endings. Instead, the peptidergic neuron's terminal requires the continuous delivery, by axonal transport, of secretory vesicles containing *de novo* synthesized peptides. Hence, the secretory vesicle is the only intracellular organelle which is involved in both peptide biosynthesis and secretion, and is found in all three topographical regions of the nerve cell. For this reason, we have focused on the nature of this organelle and the posttranslational biosynthetic processes that are located in it (Gainer *et al.*, 1985).

Given the above information about the nature of peptide diversity, it is essential for neuropharmacological studies using peptides, to know for each specific presynaptic and postsynaptic configuration under study: (1) Where are the peptides localized in secretory terminals in the CNS? (2) What are the specific molecular forms of the peptides in these terminals? (3) Are the peptides found in secretory vesicles in these terminals? (4) Do the putative postsynaptic cells contain receptors to any of those specific peptide forms? (For discussion of this last point, see Beaudet *et al.* and Quirion, this volume.) Resolution of these cell biological issues is a prerequisite for complete understanding of the physiological significance of a peptide's action on any specific neuron in the CNS. This chapter will deal with recent progress which has been made in our understanding of peptide precursor processing, neurosecretory vesicle properties, and their relevance to peptide diversity.

2. General Cell Biological Mechanisms of Peptide Biosynthesis

All peptides destined for secretion are initially synthesized as larger precursor proteins, which are subsequently proteolytically cleaved and enzymatically modified to yield the final biologically active peptide products (for reviews see Douglass *et al.*, 1984; Loh *et al.*, 1984). The manifold steps which underlie this process are listed in Table I, along with their intracellular locations and the mechanistic sources of peptide diversity. The first step is the expression of the specific gene coding for the peptide precursor. Gene expression (i.e., synthesis of a specific RNA transcript) is the principal determinant of a cell's potential for synthesizing a specific peptide, and all subsequent activities by the cell to model the exact form of the peptide to be secreted are predicated upon this choice of gene to be transcribed. However, this event is not the *sine qua non* of specific peptide expression by the cell. Several other steps shown in Table I can also be critical in this decision. These include posttranscriptional and posttranslational modifications. For example, the gene for calcitonin also expresses a calcitonin gene-related peptide (CGRP) sequence at the level of the primary transcript, but alternative splicing of introns causes the CGRP (and not calcitonin) to be synthesized in the brain, whereas the reverse is true in peripheral tissues (Douglass *et al.*, 1984). The precursor protein is translated from mRNA associated with ribosomes attached to the rough endoplasmic reticulum (RER) in the cell body of the neuron (the exclusive site of protein biosynthesis in the nerve cell, with the possible exception of the dendrites), and is simultaneously translocated into the cisternae of the RER. Several posttranslational processing steps occur cotranslationally in the RER (see Koch and Richter, 1980; Zimmermann *et al.*, 1980; Farquhar and Palade, 1981; Castel *et al.*, 1984). These include: (1) removal of the signal sequence from the precursor, (2) the initial glycosylation of the glycopeptide on the arginine vasopressin (AVP) precursor on specific asparagine residues (i.e., where the sequence Asn-X-Ser/Thr is found), and (3) the formation of eight intramolecular disulfide bonds in the oxytocin (OT) and AVP precursors. This modified precursor protein is then translocated to the Golgi apparatus, where the high-mannose sugars are removed and other carbohydrates (e.g.,

Table I. Cell Biology of Neuropeptide Biosynthesis

Biosynthetic process	Intracellular location	Diversity generation mechanism
1. Gene expression (transcriptional process yields selective mRNA precursor)	Nucleus	Specific gene expressed
2. Posttranscriptional processing yields mRNA	Nucleus	Alternative splicing of introns
3. mRNA transported to cytosol and associates with ribosomes (RER)	Nuclear membrane	None
4. Translation of mRNA to yield peptide precursor protein which enters RER cistern via signal sequence on precursor	RER	None
5. Cotranslational processing (e.g., proteolytic removal of signal sequence, and initial glycosylation of precursor)	RER	Presence or absence of -Asn-X-Ser/Thr in precursor
6. Translocation to Golgi apparatus and further posttranslational modification of precursor (e.g., glycosylation, sulfation)	Golgi	Enzyme dependent
7. Enzymatic (proteolytic and nonproteolytic) processing of precursor to yield final biologically active peptides	Secretory vesicle	Alternative enzymes

sialic acid and fucose) are added during terminal glycosylation. In addition, other posttranslational processing events may occur in the Golgi such as sulfation and phosphorylation of the precursor. The Golgi apparatus serves principally to complete the modification of the precursor, and to concentrate and package the peptide precursor into membrane-bounded secretory vesicles (or granules), which are the principal transport vehicles for the peptides in neurons during their axonal transport to the nerve terminals (Castel *et al.*, 1984). In the terminals, the peptide-containing vesicles are stored, and secreted by exocytosis in response to appropriate neural signals (e.g., action potentials). All of these modifications serve to complete the precursor, but do not directly generate the individual peptide products. The endoproteolytic cleavages which excise these peptides from the precursor appear to occur distal to the Golgi, i.e., within the neurosecretory vesicle itself.

Over the last decade, the use of recombinant DNA technology has yielded valuable data on the amino acid sequences of a large number of prohormones and propeptides (Nakanishi *et al.*, 1979; Noda *et al.*, 1982; Kakidani *et al.*, 1982; Gubler *et al.*, 1982; Land *et al.*, 1982, 1983; Ruppert *et al.*, 1984; Schmale and Richter, 1984). This information was valuable in deducing the specific structural domains within the propeptides which are the sites at which processing enzymes must act. Figure 1 illustrates the peptide precursor structures for some of these, and also the cleavage sites in these precursors, which are usually represented by pairs of basic amino acid residues (Arg, or Lys) flanking the peptide sequences that are to be excised (see Table I). The most common sequence pair is Lys-Arg, although Arg-Lys, Arg-Arg, and Lys-Lys are also found at the putative cleavage sites. Another structural requirement for posttranslational processing is the presence of a glycine residue immediately distal to the amino acid to be C-terminally amidated in the biologically active peptide (Table I). This was recognized by Smyth and co-workers (Bradbury *et al.*, 1982; Bradbury and Smyth, 1983a) studying the amidating reaction and the enzyme responsible for it. The glycine residue is utilized as the amide donor in this hydroxylating monooxygenase reaction (Bradbury *et al.*, 1982; Eipper *et al.*, 1983a,b,c; Glembotski *et al.*, 1984) (further details on posttranslational processing will be described below).

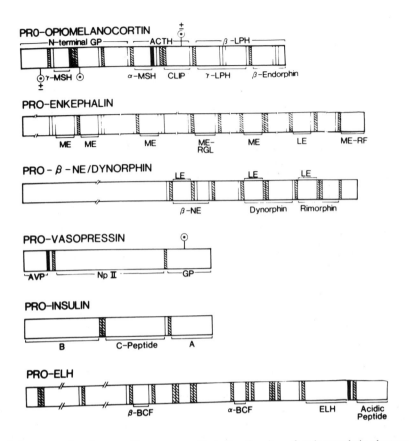

Figure 1. Structures of various peptide precursors illustrating the sites of endoproteolytic cleavage. Critical glycine, lysine, and arginine residues are represented as solid, white, and hatched bars, respectively.

3. A Cell Biological Model for Neuropeptide Biosynthesis: The Hypothalamic Magnocellular Neurons

Ever since the revolutionary morphological studies of Bargmann and Scharrer (1951), which generated the concept of neurosecretion, the magnocellular neurons in the hypothalamus have been the most intensively studied peptidergic neurons in the CNS. Excellent reviews (Castel *et al.*, 1984; Morris *et al.*, 1978; Silverman and Zimmerman, 1983; Sofroniew, 1985; Swanson and Sawchenko, 1983) as well as monographs (Schrier, 1985; Amico and Robinson, 1985; Cross and Leng, 1983) describing recent studies of immunohistochemical localizations and the putative functions of OT and AVP in the nervous system have been published, and the reader is referred to these for further information. The recent review by Sofroniew (1985) is particularly comprehensive in this regard, and is an excellent presentation of the current state of knowledge about the extrahypothalamic locations and projections of OT and AVP neurons in the CNS.

Magnocellular AVP and OT neurons are principally found in supraoptic (SON) and paraventricular (PVN) nuclei, as well as accessory groups scattered throughout the hypothalamus and nearby regions either loosely distributed or in relatively tight clusters. Aggregates of significant numbers of AVP neurons have also been found in the suprachiasmatic nucleus (SCN) and in the bed nucleus of the stria terminalis (N. interstitialis), as well as in the medial amygdala. Although recent immunocytochemical studies have extended our concepts of the locations of cell bodies containing these peptides, the relatively recently discovered extensive network of AVP and OT fibers throughout the CNS is even more impressive. Such fibers and terminals have been detected as far rostral as the olfactory bulbs and as far caudal as the spinal cord. In some cases, biosynthesis and axonal transport studies have been done to confirm these projections (Amico and Robinson, 1985). In general, AVP fibers dominate in forebrain areas, whereas OT fibers dominate in the more caudal brain stem and spinal cord.

In addition to the above distributions of OT and AVP fibers, immunocytochemical studies have indicated that these peptides may coexist with one or more different peptides (see Sofroniew, 1985). Convincing evidence exists that the magnocellular OT neurons also contain proenkephalin precursor products and CCK, and that the magnocellular AVP neurons contain prodynorphin precursor products. There is also good evidence for corticotropin releasing factor (CRF) and AVP coexistence in a subpopulation of parvocellular neurons in the PVN. In the above cases, ultrastructural immunocytochemical evidence has also been obtained showing that the peptides are colocalized in the same secretory vesicles within the fibers (Whitnall *et al.*, 1983, 1985). The function of these colocalizations in the magnocellular neurons is still unclear, although opioid effects on AVP and OT secretion from the neural lobe have been reported. The coexistence of AVP and CRF is functionally consistent with the findings of modulatory effects of AVP on ACTH secretion from the anterior pituitary (Gillies and Lowry, 1979).

4. AVP and OT Genes and Their Precursors

OT and AVP genes have been isolated and their nucleotide sequences determined for three species: cow (Ruppert *et al.*, 1984), rat (Ivell and Richter, 1984), and human (Sausville *et al.*, 1985). The structural organization of these genes is quite similar, irrespective of species; the structures of the rat genes are illustrated in Fig. 2. The OT and AVP genes contain three exons (regions in the genes which code for the amino acids in the precursors) separated by two intervening sequences (or introns). The first exon (exon A in Fig. 2) in both genes contains the nucleotide bases which encode the signal peptide, immediately followed by the nonapeptide, then a three-amino-acid spacer (Gly-Lys-Arg, which contains the signal for the endorprotease cleavage of the precursor), and finally the first nine amino acids of the N-terminus of the neurophysin in the precursor. The second exon (exon B) contains the highly conserved region of the neurophysin which encompasses amino acid positions 10–76 in this protein. The third exon (exon C) in both genes contains the remaining C-terminus of the neurophysin, followed in the AVP precursor by a single Arg separating the neurophysin from a C-terminal 39-amino-acid glycopeptide. The OT precursor contains only an extra Arg (in the rat) or a His (in the cow) following the neurophysin sequence. Thus, the only apparent structural distinction between the OT and AVP genes is the presence of the glycoprotein sequence in the latter. The function of this highly conserved AVP-associated glycoprotein remains unclear. A similar structure has been found for the human genes, where the terminal amino acid in the OT precursor is Arg, similar to the rat. Restriction analysis of the genomic DNAs has revealed only one copy each of the OT and AVP genes. Studies in the human have shown that the OT and AVP genes are physically linked on the same chromosome, separated by about 12 kilobases. However, these genes are present with an inverted arrangement of their coding strands (i.e., they have opposite transcriptional orientations). Sausville *et al.* (1985) point out that to explain the evolution of these two structural genes from a common ancestor, both gene duplication and inversion would be required, and speculate that such an inverted arrangement of related genes could influence transcriptional regulation, chromatin protein binding, and could decrease recombination efficiency. In all species studied, the expressed AVP and OT mRNAs appear to be processed to mature mRNAs with no evidence thus far for alternative splicing mechanisms. The amino acid sequences in the OT and AVP precursors appear to be directly related to the positions of the structural codons found in the genes.

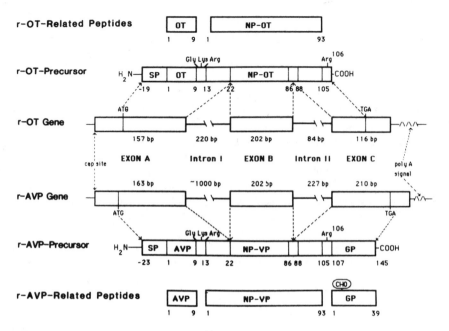

Figure 2. Organization of the AVP (r-AVP) and OT (r-OT) genes in the rat, and the relationships of these genes to their respective precursors (preprohormones) and final peptide products. Both genes are composed of three exons (A, B, and C) shown as open rectangles, separated by two introns (shown as disconnected lines between exons). The "cap site" represents the site of transcription initiation, and the ATG signal the site of translation initiation. The TGA signal on the gene represents the site of translational termination. The number of nucleotides in each gene component is illustrated (bp). The broken arrows illustrate the amino acid sequences in the precursors which are represented by the codons in the genes. Also indicated in the precursor structures are the amino acids in the precursors which are posttranslationally modified to produce the peptide products (see text). Abbreviations: SP, signal peptide; NP-OT, oxytocin-associated neurophysin; NP-VP, vasopressin-associated neurophysin; GP, glycopeptide; CHO, carbohydrate moiety on glycopeptide; bp, base pairs. (Data from Ivell and Richter, 1984; Ruppert *et al.*, 1984; Schmale *et al.*, 1983.)

The nucleotide sequences encoding the OT and AVP precursors are highly homologous; specifically, part of the first intron and exon B are exceptionally conserved between precursors and species. The high homology in this region was useful in a technical sense for cloning both genes in all the species. There are also important homologies in the nontranslated portions of the genes, i.e., in the so-called "5' flanking promoter" regions and "upstream" from the ATG translational initiation signal shown in Fig. 2 (the 5' flanking region is to the left of the ATG, and the 3' untranslated region is to the right of the TGA translational termination signal in Fig. 2). Eukaryotic genes usually have two control signals in the 5'-upstream region, a "TATA" and a "CAT" box. The TATA box is an AT-rich region usually about 25–30 bases upstream from the translational initiation signal, which is believed to direct the RNA polymerase II to the correct initiation site for transcription. The CAT box is a sequence (CAAT) which is usually 70–80 bases upstream and is believed to be a binding site for RNA polymerase II. The AVP and OT genes do not appear to contain CAT boxes, but do contain distinct but atypical TATA boxes. In addition, the genes have "cap" sites (shown in Fig. 2) which are signals for capping the 5' ends of eukaryotic mRNAs by the addition of m7Gppp (i.e., 7-methylguanoside residues joined to the mRNAs by triphosphate linkages) during transcription. At the 3' end of many eukaryotic genes there is a polyadenylation signal (Fig. 2) usually composed of the nucleotide sequence AATAAA. This codes for an mRNA sequence, AAUAAA, which is a signal for a nuclease to clip the nascent mRNA about 10–15 bases downstream. A second enzyme, poly-A synthetase, then adds the 100- to 200-base-long poly-A tail. The functions of the "capping" and poly-A tail are unknown, but some believe these modifications may protect the mRNA against degradative processes.

The main point is that there are other extensive interspecies homologies in the 5'-flanking sequences among the OT and AVP genes. OT genes in different species have distinct homologies in the 5' region, whereas OT and AVP genes, even in the same species, have little homology in the 5' region. This is significant since one would expect the 5'-flanking regions to contain conserved nucleotide sequences (i.e., promoters and enhancers) which would be responsible for the tissue- and cell-specific expression of either the AVP or OT gene. It is still not known which of these sequences, if any, are involved in the differential expression of these hormones in specific cells. However, despite these uncertainties about the mechanisms of gene regulation, knowledge of the gene structures provides access to the precursor amino acid sequences, and to the generation of either synthetic or cloned cDNA probes which are of great value for the analysis of specific gene expression (see Fuller *et al.*, 1985; Nojiri *et al.*, 1985; Burbach *et al.*, 1984; Sherman *et al.*, 1985; Uhl and Reppert, 1986; Uhl *et al.*, 1985; Majzoub, 1985; Majzoub *et al.*, 1983, 1984; Wolfson *et al.*, 1985).

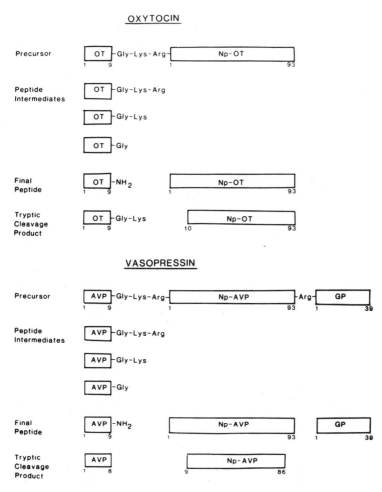

Figure 3. Illustration of OT and AVP precursors and theoretical peptide intermediates of posttranslational modifications of these precursors.

Given the amino acid sequences of the final peptide products (AVP and OT) and their respective precursors (Fig. 2), it is possible to deduce the signals for the putative enzymatic modifications. The processing steps which are necessary to transform the OT and AVP precursors to peptide products include endopeptidase cleavages at Lys-Arg residues which separate both of the peptides (located at the N-termini of their respective precursors) from their carrier proteins (the neurophysins), and another endopeptidase cleavage at a single Arg residue which separates the AVP-associated neurophysin from a 39-amino-acid glycoprotein at the C-terminal end of the AVP precursor. Figure 3 illustrates some of the intermediates which could theoretically be formed as a result of these endopeptidase cleavages. The question is, which cleavage site is used *in vivo*, and therefore which intermediates are formed? (See below.)

5. The Intracellular Location of Processing

Various lines of experimental evidence indicate that the secretory vesicle is the site of posttranslational processing of propeptides. Early studies on the biosynthesis of insulin (Kemmler *et al.*, 1973; Steiner *et al.*, 1974) and vasopressin (Sachs *et al.*, 1969) suggested that the processing of these prohormones occurred within secretory vesicles. Axonal transport studies have indicated that the OT and AVP precursors synthesized in separate magnocellular neurons in the hypothalamo-neurohypophysial system (HNS) are rapidly transported in the axons of the median eminence (internal zone), and undergo their first endopeptidase cleavage step during axonal transport at great distances from the cell bodies (Gainer *et al.*, 1977a,b). Since the only transport vehicles for the peptides are the neurosecretory vesicles (Kent and Williams, 1974; Haddad *et al.*, 1980; Castel *et al.*, 1984), it was concluded that the initial enzymatic cleavages and subsequent processing events which converted the precursors to the peptides occurred within the neurosecretory vesicles. This notion has been generalized into the "secretory vesicle hypothesis of peptide precursor processing," and has been reviewed elsewhere (Gainer *et al.*, 1985). The essential test of this hypothesis, which states that "the initial endopeptidase cleavages which excise the nascent, biologically active peptides from their protein precursors occur primarily in secretory vesicles," requires that such an endopeptidase be demonstrated within the secretory vesicles.

In recent studies using cDNA for human proinsulin, Moore *et al.* (1983a,b) showed that injection of this cDNA into fibroblasts or ACTH-secreting AtT-20 cells resulted in two opposite results; whereas the AtT-20 cells, which normally process and secrete ACTH, were able to process proinsulin into insulin-like peptides, the fibroblasts secreted unprocessed proinsulin. The fibroblasts, which do not have the cellular apparatus to package and store secretory products for regulated secretion, secreted proinsulin via a nonregulated, constitutive pathway. These elegant experiments suggested that packaging mechanisms and processing enzymes in the tumor cell line could sort and process proinsulin as well as proopiomelanocortin (POMC), and that the presence of the cellular machinery for secretory vesicle formation was necessary for prohormone processing. Recently, in another set of experiments using a preproglucagon gene, Drucker *et al.* (1986) found that when a metallothionein–glucagon fusion gene was introduced into a fibroblast cell line, the cells secreted unprocessed proglucagon. However, when the same construct was introduced into two endocrine cell lines (GH4, pituitary; RN38, islet cells), the cells were able to process the propeptide to varying degrees. Almost complete processing occurred in the islet cell line.

The secretory vesicle would be a biologically advantageous site to localize the apparatus for processing precursors to secretory peptides for the following reasons: First, it would simplify the packaging process in the Golgi. Instead of having separate concentrating and packaging mechanisms for each peptide in a precursor, only one mechanism for the precursor would be necessary. Second, it would ensure that the stoichiometric relationships between the diverse peptides found in the precursor determined at the gene level would be faithfully maintained during exocytosis. Third, since the secretory vesicle membrane is highly impermeant to small molecules, small peptide products (such as the tripeptide, TRH, and the dipeptide, Gly-Gln) would likely be retained in the vesicle for secretion. Finally, the low permeability of the vesicle membrane to H^+ would allow the ATPase in the membrane to generate a pH gradient and an acidic intravesicular environment, which appears necessary for the proteolytic processing enzymes.

To date, there have been no reports of studies directed at elucidating the natures of the OT and AVP peptide intermediates (Fig. 3) *in vivo*. This issue is of some biological significance since: (1) information about the intermediates formed *in vivo* would provide an important criterion for the evaluation of putative processing endopeptidases, and (2) it would indicate a possible alternative form of the biologically active peptide, if the intermediate was a stable and secretable product under some experimental circumstances. As discussed earlier, the AVP precursor requires an additional endopeptidase action, i.e., a cleavage at the single Arg between the neurophysin and the glycopeptide. Several workers have detected glycopeptide-extended forms of neurophysin in the HNS (North *et al.*, 1983; Robinson and Jones, 1983; Gordon-Weeks *et al.*, 1983; Jones *et al.*, 1984), and in the guinea pig this appears to be a stable and secreted intermediate form. The authors thus conclude that the peptide (AVP) is cleaved first and that the single Arg cleavage occurs second in this precursor (in the case of the guinea pig the latter cleavage seems to be significantly absent). The biological significance of this glycopeptide-extended neurophysin is still unclear. A clue to the peptide cleavage (at the Lys-Arg pair in Fig. 3) was obtained by Dr. M. Altstein in our laboratory, who found that in fetal and early postnatal rats the predominant form of stable OT in the hypothalamus was OT-Glys-Lys-Arg$_{12}$ with a small amount of OT-Gly$_{10}$-Lys$_{11}$ also produced (unpublished data). This suggests that *in vivo* the endopeptidase cleaves primarily on the carboxyl side of the Arg and possibly (to a small extent) in between the Lys-Arg pair in the precursor (see Fig. 3).

6. Enzymatic and Membrane Properties of the Secretory Vesicle

One of the features of the HNS which makes it a particularly efficacious model for the study of neuropeptide processing is the availability of large numbers of nerve terminals containing neurosecretory vesicles in the neurohypophysis. Figure 4 illustrates neurosecretosomes, which are pinched-off nerve endings from the neurohypophysis derived by a gentle homogenization in isotonic sucrose and density gradient centrifugation. These isolated nerve endings are physiological models for studies of nerve terminal secretion and contain, in addition to various membrane-bounded organelles, abundant neurosecretory vesicles. By a variant of these homogenization and subcellular fractionation procedures (Russell, 1981) it is possible to isolate highly enriched neurosecretory vesicles (Fig. 5). These vesicles are enriched in OT, AVP, and neurophysins (Nps), and most significantly do not contain lysosomal hydrolases. The significance of the latter point is that since we wanted to examine whether these vesicles contained endopeptidases that would cleave at Lys-Arg bonds in the precursor, we wanted to be sure that an enzyme which could do this, cathepsin B, but was located in the lysosome was not present in the neurosecretory vesicle preparation.

Using such secretory vesicle preparations, Dr. Y. Peng Loh and her colleagues in our laboratory have succeeded in purifying to apparent homogeneity a paired basic residue-specific endopeptidase from highly purified secretory vesicles derived from the intermediate lobe of the pituitary, which selectively cleaves at such residues in POMC and proinsulin (Loh *et al.*, 1985). This enzyme appears to be an aspartyl protease with an acidic pH maximum of activity, and is a glycoprotein of 70,000 daltons (on SDS-PAGE). Analysis of the cleavage products *in vitro* indicated that this enzyme cleaves half of the time between Lys-Arg residues and about half of the time on the carboxyl side of the Arg residue in the POMC precursor. A similar tendency to cleave

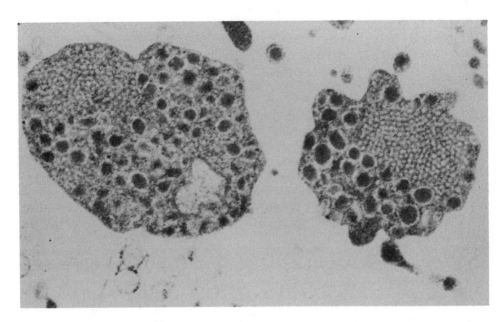

Figure 4. Electron micrograph of nerve terminals (neurosecretosomes) isolated from the bovine neurohypophysis. (J. T. Russell and M. H. Whitnall, unpublished.)

between the Lys-Arg residues (> 50%) was observed when β-lipotropin was studied using this purified enzyme preparation (Loh, 1986).

Similar studies using a highly purified neurosecretory vesicle preparation from the neural lobe, have also led to the purification of a virtually identical enzyme from the AVP- and OT-containing neurosecretory vesicles (Parish *et al.,* 1986). The neural lobe-derived enzyme is also an aspartyl glycoprotein endopeptidase (ca. 70,000 daltons) which is specific for Lys-Arg residues and can cleave POMC and proinsulin appropriately. Analysis of the cleavage products when the AVP precursor was used as a substrate also indicated a specificity for Lys-Arg residues. However, the cleavage in the AVP precursor *in vitro* occurred primarily (80%) on the carboxyl side of the Arg in the Lys-Arg pair, and only about 20% between these residues (Parish *et al.,* 1986). A similar enzyme activity has been reported using a cruder enzyme preparation from neurosecretory vesicles and a synthetic OT precursor-like peptide (amino acids 1–18 amide) substrate (Clamargirand *et al.,* 1986).

The above data provide tentative biochemical support for the "secretory vesicle hypothesis." However, it still is necessary to demonstrate by ultrastructural immunocytochemistry that these putative converting enzymes are located intravesicularly. The fact that these enzymes can cleave between the Lys-Arg residues (albeit under *in vitro* conditions, and to different extents in POMC and pro-AVP) suggests that at least two exopeptidase actions (i.e., carboxypeptidase B-like and aminopeptidase B-like enzyme activities) are necessary to remove the N- and C-terminal basic residues from the cleaved peptides (Gainer *et al.,* 1984, 1985). In addition, since OT and AVP are both amidated at their C-termini, the transformation of their C-terminal glycines into amide groups by a peptidyl-glycine-α-amidating monooxygenase would also be required in the neurosecretory vesicles. All of these enzymatic activities have been detected in secretory vesicles obtained from neural lobe nerve endings, and in a number of cases the enzymes have been purified and characterized (see Table II). In addition, the secretory vesicle membrane contains two types of proteins which by their membrane transport functions serve to regulate the internal

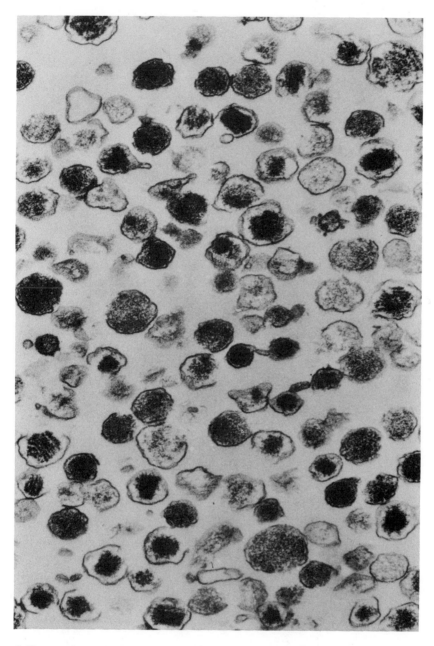

Figure 5. Electron micrograph of neurosecretory vesicles isolated from the bovine neurohypophysis. (J. T. Russell and M. H. Whitnall, unpublished.)

state of the vesicular environment. These include a cytochrome b_{561} which appears to transport electrons into the vesicle in order to maintain the intravesicular ascorbate in a reduced state, and a proton-transporting ATPase which serves to maintain the intravesicular pH between 5 and 6 (Gainer *et al.*, 1985; Russell, 1984; Russell and Holz, 1981; Duong *et al.*, 1984). In the above commentary, we have focused on the enzymatic mechanisms which are common to both the AVP

Table II. Some Peptide Precursor Processing Enzymes Found in Secretory Vesicles

Enzyme	Reaction	Molecular weight[a]	Cofactors	pH max in vitro	Inhibitors	Reference
Prohormone converting enzyme[b] (paired basic residue-specific endopeptidase)	Peptide[1]-Lys-Arg-Peptide[2] → Peptide[1]-Lys + Arg-Peptide[2] or Peptide[1]-Lys-Arg + Peptide[2]	70,000 (M, S)	—	4.0–4.5	Pepstatin	Loh et al. (1985), Loh (1986), Parish et al. (1986)
Carboxypeptidase B-like enzyme[b] (carboxypeptidase E)	Peptide-Lys-Arg→ Peptide + Lys + Arg	52,000 (M) 50,000 (S)	Co^{2+}	5.4–5.8	Cu^{2+}, Cd^{2+} PCMB EDTA	Fricker and Snyder (1982, 1983) Gainer et al. (1984, 1985)
Aminopeptidase B-like enzyme	Arg-Peptide→ Peptide + Arg	? (M)	Co^{2+} Zn^{2+}	6.0		
Peptidyl glycine α-amidating monooxygenase (PAM)[b]	Peptide-Gly→ Peptide-NH_2 + OHC-COOH	48,000 (PAM A) 42,000 (PAM B) 37,000 (S)	Cu^{2+} Ascorbic acid O_2	7.0–8.0	Diethyldithiocarbonate (reversed by $CuSO_4$)	Bradbury et al. (1982), Bradbury and Smyth (1983b), Murthy et al. (1986)
Peptide acetyltransferase	NH_2-Peptide→ CH_3-C-NH-Peptide (C=O)	? (S)	Acetyl CoA	7.0		Glembotski (1981, 1982)

[a]M, membrane associated; S, soluble.
[b]Purified to apparent homogeneity.

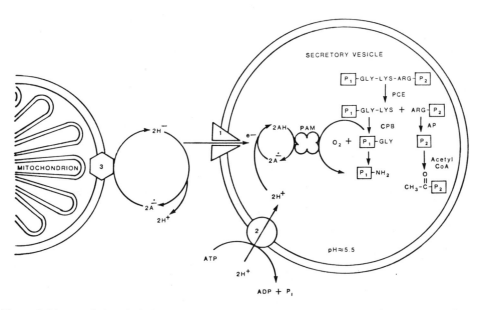

Figure 6. Diagram of a hypothetical secretory vesicle illustrating intravesicular processing enzymes, extravesicular processes, and vesicle membrane enzymes currently believed to be involved in precursor processing. Abbreviations for processing enzymes: PCE, dibasic residue-specific prohormone converting enzyme; CPB, carboxypeptidase B; AP, aminopeptidase; PAM, peptidyl glycine α-amidating monooxygenase; 1, cytochrome b_{561}; 2, H^+-translocating Mg^{2+}ATPase; 3, mitochondrial NADH:semidehydroascorbate oxidoreductase. P1 and P2 represent model peptides. AH, ascorbate; A^-, semidehydroascorbate. See text and Table II for other cofactor requirements for the different processing enzymes. (Adapted from Gainer *et al.*, 1985.)

and OT precursors. However, the AVP precursor also required another endopeptidase action at the single Arg residue separating the neurophysin from the 39-amino-acid glycopeptide. The enzyme we have purified from the neural lobe vesicle does not appear to produce this cleavage (Parish *et al.*, 1986). This would suggest that another enzyme in the vesicle is responsible for this proteolytic event. A hypothetical model illustrating the general elements of the "secretory vesicle hypothesis" is shown in Fig. 6.

7. Ionic Permeabilities of Secretory Vesicle Membranes

Since secretory vesicles have membranes which will fuse with nerve terminal membranes during exocytosis, the permeability characteristics of these membranes may be of interest to neuropharmacologists. Secretory vesicle membranes are virtually impermeant to H^+, K^+, Na^+, and Mg^{2+} (Johnson and Scarpa, 1976). Recently, evidence has been obtained for a $Ca^{2+}-Na^+$ transport system in both chromaffin and neurosecretory vesicles, the functional significance of which, however, has not been identified (Krieger-Brauer and Gratzl, 1983). Anion permeability of chromaffin vesicles determined by the measurement of vesicle swelling (optical density changes), or lysis in the presence of Mg^{2+}ATP, follows the order $SCN^- > I^- > CCl_3CO_2^- > Br^- > Cl^- > SO_4^{2-} > CH_3CO_2^-$, F^-, PO_4^{3-} (Casey *et al.*, 1976; Phillips, 1977). The Cl^- conductance calculated from these experiments is approximately 3×10^{-7} siemens/cm², which is similar to the Cl^- conductances found in artificial phospholipid bilayer membranes. Neurosecretory vesicles exhibit identical anion permeability characteristics (Russell, 1984). Both isolated chromaffin and neurosecretory vesicles are relatively stable in isoosmotic KCl, or NaCl solutions in the absence of MgATP (Johnson and Scarpa, 1976). However, when incubated in solutions containing potassium salts in the presence of the potassium ionophore valinomycin, both vesicles lyse and release their contents (Dolais-Kitabgi and Perlman, 1975; Russell, 1984). Recently, the presence of both cation and anion channels on secretory vesicles has been identified. Isolated secretory vesicles are relatively stable in isotonic (300 mosm) sucrose solutions suggesting that the membrane is impermeant to sucrose, but undergo lysis when the osmolarity is lowered to 200 mosm (Holz, 1986; Nordmann and Morris, 1982). However, chromaffin vesicles lyse rapidly in isoosmolar solutions of other nonelectrolytes like erythreitol, arabitol, and glucose. Thus, nonelectrolytes smaller than sucrose seem to be more permeant across the vesicle membrane (Holz, 1986).

It has recently been proposed that the secretory vesicle membrane may contain ionic channels, some of which may be gated by Ca^{2+} (Stanley and Ehrenstein, 1985). According to this model the function of Ca^{2+} in initiation of secretion is to open Ca-activated cation channels present on the vesicle membrane. The opening of these channels results in an influx of cations, followed by anions via anion channels in order to preserve electroneutrality. Consequently, the vesicle core osmotic activity is altered due to the increased ion concentrations or by interfering with the organization of the vesicle core. According to this model, it is this osmolarity increase that is the rate-limiting step for Ca-dependent exocytosis (see Stanley and Ehrenstein, 1985). This model is largely consistent with the experimental evidence available and can explain very rapid secretory events, and facilitation of neurotransmitter release in nerve endings. The presence of a Ca-activated cation channel with large conductances (> 400 pS) and calcium activation at submicromolar concentration ranges has been identified in isolated neurosecretory vesicles from the posterior pituitary in lipid bilayer incorporation experiments (Stanley et al., 1986). Furthermore, an anion channel also has been identified in similar experiments in neurosecretory vesicle membranes (Stanley and Russell, personal communication). In a series of experiments using chromaffin vesicles fused with large liposomes, patch clamp data showed the presence of ionic channels with large conductances on the order of 100 to 500 pS (Picaud et al., 1984). Biochemical evidence for the presence of anion channels on both chromaffin vesicles and neurosecretory vesicles has existed for some time (Casey et al., 1976, 1977; Pazzoles et al., 1980; Pazzoles and Pollard, 1978).

As mentioned earlier, the secretory mechanism may utilize the large potential osmotic energy in secretory vesicles in the exocytotic secretory process, and it is conceivable that the ionic channels may function to trigger such an event. Secretion from intact chromaffin cells initiated by acetylcholine (Hampton and Holz, 1983; Pollard et al., 1981; Holz, 1986), and in permeabilized cells initiated by increasing pCa (Knight and Baker, 1982; Knight, 1986) is inhibited by increasing the osmolarity of the bathing medium, suggesting a possible role for osmotic changes during the secretory process. In these experiments, one caveat is that the increased osmolarity also causes shrinkage of the cells themselves, and not only the chromaffin vesicles. However, experiments using high-molecular-weight polysaccharides which do not cause cell shrinkage also prevented secretion (for review see Holz, 1986). It should be pointed out here that in some experiments secretion seems to proceed in media deficient in permeant ionic species (e.g., sucrose solutions; Knight and Baker, 1982; Knight, 1986). Furthermore, additional experiments are needed to unequivocally demonstrate that the vesicle membrane, in fact, is the source of the ionic channels identified in lipid bilayer experiments of Stanley et al. (1986). It is also not inconceivable that the ionic channels on vesicle membranes provide a mechanism for regulating the intravesicular environment, e.g., pH or ionic concentrations, and thereby regulate the activities of processing enzymes involved in the posttranslational processing of propeptides.

8. Insights into Peptide Regulation from Studies of the Magnocellular Neurons

The homozygous Brattteboro rat (*di/di* rat) contains the normal complement of hypothalamic AVP neurons, but these neurons do not contain AVP, thereby leading to diabetes insipidus (Valtin *et al.*, 1974). It is also known that these neurons do not synthesize the AVP precursor (Brownstein and Gainer, 1977). Recent recombinant DNA studies by Schmale and Richter (1984) have located the genetic defect in the *di/di* rat. The mutant AVP gene has a single nucleotide base (guanosine) deletion in the second exon which encodes the highly conserved region of neurophysin. The consequences of this single base deletion would be profound, i.e., it would cause a shift in the reading frame of the AVP precursor altering the amino acid sequence from position 64 in the AVP-associated neurophysin to the C-terminus of the precursor. The result would be the loss of 5 of 14 of the cysteines in the precursor, the absence of a stop codon in the mRNA, the loss of the spacer arginine (cleavage site) between the neurophysin and the glycopeptide, and the absence of the Asn-Ala-Thr sequence in the C-terminus region of the precursor (which acts as a signal for glycosylation). The nature of this genetic defect in the *di/di* AVP gene, however, would not preclude transcription or normal mRNA processing. Indeed, Northern blots of the *di/di* hypothalamic mRNA revealed a normal-sized AVP mRNA of about 2300 nucleotides (Schmale and Richter, 1984), and *in situ* hybridization studies showed that the AVP mRNA is correctly located in the homozygous Brattleboro rat hypothalamus (Uhl *et al.*, 1985; Majzoub *et al.*, 1984; Majzoub, 1985; Fuller *et al.*, 1984). Given these data, it is likely that the major consequence of the genetic defect is at the translational and not at the transcriptional level. Recent cell-free translational studies comparing the translation of the normal AVP mRNA with that of the *di/di* AVP mRNA, and transfection studies using the normal and *di/di* AVP gene, have demonstrated that only the normal mRNA is insignificantly translated (Schmale *et al.*, 1984). It has been proposed (Schmale *et al.*, 1984) that the absence of the stop codon on the defective mRNA would eliminate the signal for the dissociation of the mRNA–ribosome complex, and hence the effective reinitiation of the mRNA for further translation. It is also possible that the loss of 5 of 14 cysteines of the neurophysin in the precursor would lead to abnormal folding of the precursor and, hence, immediate degradation.

In addition to providing an interesting analysis of a genetic defect, the above observations also introduce a caveat into the contemporary notion that mRNA hybridization studies are sufficient to demonstrate the existence of a biologically active peptide in a cell or tissue. Clearly the *di/di* rat hypothalamus contains AVP mRNA (albeit defective) containing the normal AVP sequence, but no AVP. Therefore, the availability of cDNA probes and hybridization techniques does not preclude also demonstrating the presence of the final processed peptides by more conventional immunological and chromatographic techniques.

In recent studies on the development of OT and AVP expression in the rat hypothalamus, Dr. M. Altstein in our laboratory has found that during E18–21 no completely processed (amidated) OT is present in the HNS. However, significant amounts of $OT\text{-}Gly_{10}Lys_{11}Arg_{12}$ could be detected at these stages, which indicated that the Lys-Arg-specific endopeptidase was present and functional in the OT neurons. The AVP peptides, on the other hand, were substantially processed to amidated AVP at these stages (M. Altstein, unpublished data). Although these data are still preliminary, two conclusions are immediately apparent. First, the presence of a stable form of $OT\text{-}Gly_{10}Lys_{11}Arg_{12}$ in these studies indicates that the cleavage of the AVP precursor to primarily $AVP\text{-}Gly_{10}Lys_{11}Arg_{12}$ by the purified endopeptidase *in vitro* (see above) is likely to be the correct cleavage product for the neurohypophysial peptides *in vivo*. It should be noted that some $OT\text{-}Gly_{10}Lys_{11}$ peptides were also detected *in vivo* comparable to the $AVP\text{-}Gly_{10}Lys_{11}$ product *in vitro*, but unlike the *in vitro* case, we cannot be sure that this was due only to endopeptidase cleavages between the Lys-Arg bond *in vivo* since a partial carboxypeptidase B-like activity could also account for these data. The second conclusion is that expression of prohormone and final biologically active peptide product is independently regulated during development. Clearly, the OT precursor is being expressed during E18–21, but no amidated OT is generated at these ages. The block in processing appears to be at the carboxypeptidase B-like enzymatic step, thereby resulting primarily in an OT-$Gly_{10}Lys_{11}Arg_{12}$ "final" product.

9. Conclusions

Because of the large numbers of subsequent events which determine whether the expression of a gene coding for a specific precursor will lead to the formation of a specific peptide in any given cell, it becomes apparent that localization of the appropriate mRNA in a neuron is a necessary but not sufficient criterion to prove that the neuron is of a specific peptidic character. In addition to the well-known example of alternative POMC processing in intermediate and anterior pituitary cells, which leads to different peptide messengers in these cells derived from an identical expressed gene, we see in the developing OT neurons that a selective deletion of a processing enzyme activity (e.g., carboxypeptidase B) can also determine the form of the peptide. Given that the OT precursor is accessible to secretory vesicle processing in early embryological stages, but is incompletely processed to an OT-$Gly_{10}Lys_{11}Arg_{12}$ product, one must wonder whether this has some biological significance. Assuming that this immature peptide product is present in vesicles capable of exocytosis, then this immature form of OT may play a special role during embryogenesis (e.g., as a secreted trophic factor). Alternatively, the early expression of the amidated AVP peptide vis-à-vis the OT peptide might also suggest a developmental role for the former. In any case, it is apparent that the posttranslational modifications of these two peptides are being differentially regulated during development. The biological significance of this differential development of OT and AVP neurons remains to be elucidated.

References

Amico, J. A., and Robinson, A. G. (eds.), 1985, *Oxytocin: Clinical and Laboratory Studies,* Excerpta Medica, Amsterdam.

Bargmann, W., and Scharrer, E., 1951, The origin of the posterior pituitary hormones, *Am. Sci.* **39:**255–259.

Bradbury, A. F., and Smyth, D. G., 1983a, Amidation of synthetic peptides by a pituitary enzyme: Specificity and mechanisms of the reaction, in: *Peptides 1982* (K. Blaha and P. Mahlon, eds.), de Gruyter, Berlin, pp. 383–386.

Bradbury, A. F., and Smyth, D. G., 1983b, Substrate specificity of an amidating enzyme in porcine pituitary, *Biochem. Biophys. Res. Commun.* **112:**372–377.

Bradbury, A. F., Finnie, M. D. A., and Smyth, D. G., 1982, Mechanism of C-terminal amide formation by pituitary enzymes, *Nature* **298:**686–688.

Brownstein, M. J., and Gainer, H., 1977, Neurophysin biosynthesis in normal rats and in rat with hereditary diabetes insipidus, *Proc. Natl. Acad. Sci. USA* **74:**259–261.

Burbach, J. P., De Hoop, M. J., Schmale, H., Richter, D., De Kloet, E. R., Ten Haaf, J. A., and De Wied, D., 1984, Differential responses to osmotic stress of vasopressin-neurophysin mRNA in hypothalamic nuclei, *Neuroendocrinology* **39:**582–584.

Casey, R. P., Njus, D., Radda, G. K., and Sehr, P. A., 1976, Adenosine triphosphate-evoked catecholamine release in chromaffin granules, osmotic lysis as a consequence of proton translocation, *Biochem. J.* **158:**583–588.

Casey, R. P., Njus, D., Radda, G. K., and Sehr, P. A., 1977, Active proton uptake by chromaffin granules: Observation by amine distribution and phosphorus-31 nuclear magnetic resonance techniques, *Biochemistry* **16:**972–977.

Castel, M., Gainer, H., and Dellmann, H. D., 1984, Neuronal secretory systems, *Int. Rev. Cytol.* **88:**303–459.

Clamagirand, C., Camier, M., Bousetta, H., Fahy, C., Morel, A., Nicholas, P., and Cohen, P., 1986, An endopeptidase associated with bovine neurohypophysis secretory granules cleaves pro-oxytocin/neurophysin peptide at paired basic residues, *Biochem. Biophys. Res. Commun.* **134**:1190–1196.

Cross, B. A., and Leng, G. (eds.), 1983, *The Neurohypophysis: Structure, Function and Control,* Elsevier, Amsterdam.

Dolais-Kitabgi, J., and Perlman, R. L., 1975, The stimulation of catecholamine release from chromaffin granules by valinomycin, *Mol. Pharmacol.* **11**:745–750.

Douglass, J., Civelli, O., and Herbert, E., 1984, Polyprotein gene expression: Generation of diversity of neuroendocrine peptides, *Annu. Rev. Biochem.* **53**:665–715.

Drucker, D. J., Mojsov, S., and Habener, J. F., 1986, Cell-specific posttranslational processing of preproglucagon expressed from a metallothionein–glucagon fusion gene, *J. Biol. Chem.* **261**:9637–9643.

Duong, L., Fleming, P. J., and Russell, J. T., 1984, An identical cytochrome b_{561} is present in ovine adrenal chromaffin vesicles and posterior pituitary neurosecretory vesicles, *J. Biol. Chem.* **259**:4885–4889.

Eipper, B. A., Glembotski, C. C., and Mains, R. E., 1983a, Bovine intermediate pituitary α-amidation enzyme: Preliminary characterization, *Peptides* **4**:921–928.

Eipper, B. A., Mains, R. E., and Glembotski, C. C., 1983b, Identification in pituitary tissue of a peptide α-amidation activity that acts on glycine-extended peptides and requires molecular oxygen, copper, and ascorbic acid, *Proc. Natl. Acad. Sci. USA* **80**:5144–5148.

Eipper, B. A., Myers, A. C., and Mains, R. E., 1983c, Selective loss of α-melanotropin-amidating enzyme activity in primary cultures of rat intermediate pituitary cells, *J. Biol. Chem.* **258**:7292–7298.

Farquhar, M. G., and Palade, G. E., 1981, The Golgi apparatus (complex)—(1954–1981)—From artifact to center stage, *J. Cell Biol.* **91**:77s–103s.

Fricker, L. D., and Snyder, S. H., 1982, Enkephalin convertase: Purification and characterization of a specific enkephalin-synthesizing carboxypeptidase localized to adrenal chromaffin granules, *Proc. Natl. Acad. Sci. USA* **79**:3886–3890.

Fricker, L. D., and Snyder, S. H., 1983, Purification and characterization of enkephalin convertase, and enkephalin-synthesizing carboxypeptidase, *J. Biol. Chem.* **258**:10950–10955.

Fuller, P. J., Clements, J. A., Lolait, S. J., and Funder, J. W., 1984, Expression of the gene for arginine vasopressin in Brattleboro rats, *J. Hyperten.* **2**:305–307.

Fuller, P. J., Clements, J. A., and Funder, J. W., 1985, Localization of arginine-vasopressin-neurophysin II messenger ribonucleic acid in the hypothalamus of control and Brattleboro rats by hybridization histochemistry with a synthetic pentadecamer oligonucleotide probe, *Endocrinology* **116**:2366–2388.

Gainer, H., Sarne, Y., and Brownstein, M. J., 1977a, Neurophysin biosynthesis: Conversion of a putative precursor during axonal transport, *Science* **195**:1354–1356.

Gainer, H., Sarne, Y., and Brownstein, M. J., 1977b, Biosynthesis and axonal transport of rat neurohypophysial proteins and peptides, *J. Cell Biol.* **73**:366–381.

Gainer, H., Russell, J. T., and Loh, Y. P., 1984, An aminopeptidase activity in bovine pituitary secretory vesicles that cleaves the N-terminal arginine from β-lipotropin$_{60-65}$, *FEBS Lett.* **175**:135–139.

Gainer, H., Russell, J. T., and Loh, Y. P., 1985, The enzymology and intracellular organization of peptide precursor processing: The secretory vesicle hypothesis, *Neuroendocrinology* **40**:171–184.

Gillies, G., and Lowry, P., 1979, Corticotropin releasing factor may be modulated by vasopressin, *Nature* **278**:463–464.

Glembotski, C. C., 1981, Subcellular fractionation studies on the posttranslational processing of pro-adrenocorticotropic hormone/endorphin in rat intermediate pituitary, *J. Biol. Chem.* **256**:7433–7439.

Glembotski, C. C., 1982, Characterization of the peptide acetyltransferase activity in bovine and rat intermediate pituitaries responsible for the acetylation of β-endorphin and α-melanotropin, *J. Biol. Chem.* **257**:10501–10509.

Glembotski, C. C., Eipper, B. A., and Mains, R. E., 1984, Characterization of a peptide α-amidation activity from rat anterior pituitary, *J. Biol. Chem.* **259**:6385–6392.

Gordon-Weeks, R., Jones, P. M., and Robinson, I. E., 1983, Characterization of an intermediate in neurophysin biosynthesis in the guinea pig, *FEBS Lett.* **163**:324–328.

Gubler, U., Seeburg, P., Hoffman, B. J., Gage, L. P., and Udenfriend, S., 1982, Molecular cloning establishes pro-enkephalin as precursor of enkephalin-containing peptides, *Nature* **295**:206–208.

Haddad, A., Guaraldo, S. P. M., Pelletier, G., Brasiliero, I. L. G., and Marchi, F., 1980, Glycoprotein secretion in the hypothalamoneurohypophysial system of the rat, *Cell Tissue Res.* **209**:399–422.

Hampton, R. Y., and Holz, R. W., 1983, The effects of osmolality on the stability and function of cultured chromaffin cells and the role of osmotic forces in exocytosis, *J. Cell Biol.* **96**:1082–1088.

Holz, R. W., 1986, The role of osmotic forces in exocytosis from adrenal chromaffin cells, *Annu. Rev. Physiol.* **48**:175–189.

Ivell, R., and Richter, D., 1984, Structure and comparison of the oxytocin and vasopressin genes from rat, *Proc. Natl. Acad. Sci. USA* **81**:2006–2010.

Johnson, R. G., and Scarpa, A., 1976, Ion permeability of isolated chromaffin vesicles, *J. Gen. Physiol.* **68**:601–631.

Jones, M., Saermark, T., and Robinson, I. C., 1984, Conversion and release of an intermediate in vasopressin-neurophysin biosynthesis in the guinea pig, *J. Endocrinol.* **103**:347–354.

Kakidani, H., Furutani, Y., Takahashi, H., Noda, M., Morimoto, Y., Hirose, T., Asai, M., Inayama, S., Nakanashi, S., and Numa, S., 1982, Cloning and sequence analysis of cDNA for porcine β-endorphin/dynorphin precursor, *Nature* **298**:245–249.

Kemmler, W., Steiner, D. F., and Borg, J., 1973, Studies on the conversion of proinsulin to insulin, *J. Biol. Chem.* **248**:4544–4551.

Kent, C., and Williams, M. A., 1974, The nature of the hypothalamo-neurohypophysial neurosecretion in rat: A study by light- and electron microscope autoradiography, *J. Cell Biol.* **60**:554–570.

Knight, D. E., 1986, Calcium and exocytosis, *Ciba Found. Symp.* **122**:250–269.

Knight, D. E., and Baker, P. F., 1982, Calcium-dependence of catecholamine release from bovine adrenal medullary cells after exposure to intense electric fields, *Membr. Biol.* **68**:107–140.

Koch, G., and Richter, D. (eds.), 1980, *Biosynthesis, Modification, and Processing of Cellular and Viral Polyproteins,* Academic Press, New York.

Krieger-Brauer, H., and Gratzl, M., 1983, Effects of monovalent and divalent cations on Ca^{++} fluxes across chromaffin secretory membrane vesicles, *J. Neurochem.* **41**:1269–1276.

Land, H., Schutz, G., Schmale, H., and Richter, D., 1982, Nucleotide sequence of cloned cDNA encoding bovine arginine vasopressin-neurophysin II precursor, *Nature* **295**:299–303.

Land, H., Grez, M., Ruppert, S., Schmale, H., Rehbein, M., Richter, D., and Schutz, G., 1983, Deduced amino acid sequence from the bovine oxytocin-neurophysin 1 precursor cDNA, *Nature* **302**:342–344.

Loh, Y. P., 1986, Kinetic studies on the processing of β_h-lipoprotein by bovine pituitary intermediate lobe pro-opiomelanocortin converting enzyme, *J. Biol. Chem.* **261**:11949–11952.

Loh, Y. P., Brownstein, M. J., and Gainer, H., 1984, Proteolysis in neuropeptide processing and other neural functions, *Annu. Rev. Neurosci.* **7**:189–222.

Loh, Y. P., Parish, D. C., and Tuteja, R., 1985, Purification and characterization of a paired basic residue-specific pro-opiomelanocortin converting enzyme from bovine pituitary intermediate lobe secretory vesicles, *J. Biol. Chem.* **260**:7194–7205.

Majzoub, J. A., 1985, Vasopressin biosynthesis, in: *Vasopressin* (R. W. Schrier, ed.), Raven Press, New York, pp. 465–474.

Majzoub, J. A., Rich, A., Van Boom, J., and Habener, J., 1983, Vasopressin and oxytocin mRNA regulation in the rat assessed by hybridization with synthetic oligonucleotides, *J. Biol. Chem.* **258**:14061–14064.

Majzoub, J. A., Pappey, A., Burg, R., and Habener, J., 1984, Vasopressin gene is expressed at low levels in the hypothalamus of the Brattleboro rat, *Proc. Natl. Acad. Sci. USA* **81**:5296–5299.

Moore, H. P., Gumbiner, B., and Kelley, R. B., 1983a, Chloroquine diverts ACTH from a regulated to a constitutive pathway in AtT-20 cells, *Nature* **302**:434–436.

Moore, H. P., Walker, M., Lee, F., and Kelley, R. B., 1983b, Expressing a human proinsulin cDNA in a mouse ACTH secreting cell: Intracellular storage, processing, and secretion on stimulation, *Cell* **35**:531–538.

Morris, J. F., Nordmann, J. J., and Dyball, R. E. J., 1978, Structure–function correlation in mammalian neurosecretion, *Int. Rev. Exp. Pathol.* **18**:1–95.

Murthy, A. S. N., Mains, R. E., and Eipper, B. A., 1986, Purification and characterization of peptidylglycine-α-amidating monooxygenase from bovine neurointermediate pituitary, *J. Biol. Chem.* **261**:1815–1822.

Nakanishi, S., Inoue, A., Kita, T., Nakamura, M., Chang, A. C. Y., Cohen, S. N., and Numa, S., 1979, Nucleotide sequence of cloned cDNA for bovine corticotropin-β-lipotropin precursor, *Nature* **278**:423–427.

Noda, M., Teranishi, Y., Takahashi, H., Toyosato, M., Notake, M., Nakanishi, S., and Numa, S., 1982, Isolation and structural organization of the human preproenkephalin gene, *Nature* **297**:432–434.

Nojiri, H., Sato, M., and Urano, A., 1985, *In situ* hybridization of the vasopressin mRNA in the rat hypothalamus by use of a synthetic oligonucleotide probe, *Neurosci. Lett.* **58**:101–105.

Nordmann, J. J., and Morris, J. F., 1982, Neurosecretory granules, in: *Neurotransmitter Vesicles* (R. L. Klein, H. Lagercrantz, and H. Zimmerman, eds.), Academic Press, New York, pp. 41–64.

North, W. G., Mitchell, T., and North, G. M., 1983, Characteristics of a precursor to vasopressin-associated bovine neurophysin, *FEBS Lett.* **152**:29–34.

Parish, D. C., Tutega, R., Altstein, M., Gainer, H., and Loh, Y. P., 1986, Purification and characterization of a paired-basic residue specific prohormone converting enzyme from bovine pituitary neural lobe secretory vesicles, *J. Biol. Chem.* **261**:14392–14397.

Pazzoles, C. J., and Pollard, H. B., 1978, Evidence for stimulation of anion transport in ATP-evoked transmitter release from isolated secretory vesicles, *J. Biol. Chem.* **253**:3962–3969.

Pazzoles, C. J., Creutz, C. E., Ramu, A., and Pollard, H. B., 1980, Permeant anion activation of MgATPase activity in chromaffin granules, *J. Biol. Chem.* **255**:7863–7869.

Phillips, J. H., 1977, Passive ion permeability of the chromaffin granule membrane, *Biochem. J.* **186**:289–297.

Picaud, S., Marty, A., Trautmann, O. G.-W., and Henry, J.-P., 1984, Incorporation of chromaffin granule membranes into large-size vesicles suitable for patch-clamp recording, *FEBS Lett.* **178**:20–24.

Pollard, H. B., Pazoles, C. J., and Creutz, C. E., 1981, Mechanism of calcium action and release of vesicle-bound hormones during exocytosis, *Recent Prog. Horm. Res.* **37**:299–332.

Robinson, I. C., and Jones, P. M., 1983, An intermediate in the biosynthesis of vasopressin and neurophysin in the guinea pig posterior pituitary, *Neurosci. Lett.* **39**:273–278.

Ruppert, S. D., Scherer, G., and Schutz, G., 1984, Recent gene conversion involving bovine vasopressin and oxytocin precursor genes suggested by nucleotide sequence, *Nature* **308**:554–557.

Russell, J. T., 1981, Isolation of purified neurosecretory vesicles from bovine neurohypophyses using isoosmolar density gradients, *Anal. Biochem.* **113**:229–238.

Russell, J. T., 1984, ΔpH, H$^+$ diffusion potentials, and Mg^{++} ATPase in neurosecretory vesicles isolated from bovine neurohypophyses, *J. Biol. Chem.* **259**:9496–9507.

Russell, J. T., and Holz, R., 1981, Measurement of ΔpH and membrane potential in isolated neurosecretory vesicles from bovine neurohypophyses, *J. Biol. Chem.* **256**:5950–5953.

Sachs, H., Fawcett, P., Takabatake, Y., and Portanova, R., 1969, Biosynthesis and release of vasopressin and neurophysin, *Recent Prog. Horm. Res.* **25**:447–491.

Sausville, E., Carney, D., and Battey, J., 1985, The human vasopressin gene is linked to the oxytocin gene and is selectively expressed in a cultured lung cancer cell line, *J. Biol. Chem.* **260**:10236–10241.

Schmale, H., and Richter, D., 1984, Single base deletion in the vasopressin gene is the cause of diabetes insipidus in Brattleboro rats, *Nature* **308**:705–709.

Schmale, H., Heinsohn, S., and Richter, D., 1983, Structural organization of the rat gene for the arginine-vasopressin-neurophysin precursor, *EMBO J.* **2**:763–767.

Schmale, H., Ivell, R., Breindel, M., Darmer, D., and Richter, D., 1984, The mutant vasopressin gene from diabetes insipidus (Brattleboro) rats is transcribed but the message is not efficiently translated, *EMBO J.* **3**:3289–3293.

Schrier, R. W. (ed.), 1985, *Vasopressin,* Raven Press, New York.

Sherman, T. G., Akil, H., and Watson, S. J., 1985, Vasopressin mRNA expression: A Northern and *in situ* hybridization analysis, in: *Vasopressin* (R.W. Schrier, ed.), Raven Press, New York, pp. 475–484.

Silverman, A., and Zimmerman, E. A., 1983, Magnocellular neurosecretory system, *Annu. Rev. Neurosci.* **6**:357–380.

Sofroniew, M. V., 1985, Vasopressin, oxytocin and their related neurophysins, in: *Handbook of Chemical Neuroanatomy,* Vol. 4, Part I (A. Bjorklund and T. Hökfelt, eds.), Elsevier, Amsterdam, pp. 93–165.

Stanley, E. F., and Ehrenstein, G., 1985, A model for exocytosis based on the opening of calcium-activated potassium channels in vesicles, *Life Sci.* **37**:1985–1995.

Stanley, E. F., Ehrenstein, G., and Russell, J. T., 1986a, Evidence for calcium-activated potassium channels in vesicles of pituitary cells, *Biophys. J.* **49**:19a.

Steiner, D. F., Kemmier, W., Tager, H. S., and Peterson, J. D., 1974, Proteolytic processing in the biosynthesis of insulin and other proteins, *Fed. Proc.* **33**:2105–2115.

Swanson, L. W., and Sawchenko, P. E., 1983, Hypothalamic integration: Organization of the paraventricular and supraoptic nuclei, *Annu. Rev. Neurosci.* **6**:269–324.

Uhl, G. R., and Reppert, S. M., 1986, Suprachiasmatic nucleus vasopressin messenger RNA: Circadian variation in normal and Brattleboro rats, *Science* **232**:390–393.

Uhl, G. R., Zingg, H. H., and Habener, J. F., 1985, Vasopressin mRNA *in situ* hybridization: Localization and regulation studied with oligonucleotide cDNA probes in normal and Brattleboro rat hypothalamus, *Proc. Natl. Acad. Sci. USA* **82**:5555–5559.

Valtin, H., Stewart, J., and Sokol, H. W., 1974, Genetic control of the production of posterior pituitary principles, in: *Handbook of Physiology,* Section 7, Vol. IV, Part I (R. O. Gree and E. B. Astwood, eds.), American Physiological Society, Washington, D.C., pp. 131–171.

Whitnall, M. H., Gainer, H., Cox, B. M., and Molineaux, C. J., 1983, Dynorphin-A-(1-8) is contained within vasopressin neurosecretory vesicles in rat pituitary, *Science* **222**:1137–1139.

Whitnall, M. H., Mezey, E., and Gainer, H., 1985, Co-localization of corticotropin releasing factor and vasopressin in median eminence neurosecretory vesicles, *Nature* **317:**248–250.

Wolfson, B., Manning, R. W., Davis, L. G., Arentzen, R., and Baldino, F., Jr., 1985, Co-localization of corticotropin releasing factor and vasopressin mRNA in neurons after adrenalectomy, *Nature* **315:**59–61.

Zimmerman, M., Mumford, R. A., and Steiner, D. F., 1980, Precursor processing in the biosynthesis of proteins, *Ann. N.Y. Acad. Sci.* **343:**1–449.

35

Autoradiographic Localization of Brain Peptide Receptors at the Electron Microscopic Level

A. Beaudet, E. Hamel, K. Leonard, M. Vial, E. Moyse, P. Kitabgi, J. P. Vincent, and W. Rostène

1. Introduction

Neurotransmitters and related drugs exert their biochemical, electrophysiological, and, ultimately, behavioral effects by acting upon specific receptor molecules embedded in neuronal and, in some cases, perhaps also glial plasma membranes. This interaction involves: (1) recognition of a specific binding site on the surface of the receptor and (2) translation of the recognition information into a response signal. Pioneering studies by Clark (1933) demonstrated that the binding of drugs (ligands) to receptors was reversible, obeyed the law of mass action, and occurred at very low concentrations of ligand. Considerable progress in our understanding of receptor mechanisms was later to emerge from the development of sensitive methods for measuring the receptor-specific binding of radiolabeled ligand probes (Snyder and Bennett, 1976). Not only did the availability of such methods greatly facilitate the biophysical, pharmacological, and molecular characterization of receptors for neurotransmitters, but it also made possible their localization *in situ*, using autoradiographic techniques.

The autoradiographic visualization of neurotransmitter receptors involves: (1) selective labeling of the receptor of interest with a radioligand (agonist or antagonist) and (2) detection of the bound ligand molecules in tissue sections, by putting the latter in contact with a photographic emulsion. Early studies in the CNS relied upon *in vivo* administration of radiolabeled drugs and subsequent autoradiographic processing of unfixed, frozen brain sections according to techniques developed for the localization of diffusible substances (Kuhar and Yamamura, 1974; Pert *et al.*, 1976; Schubert *et al.*, 1975). An *in vitro* approach, conceptually similar to that used on brain homogenates, was introduced at approximately the same time, to examine the distribution of α-bungarotoxin (Polz-Tejera *et al.*, 1975) and of muscarinic (Rotter *et al.*, 1977) binding sites in the CNS. This method, which was later perfected by Young and Kuhar (1979a) and Herkenham and

A. Beaudet, E. Hamel, K. Leonard, and E. Moyse • Montreal Neurological Institute, McGill University, Montreal, Quebec H3A 2B4, Canada. *M. Vial and W. Rostène* • INSERM U-55, Hôpital St. Antoine, 75012 Paris, France. *P. Kitabgi and J. P. Vincent* • Centre de Biochimie du CNRS, Université de Nice, 06034 Nice Cedex, France.

Pert (1982), is based on the incubation of either unfixed or lightly prefixed frozen sections in the presence of the radioligand, followed by autoradiographic processing of the labeled sections by apposition of nuclear emulsion-precoated coverslips (Young and Kuhar, 1979a) or tritium-sensitive film (Palacios *et al.*, 1981), or by using conventional dipping techniques, after securing the bound ligand molecules in tissue by appropriate fixation (Herkenham and Pert, 1982; Hamel and Beaudet, 1984a).

The easy accessibility and wide applicability of these methodologies have given tremendous impetus to research in the field and generated a wealth of information on the regional distribution of a variety of neurotransmitter receptor subtypes in the brain. They have also led to the development of high-resolution autoradiographic procedures applicable to the visualization of those sites at the electron microscopic level. Autoradiographic data have thus been obtained on the fine structural localization of muscarinic (Kuhar *et al.*, 1981), putative nicotinic (Hunt and Schmidt, 1978; Arimatsu *et al.*, 1978; Miller *et al.*, 1987), and benzodiazepine (Mohler *et al.*, 1981) receptors, labeled *in vivo* following administration of irreversible ligands or photoaffinity probes. The availability of specific antibodies later made it possible to localize by electron microscopic immunocytochemistry glycine receptors in the spinal cord (Triller *et al.*, 1985) and the cochlear nucleus of the rat (Altschuler *et al.*, 1986), benzodiazepine–GABA receptor complexes in the substantia nigra and globus pallidus of the rat (Richards *et al.*, 1987), and β-adrenergic receptors in the hippocampus of the frog and the cerebellum of the rat (Strader *et al.*, 1983). Until very recently, however, there was no information available concerning the ultrastructural localization of receptors for what has come to be recognized as a major group of signaling molecules in the brain, the neuropeptides. Yet, precise knowledge of the cellular and subcellular distribution of these sites is essential to a proper understanding of the mechanisms of action of neuropeptides and their analogues in the CNS.

In 1979, we proposed the use of FK 33-824 (FK), a synthetic Met-enkephalin analogue (Roemer *et al.*, 1977), for electron microscopic autoradiographic visualization of opioid binding sites in the CNS (Beaudet *et al.*, 1979). This compound offered the triple advantage of (1) being resistant to metabolic degradation (Roemer *et al.*, 1977); (2) binding selectively and with high affinity to, and dissociating at a slow rate form, mu opioid receptors (Chang *et al.*, 1979; Trémeau *et al.*, 1981; Moyse *et al.*, 1986); and (3) being endowed on its tyrosine residue with a free primary amino group through which it could be covalently cross-linked to tissue proteins by divalent aldehydes (Hamel and Beaudet, 1984a). Using monoiodinated FK, we later developed an *in vitro* labeling approach (Hamel and Beaudet, 1984a), which we applied to the analysis of the fine structural distribution of mu opioid receptors in rat neostriatum (Hamel and Beaudet, 1984b, 1987). In the present chapter, these results are reviewed and compared to more recent data on the autoradiographic distribution of neurotensin receptors in rat substantia nigra (Moyse *et al.*, 1985; Beaudet *et al.*, 1987). Neurotensin receptors were labeled by the same *in vitro* approach, using monoiodo ([^{125}I]-Tyr$_3$) neurotensin, a highly selective, "cross-linkable" compound as radioligand (Sadoul *et al.*, 1984). From this comparison, a few conclusions are drawn on what might constitute some of the distributional features of neuropeptide receptors in the CNS.

2. Methodology

2.1. Principles of the Technique

The high-resolution autoradiographic technique used in the present studies relies on the incubation of lightly prefixed brain slices with low concentrations of radioactive ligand in the absence (total binding), or in the presence (nonspecific binding), of an excess of nonradioactive competitor. At the end of incubation, the bound radioligand molecules are cross-linked to tissue proteins through the use of a divalent fixative agent. The slices are subsequently postfixed, dehydrated, and flat-embedded in plastic. Semithin and thin sections are then cut from the surface of each slice, and respectively processed for light and electron microscopic autoradiography according to conventional dipping techniques.

2.2. Experimental Procedures

2.2.1. Preparation of Brain Slices

The brains were first prefixed by intraaortic arch perfusion of an ice-cold mixture of 0.75% paraformaldehyde, 0.1% glutaraldehyde, and 1% tannic acid in 0.1 M PO_4 buffer. This prefixation procedure was shown to be without effect on the binding capacity of either [^{125}I]-FK (Hamel and Beaudet, 1984a) or [^{125}I]neurotensin (Dana et al., 1985). It did, however, greatly facilitate tissue sectioning, and proved essential for subsequent preservation of tissue morphology. Immediately after perfusion, the brains were removed from the skull and the region of interest blocked on ice and mounted on a vibratome stage. Slices, 50–75 μm thick, were cut in ice-cold 0.1 M PO_4 buffer and immediately transferred to the incubation medium.

2.2.2. Radiolabeling Brain Slices

For the labeling of mu opioid receptors, slices from the neostriatum were incubated with 1 nM [^{125}I]-FK (150 Ci/mmole) in 0.05 M Tris-HCl (pH 7.4) containing 0.25 M sucrose for 30 min at room temperature. Blanks were run through the same incubation medium, after adding a thousandfold excess of nonradioactive FK or naloxone.

For the labeling of neurotensin receptors, slices from the midbrain tegmentum were incubated with 0.1 nM ([^{125}I]-Tyr$_3$)neurotensin (2000 Ci/mmole) in 0.05 M Tris-HCl (pH 7.4) containing 0.25 M sucrose, 0.005 M $MgCl_2$, 0.2% bovine serum albumin, and 2×10^{-5} M bacitracin for 60 min at 4°C. For assessment of nonspecific binding, sections were incubated with [^{125}I]neurotensin as above, but in the presence of 500 nM nonradioactive neurotensin.

All incubations were terminated by transferring the slices through serial 5-min buffer rinses at 4°C. FK and neurotensin were iodinated using chloramine-T and lactoperoxidase, respectively, and purified by HPLC or on ion-exchange columns as previously described (Miller et al., 1978; Seidah et al., 1980; Sadoul et al., 1984).

2.2.3. Histological and Autoradiographic Processing

After washing, the slices were fixed by immersion in a solution of 4% glutaraldehyde in 0.05 M PO_4 buffer at 4°C. This postfixation step served a double purpose: (1) to cross-link ligand molecules onto their binding sites and (2) to ensure fine structural preservation of the tissue. Concentrations of glutaraldehyde ranging between 3.5 and 6% were found to provide equally good retention of the bound radioligand (Hamel and Beaudet, 1984a; Moyse et al., 1987). Concentrations of 3.5–4%, however, yielded the best morphological results (Hamel and Beaudet, 1984a). The fixation was carried out at 4°C to minimize dissociation of the bound molecules, and thereby prevent cross-linking at nonreceptor sites.

After fixation, alternate slices were mounted onto gelatin-coated glass slides and autoradiographed by apposition to tritium-sensitive film, both to monitor the outcome of the binding experiment and to assess the overall distribution of the bound molecules. These film autoradiographs were exposed for 4 days inside X-ray cassettes and developed with Kodak X-ray film developer (5 min at 13°C).

The remaining slices were transferred to a 2% OsO_4 PO_4-buffered solution containing 7% dextrose, dehydrated in graded ethanols, and flat-embedded in Epon between two plastic coverslips. They were then polymerized, trimmed, and blocked for light and electron microscopic autoradiographic processing. The entire postfixation/dehydration sequence was shown to ensure regionally proportional retention of 50–60% of bound [^{125}I]-FK in slices of the neostriatum (Hamel and Beaudet, 1984a) and of approximately 70% of bound [^{125}I]neurotensin in sections of the midbrain tegmentum (Moyse *et al.*, 1987).

For light microscopy, semithin sections (1 μm thick) were cut from the surface of each block, coated by dipping in Kodak NTB-2 emulsion, and developed 6 weeks later with D-19 (4 min at 17°C). For electron microscopy, thin sections (80 nm thick) were cut from the same blocks, autoradiographed with Ilford L-4 emulsion, and developed in D-19 (1 min at 20°C) after 8 to 12 weeks of exposure. (For details on these autoradiographic procedures, see Descarries and Beaudet, 1983.)

2.3. Analysis of Electron Microscopic Autoradiographs

In electron microscopic autoradiographs, bound radioligand molecules are detected in the form of stray silver grains scattered over the neuropil. Because of the relatively limited resolution of the autoradiographic method, statistical analysis of silver grain distribution is essential to accurately assess the location of radioactive sources within the tissue. We have resorted to a combination of two methods to analyze the distribution of labeled mu opioid receptors (Hamel and Beaudet, 1984b) and neurotensin binding sites (Beaudet *et al.*, 1987; Dana *et al.*, 1987) in the CNS. In a first step, each grain was scored by probability circle (Williams, 1969). In a second step, grains categorized as "shared" (see below) in the first analysis were subjected to a "line source" analysis, comparable to that previously used to resolve the distribution of [^{125}I]α-bungarotoxin binding sites at the neuromuscular junction (Porter *et al.*, 1973).

For probability circle analysis, the material was systematically scanned and every labeled site photographed at a magnification of 10,000. Fifty percent probability circles (diameter: 3.4 × half distance; see Blackett and Parry, 1977), drawn on a transparent overlay, were centered over each grain and the structure (exclusive grains) or combination of structures (shared grains) included within the circle were recorded and tabulated. The distribution of specific binding was determined by subtracting nonspecific from total binding as follows. First, the number of silver grains recorded in sections incubated in the presence of competitive drug (nonspecific binding) was proportionally adjusted within each tissue compartment according to nonspecific over total binding ratios (as determined by measuring the radioactivity content of the whole slice prior to embedding). The resulting figures were then subtracted from the number of grains recorded within the corresponding compartments in sections incubated with the radioactive ligand alone (total binding). Finally, the resulting distribution (specific binding) was normalized to one hundred.

To assess the relative enrichment of the different labeled compartments, the distribution of "specific" grains was subsequently compared to that of a population of randomly distributed, "hypothetical" grains. These hypothetical grains were generated by superimposing over each micrograph a regular array of resolution circles of the same diameter and by recording and tabulating the structures or combination of structures included therein.

To reduce the number of compartments in the analysis, two operations were performed. The first consisted in regrouping in a single category (miscellaneous) all grains from compartments originally containing less than 1% of the total. The second consisted in redistributing grains overlying more than two structures within compartments that contained only two, according to the labeling frequency of each pair of structures seen within the circle.

For line source analysis, the distance separating the center of each grain from the closest plasma membrane was measured and expressed in half distance units. A frequency distribution histogram was then generated by plotting the number of silver grains as a function of their distance from the closest plasma membrane. This frequency distribution was subsequently compared to that of silver grains originating from an ^{125}I line source (Salpeter *et al.*, 1978).

3. Distribution of Mu Opioid Receptors in the Neostriatum

3.1. Light Microscopy

The topographic distribution of labeled [^{125}I]-FK binding sites, as revealed by film auto-radiographs of 50- to 75-μm-thick slices from rat neostriatum incubated with the radioactive ligand alone, was characterized by the presence of multiple dense labeling foci ("patches"), prominent against a moderately labeled matrix (Fig. 1'). This distribution was similar to that previously observed by us (Hamel and Beaudet, 1984a; Moyse et al., 1986; Fig. 1) and others (Goodman et al., 1980; McLean et al., 1986) in 20-μm-thick frozen sections of rat brain incubated with [^{125}I]-FK. It also conformed with earlier descriptions of the distribution of mu opioid receptors in the neostriatum (for references, see Hamel and Beaudet, 1987), as expected from the reported selectivity of [^{125}I]-FK for this class of binding sites (Miller et al., 1978; Moyse et al., 1986).

Approximately 80% of total [^{125}I]-FK labeling was displaceable with 1 μM nonradioactive FK or naloxone. The remaining 20% (nonspecific binding) appeared fairly homogeneously distributed throughout the section.

In semithin (1 μm thick) sections taken from the surface of striatal slices incubated with [^{125}I]-FK alone (total binding), the majority of silver grains were detected over the neuropil (Fig. 2). A small amount occurred over myelinated fascicles, neuronal perikarya, or blood vessels (for details, see Hamel and Beaudet, 1987). Comparable distributions prevailed within and outside patches, except over neuronal perikarya, which contained a higher proportion of grains within than outside patches. In fact, after subtraction of nonspecific binding, nerve cell bodies were found to be on average six times more heavily labeled in the patches than in the matrix. Many of the grains associated with nerve cell bodies appeared to directly overlie the neuronal plasma membrane (Fig. 2). Others, however, were clearly inside the perikaryon. These intracellular binding sites presumably correspond to sites of synthesis, transport, and/or internalization of the receptors. The clear-cut predominance of these receptors within patches would suggest that opioceptive neurons are mainly concentrated within the so-called "striosomal" compartments of the neostriatum.

3.2. Electron Microscopy

In electron microscopic autoradiographs, [^{125}I]-FK-labeled binding sites are detected in the form of individual silver grains scattered over both neuropil and perikarya. Probability circle analysis revealed statistically significant differences (χ^2 test; $p < 0.0005$) between the distribution of these grains in sections incubated with [^{125}I]-FK alone (total binding) and in sections incubated with a thousandfold concentration of nonradioactive FK or naloxone (nonspecific binding). These two distributions were in turn significantly different from that of a random population of hypo-thetical grains ($p < 0.0005$).

In keeping with light microscopic observations, silver grains corresponding to specific binding sites predominated over the neuropil. Approximately 13% were found over neuronal perikarya, where they overlaid both the nucleus and the perikaryon. Little further information could be obtained on the precise subcellular repartition of these intraperikaryal sites, the number of grains in each cellular compartment being too low to permit adequate statistical analysis.

The vast majority of grains detected over the neuropil overlaid two neuronal profiles or more ("shared" grains). It was found by line source analysis that most if not all of these shared grains originated from radioactive sources associated with the plasma membrane(s) of these contiguous elements (see Hamel and Beaudet, 1987). However, because of limitations inherent to the autoradiographic technique, it was not possible to determine to which one of the apposed plasma membranes these radioactive sources were actually linked. Neither was it possible to ascribe those

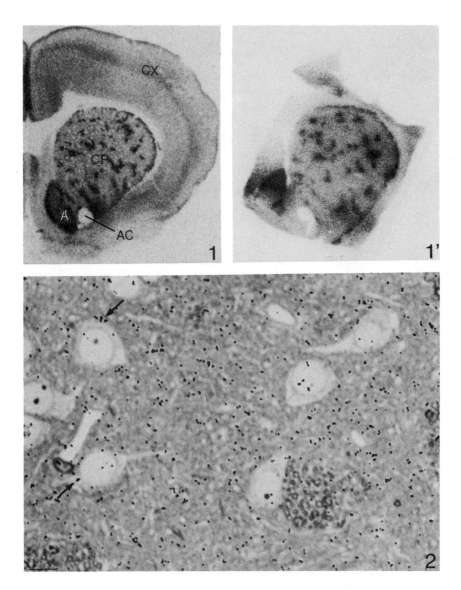

Figures 1, 1'. Film autoradiographs of 20-μm-thick cryostat- (Fig. 1) and 75-μm-thick vibratome-cut (Fig. 1')
sections from rat neostriatum incubated with the monoiodinated Met-enkephalin analogue [^{125}I]-FK 33-824. The
section in Fig. 1' was fixed with glutaraldehyde and dehydrated in graded ethanols at the end of the incubation
period. Both cryostat- and vibratome-cut sections exhibit, within the caudate putamen (CP), the typical mu opioid
mosaic labeling pattern. Note the intense labeling in the nucleus accumbens (A) and in cortical layer IV (CX), as
well as the sparing of the anterior commissure (AC).

Figure 2. Light microscopic autoradiograph of a 1-μm-thick Epon-embedded section cut from the surface of a
striatal slice incubated with [^{125}I]-FK. Silver grains are scattered throughout the neuropil. A few appear to be
associated with perikaryal plasma membranes (arrows). Bar = 10 μm.

sources to cell surface rather than to internal membrane components. Nonetheless, the distribution of shared grains could be assumed to accurately reflect the distribution of membrane-bound [125I]-FK binding sites and, by way of consequence, the real over hypothetical grain ratio taken as an index of the relative enrichment of the different membrane compartments.

As seen in Table I, the majority of shared grains corresponding to specifically bound [125I]-FK molecules were associated with axodendritic interfaces. In most instances, such interfaces were characterized by a close apposition of axonal and dendritic plasma membranes, without any apparent membrane thickening at the point of contact (Figs. 3 and 6). In a few cases (7% of the total number of grains), labeled contacts exhibited asymmetrical (Fig. 4), or symmetrical (Fig. 5), synaptic specializations.

A few dendritic profiles were labeled at more than one contact point along their plasma membranes. This observation suggests that a proportion of opioid binding sites associated with axodendritic interfaces are actually on the dendritic rather than on the axonal plasma membrane. The occurrence of dendritic receptors would conform to the demonstration of opioceptive nerve cell bodies within the neostriatum. It would also be in keeping with the drop in mu opioid binding observed in the neostriatum following local injections of the cytotoxic drug, kainic acid (Antkiewicz-Michaluk et al., 1984).

Axosomatic interfaces showed the same enrichment in labeled opioid receptors as axo-dendritic ones, even though they accounted for a considerably smaller proportion of shared grains (Table I). This suggests that mu opioid receptors synthesized in neurons of the neostriatum are incorporated into somatic as well as dendritic plasma membranes. Labeled axosomatic contacts, as their axodendritic counterparts, only rarely exhibited synaptic differentiations.

An important proportion of shared grains were associated with axoaxonic appositions (Table I). Included within this category were appositions involving either two axon terminals or one axon terminal and one or more unmyelinated axonal process. Synaptic densities were never observed at the site of labeling, but a streaming of synaptic vesicles toward the apposed membranes was apparent in some of the terminals involved. The enrichment of axoaxonic interfaces in mu opioid receptors supports the view that endogenous opioids may act presynaptically in the neostriatum (for review see Cuello, 1983). Biochemical and autoradiographic evidence derived from lesion experiments suggest that these presynaptic effects may be exerted on dopaminergic axons origi-nating from the substantia nigra (Bowen et al., 1982; Gardner et al., 1980; Murrin et al., 1980; Pollard et al., 1978; Reisine et al., 1979), presumptive glutamate axons originating from the cerebral cortex (Childers et al., 1978), serotonin axons originating from the raphe nuclei (Parenti et al., 1983), or local circuit axons (Antkiewicz-Michaluk et al., 1984; Childers et al., 1978; Murrin et al., 1980; Pollard et al., 1978).

Table I. Distribution of "Shared" Grains[a] in Autoradiographs from Sections of Rat Neostriatum Incubated with [125I]-FK

Included within probability circle[b]	Real grains[c] (specific binding)	Hypothetical grains[d]	Real/hypothetical
Axon[e]/dendrite			
Junctional	7.1 ± 0.5	3.1	2.3
Nonjunctional	45.8 ± 3.7	13.0	3.5
Axon/axon	17.6 ± 1.3	9.2	1.9
Axon/soma	3.2 ± 1.1	1.0	3.2
Dendrite/dendrite	1.9 ± 0.5	6.1	0.3

[a]Expressed as percent of total.
[b]Categories containing more than 1% of total number of grains.
[c]2460 grains counted.
[d]10,039 grains counted.
[e]Includes axon terminals and unmyelinated axons.

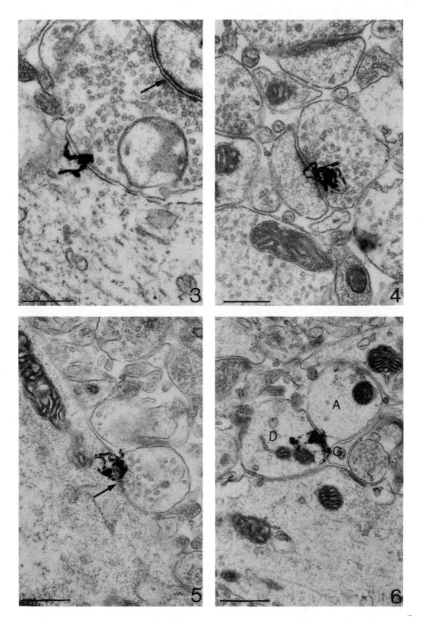

Figures 3–6. Electron microscopic autoradiographs from sections incubated with 1 nM [^{125}I]-FK: Labeled axodendritic interfaces. Bars = 0.5 μm.

Figure 3. A silver grain overlies the juxtaposed plasma membranes of a longitudinally sectioned dendrite and of a large axon terminal filled with small round electronlucent synaptic vesicles. The axon terminal is in synaptic contact with a dendritic spine (arrow) but shows no synaptic density at the site of labeling.

Figure 4. This silver grain is associated with an asymmetrical synaptic junction established on a cross-sectioned dendritic spine.

Figure 5. Several vesicle-filled axon terminals abut a large, spinous dendrite. The label is visible over a symmetrical contact established by one of these terminals on the shaft of the dendrite (arrow).

Figure 6. The probability circle associated with this silver grain includes an axon terminal (A) containing a sparse contingent of synaptic vesicles, a cross-sectioned dendritic branch (D), and a thin glial leaflet (G). No junctional specialization is present at the site of labeling.

4. Distribution of Neurotensin Receptors in the Substantia Nigra

4.1. Light Microscopy

In film autoradiographs from slices of rat midbrain tegmentum incubated with [125I]neuro-tensin, high concentrations of radioactivity were apparent throughout the ventral tegmental area and pars compacta of the substantia nigra (Fig. 7'). This labeling pattern conformed to that previously observed in 30-μm-thick frozen sections from the same region incubated with [125I]neurotensin (Fig. 7; also see Moyse et al., 1987) or [3H]neurotensin (Young and Kuhar, 1979b, 1981; Uhl, 1982; Quirion et al., 1982). Slices incubated in the presence of an excess of nonradioactive neurotensin (to assess nonspecific binding) contained 70–85% less radioactivity than the ones incubated with [125I]neurotensin alone, and exhibited an autoradiographic labeling that appeared fairly homogeneous at that level of resolution.

In light microscopic autoradiographs of 1-μm-thick sections taken from the substantia nigra in slices incubated with [125I]neurotensin, most of the label was detected over the neuropil. A few silver grains overlaid myelinated axons or were associated with endothelial cells and pericytes surrounding intraparenchymal capillaries. Approximately 11% of the grains were found over neuronal perikarya. Some of these overlaid the cytoplasm or nucleus of the cells, but others were clearly aligned along their plasma membrane, sometimes extending over proximal dendrites (Fig. 8). This observation suggests that not only may neurotensin receptors be synthesized in pars compacta neurons, but that they are also likely to be inserted into the latter's perikaryal plasma membrane. In light of recent results from combined autoradiographic and immunohistochemical investigations (Szigethy et al., 1986), it would appear that most if not all of these putative "neurotensinoceptive" neurons are dopaminergic. This interpretation is also in keeping with the substantial decrease in neurotensin binding observed in the substantia nigra after local injection of the neurotoxin 6-hydroxydopamine (Palacios and Kuhar, 1981; for review, see Quirion, 1983).

In semithin sections from brain slices incubated in the presence of an excess of nonradioac-tive neurotensin, silver grains were sparse except over capillary walls and pericytes which appeared as selectively and strongly labeled as in sections incubated with [125I]neurotensin alone. This finding indicates that most if not all of the neurotensin binding associated with endothelial cells and pericytes corresponds to nonspecific binding.

4.2. Electron Microscopy

Probability circle analysis of electron microscopic autoradiographs indicated that the dis-tribution of silver grains in sections incubated with [125I]neurotensin alone (total binding) was significantly different (χ^2 test; $p < 0.0001$) from that in sections incubated with an excess of nonradioactive neurotensin (nonspecific binding). Both of these distributions were in turn signifi-cantly different from that of randomly generated hypothetical grains. In conformity with light microscopic observations, most of the silver grains corresponding to specifically bound neuroten-sin molecules were associated with elements of the neuropil. Approximately 10% overlaid nerve cell bodies, including those overlapping perikaryal plasma membranes.

As in the case of opioid labeling in the striatum, most of neuropil-bound specific grains were shared, i.e., overlaid more than one cellular profile. Analysis of this population of shared grains by the line source method indicated that it originated from membrane-bound radioactive sources. The distribution of these shared grains could therefore be surmised to accurately reflect the relative repartition of membrane-bound neurotensin receptors.

As seen in Table II, the majority of shared grains corresponding to specifically bound [125I]-neurotensin molecules was associated with axodendritic appositions. Most of these appositions were devoid of junctional specialization (Fig. 9), but a few (2% of labeled sites) exhibited well-differentiated, asymmetrical synaptic densities (Fig. 10).

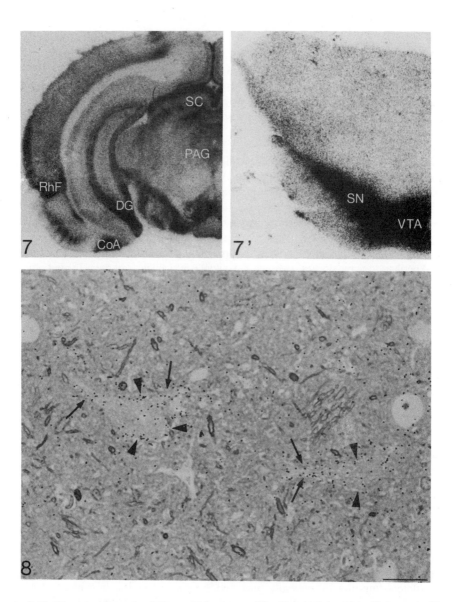

Figures 7, 7'. Film autoradiographs of 20-μm-thick cryostat- (Fig. 7) and 75-μm-thick vibratome-cut (Fig. 7')
sections from rat midbrain tegmentum incubated with [^{125}I]neurotensin. In both cases, an intense labeling is
apparent over the substantia nigra, pars compacta (SN), and the ventral tegmental area (VTA). Also note, in Fig. 7,
the dense labeling within the superior colliculus (SC), periaqueductal gray (PAG), ventral dentate gyrus (DG),
posterior cortical nucleus of the amygdala (CoA), and rhinal fissure (RhF).

Figure 8. Light microscopic autoradiograph of a 1-μm-thick, Epon-embedded section of the substantia nigra taken
from the surface of a tegmental slice incubated with [^{125}I]neurotensin. Two perikaryal profiles are outlined by
discrete silver grain alignments (arrowheads). Note that silver grains also appear to be associated with the plasma
membrane of proximal dendrites (arrows). Bar = 30 μm.

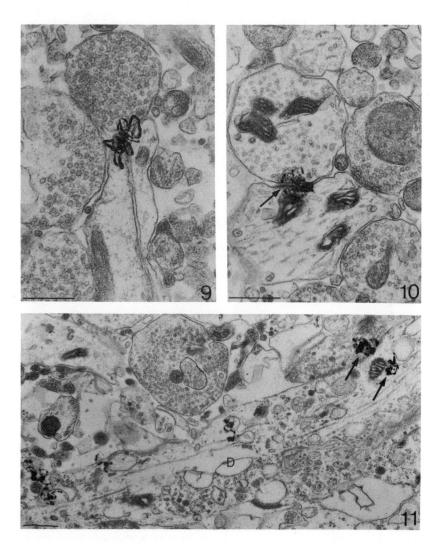

Figures 9–11. Electron microscopic autoradiographs from sections of the substantia nigra incubated with [^{125}I]neurotensin.

Figure 9. This silver grain is associated with two axon terminals, both filled with clear, round agranular synaptic vesicles, and abutting a longitudinally sectioned dendritic branch. Neither of these two boutons exhibits a membrane differentiation suggestive of synaptic specialization. Bar = 0.5 μm.

Figure 10. This silver grain directly overlies an asymmetrical synapse (arrow) established on a dendritic branch by an axon terminal containing a sparse population of synaptic vesicles. Bar = 0.5 μm.

Figure 11. This large proximal dendrite (D) is labeled at four different loci along its plasma membrane. Note that only two of the silver grains (arrows) are located opposite an abutting axon terminal. Bar = 0.75 μm.

Not all of the silver grains associated with dendritic membranes, however, were found opposite axon terminals. This was most apparent in certain favorable cross-sectional planes in which silver grains appeared haphazardly distributed along the plasma membrane of longitudinally cut dendrites (Fig. 11). Dendrodendritic, dendrosomatic, and dendroglial compartments, even though comprising a smaller proportion of the total number of grains, indeed showed a

Table II. Distribution of "Shared" Grains[a] in Autoradiograph from Sections of Rat Substantia Nigra Incubated with [[125I]-NT

Included within probability circle[b]	Real grains[c] (specific binding)	Hypothetical grains[d]	Real/hypothetical
Axon[e]/dendrite			
Junctional	1.8 ± 0.4	1.0 ± 0.5	1.8
Nonjunctional	18.7 ± 3.3	7.6 ± 0.5	2.5
Axon/axon	8.5 ± 0.6	12.2 ± 0.5	0.7
Axon/soma	2.0 ± 0.8	0.3 ± 0.2	6.7
Axon/glia	5.1 ± 0.6	5.5 ± 0.8	0.9
Dendrite/dendrite	1.9 ± 0.6	0.3 ± 0.2	6.3
Dendrite/soma	1.0 ± 0.5	0.1 ± 0.0	10.0
Dendrite/glia	2.7 ± 0.6	1.9 ± 0.4	1.4

[a]Expressed as percent of total.
[b]Categories containing more than 1% of total number of grains.
[c]2232 grains counted.
[d]9923 grains counted.
[e]Includes axon terminals and unmyelinated axons.

labeling index that was as high as, if not higher than, axodendritic interfaces when compared to uniformly distributed hypothetical grains (Table II). Two conclusions may be drawn from these observations: (1) silver grains associated with neuronal interfaces involving dendritic profiles are more likely to arise from the membrane of the dendrite itself than from the membrane of adjoining structures; (2) neurotensin receptors associated with dendritic membranes do not appear to be concentrated opposite abutting axon terminals, but rather to be dispersed throughout the membrane surface.

The high labeling indexes of compartments involving perikaryal plasma membranes (i.e., axosomatic, dendrosomatic, and gliosomatic interfaces; Table II) indicate that neurotensin receptors are present on the membrane of the perikaryon as well as on that of the dendrites of pars compacta neurons. As much could be surmised from the observation of pericellular grain arrangements at the light microscopic level. Electron microscopic data further suggest, however, that as in the case of dendritic membranes, labeled receptors are not concentrated opposite abutting axon terminals.

Finally, approximately 8.5% of specific grains were associated with axoaxonic interfaces within the substantia nigra (Table II). These axoaxonic appositions involved either two axon terminals or an axon terminal and one or several cross-sectioned unmyelinated axonal processes. As a whole, axoaxonic interfaces were not as enriched as interfaces that involved dendritic or somatic membranes, suggesting that neurotensin's primary site of action in the substantia nigra is not presynaptic.

5. Junctional versus Extrajunctional Neuropeptide Receptors: Functional Significance

A major distributional feature of both mu opioid and neurotensin receptors in the rat neostriatum and substantia nigra is their infrequent association with synaptic junctions. The proportion of labeled synaptic densities was for each of these markedly lower than that reported for muscarinic (Kuhar et al., 1981), putative nicotinic (Arimatsu et al., 1978; Hunt and Schmidt, 1978; Lentz and Chester, 1977; Miller et al., 1987), GABAergic (Mohler et al., 1981; Richards et al., 1987), or glycinergic (Triller et al., 1985; Altschuler et al., 1986) receptors in the CNS.

The low incidence of synaptic labeling observed with monoiodinated neuropeptides is unlikely to be due to poor diffusion of iodine into the synaptic cleft, since considerably larger molecules, such as horseradish peroxidase-conjugated antibodies, have been shown to enter the cleft and to label postsynaptic membranes (Jacob and Berg, 1983). It could be argued that the *in vitro* incubation conditions used in the present study are deleterious to morphological preservation of synaptic differentiations. If this were the case, however, one would expect synaptic junctions that are not affected by the incubation to show a higher labeling index than nonsynaptic compartments. One would also expect a higher proportion of silver grains to be associated with axodendritic and axosomatic interfaces, which are the most likely to be endowed with synaptic specializations. Admittedly, since agonists are being used as radioligands, the possibility that synaptic binding sites correspond to low-affinity states of the receptor, and may therefore not be effectively labeled, cannot be excluded. Neither can we be certain that the distribution of the labeled binding sites would be identical if the labeling had been carried out *in vivo* instead of *in vitro*. Opioid receptors have been shown to form clusters in the presence of enkephalins on the surface of neuroblastoma cells *in vivo* (Hazum *et al.*, 1980). The high-affinity conformational state of these receptors has also been claimed to be different under ionic conditions prevailing *in vivo* (Demoliou-Mason and Barnard, 1986). Still, the similarity between topographic distributions of opioid binding sites labeled *in vivo* and *in vitro* in rat brain (Pert *et al.*, 1976; Atweh and Kuhar, 1977; Herkenham and Pert, 1982; McLean *et al.*, 1986) suggests that, at least in the case of opioid receptors, the distribution observed *in vitro* provides an accurate reflection of that prevailing *in vivo*. The excellent correlation between the pharmacological effects of opioid and neurotensin and their *in vivo* (Hollt and Herz, 1978) or *in vitro* (Herkenham, 1984; Kitabgi *et al.*, 1980) binding potencies in the CNS further suggests that the specific binding sites labeled in the present study correspond to functional receptors. The fact that these binding sites are predominantly extrajunctional does not preclude such an interpretation, since it has long been recognized that certain receptor-mediated effects can be exerted in the absence of junctional specialization. Presynaptic inhibition is a good case in point, axoaxonic synapses being only infrequently encountered in the CNS.

The question then arises as to the site of release of endogenous ligands acting upon the labeled (junctional as well as extrajunctional) receptors. In the case of mu-opioid binding sites, their frequent occurrence opposite (or onto) axon terminals would suggest that the endogenous ligand(s) is released by the labeled terminals themselves. Axon terminals containing derivatives of proenkephalin and prodynorphin, which could play the role of endogenous ligands at the mu receptor, have both been immunohistochemically demonstrated in rat neostriatum (for review, see Hamel and Beaudet, 1987). There seems to be little correspondence, however, between the distribution of these opioid peptides and that of mu-opioid binding sites labeled in the neostriatum (Lewis *et al.*, 1985; Herkenham and McLean, 1986). It is therefore possible that as previously postulated for monoamines (Descarries *et al.*, 1975; Beaudet and Descarries, 1978) and peptides (Jan and Jan, 1983; Cuello, 1983; for review, see Schmidt, 1984) in the CNS, endogenous opioids are actually released at a distance from their receptor sites and must diffuse in the extracellular space to reach their receptive target.

Such a paracrine mode of action is even more likely in the case of neurotensin, whose receptors are found to be almost evenly distributed along the plasma membrane of the perikarya and dendrites of certain nigral neurons. Here again, it would be important to know if neurotensin, or any of the other endogenous peptides susceptible to act upon neurotensin receptors, such as Neuromedin-N or Lant 6 (see Kitabgi *et al.*, 1985), are released by terminals directly abutting these presumptive neurotensinoceptive neurons, or by axon terminals located at a distance from their plasma membrane. Light microscopic immunohistochemical studies by Hökfelt *et al.* (1984) have revealed the presence of a medium to dense network of neurotensin-immunoreactive fibers surrounding the dopamine cell bodies in the zona compacta and pars lateralis of the substantia nigra. Double labeling experiments at the electron microscopic level will be needed, however, to determine whether these neurotensin-containing axons actually contact the perikaryon and/or dendrites of dopamine cells.

6. Conclusion

In summary, the present study indicates that neuropeptide binding sites labeled *in vitro* in rat brain slices may be either intracellular or membrane-bound.

Intracellular binding sites presumably correspond to sites of synthesis, storage, and/or transport of the receptors. Some might also represent receptor molecules that are being degraded and/or recycled. It is important to recall in this context that both opioid and neurotensin receptors have been shown to undergo bidirectional axonal transport in CNS neurons (Young *et al.*, 1980; Kessler *et al.*, 1986). Clearly, the radioactive molecules found inside neuronal perikarya were not themselves internalized since (1) the tissue was prefixed at the time of incubation, and (2) the incubations were carried out at a low temperature, and in the absence of ions and oxygen supply. Several lines of evidence, however, suggest that *in vivo,* both opioids and neurotensin may be internalized (Van Loon and George, 1983; Kitabgi *et al.*, unpublished).

Correlative biochemical and pharmacological evidence suggests that most, if not all, membrane-bound binding sites correspond to functional receptors. In the neostriatum, opioid receptors are mainly associated with axodendritic, axosomatic, and axoaxonic neuronal interfaces, indicating that endogenous, as well as exogenous opioids may act both pre- and postsynaptically in this region of the brain. In the substantia nigra, neurotensin receptors are predominately found on the perikaryal and dendritic plasma membranes of presumptive dopaminergic pars compacta neurons. These receptors provide a substrate through which neurotensin may regulate the activity of nigrostriatal dopamine neurons (for review, see Quirion, 1983).

In both cases, the ultrastructural distributional pattern of the labeled binding sites clearly favors an extrajunctional if not outright paracrine mode of action for these neuropeptides. Such a mode of action has already been invoked as a possible explanation for apparent mismatches between concentrations of different transmitters and their receptors in the CNS (Herkenham and McLean, 1986). Further electron microscopic studies aimed at determining the relationship between neuropeptide receptors and the sites of release of their endogenous ligand(s) are clearly needed to help assess the extent to which such "parasynaptic" mechanisms might account for the effects of neuropeptides in the CNS.

ACKNOWLEDGMENTS. This work was supported by grants from the Medical Research Council of Canada (MT-7375), the Parkinson Foundation of Canada, and a France–Quebec exchange program. The authors are indebted to Beverley Lindsay for clerical assistance, Charles Hodge for photographic work, and Barbara E. Jones and Maya Frankfurt for their critical review of the manuscript.

References

Altschuler, R. A., Betz, H., Parakkal, M. H., Reeks, K. A., and Wenthold, R. J., 1986, Identification of glycinergic synapses in the cochlear nucleus through immunocytochemical localization of the postsynaptic receptor, *Brain Res.* **369**:316–320.
Antkiewicz-Michaluk, L., Havemann, U., Vetulani, J., Wellstein, A., and Kuschinsky, K., 1984, Opioid-specific recognition sites of the mu- and the delta-type in rat striatum after lesions with kainic acid, *Life Sci.* **35**:347–355.
Arimatsu, Y., Seto, A., and Amano, T., 1978, Localization of α-bungarotoxin binding sites in mouse brain by light and electron microscopic autoradiography, *Brain Res.* **147**:165–169.

Atweh, S. F., and Kuhar, M. J., 1977, Autoradiographic localization of opiate receptors in rat brain. III. The telencephalon, *Brain Res.* **134**:393–405.

Beaudet, A., and Descarries, L., 1978, The monoamine innervation of rat cerebral cortex: Synaptic and nonsynaptic axon terminals, *Neuroscience* **3**:851–860.

Beaudet, A., Trémeau, O., Ménez, A., and Droz, B., 1979, Visualisation des récepteurs aux opiacés dans le locus coeruleus du rat: Étude radioautographique à haute résolution après administration d'un analogue tritié de la met-enképhaline, *C.R. Acad. Sci.* **289**:591–594.

Beaudet, A., Leonard, K., Vial, M., Moyse, E., Kitabgi, P., Vincent, J. P., and Rostene W., 1987, Electron microscopic localization of neurotensin receptors in the substantia nigra of the rat, *Soc. Neurosci. Abstr.* **13**:563.

Blackett, N. M., and Parry, D. M., 1977, A simplified method of "hypothetical grain" analysis of electron microscope autoradiographs, *J. Histochem. Cytochem.* **25**:206–214.

Bowen, W. D., Pert, C. B., and Pert, A., 1982, Nigral 6-hydroxydopamine lesions equally decrease μ and δ opiate binding to striatal patches: Further evidence for a conformationally malleable type 1 opiate receptor, *Life Sci.* **31**:1679–1682.

Chang, K. J., Cooper, B. R., Hazum, E., and Cuatrecasas, P., 1979, Multiple opiate receptors: Different regional distribution in the brain and differential binding of opiates and opioid peptides, *Mol. Pharmacol.* **16**:91–104.

Childers, S. R., Schwarcz, R., Coyle, J. T., and Snyder, S. H., 1978, Radioimmunoassay of enkephalins: Levels of methionine- and leucine-enkephalin in morphine dependent and kainic acid lesioned rat brains, in: *Advances in Biochemical Psychopharmacology*, Vol. 18 (E. Costa and M. Trabucchi, eds.), Raven Press, New York, pp. 161–173.

Clark, A. J., 1933, *The Mode of Action of Drugs on Cells*, Arnold, London.

Cuello, A. C., 1983, Nonclassical neuronal communication, *Fed. Proc. Fed. Am. Soc. Exp. Biol.* **42**:2912–2922.

Dana, C., Vial, M., Kitabgi, P., Leonard, K., Beaudet, A., and Rostène, W., 1985, Distribution radioautographique et ultrastructurale des sites de liaison de la neurotensine dans le cerveau de rat, *Ann. Endocrinol.* **46**:16N.

Dana, C., Leonard, K., Vial, M., Rostene, W., and Beaudet, A., 1987, Autoradiographic localization of neurotensin binding sites in rat ventral tegmental area at the electron microscopic level, *Neuroscience* **22**:5785.

Demoliou-Mason, C. D., and Barnard, E. A., 1986, Distinct subtypes of the opioid receptor with allosteric interactions in brain membranes, *J. Neurochem.* **46**:1118–1128.

Descarries, L., and Beaudet, A., 1983, The use of radioautography for investigating transmitter-specific neurons, in: *Handbook of Chemical Neuroanatomy*, Vol. 1 (A. Bjorklund and T. Hökfelt, eds.), Elsevier, Amsterdam, pp. 286–364.

Descarries, L., Beaudet, A., and Watkins, K. C., 1975, Serotonin nerve terminals in adult rat neocortex, *Brain Res.* **100**:563–588.

Gardner, E. L., Zukin, S. R., and Makman, M. H., 1980, Modulation of opiate receptor binding in striatum and amygdala by selective mesencephalic lesions, *Brain Res.* **194**:232–239.

Goodman, R. R., Snyder, S. H., Kuhar, M. J., and Young, W. S., III, 1980, Differentiation of delta and mu opiate receptor localizations by light microscopic autoradiography, *Proc. Natl. Acad. Sci. USA* **77**:6239–6243.

Hamel, E., and Beaudet, A., 1984a, Localization of opioid binding sites in rat brain by electron microscopic radioautography, *J. Electron Microsc. Tech.* **1**:317–329.

Hamel, E., and Beaudet, A., 1984b, Electron microscopic autoradiographic localization of opioid receptors in rat neostriatum, *Nature* **312**:155–157.

Hamel, E., and Beaudet, A., 1987, Opioid receptors in rat neostriatum: Radioautographic distribution at the electron microscopic level, *Brain Res.* **401**:239–257.

Hazum, E., Chang, K.-J., and Cuatrecasas, P., 1980, Cluster formation of opiate (enkephalin) receptors in neuroblastoma cells: Differences between agonists and antagonists and possible relationships to biological functions, *Proc. Natl. Acad. Sci. USA* **77**:3038–3041.

Herkenham, M., 1984, Autoradiographic demonstration of receptor distributions, in: *Brain Receptor Methodologies*, Part A (P. J. Marangos, I. C. Campbell, and R. M. Cohen, eds.), Academic Press, New York, pp. 127–152.

Herkenham, M., and McLean, S., 1986, Mismatches between receptor and transmitter localizations in the brain, in: *Quantitative Receptor Autoradiography*, Vol. 19 (C. A. Boast, E. A. Snowhill, and C. A. Altar, eds.), Liss, New York, pp. 137–171.

Herkenham, M., and Pert, C.B., 1982, Light microscopic localization of brain opiate receptors: A general autoradiographic method which preserves tissue quality, *J. Neurosci.* **2**:1129–1149.

Hökfelt, T., Everitt, B. J., Theodorsson-Norheim, E., and Goldstein, M., 1984, Occurrence of neurotensinlike immunoreactivity in subpopulations of hypothalamic, mesencephalic, and medullary catecholamine neurons, *J. Comp. Neurol.* **222**:543–559.

Hollt, V., and Herz, A., 1978, In vivo receptor occupation by opiates and correlation to the pharmacological effect, *Fed. Proc. Fed. Am. Soc. Exp. Biol.* **37**:158–161.

Hunt, S. P., and Schmidt, J., 1978, The electron microscopic autoradiographic localization of α-bungarotoxin binding sites within the central nervous system of the rat, *Brain Res.* **142**:152–159.

Jacob, M. H., and Berg, D. K., 1983, The ultrastructural localization of α-bungarotoxin binding sites in relation to synapses on chick ciliary ganglion neurons, *J. Neurosci.* **3**:260–271.

Jan, Y. N., and Jan, L. Y., 1983, A LHRH-like peptidergic neurotransmitter capable of 'action at a distance' in autonomic ganglia, *Trends Neurosci.* **6**:320–325.

Kessler, J. P., Kitabgi, P., and Beaudet, A., 1986, High affinity neurotensin binding to afferent and efferent components of the vagal complex, *Soc. Neurosci. Abstr.* **12**:811.

Kitabgi, P., Poustis, C., Granier, C., Van Rietschoten, J., Rivier, J., Morgat, J. L., and Freychet, P., 1980, Neurotensin binding to extraneuronal and neural receptors: Comparison with biological activity and structure activity relationships, *Mol. Pharmacol.* **18**:11–19.

Kitabgi, P., Checler, F., Mazella, J., and Vincent, J. P., 1985, Pharmacology and biochemistry of neurotensin receptors, *Rev. Clin. Basic Pharmacol.* **5**:397–486.

Kuhar, M. J., and Yamamura, H. I., 1974, Light microscopic autoradiographic localization of cholinergic muscarinic sites in rat brain, *Proc. Soc. Neurosci.* **4**:29.

Kuhar, M. J., Taylor, M., Wamsley, J. K., Hulme, E. C., and Birdsall, N. J. M., 1981, Muscarinic cholinergic receptor localization in brain by electron microscopic autoradiography, *Brain Res.* **216**:1–9.

Lentz, T. L., and Chester, J., 1977, Localization of acetylcholine receptors in central synapses, *J. Cell Biol.* **75**:258–267.

Lewis, M. E., Khachaturian, H., and Watson, S. J., 1985, Combined autoradiographic–immunocytochemical analysis of opioid receptors and opioid peptide neuronal systems in brain, *Peptides* **6**:37–47.

McLean, S., Rothman, R. B., and Herkenham, M., 1986, Autoradiographic localization of μ- and δ-opiate receptors in the forebrain of the rat, *Brain Res.* **378**:49–60.

Miller, M. M., Billiar, R. B., and Beaudet, A., 1987, Ultrastructural distribution of alpha-bungarotoxin binding sites in the suprachiasmatic nucleus of the rat hypothalamus, *Cell Tissue Res.* (in press).

Miller, R. J., Chang, K.-J., Leighton, J., and Cuatrecasas, P., 1978, Interaction of iodinated enkephalin analogs with opiate receptors, *Life Sci.* **22**:379–388.

Mohler, H., Richards, J. G., and Wu, J.-Y., 1981, Autoradiographic localization of benzodiazepine receptors in immunocytochemically identified γ-aminobutyrergic synapses, *Proc. Natl. Acad. Sci. USA* **78**:1935–1938.

Moyse, E., Vial, M., Leonard, K., Kitabgi, P., Vincent, J. P., Rostène, W., and Beaudet, A., 1985, Electron microscopic visualization of neurotensin binding sites in rat substantia nigra, *Soc. Neurosci. Abstr.* **11**:415.

Moyse, E., Pasquini, F., Quirion, R., and Beaudet, A., 1986, ^{125}I-FK 33-824: A selective probe for radioautographic labeling of μ opioid receptors in the brain, *Peptides* **7**:351–355.

Moyse, E., Rostène, W., Vial, M., Leonard, K., Mazella, J., Kitabgi, P., Vincent, J. P., and Beaudet, A., 1987, Regional distribution of neurotensin binding sites in rat brain: A light microscopic radioautographic study using monoiodo ^{125}I-Tyr$_3$-neurotensin, *Neuroscience* **22**:525–536.

Murrin, L. C., Coyle, J. T., and Kuhar, M. J., 1980, Striatal opiate receptors: Pre- and post-synaptic localization, *Life Sci.* **27**:1175–1183.

Palacios, J. M., and Kuhar, M. J., 1981, Neurotensin receptors are located on dopamine-containing neurons in rat midbrain, *Nature* **294**:587–589.

Palacios, J. M., Niehoff, D. L., and Kuhar, M. J., 1981, Receptor autoradiography with tritium-sensitive film: Potential for computerized densitometry, *Neurosci. Lett.* **25**:101–105.

Parenti, M., Titrone, F., Olgiati, V. R., and Gropetti, A., 1983, Presence of opiate receptors on striatal serotoninergic nerve terminals, *Brain Res.* **280**:317–322.

Pert, C. B., Kuhar, M. J., and Snyder, S. H., 1976, Opiate receptors: Autoradiographic localization in rat brain, *Proc. Natl. Acad. Sci. USA* **73**:3729–3733.

Pollard, H., Llorens, C., Schwartz, J. C., Gros, C., and Dray, F., 1978, Localization of opiate receptors and enkephalins in the rat striatum in relationship with nigrostriatal dopaminergic system: Lesion studies, *Brain Res.* **151**:392–398.

Polz-Tejera, G., Schmidt, J., and Karten, H. J., 1975, Autoradiographic localization of α-bungarotoxin-binding sites in the central nervous system, *Nature* **258**:349–351.

Porter, C., Barnard, E. A., and Chiu, T. H., 1973, The ultrastructural localization and quantitation of cholinergic receptors at the mouse motor endplate, *J. Membr. Biol.* **14**:383–402.

Quirion, R., 1983, Interactions between neurotensin and dopamine in the brain: An overview, *Peptides* **4**:609–615.

Quirion, R., Gaudreau, P., St. Pierre, S., Rioux, F., and Pert, C. B., 1982, Autoradiographic distribution of [3H]neurotensin receptors in rat brain: Visualization by tritium sensitive film, *Peptides* **3**:757–763.

Reisine, T. D., Nagy, J. I., Beaumont, K., Fibiger, H. C., and Yamamura, H. I., 1979, The localization of receptor binding sites in the substantia nigra and striatum of the rat, *Brain Res.* **177:**241–252.

Richards, J. G., Schoch, P., Häring, P., Takacs, B., and Möhler, H., 1987, Resolving $GABA_A$/benzodiazepine receptors: cellular and subcellular localization in the CNS with monoclonal antibodies, *J. Neurosci.* **7:**1866–1886.

Roemer, D., Buescher, H. H., Hill, R. C., Pless, J., Bauer, W., Cardinaux, F., Closse, A., Hauser, D., and Huguenin, R., 1977, A synthetic enkephalin analogue with prolonged parenteral and oral analgesic activity, *Nature* **268:**547–549.

Rotter, A., Birdsall, N. J. M., Burgen, A. S. V., Field, P. M., and Raisman, G., 1977, Axotomy causes loss of muscarinic receptors and loss of synaptic contacts in the hypoglossal nucleus, *Nature* **266:**734–735.

Sadoul, J. L., Mazella, J., Amar, S., Kitabgi, P., and Vincent, J. P., 1984, Preparation of neurotensin selectively iodinated on the tyrosine 3 residue: Biological activity and binding properties on mammalian neurotensin receptors, *Biochem. Biophys. Res. Commun.* **120:**812–819.

Salpeter, M. M., McHenry, F. A., and Salpeter, E. E., 1978, Resolution in electron microscope autoradiography. IV. Application to analysis of autoradiographs, *J. Cell Biol.* **76:**127–145.

Schmidt, F. O., 1984, Molecular regulators of brain function: A new view, *Neuroscience* **13:**991–1001.

Schubert, P., Höllt, V., and Herz, A., 1975, Autoradiographic evaluation of the intracerebral distribution of ^{3}H-etorphine in the mouse brain, *Life Sci.* **16:**1855–1856.

Seidah, N. G., Dennis, M., Corvol, R., Rochemont, J., and Chrétien, M., 1980, A rapid high-performance liquid chromatography purification method of iodinated polypeptide hormones, *Anal. Biochem.* **109:**185–191.

Snyder, S. H., and Bennett, J. P., Jr., 1976, Neurotransmitter receptors in the brain: Biochemical identification, *Annu. Rev. Physiol.* **38:**153–175.

Strader, C. D., Pickel, V. M., Joh, T. H., Strohsacker, M. W., Shorr, R. G. L., Lefkowitz, R. J., and Caron, M. G., 1983, Antibodies to the α-adrenergic receptor: Attenuation of catecholamine-sensitive adenylate cyclase and demonstration of postsynaptic receptor localization in brain, *Proc. Natl. Acad. Sci. USA* **80:**1840–1844.

Szigethy, E., Kitabgi, P., and Beaudet, A., 1986, Localization of neurotensin binding sites to dopaminergic and putative cholinergic neurons in rat central nervous system, *Soc. Neurosci. Abstr.* **12:**1003.

Trémeau, O., Faure, G., Boulain, J. C., Bouet, F., Ménez, A., Lecocq, G., Morgat, J. L., and Fromageot, P., 1981, Liaison d'un analogue enképhalinergique (FK 33-824) tritié à une fraction mitochondriale de cerveau de rat, *Biochimie* **63:**477–484.

Triller, A., Cluzeaud, F., Pfeiffer, F., Betz, H., and Korn, H., 1985, Distribution of glycine receptors at central synapses: An immunoelectron microscopy study, *J. Cell Biol.* **101:**683–688.

Uhl, G. R., 1982, Distribution of neurotensin and its receptors in the central nervous system, *Ann. N.Y. Acad. Sci.* **400:**132–149.

Van Loon, G. R., and George, S. R., 1983, Uptake/internalization of met-enkephalin by brain synaptosomes, *Life Sci.* **33:**145–148.

Williams, M. A., 1969, The assessment of electron microscopic autoradiography, in: *Advances in Optical and Electron Microscopy*, Vol. 3 (R. Barer and V. E. Cosslett, eds.), Academic Press, New York, pp. 219–272.

Young, W. S., III, and Kuhar, M. J., 1979a, A new method for receptor autoradiography: [^{3}H]opioid receptors in rat brain, *Brain Res.* **179:**255–270.

Young, W. S., III, and Kuhar, M. J., 1979b, Neurotensin receptors: Autoradiographic localization in rat CNS, *Eur. J. Pharmacol.* **59:**161–163.

Young, W. S., III, and Kuhar, M. J., 1981, Neurotensin receptor localization by light microscopic autoradiography in rat brain, *Brain Res.* **206:**272–285.

Young, W. S., Wamsley, J. K., Zarbin, M. A., and Kuhar, M. J., 1980, Opioid receptors undergo axonal transport, *Science* **210:**76–77.

36

Neuropeptide Receptors in the Brain
Possible Relevance to Function

Remi Quirion

1. Introduction

Over the last decade, the existence of multiple brain neuropeptide systems has been demonstrated. However, the precise physiological role of each of these neuropeptides is almost totally unknown except for their effects on the release of hypophysial hormones and the role of opioid peptides in pain transmission (Akil *et al.*, 1984; Quirion, 1984).

One of the first steps toward identifying a possible function for a given neuropeptide is to characterize its distribution in brain using highly sensitive and specific radioimmunoassays and immunohistochemical techniques. For example, the high densities of immunoreactive fibers in the periaqueductal gray matter may suggest a possible role for the peptide in nociception. Another useful technique is to study the distribution of its receptor sites. The concentration of receptor binding sites in a given region (e.g., substantia nigra) may suggest that a peptide modulates certain brain functions (e.g., activity of the dopaminergic system). In this chapter I will illustrate the usefulness of the receptor autoradiographic method (Kuhar, 1985; Herkenham and McLean, 1986) for identifying neuropeptide binding sites using substance P and neurokinins, atrial natriuretic factors and angiotensin II, and neuropeptide Y as examples.

2. Substance P and Tachykinins

It is now known that three mammalian tachykinins, namely substance P (SP), neurokinin A (NKA), and neurokinin B (NKB) (Chang and Leeman, 1970; Kangawa *et al.*, 1983; Kimura *et al.*, 1984; Maggio *et al.*, 1983), are found in brain and peripheral tissues. These peptides are characterized by the amino acid sequence Phe-X-Gly-Leu-Met-NH$_2$ at the C-terminus, where X represents a hydrophobic or aromatic residue (Quirion, 1985).

The isolation of two mammalian tachykinin precursors has recently been reported (Nawa *et al.*, 1983). α-Preprotachykinin contains only one copy of SP while β-preprotachykinin contains

Remi Quirion • Douglas Hospital Research Centre and Department of Psychiatry, Faculty of Medicine, McGill University, Verdun, Quebec H4H 1R3, Canada.

one copy each of SP and NKA. The characterization of a third precursor responsible for the generation of NKB has yet to be reported. Moreover, Nawa *et al.* (1984b) have shown that the α/β preprotachykinin ratio varies markedly between tissues. This suggests that in certain tissues, SP is the most likely active tachykinin while in others, both SP and NKA could have important and maybe even opposite effects. Thus, biological effects thought to be mediated by SP will have to be reevaluated in light of these findings showing multiple mammalian tachykinins.

2.1. Multiple Biological Actions in Brain

SP has been postulated to be "the" pain neurotransmitter (Henry, 1977; Pernow, 1983). Peripheral nervous system pathways containing SP appear to be involved in the perception and transmission of nociceptive stimuli. Following trauma, SP is released under conditions that generate painful sensations as well as when noxious information is relayed to higher centers. Thus, peripheral SP systems could mediate information about noxious stimuli, while certain central SP pathways could be responsible for the integration and analysis of related information (Henry, 1977; Pernow, 1983). Moreover, SP and/or related tachykinins could be involved in the process of tissue repair (Pernow, 1983). For example, it is known that SP is involved in the initial massive protein extravasation and subsequent development of edema following injury. All these biological effects strongly suggest that SP and/or related tachykinins may serve important functions in pain transmission.

Probably tachykinins are also involved in the modulation of brain dopaminergic systems. The highest densities of SP-like nerve fiber terminals in the brain are found in the substantia nigra. Their cell bodies are located in the striatum (striatonigral pathway) (Brownstein *et al.*, 1976, 1977; Cuello and Kanazawa, 1978; Ljungdahl *et al.*, 1978). Fairly high concentrations of SP stimulate the synthesis and release of dopamine in the substantia nigra (Cheramy *et al.*, 1977; Michelot *et al.*, 1979; Waldmeier *et al.*, 1978). Moreover, direct injections of SP into the substantia nigra and the ventral tegmental area (VTA) elicit behavioral effects similar to those produced by stimulation of dopaminergic pathways (Kelley and Iversen, 1978, 1979; Kelley *et al.*, 1979; Stinus *et al.*, 1978). Chronic neuroleptic treatments reduce SP-like immunoreactivity in the striatum and substantia nigra probably through the blockade of the dopamine D2 receptor subtype (Hanson *et al.*, 1981; Hong *et al.*, 1979; Oblin *et al.*, 1984). However, recent evidence indicates that other tachykinins are more effective modulators of dopaminergic systems (see below), suggesting that the comparative effects of SP, NKA, and NKB on dopaminergic innervation should be investigated.

SP and related tachykinins have other effects in the brain. For example, SP excites certain cortical neurons and various nuclei involved in the control of respiratory and cardiovascular parameters, and stimulates the release of growth hormone and prolactin (Pernow, 1983). However, the exact physiological significance of these various effects remains to be established.

2.2. Brain SP Receptor Sites

Several classes of tachykinin receptors exist in mammalian tissues (for reviews: Regoli *et al.*, 1984; Quirion, 1985; Quirion and Dam, 1985b; Watson, 1984). In peripheral tissues, Lee *et al.* (1982) were among the first to suggest the existence of two SP receptor subtypes, SP-P and SP-E. On the SP-P receptor subtype, the compounds SP, physalaemin, eledoisin, and kassinin are more or less equipotent, while the last two are much more active than SP on the SP-E receptor. Since then, it has been demonstrated in various assays that NKA and NKB are more active on the putative SP-E subtype (Hunter and Maggio, 1984; Nawa *et al.*, 1984a; Quirion and Pilapil, 1984; Torrens, *et al.*, 1984).

However, the demonstration of highly specific receptor binding sites for SP and related tachykinins has been more difficult than expected. It is only over the past 3 to 4 years that various groups have succeeded in demonstrating the presence of highly specific and selective SP receptor binding sites in mammalian brain (Cascieri and Liang, 1983; Park *et al.*, 1984; Torrens *et al.*, 1983; Viger *et al.*, 1983). In 1982–1983, our group was the first to report on the discrete distribution of SP receptor binding sites in mammalian brain using an *in vitro* autoradiographic technique (Shults *et al.*, 1982; O'Donohue *et al.*, 1983; Quirion *et al.*, 1983a,b). We clearly demonstrated the existence in rat brain sections of an apparent single class of high-affinity binding sites for either [³H]SP, [¹²⁵I]Bolton–Hunter SP or [¹²⁵I]physalaemin (Quirion *et al.*, 1983a,b Shults *et al.*, 1984; Wolf *et al.*, 1985). The ligand selectivity pattern was very similar using either of the radioligands, suggesting that each was binding to the same population of receptor sites (Table I).

The identical autoradiographic distributions of binding sites for these radioligands also supported this hypothesis. High densities of SP binding sites were found in various brain areas including the striatum, olfactory bulb, locus coeruleus, inferior olive, and superficial layers of the dorsal horn of the spinal cord (Mantyh *et al.*, 1984a; Quirion *et al.*, 1983a,b; Rothman *et al.*, 1984a; Shults *et al.*, 1984). Surprisingly, very low densities of sites were present in the substantia nigra, zona compacta, and reticulata (Fig. 1). As mentioned above, the substantia nigra is the brain region containing the highest density of SP-like nerve fiber terminals (Brownstein *et al.*, 1977; Cuello and Kanazawa, 1978). Thus, it was expected that this structure would at least be moderately rich in SP binding sites, especially since it had been shown that SP (even at high concentrations) was inducing various biological effects following intranigral injections (Cheramy *et al.*, 1977; Kelley *et al.*, 1979; Stinus *et al.*, 1978). However, it must be remembered that most electrophysiological studies had failed to demonstrate a direct action of SP on nigral neurons (Guyenet and Aghajanian, personal communication; Innis *et al.*, 1985).

The quasi-absence of SP binding sites intrigued us and we performed a series of experiments to make sure that it was not related to technical problems. First, we performed membrane binding assays with either [³H]-SP or [¹²⁵I]-Bolton-Hunter SP using micropunched substantia nigra. Again, it was not possible to demonstrate significant SP binding in nigral membrane preparations (unpublished results). Torrens *et al.* (1983) reported similar results. Thus, autoradiographic data were confirmed by membrane binding assays. In a second series of experiments, destruction of the striatonigral SP pathway was performed according to Brownstein *et al.* (1977). This manipulation induced a 90–95% depletion in the content of the nigral SP-like immunoreactivity, without increasing SP binding (unpublished results). Thus, the apparent absence of SP binding in the substantia nigra was not due to the presence of high concentrations of endogenous ligand in these structures. Finally, various other species were studied (guinea pig, pigeon, monkey, human) and in all of them, very low densities of SP binding sites were found in the substantia nigra (Dam

Table I. Comparative Potency of Various Mammalian and Nonmammalian Tachykinins on [¹²⁵I]-BH Substance P and [¹²⁵I]-BH Neurokinin A Binding Sites in Guinea Pig Brain[a]

Tachykinin	Relative potency	
	[¹²⁵I]-BH substance P	[¹²⁵I]-BH neurokinin A
Substance P	100	0.33
Neurokinin A	0.11	100
Neurokinin B	<0.01	10.4
Kassinin	0.08	24.4
Eledoisin	1.35	4.1
Physalaemin	29.8	0.16

[a]Modified from Quirion and Dam (1985a).

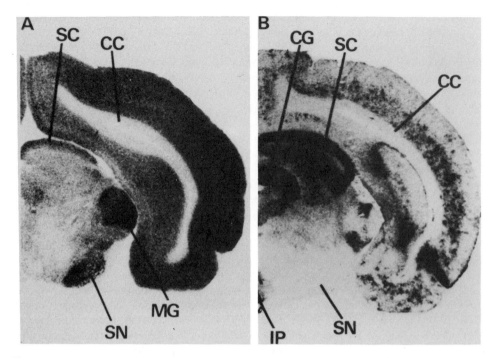

Figure 1. Comparative distribution of (A) [^{125}I]-Bolton–Hunter neurokinin A and (B) [^{125}I]-Bolton–Hunter substance P binding sites at the level of the guinea pig substantia nigra. CC, corpus callosum; CG, central gray; IP, interpeduncular nucleus; MG, medial geniculate nucleus; SC, superior colliculus; SN, substantia nigra. (From Quirion, 1985.)

and Quirion, 1986; Quirion *et al.*, 1987; R. Quirion, unpublished results). At about the same time, various groups reported on the existence of other mammalian tachykinins (NKA and NKB) in the brain. This eventually provided an alternative hypothesis on the apparent mismatch between the nigral content in SP-like immunoreactivity and the density of receptor binding sites in this region (see below).

2.3. Multiple Tachykinin/Neurokinin Receptor Classes

The presence of other tachykinins in mammalian brain (neurokinin A, neurokinin B) suggested the possible existence of multiple classes of tachykinin/neurokinin receptor classes now labeled as neurokinin-1 (NK-1), NK-2, and NK-3 receptors (as adopted at the Montreal Substance P Symposium, July, 1986).

This hypothesis is now supported by various findings. First, it was shown, shortly after the isolation of these new tachykinins, that NKA and NKB were poorly active on SP receptors, suggesting that they were probably binding to different sites to induce their biological effects (Hunter and Maggio, 1984; Nawa *et al.*, 1984a; Quirion and Pilapil, 1984). Later, it was shown that the relative potencies of various tachykinins on SP, NKA, and NKB binding sites were very different (Quirion and Dam, 1985a,b; Torrens *et al.*, 1984; Beaujouan *et al.*, 1984; Cascieri and Liang, 1984; Buck *et al.*, 1984). As shown in Table I, SP and physalaemin are potent competitors of [^{125}I]-BH SP binding but not of [^{125}I]-BH NKA binding in guinea pig brain membrane preparations. On the other hand, NKA, NKB, and kassinin demonstrated high affinities for [^{125}I]-BH NKA binding sites but comparatively low affinities for [^{125}I]-BH SP sites (Table I). Comparable results have been obtained in various peripheral tissues (Hunter and Maggio, 1984; Nawa *et al.*, 1984a). Moreover, the respective distribution of SP, NKA, and NKB (using eledoisin as ligand) binding sites is different as demonstrated by membrane binding assays (Beaujouan *et al.*, 1984; Cascieri and Liang, 1984; Buck *et al.*, 1984).

The autoradiographic distribution of SP, NKA, and NKB binding sites is also markedly very different, both in brain (Mantyh *et al.*, 1984b; Quirion, 1985; Quirion and Dam, 1985a,b; Rothman *et al.*, 1984b; Shults *et al.*, 1985a) and peripheral tissues (Burcher *et al.*, 1986). The differential distribution of these various tachykinin binding sites at the level of the substantia nigra, VTA, and spinal cord is of special interest (Quirion and Dam, 1985a,b; Rothman *et al.*, 1984b; Kalivas *et al.*, 1985; Ninkovic *et al.*, 1985). As shown in Fig. 1, the guinea pig substantia nigra is enriched in NKA binding sites but devoid of SP receptors. Similar results have been observed in the rat substantia nigra (Mantyh *et al.*, 1984b) and VTA (Kalivas *et al.*, 1985).

2.4. Possible Relevance to Function

This could be highly relevant for the apparent mismatch between nigral SP-like immunoreactivity and the lack of SP receptor binding sites in this structure (Quirion, 1985). Since SP and NKA are similarly distributed in brain (Maggio and Hunter, 1984; Shults *et al.*, 1985b) and are most likely derived from the same precursor (Nawa *et al.*, 1983), it suggests that NKA could be the most relevant tachykinin in the striatonigral pathway and in the VTA. Already, this hypothesis is supported by various recent findings including (1) the presence of high densities of NKA binding sites in these two areas (Mantyh *et al.*, 1984b; Quirion, 1985; Kalivas *et al.*, 1985), (2) the potent electrophysiological effect of NKA (versus SP) on dopaminergic and nondopaminergic neurons in the rat substantia nigra (Innis *et al.*, 1985), (3) the higher potency of NKA (10 times that of SP) in producing an increase in motor activity (Kalivas *et al.*, 1985; Deutch *et al.*, 1985; Takano *et al.*, 1985) when injected into the VTA, (4) the differential effect of SP and NKA on dopaminergic metabolism in the mesencephalon (McQuade *et al.*, 1986; Baruch *et al.*, 1987), and (5) the differential effect of neuroleptic treatments on SP and NKA-like immunoreactivity in rat brain (Lindefors *et al.*, 1986). This suggests that NKA is probably more potent than SP in stimulating dopaminergic cells in the mesencephalon. However, it does not mean that SP is totally devoid of activity in this area. SP could even act on NKA receptors to induce its effects since none of the putative tachykinin receptor classes are totally selective for any given endogenous ligand (Table II).

Similarly, $[^{125}I]$-BH SP and $[^{125}I]$-BH eledoisin receptor binding sites are differentially

Table II. Putative Classes of Neurokinin Receptors[a]

	NK-1 (substance P)	NK-2 (neurokinin A)	NK-3 (neurokinin B)
Potency of homologues	SP > Phy > NKA > NKB[b]	NKA > NKB > SP > Phy	NKB > Phy > NKA > SP
Endogenous agonist	SP	NKA	NKB
Selective antagonist	n.a.[c]	n.a.	n.a.
Localization in the brain	Olfactory bulb Striatum Hippocampus Locus coeruleus	Frontal cortex Striatum Septum Hippocampus Substantia nigra Ventral tegmental area	Cortex Hippocampus Interpeduncular nucleus Laminae I–II of the spinal cord

[a]Nomenclature according to discussion held at the International Meeting on Substance P and Neurokinins held in Montreal, July 20–23, 1986. Modified from Quirion (1985) with permission.
[b]Abbreviations: NKA, neurokinin A; NKB, neurokinin B; Phy, physalaemin; SP, substance P.
[c]Highly selective antagonists are not available (n.a.) as yet.

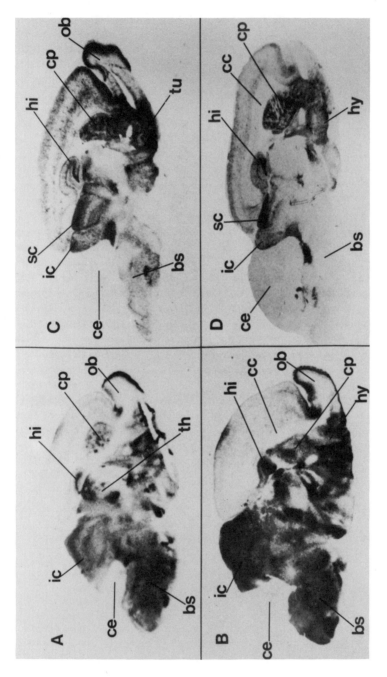

Figure 2. Photomicrographs of the autoradiographic distribution of brain substance P receptor binding sites in sagittal sections from (A) 1-, (B) 4-, and (C) 21-day-old rats, and (D) adult (3-month-old) rats. bs, brain stem; cc, corpus callosum; ce, cerebellum; cp, caudate–putamen; hi, hippocampus; hy, hypothalamus; ic, inferior colliculus; ob, olfactory bulb; sc, superior colliculus; th, thalamus; tu, olfactory tubercle. (From Quirion and Dam, 1986.)

distributed in the rat spinal cord (Ninkovic et al., 1985). The eledoisin binding sites are concentrated in superficial laminae of the dorsal horn while SP sites are found within the dorsal and ventral horns of the spinal cord. Since [125I]-BH eledoisin most likely labels NKB receptor sites in brain (Quirion, 1985; Torrens et al., 1984; Buck et al., 1984), it demonstrates the differential distribution of SP and NKB receptors in the CNS. Moreover, it reveals that biological effects assumed to be mediated by the release of SP should be reevaluated in light of the discovery of NKA and NKB, especially since they are most likely derived from common precursors (Nawa et al., 1983) and are similarly distributed in the brain (Maggio and Hunter, 1984; Shults et al., 1985b).

In summary, recent data strongly suggest the existence of three different classes of tachykinin/neurokinin receptors. As shown in Table II, the neurokinin-1 (NK-1) receptor site preferentially binds SP while the neurokinin-2 (NK-2) and neurokinin-3 (NK-3) receptor binding sites are fairly selective for NKA and NKB, respectively. Moreover, the distribution of each receptor type is unique in both peripheral tissues and brain. This will probably determine ultimately the respective physiological function of each neurokinin.

2.5. Ontogeny of Brain SP Receptors

The possible role of neuropeptides as neurotropic factors during brain development has recently generated much interest. For example, it has been shown that SP stimulates neurite outgrowth (Narumi and Fujita, 1978; Narumi and Maki, 1978), counteracts neurotoxin-induced damage of noradrenaline and serotonin neurons during ontogeny (Nakai and Kasamatsu, 1984; Jonsson and Hallman, 1982a,b, 1983a,b), and activates connective tissue cell growth (Nilsson et al., 1985). These findings prompted us to study the development of SP receptor binding sites in rat brain (Quirion and Dam, 1986).

Our findings demonstrated that SP receptor binding sites appear very early, reach a maximal density 1 day before birth, and decrease thereafter to reach adult values by 14 days after birth (Quirion and Dam, 1986). However, more importantly, the distribution of SP binding sites undergoes major modifications during this period. For example, very high densities of SP binding sites are present in most brain stem nuclei early after birth while this is not the case in adults (Fig. 2). This difference may be relevant to the possible role of SP as a neurotrophic factor during brain development, especially since SP has been shown to protect noradrenaline and serotonin neurons against neurotoxin-induced damage (Jonsson and Hallman, 1982a,b, 1983a,b). Thus, further studies on the comparative ontogeny of the various tachykinin receptor classes should be performed. Moreover, the characterization of their putative respective roles in brain development certainly warrants further investigation.

3. Atrial Natriuretic Factors (ANF) and Angiotensin II (AT$_{II}$)

Over the last 10 years, the existence of a brain angiotensin system has been demonstrated (Lang, et al., 1983; Phillips et al., 1978). Moreover, recent data suggest the presence of ANF in the brain (Quirion et al., 1984, 1986).

3.1. ANF and ANF Receptors in Brain

The detailed neuroanatomical distribution of ANF-like peptides in rat brain has just been reported by two independent laboratories (Kawata et al., 1985; Skofitsch et al., 1985). Perikarya containing immunoreactive ANF neurons are found mostly in the lateral septal nucleus, periventricular preoptic nucleus, bed nucleus of the stria terminalis, periventricular and dorsal parts of the paraventricular hypothalamic nuclei, ventromedial nucleus, dorsomedial nucleus, arcuate nucleus, mammillary nucleus, habenular nuclei, and the periaqueductal gray matter. Fewer immunoreactive cell bodies are present in the cingulate cortex, endopiriform nucleus, lateral hypothalamic area, pretectal and dorsal thalamic areas. High densities of immunoreactive *fibers* are found in the above-mentioned areas as well as in the olfactory bulb, median eminence, interpeduncular nucleus, medial and central amygdaloid nuclei, dorsal raphe, locus coeruleus, vagal dorsal motor nucleus, and solitary nucleus. Circumventricular organs such as the subfornical organ, organum vasculosum laminae terminalis, and area postrema are also enriched in ANF-immunoreactive varicose fibers. Radioimmunoassay data agree with the observed immunohistochemical distribution of ANF-like peptides in rat brain (Zamir *et al.*, 1986). Interestingly, the density of ANF-immunoreactive perikarya and varicose fibers is not altered in either dehydrated or homozygous Brattleboro rats (Kawata *et al.*, 1985). This could be relevant to the possible effect of ANF peptides on water and salt intake (see below).

The recent demonstration of the release of ANF-like immunoreactive materials from rat hypothalamic slices (Tanaka and Inagami, 1986) is also of major importance in relation to the possible role of ANF as a neurotransmitter or neuromodulator. Tanaka and Inagami (1986) have shown that ANF-like material is released, in a calcium-dependent manner, from rat hypothalamus by a depolarizing concentration of potassium. This fulfills one of the most important criteria for the consideration of any neuropeptide as a neurotransmitter or neuromodulator.

Another very important criterion is the presence of highly specific and selective receptor sites for ANF peptides in brain. In our initial study (Quirion *et al.*, 1984), we described the autoradiographic distribution of [^{125}I]-ANF binding sites in rat brain. More recently, we reported on the affinity, capacity, and ligand selectivity pattern of ANF binding sites in two areas of the guinea pig brain (Quirion *et al.*, 1986). These sites demonstrated very high affinity (picomolar range) and low capacity (low femtomoles per milligram protein) for ANF-like peptides. Moreover, their ligand selectivity is very similar to various peripheral tissues including the kidney, adrenals, and blood vessels (Cantin and Genest, 1985). This strongly suggests that these binding sites are relevant ANF receptors and that ANF receptors have similar structural requirements in brain and peripheral tissues.

The brain distribution of ANF receptor binding sites is very discrete, and autoradiographic studies performed in at least five independent laboratories have reported similar results (Quirion *et al.*, 1984, 1986; Mantyh *et al.*, 1985; Gibson *et al.*, 1986; Saavedra *et al.*, 1986; Lynch *et al.*, 1986). In the rat brain, high densities of sites are found in the olfactory bulb, subfornical organ (Fig. 3A), habenular nucleus, and area postrema. In the guinea pig brain, the distribution of ANF binding sites is more extensive with high densities in the olfactory apparatus, subfornical organ, various thalamic nuclei, hippocampal formation (Fig. 3B), area postrema, and cerebellum (Quirion *et al.*, 1986). The monkey cerebellum is also relatively enriched in ANF binding sites (Quirion *et al.*, 1986). This clearly demonstrates the differential distribution of ANF receptor binding sites in various species. Similar results have been observed for other neuropeptide receptors such as the opiates (Quirion *et al.*, 1983c). It has also been shown that the density of ANF binding sites is altered in the brain of hypertensive rats (Saavedra *et al.*, 1986).

The high densities of ANF receptor binding sites in some circumventricular organs such as the subfornical organ and the area postrema correlate well with the high concentrations of ANF-immunoreactive varicose fibers found in these areas (Kawata *et al.*, 1985; Skofitsch *et al.*, 1985), even if bloodborne ANF-like substances could have access to those brain regions. In rat brain, good correlations between the distribution of ANF and its receptor binding sites are also observed in the olfactory bulb, most cortical areas, habenula, hippocampus, striatum, thalamus, and most brain stem areas. Similar comparisons cannot be drawn for guinea pig and monkey brain since the distribution of ANF-like immunoreactive materials is unknown in these species.

However, there are various regions of the rat brain containing high concentrations of ANF-like substances (e.g., hypothalamus, septum) but only a very limited density of binding sites, and vice versa. Such "apparent" mismatches are frequent and have been observed for various

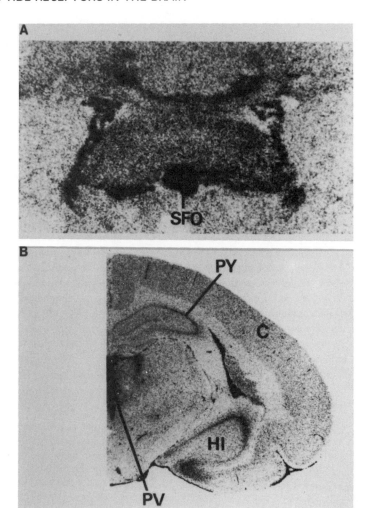

Figure 3. Photomicrographs of the autoradiographic distribution of [^{125}I]-atrial natriuretic peptide (ANP) binding sites in the rat subfornical organ (SFO) (A) and the guinea pig brain at the level of the hippocampus (B). C, cortex; HI, hippocampus; PV, paraventricular nucleus of the thalamus; PY, pyramidal cell layer of the hippocampus. Sections were prepared and incubated as described by Quirion *et al.* (1984, 1986).

neuropeptides and neurotransmitters (Kuhar, 1985; Herkenham and McLean, 1986). This may only reflect our current ignorance on the release of the various active peptides from the same precursor as well as on the existence of receptor subtypes (Quirion, 1985). In any case, it is certainly too early to claim that a given region should be enriched in receptors because it contains ANF-like immunoreactive materials. Moreover, it remains to be demonstrated if the immunoreactive material is identical to ANF as well as if it is released following physiological stimuli. Thus, the identification of receptors on "suitable target neurons" should not necessarily be expected, especially since so little is currently known on the effect of ANF-like peptides in brain.

Finally, we have recently obtained additional evidence that brain ANF binding sites are relevant ANF receptors. We have found that the regional stimulation of cGMP levels by ANF correlates very well (*r* = 0.85) with the discrete distribution of ANF binding sites in both rat and guinea pig brain (Quirion *et al.*, 1988). This strongly suggests that ANF must bind to its receptors to stimulate a biochemical event in a receptor density-dependent manner. Similar results have been obtained by others (Takayanagi *et al.*, 1986). It is also well known that the activation of ANF receptors is coupled with the production of cGMP in peripheral tissues (Hamet *et al.*, 1984) as well as in brain cell cultures (Friedl *et al.*, 1986). Thus, the presence of highly specific brain receptor sites for ANF-like substances has been demonstrated.

3.2. Possible Relevance to Function

The presence of ANF-like substances and receptors in brain tissues suggests that these new peptides could have various biological effects in the CNS. Already it has been shown that intracerebroventricular injections of ANF-related peptides inhibit osmotic and angiotensin-stimulated drinking (Antunes-Rodrigues *et al.*, 1985; Nakamura *et al.*, 1985; Katsuura *et al.*, 1986; Nakamaru *et al.*, 1986), reduce salt appetite (Fitts *et al.*, 1985), and suppress the release of vasopressin stimulated by dehydration, hemorrhage, and AT_{II} (Samson, 1985; Yamada *et al.*, 1986). Also, microinjections of ANF into the preoptic suprachiasmatic nucleus increase heart rate and blood pressure in the rat (Sills *et al.*, 1985). Moreover, electrophysiological studies have shown that ANF is capable of modulating the membrane excitability of rat forebrain neurons (Wong *et al.*, 1986). These results strongly suggest that brain ANF-containing pathways could have a major role in the central integration of various cardiovascular parameters. However, the presence of ANF-like immunoreactive materials and ANF receptor binding sites in other brain regions such as the olfactory system, cortex, hippocampus, and thalamus indicates that possible functions of ANF-like peptides in brain are probably not limited to the central regulation of the cardiovascular system.

3.3. Angiotensin Receptors in Brain

The presence of brain angiotensin, renin, and angiotensin-converting isoenzyme systems has been clearly demonstrated (for reviews, see Lang *et al.*, 1983; Lind *et al.*, 1985). Moreover, specific AT_{II} brain receptor sites have been shown using membrane binding assays (Baxter *et al.*, 1980; Bennett and Snyder, 1976; Harding *et al.*, 1981; Sirett *et al.*, 1977). More recently, the *in vitro* receptor autoradiographic technique has allowed the demonstration of the discrete distribution of highly specific AT_{II} receptor binding sites in mammalian brain (Gehlert *et al.*, 1984; Mendelsohn *et al.*, 1983, 1984a,b).

Using ^{125}I [Sar^1]-AT_{II} (Mendelsohn *et al.*, 1984a) or ^{125}I [Sar^1,Leu^8]-AT_{II} (R. Quirion, unpublished results), we found that AT_{II} receptor binding sites are heterogeneously distributed in rat brain. Very high densities of sites are found in the subfornical organ (Fig. 4A), paraventricular and periventricular hypothalamic nuclei (Fig. 4B), nucleus of the tractus solitarius, area postrema, and organum vasculosum of the lamina terminalis.

High densities of AT_{II} receptors are present in the lateral olfactory tract, olfactory tubercle, suprachiasmatic nucleus of the hypothalamus, subthalamic nucleus, locus coeruleus, and inferior olivary nuclei. Moderate concentrations of sites are seen in the median eminence, medial habenula, hippocampus, lateral septum, medial geniculate nucleus, and spinal trigeminal nerve tract. Low concentrations of sites are found in most remaining areas including the caudate putamen, nucleus accumbens, amygdala, cerebellum, and various cortical areas (Mendelsohn *et al.*, 1984a).

3.4. Possible Relevance to Function

The discrete distribution of AT_{II} receptor binding sites in rat brain is likely to be relevant to function. Multiple electrophysiological studies have identified AT_{II}-sensitive neurons in various brain structures enriched in AT_{II} sites such as the subfornical organ, lateral and medial septum,

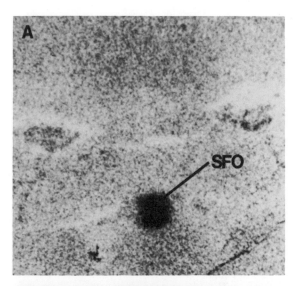

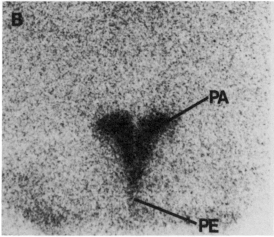

Figure 4. Photomicrographs of the autoradiographic distribution of [^{125}I]-sarcosine^1-angiotensin II binding sites in rat brain at the level of the subfornical organ (SFO) (A) and the hypothalamus (B). PA, paraventricular nucleus of the hypothalamus; PE, periventricular nucleus of the hypothalamus. Brain sections were prepared and incubated as described by Mendelsohn *et al.* (1984a).

and periventricular and supraoptic nuclei (Felix and Akert, 1974; Renaud and Padjen, 1978; Sakai *et al.*, 1974). Moreover, AT$_{II}$ receptor binding sites are localized in areas where AT$_{II}$ is known to exert various biological actions. For example, the moderate to high densities of sites in the subfornical organ, organum vasculosum of the lamina terminalis, and medial preoptic area correlate with the effect of AT$_{II}$ on water intake (Simpson, 1980; Mangiapane *et al.*, 1983). The release of vasopressin induced by AT$_{II}$ correlates well with the high densities of sites found in the paraventricular and suprachiasmatic nuclei of the hypothalamus (Lang *et al.*, 1983).

Similarly, the presence of AT$_{II}$ binding sites in the nucleus tractus solitarius, locus coeruleus, median preoptic nucleus, and area postrema may be related to actions of AT$_{II}$ in the central regulation of blood pressure (Mangiapane *et al.*, 1983; Fitzsimmons, 1979). Moreover, the presence of high densities of receptors in the olfactory system suggests a role(s) for AT$_{II}$ in the pathway. However, AT$_{II}$ binding sites are also concentrated in areas (e.g., subthalamic nucleus, superior colliculus) for which no AT$_{II}$ actions have been demonstrated thus far. This suggests that further studies on the characterization of possible actions of AT$_{II}$ in these regions should be considered.

*Table III. Comparative Characteristics of ANF and AT$_{II}$
Brain Systems*

	ANF	AT$_{II}$
Presence in brain	Yes	Yes
Synthesis from brain precursor	Yes	Yes
Maturation enzyme in brain	—	Yes
Specific receptors in brain	Yes	Yes
Concentration of peptides and receptors in cardiovascular-related areas	Yes	Yes
Effects of water and salt intake	Yes	Yes
Alterations in hypertensive animals	Yes	Yes
Electrophysiological effects in brain	Yes	Yes
Effects on release of pituitary hormones	Yes	Yes

3.5. ANF–AT$_{II}$—Physiological Antagonists?

In the periphery, ANF and AT$_{II}$ often have opposite actions. For example, ANF stimulates salt and water excretion while AT$_{II}$ leads to retention. Similarly, ANF lowers blood pressure and dilates arteries while AT$_{II}$ is a hypertensive and vasoconstrictive agent (Cantin and Genest, 1985).

In the brain, the respective distribution of their receptor sites is similar in many brain regions such as the subfornical organ, nucleus tractus solitarius, and area postrema (Table III). These regions are most likely involved in the regulation of salt and water intake, and in the control of blood pressure (Table III). It is also known that intracerebroventricular injections of ANF and AT$_{II}$ exert opposite effects on these three parameters (see Sections 3.2 and 3.4) and ANF blocks AT$_{II}$-induced vasopressin release. Moreover, brain ANF, AT$_{II}$, and their respective receptor sites are possibly altered in hypertensive animals (Cantin and Genest, 1985; Lang et al., 1983; Saavedra et al., 1986). Thus, we have recently suggested that brain ANF and AT$_{II}$ systems could be acting as physiological antagonists to ensure appropriate regulation of various cardiovascular parameters (Quirion et al., 1984). However, this does not exclude that a possible effect of a given peptide could be independent from the other (e.g., AT$_{II}$ in subthalamic nucleus; ANF in hippocampus).

In summary, it appears that complete ANF and AT$_{II}$ systems are present in the mammalian brain. Further studies should provide more insight on their comparative physiological significance.

4. Neuropeptide Y

Neuropeptide Y (NPY) is a recently isolated member of the pancreatic polypeptide family (Tatemoto, 1982a,b). In the brain, NPY is one of the most highly concentrated peptides. It is widely distributed but found especially in hypothalamic and cortical areas (Adrian et al., 1983; Allen et al., 1983; Chronwall et al., 1985; O'Donohue et al., 1985). NPY induces various biological effects including stimulation of feeding behavior (Clark et al., 1984; Levine and Morley, 1984; Stanley and Leibowitz, 1984), alteration of the release of pituitary hormones (Kalra and Crowley, 1984; O'Donohue et al., 1985), and modulation of the central regulation of cardiovascular parameters (Lundberg and Tatemoto, 1982; Lundberg et al., 1984). Moreover, the colocalization of NPY and catecholamines in various noradrenergic and adrenergic cell groups suggests important functions for this peptide in the control of the autonomic nervous system (O'Donohue et al., 1985; Emson and DeQuidt, 1984). Thus, the high concentrations of NPY in multiple brain regions and its various biological effects strongly suggest the existence of specific receptors for this peptide in the CNS.

4.1. Brain NPY Receptors

The multiple actions of NPY in the brain are most likely initiated by binding to high-affinity receptor sites. To date, only a few reports have described the existence of such sites using membrane binding assays (Unden and Bartfai, 1984; Unden et al., 1985; Chang et al., 1985; Saria et al., 1985). Recently, we have demonstrated the presence in rat brain of highly specific NPY receptor binding sites using in vitro receptor autoradiography (Martel et al., 1986).

Our data clearly demonstrated the existence of high-affinity binding sites for either [³H]-NPY or [¹²⁵I]-BH NPY in rat brain. The relative potency of various NPY homologues, fragments, and analogues in the binding assays correlates well with their respective activity in peripheral bioassays (Martel et al., 1986). This strongly suggests that NPY receptors possess similar structural requirements in brain and peripheral tissues. However, the possible existence of other receptor classes for related peptides such as polypeptide YY or the pancreatic polypeptide cannot be excluded at the present time (Martel et al., 1986).

The autoradiographic distribution of NPY receptor binding sites is unique (Fig. 5; Martel et al., 1986). Very high densities of NPY binding sites are found in the hippocampus, especially in the oriens layer and stratum radiatum (Fig. 5). Other areas enriched in NPY binding sites include the superficial layers of the cortex, anterior olfactory nucleus, lateral septum, stria terminalis, various thalamic nuclei, substantia nigra, VTA, lateral geniculate nucleus, and area postrema. Moderate densities of sites are seen in the olfactory tubercle, certain hypothalamic nuclei, medial geniculate nuclei, inferior colliculus, and inferior olive. Low to moderate densities of sites are present in the striatum (Fig. 5), amygdala, and spinal cord. Low densities are observed in most hypothalamic nuclei, globus pallidus, superior colliculus, and cerebellum (Fig. 5).

4.2. Possible Relevance to Function

The respective distribution of NPY receptor binding sites and NPY-like immunoreactivity demonstrates striking similarities and differences (mismatch) (Martel et al., 1986; Chronwall et

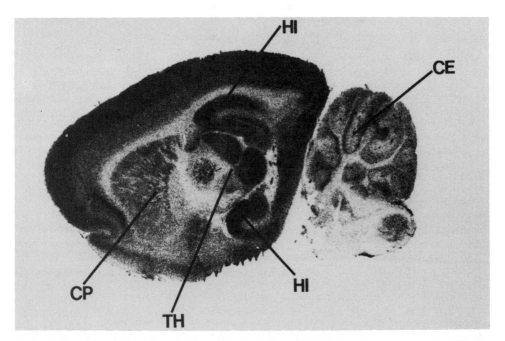

Figure 5. Photomicrograph of the autoradiographic distribution of [¹²⁵I]-Bolton–Hunter neuropeptide Y binding sites in the rat brain (sagittal section). The incubation was performed as described by Martel *et al.* (1986). CE, cerebellum; CP, caudate–putamen; HI, hippocampus; TH, thalamus.

al., 1985). Such observations are generalized and have been reported for various neuropeptides, monoamines, and amino acids (Quirion *et al.*, 1983a; Kuhar, 1985; Herkenham and McLean, 1986). Various hypotheses have been proposed to explain these mismatches including the existence of multiple receptor classes, the lack of correspondence between binding sites and physiologically relevant receptors, the lack of sensitivity of immunohistochemical techniques, the diffusion of endogenous ligands from their site of release to reach target sites, the plasticity of receptor expressions, and so on. However, in the case of NPY as for many others, our current knowledge on the processing of the NPY precursor, as well as the possible release of other active peptides from this precursor, is very limited. The development of better ligands (high-affinity agonists and antagonists) might help to resolve these apparent mismatches, which may disappear with improved techniques.

In any case, the high densities of NPY receptor binding sites present in the hippocampus, cortex, and septum could indicate that this peptide has an important modulatory role on cholinergic innervation. It is well known that these brain regions are enriched in cholinergic cell bodies and nerve fiber terminals and this could be most relevant in relation to possible roles of NPY in higher cognitive functions and pathologies such as Alzheimer's disease. Already, several reports have shown that the cortical distribution of NPY-like immunoreactivity is altered in this disease (Chan-Palay *et al.*, 1985; Emson and DeQuidt, 1984; O'Donohue *et al.*, 1985). Thus, further studies on the effects of NPY on cholinergic innervation are certainly most relevant. Moreover, it has recently been shown that NPY modulates excitatory transmission in the hippocampus via a presynaptic mechanism (Colmers *et al.*, 1985) and the possible participation of the cholinergic innervation to that effect should be carefully monitored.

The high densities of NPY receptor binding sites in brain regions involved in the central regulation of cardiovascular parameters such as the area postrema suggest that NPY could modulate these functions. Already, it has been shown that NPY induces cardiovascular effects following central and peripheral injections (Lundberg *et al.*, 1984; Lundberg and Tatemoto, 1982; O'Donohue *et al.*, 1985).

In summary, brain NPY receptor sites are widely distributed with high densities of sites being present in cortical, hippocampal, and thalamic areas. However, the precise significance and role of these NPY receptors in the brain remain to be determined.

5. Conclusion

An ever-increasing diversity of neuropeptides is being demonstrated by recent work. Using approaches such as immunohistochemistry, *in situ* hybridization, and retrograde tracing methods, it has been possible to establish with more or less certainty (depending on each peptide family) the anatomical distribution and detailed organization of various peptidergic systems. The recent development of autoradiographic approaches to characterize the precise distribution of neuropeptide receptor sites has generated much interest and has already indicated new avenues for investigation. In this brief review, I have given a few examples that demonstrate the usefulness of this approach in revealing directions for further research, either electrophysiological, neurochemical, and/or behavioral. Naturally, brain functions for any given neuropeptide cannot be solely based on the distribution of its receptors. However, that distribution certainly constitutes a most valuable and powerful piece of information that generates multiple hypotheses on the possible roles of peptides in the CNS.

ACKNOWLEDGMENTS. This research was supported by the Medical Research Council of Canada and the Scottish Rite Foundation for Research on Schizophrenia (USA). The author is Chercheur-Boursier of the Fonds de la recherche en santé du Québec. The expert secretarial assistance of Mrs. Joan Currie and Mrs. Dawn Vetro is acknowledged.

References

Adrian, T. E., Allen, J. M., Bloom, S. R., Ghatei, M. A., Rossor, M. N., Roberts, G. W., Crow, T. J., Tatemoto, K., and Polak, J. M., 1983, Neuropeptide Y distribution in human brain, *Nature* **306**:584–586.

Akil, H., Watson, S. J., Young, E., Lewis, M. E., Khachaturian, H., and Walker, J. M., 1984, Endogenous opioids: Biology and function, *Annu. Rev. Neurosci.* **7**:223–255.

Allen, Y. S., Adrian, T. E., Allen, J. M., Tatemoto, K., Crow, T. J., Bloom, S. R., and Polak, J. M., 1983, Neuropeptide Y distribution in the rat brain, *Science* **221**:877–879.

Antunes-Rodrigues, A., McCann, S. M., Rogers, L. C., and Samson, W. K., 1985, Atrial natriuretic factor inhibits dehydration and angiotensin II-induced water intake in the conscious, unrestrained rat, *Proc. Natl. Acad. Sci. USA* **82**:8720–8723.

Baruch, P., Petit, F., Artaud, F., Basbeits, L., Godeheu, G., Cheramy, A., and Glowinski, J., 1987, Effects of tachykinins on dopamine release in the striatum: In vitro and in vivo studies, in: *Substance P and Neurokinins* (J. Henry, R. Couture, A. C. Cuello, G. Pelletier, R. Quirion, and D. Regoli, eds.), Springer-Verlag, Berlin pp. 308–310.

Baxter, C. R., Horvath, J. S., Duggin, G. G., and Tiller, D. J., 1980, Effect of age on specific angiotensin II-binding sites in rat brain, *Endocrinology* **106**:995–999.

Beaujouan, J. C., Torrens, Y., Viger, A., and Glowinski, J., 1984, A new type of tachykinin binding sites in the rat brain characterized by specific binding of a labelled eledoisin derivative, *Mol. Pharmacol.* **26**:248–254.

Bennett, J. P., and Snyder, S. H., 1976, Angiotensin II binding to mammalian brain membranes, *J. Biol. Chem.* **251**:7423–7430.

Brownstein, M. J., Mroz, E. A., Kizer, J. S., Palkovits, M., and Leeman, S. E., 1976, Regional distribution of substance P in the brain of the rat, *Brain Res.* **116**:299–305.

Brownstein, M. J., Mroz, E. A., Tappaz, M. L., and Leeman, S. E., 1977, On the origin of substance P and glutamic acid decarboxylase (GAD) in the substantia nigra, *Brain Res.* **135**:315–323.

Buck, S. H., Burcher, E., Shults, C. W., Lovenberg, W., and O'Donohue, T. L., 1984, Novel pharmacology of substance K binding sites: A third type of tachykinin receptor, *Science* **226**:987–989.

Burcher, E., Buck, S., Lovenberg, W., and O'Donohue, T. L., 1986, Characterization and autoradiographic localization of multiple tachykinin binding sites in gastrointestinal tract and bladder, *J. Pharmacol. Exp. Ther.* **236**:819–831.

Cantin, M., and Genest, J., 1985, The heart and the atrial natriuretic factor, *Endocrine Rev.* **6**:107–127.

Cascieri, M. A., and Liang, T., 1983, Characterization of the substance P receptor in rat brain cortex membranes and the inhibition of radioligand binding by guanine nucleotides, *J. Biol. Chem.* **258**:5158–5164.

Cascieri, M. A., and Liang, T., 1984, Binding of [^{125}I]Bolton–Hunter conjugated eledoisin to rat brain cortex membranes: Evidence for two classes of tachykinin receptors in the mammalian central nervous system, *Life Sci.* **35**:179–184.

Chang, M. S., and Leeman, S. E., 1970, Isolation of sialogogic peptide from bovine hypothalamic tissue and its characterization as substance P, *J. Biol. Chem.* **245**:4784–4790.

Chang, R. S. L., Lotti, V. J., Chen, T. B., Cerino, D. J., and Kling, P. J., 1985, Neuropeptide Y (NPY) binding sites in rat brain labeled with ^{125}I-Bolton–Hunter NPY: Comparative potencies of various polypeptides on brain NPY binding and biological responses in the rat vas deferens, *Life Sci.* **37**:2111–2122.

Chan-Palay, V., Lang, W., Allen, Y. S., Haesler, U., and Polak, J. M., 1985, II. Cortical neurons immunoreactive with antisera against neuropeptide Y are altered in Alzheimer's type dementia, *J. Comp. Neurol.* **238**:390–400.

Cheramy, A., Nieoullon, A., Michelot, R., and Glowinski, J., 1977, Effects of intranigral application of dopamine and substance P on the in vivo release of newly synthesized [^{3}H]dopamine in the ipsilateral caudate nucleus of the cat, *Neurosci. Lett.* **5**:105–109.

Chronwall, B. M., DiMaggio, D. A., Massari, V. J., Pickel, V. M., Ruggiero, D. A., and O'Donohue, T. L., 1985, The anatomy of neuropeptide Y containing neurons in rat brain, *Neuroscience* **15**:1159–1181.

Clark, J. T., Kalra, P. S., Crowley, W. R., and Kalra, S. P., 1984, Neuropeptide Y and human pancreatic polypeptide stimulates feeding behavior in rats, *Endocrinology* **115**:427–429.

Colmers, W. F., Lukowiak, K., and Pittman, Q. J., 1985, Neuropeptide Y reduces orthodromically evoked population spike in rat hippocampal CA1 by a possibly presynaptic mechanism, *Brain Res.* **346**:404–408.

Cuello, A. C., and Kanazawa, I., 1978, The distribution of substance P immunoreactive fibers in the rat central nervous system, *J. Comp. Neurol.* **178**:129–156.

Dam, T. V., and Quirion, R., 1986, Characterization of substance P receptors in guinea pig brain, *Peptides* **7**:855–864.

Deutch, A. Y., Maggio, J. E., Bannon, M. J., Kalivas, P. W., Tam, S. Y., Goldstein, M., and Roth, R. H., 1985, Substance K and substance P differentially modulate mesolimbic and mesocortical systems, *Peptides,* Suppl. 2, **6**:113–122.

Emson, P. C., and DeQuidt, M. E., 1984, NPY—a new member of the pancreatic polypeptide family, *Trends Neurosci.* **7**:31–35.

Felix, D., and Akert, K., 1974, The effect of angiotensin II on neurones of the cat subfornical organ, *Brain Res.* **76**:350–353.

Fitts, D. A., Thunhorst, R. L., and Simpson, J. R., 1985, Diuresis and reduction of salt appetite by lateral ventricular infusions of atriopeptin II, *Brain Res.* **348**:118–124.

Fitzsimmons, J. T., 1979, *The Physiology of Thirst and Sodium Appetite,* Cambridge University Press, London.

Friedl, A., Harmening, C., and Hamprecht, B., 1986, Atrial natriuretic hormone raises the level of cyclic GMP in neural cell lines, *J. Neurochem.* **46**:1522–1527.

Gehlert, D. R., Speth, R. C., and Wamsley, J. K., 1984, Autoradiographic localization of angiotensin II receptors in the rat brain and kidney, *Eur. J. Pharmacol.* **98**:145–146.

Gibson, T. R., Widley, G. M., Manaker, S., and Glembotski, C. C., 1986, Autoradiographic localization and characterization of atrial natriuretic peptide binding sites in the rat central nervous system and adrenal gland, *J. Neurosci.* **6**:2004–2011.

Hamet, P., Tremblay, J., Pang, S. C., Garcia, R., Thibault, G., Gutkowska, J., Cantin, M., and Genest, J., 1984, Effect of native and synthetic atrial natriuretic factor on cyclic GMP, *Biochem. Biophys. Res. Commun.* **123**:515–527.

Hanson, G. R., Alphis, L., Wolf, W., Levine, R., and Lovenberg, W., 1981, Haloperidol-induced reduction of nigral substance P-like immunoreactivity: A probe for the interactions between dopamine and substance P neuronal systems, *J. Pharmacol. Exp. Ther.* **218**:568–574.

Harding, J. W., Stone, L. P., and Wright, J. W., 1981, The distribution of angiotensin II binding sites in rodent brain, *Brain Res.* **205**:265–274.

Henry, J. L., 1977, Substance P and pain: A possible relation in afferent transmission, in: *Substance P, Nobel Symposium 37* (U.S. von Euler and B. Pernow, eds.), Raven Press, New York, pp. 231–240.

Herkenham, M., and McLean, S., 1986, Mismatches between receptor and transmitter localizations in the brain, in: *Quantitative Receptor Autoradiography* (C. Boast, E. W. Snowhill, and C. A. Altar, eds.), Liss, New York, pp. 137–171.

Hong, J. S., Yang, H. Y. T., and Costa, E., 1979, Substance P content of substantia nigra after chronic treatment with antischizophrenic drugs, *Neuropharmacology* **17**:83–85.

Hunter, J. C., and Maggio, J. E., 1984, Pharmacological characterization of a novel tachykinin isolated from mammalian spinal cord, *Eur, J. Pharmacol.* **97**:159–160.

Innis, R. B., Andrade, R., and Aghajanian, G. K., 1985, Substance K excites dopaminergic and non-dopaminergic neurons in rat substantia nigra, *Brain Res.* **335**:381–383.

Jonsson, G., and Hallman, H., 1982a, Substance P counteracts neurotoxin damage on norepinephrine neurons in rat brain during ontogeny, *Science* **215**:75–77.

Jonsson, G., and Hallman, H., 1982b, Substance P modifies the 6-hydroxydopamine induced alteration of postnatal development of central noradrenaline neurons, *Neuroscience* **7**:2909–2918.

Jonsson, G., and Hallman, H., 1983a, Effect of substance P on the 5,7-dihydroxytryptamine induced alteration of postnatal development of central serotonin neurons, *Med. Biol.* **61**:105–112.

Jonsson, G., and Hallman, H., 1983b, Effect of substance P on neonatally axotomized noradrenaline neurons in rat brain, *Med. Biol.* **61**:179–185.

Kalivas, T. W., Deutch, A. Y., Maggio, J. E., Mantyh, P. W., and Roth, R. H., 1985, Substance K and substance P in the ventral tegmental area, *Neurosci. Lett.* **57**:241–246.

Kalra, S. P., and Crowley, W. R., 1984, Norepinephrine-like effects of neuropeptide Y on LH release in the rat, *Life Sci.* **35**:1173–1176.

Kangawa, K., Minamino, N., Fukuda, A., and Matsuo, H., 1983, Neuromedin K: A novel mammalian tachykinin identified in porcine spinal cord, *Biochem. Biophys. Res. Commun.* **114**:533–540.

Katsuura, G., Nakamura, M., Inouye, K., Kono, M., Nakao, K., and Imura, H., 1986, Regulatory role of atrial natriuretic polypeptide in water drinking in rats, *Eur. J. Pharmacol.* **121**:285–287.

Kawata, M., Nakao, K., Norii, N., Kiso, Y., Yamashita, H., Imura, H., and Sano, Y., 1985, Atrial natriuretic polypeptide: Topographical distribution in the rat brain by radioimmunoassay and immunohistochemistry, *Neuroscience* **16**:521–546.

Kelley, A. E., and Iversen, S. D., 1978, Behavioural response to bilateral injections of substance P into the substantia nigra, *Brain Res.* **158**:474–478.

Kelley, A. E., and Iversen, S. D., 1979, Substance P infusion into substantia nigra of the rat: Behavioural analysis and involvement of striatal dopamine, *Eur. J. Pharmacol.* **60**:171–179.

Kelley, A. E., Stinus, L., and Iversen, S. D., 1979, Behavioural activation induced in the rat by substance P infusion into ventral tegmental area: Implication of dopaminergic A10 neurones, *Neurosci. Lett.* **11**:335–339.

Kimura, S., Okada, M., Sugita, Y., Kanazawa, I., and Munekata, E., 1984, Novel neuropeptides, neurokinin α and β, isolated from porcine spinal cord, *Proc. Jpn. Acad. Ser. B* **59**:101–104.

Kuhar, M. J., 1985, The mismatch problem in receptor mapping studies, *Trends Neurosci.* **8**:190–191.

Lang, R. E., Unger, T., Rascher, W., and Ganten, D., 1983, Brain angiotensin, in: *Handbook of Psychopharmacology*, Vol. 16 (L. L. Iversen, S. D. Iversen, and S. H. Snyder, eds.), Plenum Press, New York, pp. 307–361.

Lee, C. M., Iversen, L. L., Hanley, M. R., and Sandberg, B. E. B., 1982, The possible existence of multiple receptors for substance P, *Naunyn-Schmiedebergs Arch. Pharmacol.* **318**:281–287.

Levine, A. S., and Morley, J. E., 1984, A potent inducer of consummatory behavior in rats, *Peptides* **5**:1025–1030.

Lind, R. W., Swanson, L. W., and Ganten, D., 1985, Organization of angiotensin II immunoreactive cells and fibers in the rat central nervous system, *Neuroendocrinology* **40**:2–24.

Lindefors, N., Brodin, E., and Ungerstedt, U., 1986, Neuroleptic treatment induces region-specific changes in the levels of neurokinin A and substance P in rat brain, *Neuropeptides* **7**:265–280.

Ljungdahl, Å., Hökfelt, T., and Nilsson, G., 1978, Distribution of substance P-like immunoreactivity in the central nervous system of the rat. I. Cell bodies and nerve terminals, *Neuroscience* **3**:861–943.

Lundberg, J. M., and Tatemoto, K., 1982, Pancreatic polypeptide family (APP, BPP, NPY and PYY) in relation to sympathetic vasoconstriction resistant to α-adrenoreceptor blockade, *Acta Physiol. Scand.* **116**:393–402.

Lundberg, J. M., Hua, S. Y., and Franco-Cereceda, A., 1984, Effects of neuropeptide Y (NPY) on mechanical activity and neurotransmission in the heart, vas deferens and urinary bladder of the guinea-pig, *Acta Physiol. Scand.* **121**:325–332.

Lynch, D. R., Braas, K. M., and Snyder, S. H., 1986, Atrial natriuretic factors in rat kidney, adrenal gland, and brain: Autoradiographic localization and fluid balance dependent changes, *Proc. Natl. Acad. Sci USA* **83**:3357–3361.

McQuade, P. S., Richard, J. W., Thakur, M. T., and Quirion, R., 1986, The effect of tyrosine hydroxylase inhibition on the changes produced in dopamine metabolism by substance P, Abstracts, *Substance P and Neurokinins,* Montreal, p. 46.

Maggio, J. E., and Hunter, J. C., 1984, Regional distribution of kassinin-like immunoreactivity in rat central and peripheral tissues and the effect of capsaicin, *Brain Res.* **307**:370–373.

Maggio, J. E., Sandberg, B. E. B., Bradley, C. V., Iversen, L. L., Santikarn, S., Williams, B. H., Hunter, J. C., and Hanley, M. R., 1983, Substance K: A novel tachykinin in mammalian spinal cord, in: *Substance P* (P. Skrabanek and D. Powell, eds.), Boole Press, Dublin, pp. 20–21.

Mangiapane, M. L., Thrasher, T. N., Keil, L. C., Simpson, J. B., and Ganong, W. F., 1983, Deficits in drinking and vasopressin secretion after lesions of the nucleus medianus, *Neuroendocrinology* **37**:73–77.

Mantyh, C. R., Brecha, N. C., Kruger, L., and Mantyh, P. W., 1985, Autoradiographic localization of atrial natriuretic factor binding sites in the periphery and central nervous system of the rat and guinea pig, *Soc. Neurosci. Abstr.* **11**:189.

Mantyh, P. W., Hunt, S. P., and Maggio, J. E., 1984a, Substance P receptors: Localization by light microscopic autoradiography in rat brain using [³H]SP as the radioligand, *Brain Res.* **307**:147–165.

Mantyh, P. W., Maggio, J. E., and Hunt, S. P., 1984b, The autoradiographic distribution of kassinin and substance K binding sites is different from the distribution of substance P binding sites in rat brain, *Eur. J. Pharmacol.* **102**:361–364.

Martel, J. C., St-Pierre, S., and Quirion, R., 1986, Neuropeptide Y receptors in rat brain: Autoradiographic localization, *Peptides* **7**:55–60.

Mendelsohn, F. A. O., Aguilera, G., Saavedra, J. M., Quirion, R., and Catt, K. J., 1983, Characteristics and regulation of angiotensin II receptors in pituitary, circumventricular organs and kidney, *Clin. Exp. Hypertens.* A5, 1081–1097.

Mendelsohn, F. A. O., Quirion, R., Saavedra, J. M., Aguilera, G., and Catt, K. J., 1984a, Autoradiographic localization of angiotensin II receptors in rat brain, *Proc. Natl. Acad. Sci. USA* **81**:1575–1579.

Mendelsohn, F. A. O., Quirion, R., Aguilera, G., and Catt, K. J., 1984b, Localization of angiotensin II receptors in rat brain and kidney by autoradiography, in: *Receptors, Membranes and Transport Mechanisms in Medicine* (A. E. Doyle and F. A. O. Mendelsohn, eds.), Elsevier, Amsterdam, pp. 13–25.

Michelot, R., Leviel, V., Giorguieff-Chesselet, M. F., Cheramy, A., and Glowinski, J., 1979, Effects of the unilateral nigral modulation of substance P transmission on the activity of the two nigro-striatal pathways, *Life Sci.* **24**:715–724.

Nakai, K., and Kasamatsu, T., 1984, Accelerated regeneration of central catecholamine fibers in cat occipital cortex: Effects of substance P, *Brain Res.* **323**:374–379.

Nakamura, M., Katsuura, G., Nakao, K., and Imura, H., 1985, Antidipsogenic action of α-human atrial natriuretic polypeptide administered intracerebroventricularly in rats, *Neurosci. Lett.* **5**:1–6.

Nakamura, M., Takayanegi, R., and Inagami, T., 1986, Effect of atrial natriuretic factor on central angiotensin II-induced response in rats, *Peptides* **7**:373–375.

Narumi, S., and Fujita, T., 1978, Stimulatory effects of substance P and nerve growth factor (NGF) on neurite outgrowth in embryonic chick dorsal root ganglia, *Neuropharmacology* **17**:73–76.

Narumi, S., and Maki, Y., 1978, Stimulatory effects of substance P on neurite extension and cyclic AMP levels in cultured neuroblastoma cells, *J. Neurochem.* **30**:1321–1326.

Nawa, H., Hirose, T., Takashima, H., Inayama, S., and Nakanishi, S., 1983, Nucleotide sequences of cloned cDNAs for two types of bovine brain substance P precursor, *Nature* **206**:32–36.

Nawa, H., Doteuchi, M., Igano, K., Inouye, K., and Nakanishi, S., 1984a, Substance K: A novel mammalian tachykinin that differs from substance P in its pharmacological profile, *Life Sci.* **34**:1153–1160.

Nawa, H., Kotani, H., and Nakanishi, S., 1984b, Tissue-specific generation of two preprotachykinin mRNAs from one gene by alternative RNA splicing, *Nature* **312**:729–734.

Nilsson, J., von Euler, A. M., and Dalsgaard, C. J., 1985, Stimulation of connective tissue cell growth by substance P and substance K, *Nature* **315**:61–63.

Ninkovic, M., Beaujouan, J. C., Torrens, Y., Saffroy, M., Hall, M. D., and Glowinski, J., 1985, Differential localization of tachykinin receptors in rat spinal cord, *Eur. J. Pharmacol.* **106**:463–464.

Oblin, A., Zivkovic, B., and Bartholini, G., 1984, Involvement of the D-2 dopamine receptor in the neuroleptic induced decrease in nigral substance P, *Eur. J. Pharmacol.* **105**:175–177.

O'Donohue, T. L., Shults, C. W., Quirion, R., Moody, T. W., Wolf, S. S., Jensen, R. T., and Chase, T. N., 1983, Autoradiographic localization of substance P (SP) receptors in rat brain: Anatomical comparison of the localization of SP receptors and SP, in: *Substance P* (P. Skrabranek and D. Powell, eds.), Boole Press, Dublin, pp. 57–58.

O'Donohue, T. L., Chronwall, B. M., Pruss, R. M., Mezey, J., Kiss, Z., Eiden, L. E., Massari, V. J., Tossel, R. E., Pickel, V. M., DiMaggio, D. A., Hotchkiss, A. J., Crowley, W. R., and Zukowska-Grojec, Z., 1985, Neuropeptide Y and peptide YY neuronal and endocrine systems, *Peptides* **6**:755–768.

Park, C. H., Massari, V. J., Quirion, R., Tizabi, Y., Shults, C. W., and O'Donohue, T. L., 1984, Characterization of ^{3}H-substance P binding sites in rat brain membranes, *Peptides* **5**:833–836.

Pernow, B., 1983, Substance P, *Pharmacol. Rev.* **35**:85–141.

Phillips, M. I., Quinlan, J., Keyser, C., and Phipps, J., 1978, Organum vasculosum of the lamina terminalis (OVLT) as a receptor site for ADH release, drinking and blood pressure responses to angiotensin II (AII), *Fed. Proc. Fed. Am. Soc. Exp. Biol.* **28**:438–442.

Quirion, R., 1984, Pain, nociception and spinal opioid receptors, *Prog. Neuro-Psychopharmacol. Biol. Psychiatry* **8**:571–579.

Quirion, R., 1985, Multiple tachykinin receptors, *Trends Neurosci.* **8**:183–185.

Quirion, R., and Dam, T. V., 1985a, Multiple tachykinin receptors in guinea pig brain: High densities of substance K(neurokinin A) binding sites in substantia nigra, *Neuropeptides* **6**:191–204.

Quirion, R., and Dam, T. V., 1985b, Multiple tachykinin and substance P receptors, in: *Substance P: Metabolism and Biological Actions* (C.C. Jordan and P. Oehme, eds.), Taylor & Francis, London, pp. 45–64.

Quirion, R., and Dam, T. V., 1986, Ontogeny of substance P receptor binding sites in rat brain, *J. Neurosci.* **6**:2187–2199.

Quirion, R., and Pilapil, C., 1984, Comparative potencies of substance P, substance K and neuromedin K on brain substance P receptors, *Neuropeptides* **4**:325–329.

Quirion, R., Shults, C. W., Moody, T. W., Pert, C. B., Chase, T. B., and O'Donohue, T. L., 1983a, Autoradiographic distribution of substance P receptors in rat central nervous system, *Nature* **303**:714–716.

Quirion, R., Shults, C.W., Moody, T. W., Wolf, S. S., Jensen, R. T., Pert, C. B., Chase, T. B., and O'Donohue, T. L., 1983b, Autoradiographic localization of substance P (SP) receptors in rat brain: A comparison of binding properties of [^{3}H]SP, [^{125}I]SP and [^{125}I]physalaemin, in: *Substance P* (P. Skrabranek and D. Powell, eds.), Boole Press, Dublin, pp. 55–56.

Quirion, R., Weiss, A. S., and Pert, C. B., 1983c, Comparative pharmacological properties and autoradiographic distribution of [^{3}H]ethylketocyclazocine binding sites in rat and guinea pig brain, *Life Sci.* **33**:183–186.

Quirion, R., Dalpé, M., DeLean, A., Gutkowska, J., Cantin, M., and Genest, J., 1984, Atrial natriuretic factor (ANF) binding sites in brain and related structures, *Peptides* **5**:1167–1172.

Quirion, R., Dalpé, M., and Dam, T. V., 1986, Characterization and distribution of receptors for the atrial natriuretic peptides in mammalian brain, *Proc. Natl. Acad. Sci. USA* **83**:174–178.

Quirion, R., Mount, H., Dam, T. V., Boksa, P., Buck, S. H., Burcher, E., and O'Donohue, T. L., 1987, Neurokinin receptors in human brain, in: *Substance P and Neurokinins* (J. Henry, R. Couture, A. C. Cuello, G. Pelletier, R. Quirion, and D. Regoli, eds.), Springer-Verlag, Berlin, pp. 96–98.

Quirion, R., Dalpe, M., and Delean, A., 1988, Characterization, distribution, and plasticity of atrial natriuretic factor binding sites in brain, *Can. J. Physiol. Pharmacol.*, (in press).

Regoli, D., Escher, E., and Mizrahi, J., 1984, Substance P—Structure–activity studies and the development of antagonists, *Pharmacology* **28**:301–320.

Renaud, L. P., and Padjen, A., 1978, in: *Centrally Acting Peptides* (J. Hughes, ed.), University Park Press, Baltimore, pp. 59–84.

Rothman, R.B., Herkenham, M., Pert, C. B., Liang, T., and Cascieri, M. A., 1984a, Visualization of rat brain receptors for the neuropeptide substance P, *Brain Res.* **309**:47–54.

Rothman, R. B., Danks, J. A., Herkenham, M., Cascieri, M. A., Chicchi, G. G., Liang, T., and Pert, C. B., 1984b, Autoradiographic localization of a novel peptide binding site in rat brain using the substance P analog, eledoisin, *Neuropeptides* **5**:343–349.

Saavedra, J. M., Correa, F. M. A., Plunkett, L. M., Israel, A., Kurihara, M., and Shigematsu, K., 1986, Binding of angiotensin and atrial natriuretic peptide in brain of hypertensive rats, *Nature* **320**:758–760.

Sakai, K. K., Marks, G. H., George, J., and Koestner, A., 1974, Specific angiotensin II receptors in organ-cultured canine supraoptic nucleus cells, *Life Sci.* **14**:1337–1344.

Samson, W. K., 1985, Atrial natriuretic factor inhibits dehydration and hemorrhage-induced vasopressin release, *Neuroendocrinology* **40**:277–279.

Saria, A., Theodorsson-Norheim, E., and Lundberg, J. M., 1985, Evidence for specific neuropeptide Y binding sites in rat brain synaptosomes, *Eur. J. Pharmacol.* **107**:105–107.

Shults, C. W., Quirion, R., Jensen, R. T., Moody, T. W., O'Donohue, T. L., and Chase, T. N., 1982, Autoradiographic localization of substance P receptors using [^{125}I]substance P, *Peptides* **3**:1073–1075.

Shults, C. W., Quirion, R., Cornwall, B., Chase, T. N., and O'Donohue, T. L., 1984, A comparison of the anatomical distribution of substance P and substance P receptors in the rat central nervous system, *Peptides* **5**:1097–1128.

Shults, C. W., Buck, S. H., Burcher, E., Chase, T. N., and O'Donohue, T. L., 1985a, Distinct binding sites for substance P and neurokinin A in rat brain, *Peptides* **6**:343–345.

Shults, C. W., Yajima, H., Gullner, H. G., Chase, T. N., and O'Donohue, T. L., 1985b, Demonstration and distribution of kassinin-like material (substance K) in the rat central nervous system, *J. Neurochem.* **45**:552–558.

Sills, M. A., Nguyen, K. Q., and Jacobowitz, D. M., 1985, Increases in heart rate and blood pressure produced by microinjections of atrial natriuretic factor into the AV3V region of rat brain, *Peptides* **6**:1037–1042.

Simpson, J. B., 1980, The circumventricular organs and the central actions of angiotension, *Neuroendocrinology* **32**:248–256.

Sirett, N. E., McLean, A. S., Bray, J. J., and Hubbard, J. I., 1977, Distribution of angiotensin II receptors in rat brain, *Brain Res.* **122**:299–312.

Skofitsch, G., Jacobowitz, D. M., Eskay, R. L., and Zamir, N., 1985, Distribution of atrial natriuretic factor-like immunoreactive neurons in the rat brain, *Neuroscience* **16**:917–948.

Stanley, B. G., and Leibowitz, S. P., 1984, Neuropeptide Y: Stimulation of feeding and drinking by injection into the paraventricular nucleus, *Life Sci.* **35**:2635–2642.

Stinus, L., Kelley, A. E., and Iversen, S. D., 1978, Increased spontaneous activity following substance P infusion into A10 dopaminergic area, *Nature* **276**:616–618.

Takano, Y., Takeda, Y., Yamada, K., and Kamiya, H., 1985, Substance K, a novel tachykinin injected bilaterally into the ventral tegmental area of rats increases behavioral response, *Life Sci.* **37**:2507–2514.

Takayanagi, R., Grammer, R. T., and Inagami, T., 1986, Regional increase of cyclic GMP by atrial natriuretic factor in rat brain: Markedly elevated response in spontaneously hypertensive rats, *Life Sci.* **39**:573–580.

Tanaka, I., and Inagami, T., 1986, Release of immunoreactive atrial natriuretic factor from rat hypothalamus in vitro, *Eur. J. Pharmacol.* **122**:353–356.

Tatemoto, K., 1982a, Isolation and characterization of peptide YY (PYY), a candidate gut hormone that inhibits pancreatic exocrine secretion, *Proc. Natl. Acad. Sci. USA* **79**:2514–2518.

Tatemoto, K., 1982b, Neuropeptide Y: Complete amino acid sequence of the brain peptide, *Proc. Natl. Acad. Sci. USA* **79**:5485–5489.

Torrens, Y., Beaujouan, J. C., Viger, A., and Glowinski, J., 1983, Properties of a ^{125}I-substance P derivative binding to synaptosomes from various brain structures and the spinal cord of the rat, *Naunyn-Schmiedebergs Arch. Pharmacol.* **324**:134–139.

Torrens, Y., Lavielle, S., Chassaing, G., Marquet, A., Glowinski, J., and Beaujouan, J. C., 1984, Neuromedin K, a tool to further distinguish two central tachykinin binding sites, *Eur. J. Pharmacol.* **102**:381–382.

Unden, A., and Bartfai, T., 1984, Regulation of neuropeptide Y (NPY) binding by guanine nucleotides in the rat cerebral cortex, *FEBS Lett.* **177**:125–128.

Unden, A., Tatemoto, K., Mutt, V., and Bartfai, T., 1985, Neuropeptide Y receptor in the rat brain, *Eur. J. Biochem.* **145**:525–530.

Viger, A., Beaujouan, J. C., Torrens, Y., and Glowinski, J., 1983, Specific binding of a ^{125}I-substance P derivative to rat brain synaptosomes, *J. Neurochem.* **40:**1030–1039.

Waldmeier, P. C., Kam, R., and Stocklin, K., 1978, Increased dopamine metabolism in rat striatum after infusions of substance P into the substantia nigra, *Brain Res.* **159:**223–227.

Watson, S. P., 1984, Are the proposed substance P receptor sub-types, substance P receptors? *Life Sci.* **25:**797–808.

Wolf, S. S., Moody, T. W., Quirion, R., and O'Donohue, T. L., 1985, Biochemical characterization and autoradiographic localization of central substance P receptors using [^{125}I]physalaemin, *Brain Res.* **332:**299–307.

Wong, M., Samson, W. K., Dudley, C. A., and Moss, R. L., 1986, Direct neuronal action of atrial natriuretic factor in the rat brain, *Neuroendocrinology* **44:**49–53.

Yamada, T., Nakav, K., Morii, N., Itoh, H., Shiono, S., Sakamoti, M., Sugawara, A., Saito, Y., Ohno, H., Kanai, A., Katsuura, G., Eigyo, M., Matsushita, A., and Imura, H., 1986, Central effects of atrial natriuretic polypeptide on angiotensin II-stimulated vasopressin secretion in conscious rats, *Eur. J. Pharmacol.* **125:**453–457.

Zamir, N., Skofitsch, G., Eskay, R. L., and Jacobowitz, D. M., 1986, Distribution of atrial natriuretic peptides in the rat brain, *Brain Res.* **365:**105–111.

37

Increases in Potassium Conductance
Common Mechanisms of Opiate Action in Neurons of the Central Nervous System

Daniel V. Madison and Roger A. Nicoll

1. Introduction

In the past several years, many advances, most notably the discovery of opioid peptides and the widespread use of *in vitro* brain slice techniques, have accelerated the study of opiate action in the CNS. Since much of the work on the physiological actions of opiates has been done in the hippocampus and in the locus coeruleus (LC), this paper will concentrate on these areas, using other studies when useful for illustration.

2. Inhibitory Actions

In early studies of the actions of opiates in the CNS, the most common effect observed was an inhibition of spontaneous action potentials recorded extracellularly (see Duggan and North, 1983). An example, presented in Fig. 1, shows the extracellularly recorded discharge of a neocortical neuron. Application of the opioid peptide enkephalin caused a marked slowing of the discharge frequency. This inhibition could be seen both with spontaneous discharges and also when the neurons were stimulated to discharge with the excitatory amino acid glutamate, applied by iontophoresis (Nicoll *et al.*, 1977, 1980). Similar opiate-induced inhibitions of neuronal firing could be observed in a variety of brain regions although the sensitivity of neurons in these different regions varied considerably (Nicoll *et al.*, 1977). While it was generally believed that inhibition of neuronal firing by opiates was due to a direct effect on the inhibited neuron, because of the limitations of extracellular recording, the actual mechanism is unknown.

The LC, a small nucleus located in the dorsal pons, is the largest group of noradrenergic neurons in the brains of rat and other species, containing about half of all the noradrenergic cell

Daniel V. Madison • Department of Cellular and Molecular Physiology, University of California, San Francisco, California 94143. *Roger A. Nicoll* • Department of Pharmacology, University of California, San Francisco, California 94143. *Present address of D.V.M.:* Department of Physiology, Yale University School of Medicine, New Haven, Connecticut 06510

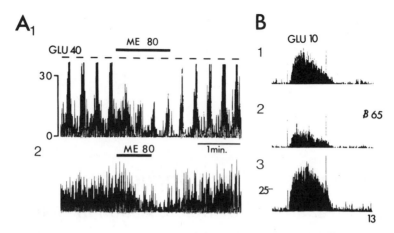

Figure 1. Opioid peptides inhibit neurons in the cerebral cortex. In A_1, methionine enkephalin (ME) inhibited the firing evoked by 40-nA ejection of glutamate from a multibarrel pipette. A_2 shows the inhibition of spontaneous firing in the same neuron. (B) Computer-generated histograms of responses evoked by glutamate. In B_2, β-endorphin was ejected during the construction of the histogram and inhibited the firing of the neuron. (From Nicoll, 1982.)

bodies in the brain. In addition, the LC has a very high density of opiate binding (Pert *et al.*, 1976). Extracellular *in vivo* recording from LC neurons indicated that opiates inhibit spontaneous action potential discharge (Korf *et al.*, 1974; Bird and Kuhar, 1977). Studies utilizing intracellular recording, particularly studies performed in the LC, have demonstrated a mechanism for opiate inhibition of CNS neurons.

Application of opiates or opioid peptides to *in vitro* slices of LC results in a large and reproducible hyperpolarization of the resting membrane potential of LC neurons (Pepper and Henderson, 1980; Williams *et al.*, 1982; North and Williams, 1985). The hyperpolarization is large enough to completely inhibit the spontaneous discharge of the neurons, and it is accompanied by a clear increase in membrane conductance (Fig. 2). This hyperpolarization is not reversed in chloride-injected cells. This suggests that opiates inhibit LC neuronal firing by an increase in resting potassium conductance. Consistent with this hypothesis is the finding that the opiate hyperpolarization can be blocked by treatments, such as barium application, which are known to block potassium currents. Confirmation of the idea that opiate inhibition of firing is caused by an increase in potassium conductance was obtained from the finding that the very negative reversal potential of the hyperpolarization (approximately -100 mV) shifts exactly as predicted by the Nernst equation when extracellular potassium concentrations are altered (North and Williams, 1985).

More recent work has dealt with the mechanism coupling the binding of a ligand to the opiate receptor and the opening of a potassium channel. In opening a potassium channel, opiates share a mechanism with another neurotransmitter, noradrenaline (NA), although the latter acts at the α_2 receptor specific for NA. While opiates and NA act on separate receptors to open potassium channels of the LC neuron, the amount of outward current generated by application of both NA and opiates together is no larger than that produced by either substance alone (Andrade and Aghajanian, 1985; North and Williams, 1985). This strongly suggests that the two putative transmitters share the same potassium channel.

It has recently been reported that the intraventricular injection of pertussis toxin, which disables the G_i and G_o subclasses of GTP binding proteins, blocks the action of both opiates and α_2 agonists (Aghajanian and Wang, 1986). This finding strongly suggests that a G protein is involved in the coupling of the receptor to the potassium channel. It is known in other systems that both opiates and α_2 agonists can decrease the levels of intracellular cAMP. Therefore, an inhibi-

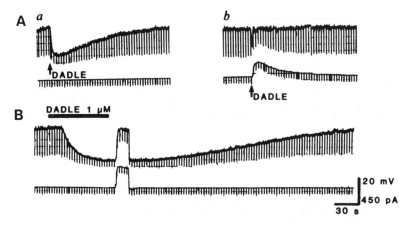

Figure 2. Enkephalin increases membrane conductance. The upper trace is the membrane potential (resting potential −67 mV); the lower trace is the transmembrane current passed by means of a bridge circuit. (A) DADLE was applied at the arrow by pressure [two 50-msec pulses, 35 kN/m² (5 psi)]. In a, DADLE hyperpolarized the membrane and reduced membrane resistance. In b, the DADLE hyperpolarization was annulled by passing inward current. (B) A similar experiment with superfusion of DADLE (1 μM) during the period indicated. The apparent delay in onset of the hyperpolarization is due to passage through the perfusion system. Restoration of the membrane potential to its control level allowed separation of the DADLE-induced resistance change and membrane rectification. (From Williams *et al.*, 1982.)

tion of adenylate cyclase might be the common step in the transduction mechanism. In support of such a mechanism, it has been reported that the responses to opiates and α_2 agonists were reversed by application of the membrane-permeant analogue of cAMP, 8-Br cAMP (Andrade and Aghajanian, 1985). On the other hand, forskolin, which stimulates adenylate cyclase and thereby increases intracellular cAMP directly, had no effect on the action of opiates (North and Williams, 1985). An attractive alternative mechanism comes from studies on muscarine inhibition of cardiac muscle. In this system, muscarinic receptor activation opens potassium channels by a pertussis toxin-sensitive and GTP-dependent mechanism (Pfaffinger *et al.*, 1985). Since diffusible second messenger systems do not appear to be involved in the response, these results suggest that the G protein may directly couple the receptor to the potassium channel. Results in hippocampal pyramidal cells also suggest that G proteins may directly link receptors to a potassium channel (Andrade *et al.*, 1986). In this system, serotonin and GABA$_B$ receptors share the same potassium channels by a mechanism that involves a G protein. In addition, known second messenger systems do not appear to be involved in the responses.

3. Disinhibitory Actions

While the action of opiates, leading to increased resting potassium conductance, is sufficient to account for their inhibitory action in many regions of the CNS, one region of the brain where opiate action is quite different is the hippocampus. Early studies indicated a strong excitatory action on the principal neurons of the hippocampus, the pyramidal cells (Nicoll *et al.*, 1977). While some later studies in the hippocampus were contradictory, the consensus is that opiates do indeed have a potent excitatory effect on pyramidal cells. This excitatory effect on extracellularly recorded firing is shown in Fig. 3. A large number of studies from several different laboratories have been aimed at determining the mechanism for this excitatory effect of opiates. These studies have been discussed in detail in a recent review (Corigall, 1983). Using extracellular recording,

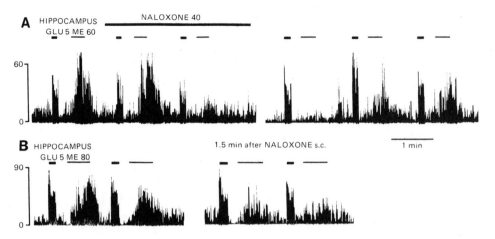

Figure 3. Naloxone antagonism of excitatory responses to the opioid peptides. (A) Iontophoresis of naloxone reversibly and selectively blocks the excitatory action of [Met⁵]enkephalin on a hippocampal neuron. The break in the record is 8.5 min. (B) A subcutaneous injection of naloxone (10 mg/kg) also selectively antagonizes the [Met⁵]enkephalin excitation of another hippocampal neuron. (From Nicoll *et al.*, 1977.)

Zieglgansberger *et al.* (1979) found that while the activity of pyramidal cells was increased by application of the opioid peptide enkephalin, the activity of presumed interneurons was decreased (see also Lee *et al.*, 1980). Thus, they proposed that the excitatory action of enkephalin might be indirect, i.e., that opiates excited pyramidal cells by the removal of the inhibitory influence of interneurons. A direct demonstration of this possibility was provided in a study from this laboratory (Nicoll *et al.*, 1980). Application of the stable enkephalin analogue D-Ala²-Met⁵-enkephalinamide (DALA) caused a large enhancement of the extracellularly recorded orthodromically elicited population spike. Since the population spike recorded in the pyramidal layer is a compound action potential, its amplitude gives an index of the number of pyramidal cells brought to threshold by an orthodromic stimulus. In addition to the increase in the amplitude of the population spike, DALA also caused the appearance of several additional population spikes following the initial single spike, a pattern not seen in the control (Fig. 4) (see also Dunwiddie *et al.*, 1980). Similar field potential profiles can be seen when hippocampal slices are treated with GABA antagonists, suggesting that multiple population spikes are produced in slices with impaired synaptic inhibition. Population spikes elicited by antidromic stimulation are unaffected by DALA, suggesting further that the effect of the opioid is on a synaptic pathway.

Intracellular recording from pyramidal neurons reveals that DALA application has a selective action on inhibitory transmission onto these neurons. Antidromic stimulation produces a single-phase IPSP, mediated by GABA, which causes an increase in somatic chloride conductance on the pyramidal cell (Alger and Nicoll, 1982a,b). Orthodromic stimulation produces a two-phase IPSP. The first phase is apparently identical to the IPSP produced by antidromic stimulation; it is GABA and chloride mediated. The second, slower phase of the IPSP is mediated by an increase in potassium conductance and has been referred to as the slow IPSP or the late hyperpolarizing potential (LHP) (Alger, 1984; Newberry and Nicoll, 1984, 1985). The slow IPSP is mediated by an increase in postsynaptic potassium conductance, a substantial portion of which may occur in the pyramidal cell dendritic region. Since the late IPSP is mimicked by application of the selective GABA$_B$ agonist baclofen, it is likely that it is also mediated by GABA acting at the GABA$_B$ receptor. Application of DALA reduces the amplitude of the antidromic IPSP and both phases of the orthodromic IPSP (Fig. 5).

Evidence obtained with intracellular recording indicates that the reduction of the IPSP occurs

Figure 4. Effect of opioid peptide (DALA) on field potentials in the hippocampal slice. The left-hand traces show the control responses recorded with an extracellular electrode in the pyramidal cell layer to antidromic (ANTI) and orthodromic (ORTHO) stimulation. The sharp downward deflections represent the synchronous firing of pyramidal cells and are termed population

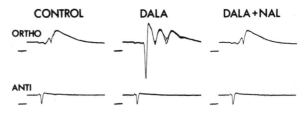

spikes. The middle traces show that exposure to 5 μM DALA greatly augments the orthodromic population spike and creates later population spikes while having no effect on the antidromic responses. Addition of naloxone (2 μM) to the DALA solution (DALA + NAL) completely reverses the effects of DALA. The calibration pulse at the beginning of each trace is 2 mV and 5 msec. (From Nicoll *et al.*, 1980.)

from an action of DALA at a site presynaptic to the pyramidal cell. This conclusion is based on the observation that the hyperpolarization caused by iontophoretic application of the IPSP transmitter GABA to pyramidal cells is not reduced by DALA. In the same cells, DALA clearly reduces the amplitude of the IPSP. Furthermore, spontaneous IPSPs, which can be recorded on the baseline of pyramidal cell resting potentials, are abolished by DALA. The resting potential and resting input resistance are not changed by DALA. The simplest explanation that can account for a reduction in IPSPs, both spontaneous and evoked, without reducing the GABA sensitivity or resting properties of the pyramidal cell is that DALA causes disinhibition at a site presynaptic to

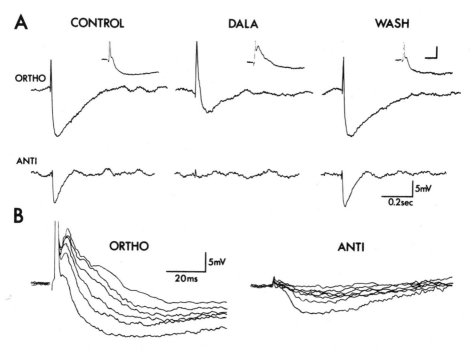

Figure 5. Enkephalin reduces IPSPs in a hippocampal pyramidal cell. (A) Intracellular chart records of responses to orthodromic (ORTHO) and antidromic (ANTI) stimulation. The inset shows film records at a faster speed. The calibration for the inset is 10 mV and 20 msec. The enkephalin analogue D-Ala²-Met⁵-enkephalinamide (DALA) was iontophoresed from an electrode positioned over the pyramidal cell layer. The electrode was filled with 10 mM DALA in 0.9% NaCl. (B) Superimposed traces of film records from the experiment in A showing the effect of DALA on the synaptic potentials. (From Nicoll, 1986.)

the pyramidal neuron. The effects of DALA described here are completely reversibly by naloxone. Interestingly, this same type of disinhibition can be recorded in mitral neurons of the olfactory bulb and this also occurs without any decrease in postsynaptic GABA sensitivity (Nicoll *et al.*, 1980).

Application of DALA causes the size of the intracellularly recorded EPSP to increase in a naloxone-reversible manner (Fig. 5; see also Dingledine, 1981). However, the rising phase of the extracellularly recorded EPSP field potential was not increased by DALA, suggesting strongly that neither the amount of excitatory transmitter released nor the sensitivity of the pyramidal cell to that transmitter is increased. Since the EPSP and IPSP overlap and the full amplitude of the intracellular EPSP is normally curtailed by the IPSP, the simplest explanation for the increase in the EPSP with enkephalin is that reduction in the IPSP allows for the full expression of the EPSP. This EPSP once released from inhibition is more likely to elicit an action potential from the cell. As the duration of the EPSP is also curtailed by the IPSP, a longer EPSP in a DALA-disinhibited cell can also elicit multiple action potentials. Thus, the disinhibitory action of enkephalin can account for both the increase in the size of the population spike and also the appearance of multiple population spikes.

Several studies of opiate action in the hippocampus are essentially in agreement with our results (Gahwiler, 1980; Robinson and Deadwyler, 1981; Siggins and Zieglgansberger, 1981; Masukawa and Prince, 1982). In cultured hippocampal neurons, presumed to be pyramidal, Gahwiler found that enkephalin caused an increase in spontaneous EPSPs and a reduction in evoked IPSPs. These effects of enkephalin were absent in synaptically isolated cells, suggesting that they were indirect. Working in hippocampal slices *in vitro*, Robinson and Deadwyler (1981) found that morphine caused reductions in IPSP amplitude. They also found that morphine at high doses could cause depolarizing shifts from the resting potential. Since the disinhibition caused by enkephalin and its analogues could occur in the absence of membrane depolarization, it seems unlikely that this depolarization can account for the excitatory effects of opioids.

To summarize, the preponderance of evidence from our own and other studies indicates that the major action of enkephalin in the hippocampus is to inhibit inhibitory synaptic transmission thereby causing an indirect excitation of pyramidal neurons. This disinhibition could occur at a number of sites presynaptic to the pyramidal cell. First, enkephalin could act at the presynaptic terminals of inhibitory interneurons to decrease release of GABA. Second, enkephalin could act directly to inhibit the action potential discharge of inhibitory interneurons. These first two possibilities are supported by the finding that enkephalin inhibits spontaneous IPSPs onto pyramidal cells. Another possibility is that enkephalin acts either pre- or postsynaptically to the interneuron to inhibit its activation by afferent excitatory input. We (Nicoll and Madison, 1984) have recently recorded from presumed inhibitory interneurons identified by the criteria of Schwartzkroin and Mathers (1978). Paired recordings of interneurons and pyramidal cells (Knowles and Schwartzkroin, 1981) have shown that stimulation of the interneuron produces an IPSP in the pyramidal cell. To be identified as an interneuron in our study, cells had to: (1) have a very short-duration action potential (approximately 0.5 msec in duration as opposed to 1–2 msec for a pyramidal cell); (2) have a fast afterhyperpolarization (AHP) following single action potentials and no slow AHP following a train of action potentials; (3) show little or no spike frequency adaptation during a current-induced train of action potentials; and (4) show spontaneous EPSPs on the baseline membrane potential recording. Interneurons were also easily identified by the very high-frequency discharge that was generated upon impalement. We find that DALA, applied in the bath, potently and reproducibly produces a large hyperpolarization of the membrane potential of interneurons. This hyperpolarization is associated with an increase in conductance as measured by constant-current hyperpolarizing pulses passed through the recording electrode. The extrapolated reversal potential of the DALA response was approximately −85 mV in 5.4 mM extracellular potassium and approximately −100 mV in 2.5 mM potassium, suggesting strongly that it was due to an increase in potassium conductance. An EPSP/IPSP sequence could be evoked in these interneurons by orthodromic stimulation in the stratum radiatum. When DALA was applied, and even when the membrane potential of the interneuron was returned to control levels by passing depolarizing current through the recording electrode, the size of the IPSP was markedly reduced and the EPSP was increased in amplitude. However, the increase in the EPSP was not sufficient to overcome the inhibitory influence of the DALA hyperpolarization and so the net effect of DALA was to inhibit the discharge of the interneuron evoked by to orthodromic stimulation.

4. Conclusion

In CNS neurons where the ionic mechanism of opiate action has been studied, the most common effect is an inhibition of neuronal discharge and this inhibition is mediated by an increase in resting potassium conductance, at least for opiate action at mu receptors. The best evidence for this comes from studies of the LC where opiate administration causes large, reproducible, and naloxone-reversible hyperpolarizations in resting membrane potential. Effects such as this could also account for another common effect of opiates, to decrease transmitter release from presynaptic terminals, although evidence from the dorsal root ganglion also suggests that calcium currents can be inhibited by opiate action at the kappa receptor (Macdonald and Werz, 1986).

In the hippocampus, unlike most other areas of the brain, the principal neurons, pyramidal cells, are excited by opiates. However, this seemingly paradoxical opiate effect can be explained in terms of the same inhibitory mechanism of opiates. Judging from their lack of responsiveness to opiate agonists, pyramidal cells do not appear to have functional opiate receptors on their membranes and thus are relatively insensitive to opiates. In contrast, inhibitory interneurons possess opiate receptors. Our results, showing that enkephalin analogues hyperpolarize interneurons, though not as completely characterized as in the LC, support this explanation and strengthen the hypothesis that opiates exert their major CNS effect by increasing neuronal potassium conductance.

Compared to pyramidal cells, there are relatively few interneurons in the hippocampus (Schwartkroin and Mathers, 1978). However, since each interneuron synaptically controls the discharge of hundreds of pyramidal cells (Somogyi et al., 1983), the actions of opiates on this minority of cells can have a widespread effect. By controlling the excitability of interneurons, opioid peptides can in an economical way control the excitability of the entire hippocampal formation.

References

Aghajanian, G. K., and Wang, Y. Y., 1986, Pertussis toxin blocks the outward currents evoked by opiate and α_2-agonists in locus coeruleus neurons, *Brain Res.* **371**:390–394.

Alger, B. E., 1984, Characteristic of a slow hyperpolarizing synaptic potential in rat hippocampal cells *in vitro, J. Neurophysiol.* **52**:892–910.

Alger, B. E., and Nicoll, R. A., 1982a, Feedforward dendritic inhibition in rat hippocampal pyramidal cells studied *in vitro, J. Physiol. (London)* **328**:105–123.

Alger, B. E., and Nicoll, R. A., 1982b, Pharmacological evidence for two kinds of GABA receptor on rat hippocampal pyramidal cells studied *in vitro, J. Physiol. (London)* **328**:125–141.

Andrade, R., and Aghajanian, G. K., 1985, Opiate and α_2 adrenoceptor-induced hyperpolarizations of locus coeruleus neurons in brain slices: Reversal by cyclic-AMP analogs, *J. Neurosci.* **5**:2359–2364.

Andrade, R., Malenka, R. C., and Nicoll, R. A., 1986, A G protein couples serotonin and GABA$_B$ receptors to the same channels in hippocampus, *Science* **234**:1261–1265.

Bird, S. J., and Kuhar, M. J., 1977, Iontophoretic application of opiates to the locus coeruleus, *Brain Res.* **122**:523–533.

Corigall, W. A., 1983, Opiates and the hippocampus: A review of the functional and morphological evidence, *Pharmacol. Biochem. Behav.* **18**:255–262.

Dingledine, R., 1981, Possible mechanisms of enkephalin action on hippocampal CA1 pyramidal neurons, *J. Neurosci.* **1:**1022–1035.

Duggan, A. W., and North, R. A., 1983, Electrophysiology of opioids, *Pharmacol. Rev.* **35:**219–282.

Dunwiddie, T., Mueller, A., Palmer, M., Stewart, J., and Hoffer, B., 1980, Electrophysiological interactions of enkephalins with neuronal circuitry in the rat hippocampus. I. Effects on pyramidal cell activity, *Brain Res.* **184:**311–330.

Gahwiler, B. H., 1980, Excitatory action of opioid peptides and opiates on cultured hippocampal pyramidal cells, *Brain Res.* **194:**193–203.

Knowles, W. D., and Schwartzkroin, P. A., 1981, Local circuit synaptic interactions in hippocampal brain slices, *J. Neurosci.* **1:**318–322.

Korf, J., Bunney, B. S., and Aghajanian, G. K., 1974, Noradrenergic neurons: Morphine inhibition of spontaneous activity, *Eur. J. Pharmacol.* **25:**165–169.

Lee, K. S., Dunwiddie, T. V., and Hoffer, B., 1980, Electrophysiological interactions of enkephalins with neuronal circuitry in the rat hippocampus. II. Effects on interneuron excitability, *Brain Res.* **184:**331–342.

Macdonald, R. L., and Werz, N. A., 1986, Dymorphin A decreases voltage-dependent calcium conductance of mouse dorsal root ganglion neurones, *J. Physiol. (London)* **377:**237–250.

Masukawa, L. M., and Prince, D. A., 1982, Enkephalin inhibition of inhibitory input to CA1 and CA3 pyramidal neurons in the hippocampus, *Brain Res.* **249:**271–280.

Newberry, N. R., and Nicoll, R. A., 1984, A bicuculline-resistant inhibitory post-synaptic potential in rat hippocampal pyramidal cells in vitro, *J. Physiol. (London)* **348:**239–254.

Newberry, N. R., and Nicoll, R. A., 1985, Comparison of the action of baclofen with gamma-aminobutyric acid on rat hippocampal pyramidal cells in vitro, *J. Physiol. (London)* **360:**161–185.

Nicoll, R. A., 1982, Responses of central neurons to opiates and opioid peptides, in: *Regulatory Peptides: From Molecular Biology to Function* (E. Costa and M. Trabucchi, eds.), Raven Press, New York, pp. 337–346.

Nicoll, R. A., 1986, The role of potassium in the action of opioid peptides in the CNS, in: *Ion Channels in Neural Membranes* (J. M. Ritchie, R. D. Keynes, and L. Bolis, eds.), Liss, New York, pp. 363–372.

Nicoll, R. A., and Madison, D. V., 1984, The action of enkephalin on interneurons in the hippocampus, *Soc. Neurosci. Abstr.* **10:**660.

Nicoll, R. A., Siggins, G. R., Ling, N., Bloom, F. E., and Guillemin, R., 1977, Neuronal actions of endorphins and enkephalins among brain regions: A comparative microiontophoretic study, *Proc. Natl. Acad. Sci. USA* **74:**2584–2588.

Nicoll, R. A., Alger, B. E., and Jahr, C. E., 1980, Enkephalin blocks inhibitory pathways in the vertebrate CNS, *Nature* **287:**22–25.

North, R. A., and Williams, J. T., 1985, On the potassium conductance increased by opioids in rat locus coeruleus neurones, *J. Physiol. (London)* **364:**265–280.

Pepper, C. M., and Henderson, G., 1980, Opiates and opioid peptides hyperpolarize locus coeruleus neurons *in vitro, Science* **209:**394–396.

Pert, C. B., Kuhar, M. J., and Snyder, S. H., 1976, The opiate receptor: Autoradiographic localization in rat brain, *Proc. Natl. Acad. Sci. USA* **73:**3729–3733.

Pfaffinger, P. J., Martin, J. M., Hunter, D. D., Nathanson, N. M., and Hille, B., 1985, GTP-binding proteins couple cardiac muscarinic receptors to a K channel, *Nature* **317:**536–538.

Robinson, J. H., and Deadwyler, S. A., 1981, Intracellular correlates of morphine excitation in the hippocampal slice preparation, *Brain Res.* **224:**375–387.

Schwartzkroin, P. A., and Mathers, L. H., 1978, Physiological and morphological identification of a nonpyramidal hippocampal cell type, *Brain Res.* **157:**1–10.

Siggins, G. R., and Zieglgansberger, W., 1981, Morphine and opioid peptides reduce inhibitory synaptic potentials in hippocampal pyramidal cell in vitro without alteration of membrane potential, *Proc. Natl. Acad. Sci. USA* **78:**5235–5239.

Somogyi, P., Smith, A. D., Nunzi, M. G., Gorio, A., Takagi, H., and Wu, J. Y., 1983, Glutamate decarboxylase immunoreactivity in the hippocampus of the cat: Distribution of immunoreactive synaptic terminals with special reference to the axon initial segment of pyramidal neurons, *J. Neurosci.* **3:**1450–1468.

Williams, J. T., Egan, T. M., and North, R. A., 1982, Enkephalin opens potassium channels on mammalian central neurones, *Nature* **299:**74–77.

Zieglgansberger, W., French, E. D., Siggins, G. R., and Bloom, F. E., 1979, Opioid peptides may excite hippocampal pyramidal neurons by inhibiting adjacent inhibitory interneurons, *Science* **205:**415–417.

38

Molecular Controls and Communication in Cerebral Cortex
An Overview

Herbert H. Jasper, Tomás A. Reader, Massimo Avoli,
Robert W. Dykes, and Pierre Gloor

1. Significance of Cortical Neurotransmitters

The contributors to the present symposium have provided many fascinating and important highlights of recent research on the many neurotransmitters or modulators which have played a leading role in the remarkable advances being made during recent years in our understanding of the chemical and molecular mechanisms involved in the organization of cortical function. In this final chapter, we shall attempt to present some of our impressions of the overall importance of these developments with an emphasis on the subtitle of this book *From Molecules to Mind.*

1.1. Amino Acids

It would seem that the only good candidates for the chemical synaptic mediation of the rapid transient transmission of excitatory and inhibitory actions in the specific information processing, cognitive, and specific motor functions of cerebral cortex are amino acids, i.e., glutamic (Glu) and aspartic (Asp) acids, which are universally excitatory, while GABA is the major, if not the only, generally active specific inhibitory substance in cerebral cortex. All of the other neuroactive substances found in cerebral cortex have slower and longer-lasting effects, modulating excitability and the action of other neurotransmitters. Some may be "cotransmitters," as shown by Jones in this volume with his immunocytochemical studies of GAD (the enzyme for GABA synthesis) and certain peptides.

It would seem to be of considerable importance that the metabolism of Glu and GABA are so

Herbert H. Jasper • Centre de Recherche en Sciences Neurologiques, Département de Physiologie, Faculté de Médecine, Université de Montréal, and Montreal Neurological Institute, McGill University, Montreal, Quebec, H3A 2B4, Canada. *Tomás A. Reader* • Centre de Recherche en Sciences Neurologiques, Département de Physiologie, Faculté de Médecine, Université de Montréal, Montreal, Quebec, H3C 3J7, Canada. *Massimo Avoli, and Pierre Gloor* • Montreal Neurological Institute and Department of Neurology and Neurosurgery, McGill University, Montreal, Quebec, H3A 2B4, Canada. *Robert W. Dykes* • Departments of Physiology, Neurology, and Neurosurgery, McGill University, Montreal, Quebec H3A 1A1, Canada.

closely interrelated; GABA being produced by the decarboxylation of Glu by means of a decar-boxylating enzyme (GAD), together with the coenzyme pyridoxine (vitamin B_6). Rate-limiting steps in the synthesis of both GABA and Glu are also closely related, as shown by Szerb in this volume.

The fact that the most important excitatory substance can be the immediate precursor of the most important inhibitory substance in the cortex suggests that these interrelationships may be relevant to the maintenance of a balance in excitatory and inhibitory controls in the synaptic mechanisms involved both in information processing as well as in integrative motor control. Defects in GABA-mediated inhibitory controls may lead to epileptic discharge, as described in this volume by Avoli, and may abolish pattern discrimination in cells of visual cortex, as shown in this book by Sillito and Murphy. Dykes et al. (this volume) have shown that blocking of GABA action by bicuculline enlarges and blurs receptive fields of single cells in somatosensory cortex. Thus, GABA may play a leading role in all higher integrative functions of cerebral cortex in which patterns of excitation are being molded by inhibition.

The specific ionic channels mediating the excitatory properties of Glu and Asp have not been clearly elucidated, but they probably involve both Na^+ and Ca^{2+} conductances. The ionic mechanism of inhibition by GABA involves chloride channels, and such GABA receptors are very closely related and couple to benzodiazepine recognition sites, as described by Lambert et al. (this volume). The barbiturates may also act, in part, via the GABA system, further increasing the importance of GABA in such physiological phenomena, and pointing to its interest in neuropharmacology.

Studying experimental focal epileptogenic lesions in animals, Ribak et al. (1979) reported that GAD-containing interneurons are selectively decreased in number, which may be one of the factors causing the focal epileptic discharge (disinhibition). However, GAD was found to be increased in the hippocampus of seizure-susceptible gerbils by the same group, so that other mechanisms may be operating in this model. There is some evidence that the accumulation of Glu, partly due to defective mechanisms for converting it into GABA, and other defects in the mechanisms for its binding or inactivation by both glial and nerve cells may also play an important role in the excess excitability which characterizes epileptogenic brain tissue.

It is of interest to compare the molecular quantity of amino acids, acetylcholine, mono-amines, and peptides in cerebral cortex. A rapid analysis (see Table I) clearly shows that the most

Table I. Neurotransmitter Levels in the Cerebral Cortex[a]

	Endogenous levels (nmoles/g tissue)	Species	Reference
Glutamic acid	8700–10,800	Human	Perry et al. (1971)
GABA	2100–2700	Monkey	Fahn and Cote (1968)
Glycine	2700	Monkey	Aprison et al. (1970)
Aspartate	1900–2600	Human	Perry et al. (1971)
Taurine	2100	Cat	Guidotti et al. (1972)
Acetylcholine	0.7 μg/g	Human	MacIntosh (1941)
	11–28	Rat	Hoover et al. (1978)
Noradrenaline	1.5–3.8	Rat	Diop et al. (1987)
Serotonin	2.0	Rat	Reader et al. (1986)
Dopamine	0.5–1.1	Cat	Reader and Quesney (1986)
Histamine	1	Human	Lipinski et al. (1973)
Substance P	0.025	Rat	Kanazawa and Jessell (1976)
Met-enkephalin	0.98 ng/mg	Rat	Hong et al. (1977)

[a]For comparative purposes, the original data were converted into nmoles/g tissue (wet weight) when required, except for acetylcholine in human cerebral cortex, which is in μg/g, and for Met-enkephalin, expressed in ng/mg protein.

abundant neurotransmitter molecules are Glu, GABA, glycine, Asp, and taurine. These amino acid neurotransmitters are present in micromolar concentrations and their specific receptors have low affinity constants (micromolar range). The biogenic amines acetylcholine, noradrenaline, serotonin, dopamine, and histamine are present in the cortex in absolute amounts which are 1000–10,000 times lower (nanomoles) than the amino acids. The specific receptors for these compounds have affinity constants in the nano- or even in the picomolar range. Finally, peptide neurotransmitters are found in picomoles and their receptors consequently seem to have affinity constants on the order of pico- or femtomoles.

The rate of liberation of amino acids from the surface of the cat cerebral cortex is related to the state of cortical activation, as determined by the electrocorticogram and behavioral signs of sleep or waking (Jasper *et al.*, 1965; Jasper and Koyama, 1969). Desynchronized EEG activation with arousal was accompanied by a marked increase in the liberation of both Glu and Asp, and with a decrease in GABA. However, an increase in the liberation of GABA was produced by stimulation of the midbrain in the vicinity of the periaqueductal gray.

It is of interest that the discovery of the inhibitory properties of GABA by Elliott and co-workers just 30 years ago (Elliott, 1958; Elliott and Jasper, 1959; Jasper, 1984) was in the course of their search for a neurochemical defect in epileptic brain tissue, and influenced by the report that infants fed prepared food lacking in pyridoxine had convulsive seizures which were promptly arrested when the essential vitamin for the production of GABA was replaced in their diet. The excitatory and inhibitory transmitter properties of Glu and GABA were then clearly established by microiontophoretic studies of single cortical cells by Krnjević and Schwartz (1967). It was then found that GABA antagonists such as picrotoxin and bicuculline are potent convulsant drugs; GABA agonists (e.g., benzodiazepines, sodium valproate) have been shown to be effective in the treatment of certain forms of epilepsy.

1.2. Acetylcholine

Acetylcholine (ACh) was the first putative neurotransmitter proposed for synapses of the CNS about 40 years ago (Feldberg, 1945). This followed the earlier demonstration that ACh was the transmitter of the inhibitory action of the vagus nerve on the heart, the transmitter of neuromuscular excitation at the motor end plate in skeletal muscle, and the synaptic transmitter in sympathetic ganglia. We learned some important lessons from these early studies of about 50 years ago: (1) The same neurotransmitter substance may be either excitatory or inhibitory depending on the nature of the receptor subtype on which it acts, (2) the same substance may be excitatory in different ways as, for example, the "nicotinic" action of ACh at the motor end plate, and its muscarinic action in sympathetic ganglia, and (3) the excitatory action of a given substance may be transformed into an inhibitory effect by activation of inhibitory interneurons, as in collateral inhibition of motoneurons via the Renshaw cells of the spinal cord.

Discovery of the presence of ACh in cerebral cortex, together with its synthetic enzyme, choline acetyltransferase, and its hydrolyzing enzyme, acetylcholinesterase, occurred just as the electroencephalogram was being developed for the study of the electrical activity of the cortex in man and experimental animals without anesthesia. It was found that application of weak solutions of ACh to the cortical surface produced a local desynchronizing activation of the EEG, similar to that seen in arousal or waking from sleep. This would proceed into a sustained rhythmic epileptic discharge with slightly higher concentrations of ACh. This excitatory action was blocked by atropine or scopolamine (Miller *et al.*, 1940). It was then found that the superfusion of the cortical surface with a solution containing eserine made it possible to measure the rate of liberation of ACh from the cortical surface not only at rest but also during various states of activation. The resting rate in cats was about 1–2 ng/cm^2 per min, and it increased to 4–5 ng/cm^2 per min during desynchronizing activation, as in arousal or by stimulation of the brain stem reticular formation (Sie *et al.*, 1965; Celesia and Jasper, 1966). Even in the state of paradoxical or REM sleep in the cat, characterized by desynchronized activation of the EEG, there was also an increased ACh liberation relative to that in slow-wave sleep, though less than that during acute arousal in the waking animals (Jasper and Tessier, 1971).

The release of ACh from cerebral cortex was first measured by MacIntosh and Oborin (1953) and confirmed in several other laboratories in addition to the work of Celesia and Jasper mentioned above (Bartolini et al., 1972; Giarman and Pepeu, 1964; Mitchell, 1963; Mullin and Phillis, 1975; Pepeu, 1973; Szerb, 1964). Atropine was found not only to block the action of ACh on cortical electrical activity, but also to increase by severalfold the rate of release from the cortical surface, presumably due to competitive blockade of ACh receptors involved in reuptake or inactivation of ACh, or possibly a blocking of presynaptic receptors involved in negative feedback.

Krnjević (this volume) described microiontophoretic studies on the nature of the excitatory action of ACh on cortical nerve cells. He concluded that ACh does not act like a classical neurotransmitter at cortical synapses. Cellular impedance is increased instead of decreased with excitation, and the resulting neuronal excitation has a slow onset and prolonged duration. The effect is thought to be due to blocking of K^+ channels, thus prolonging the action of other transmitters. It has also been suggested that a second messenger such as cGMP might be involved, acting via some form of protein phosphorylation. In any case, it would appear that ACh plays a most important role in regulating the state of reactivity of cortical cells, as in sleep and waking, and attention, as well as in the reinforcement and prolongation of cortical and hippocampal synaptic activity important in mechanisms of memory, as suggested by its deficiency in Alzheimer's disease (Whitehouse et al., 1981).

It has been shown by Dykes et al. in this symposium that ACh also may play an important role in regulating the excitability and functional organization of somatosensory cortex. This may well be a model of how it may act upon the integrative functions of cerebral cortex in general. It would seem, therefore, that ACh does not play a true transmitter role in cerebral cortex but rather functions as a modulator of neuronal excitability and can modify the response to other transmitters, while setting the stage for states of reactivity such as waking, attention, or the reinforcement of learning and facilitation of certain integrative processes as has been shown for somatosensory cortex. Cortical ACh, like cortical monoamines, is derived largely from subcortical afferent fibers originating in specific ACh-containing subcortical neuronal structures (Mesulam et al., 1983; Mesulam, this volume).

1.3. Monoamines and Cyclic Nucleotides

The monoamine innervation of cerebral cortex was recently reviewed in the Université de Montréal International Symposium series. Our chairman, Laurent Descarries, was also principal organizer and editor of the previous symposium (Descarries et al., 1984). Monoamine axonal terminals, containing either noradrenaline (NA), serotonin (5-HT), or dopamine (DA), are distributed throughout all areas of cerebral cortex, although they originate from relatively very few (a few thousand) cells located in subcortical nuclei of the brain stem. It has been said that never have so few done so much for so many!

The three monoamines are not uniformly distributed in all cortical areas, and when projection areas are overlapping they are parcellated within the cortical layers. There is also a degree of topographical organization. This is of relevance when the distribution of monoamine receptors is considered in the light of the afferent projection patterns (Diop et al., 1987; Reader et al., this volume; but see also Wamsley, 1984). On the other hand, if the release of these substances from their axonal terminals or varicosities is controlled only by action potentials in these relatively few slowly conducting and slowly firing fine nerve fibers, most of which in the cortex are collaterals of even fewer fibers of origin, severe restraints are placed upon their possible importance in discriminative or integrative cortical function. There is, however, the possibility that the monoamine-containing neurons of the brain stem serve primarily to distribute NA, 5-HT, and DA to many or most cortical areas in a relatively diffuse fashion, but that the release (or the effectiveness) of these substances may be under local control determined by locally acting neurotransmitter substances (Reader *et al.*, 1976, 1979b, 1980). Important interactions between monoamines and ACh, as well as interactions with amino acids in cerebral cortex have been reviewed elsewhere (Reader, 1983; Reader and Jasper, 1984).

Another constraint placed upon our understanding of the functional importance of monoamines in cerebral cortex is the fact that relatively few of the NA and 5-HT axonal terminals appear to be associated with the usual increased density of the postsynaptic membrane as seen in the electron microscope (Beaudet and Descarries, 1978). This suggests a more diffuse and different function as compared to the precise punctate actions of classical excitatory and inhibitory synapses on the soma or dendrites of postsynaptic cells.

Electrophysiological studies of the responses of single cortical cells to the local microiontophoretic application of the monoamines NA, DA, and 5-HT have been performed in numerous laboratories, mostly on spontaneously active neurons (for reviews see Krnjević, 1964, 1974, 1984; Phillis, 1977, 1984). Effects on sensory-evoked potentials are less consistent, sometimes depressing them, but at other times (perhaps with lower amounts of monoamine ejected) sensory-evoked potentials may appear to be enhanced, thus increasing the signal-to-noise ratio in primary sensory cortical areas (Foote *et al.*, 1975; Kolta *et al.*, 1987; Reader, 1978, 1980). The action of monoamines is characteristically of slow onset and long duration, outlasting the duration of the ejection itself. It would seem, therefore, that the monoamines act more likely as modulators than as true transmitters in cerebral cortex, i.e., regulating the synaptic action of amino acids and ACh (Reader, 1978; Reader *et al.*, 1979a). There may be other much longer-lasting effects mediated via second messengers, such as cyclic nucleotides (Greengard, 1978; Ouimet, this volume) as Libet has shown so well in synaptic transmission through the cervical ganglia (Libet, this volume; Libet *et al.*, 1975).

The importance of monoamines for cortical function has been emphasized because of their apparent significance in nervous and mental diseases. The neuroleptic and psychoactive drugs such as reserpine and chlorpromazine, the antidepressant effects of monoamine oxidase (MAO) inhibitors, and the schizophrenic-like psychosis produced by amphetamine all suggest that biogenic amines play an important role in mental disease. Recent studies on dopamine contents and receptors in brain tissue from psychotic patients (Bird *et al.*, 1979a,b; Iversen, 1975; Seeman, 1980; Seeman and Lee, 1975) reinforce the idea that monoamines play an important role in higher mental processes. The presentation in this meeting of Laurent Descarries on DA terminals in different neocortical areas (Descarries *et al.*, this volume) and that of Charles Ouimet showing the presence in cerebral cortex of DARPP-32 (Ouimet, this volume) give added impetus for future investigations on the role of dopamine in cortical function.

It is also apparent that iontophoretic microelectrodes do not tell the whole story. Possible effects on the plasticity of neuronal circuits, as suggested by the work of Kasamatsu (Kasamatsu and Pettigrew, 1976; Kasamatsu *et al.*, 1984), as well as possible trophic actions are also to be considered. The suggestion by Kety (1970) that NA might be involved in the reinforcement of neuronal circuits during the establishment of conditioned responses in learning and memory has not received definite support by the careful work of Susan Iversen (Iversen, 1984). Perhaps, as modulators of activity in amino acid and cholinergic synaptic circuits, they may exert critical controls on the higher integrative functions of cerebral cortex.

1.4. Peptides

After the initial description by von Euler and Gaddum (1931) of a neuroactive substance (substance P), the discovery and localization of over 60 neuropeptides, together with their specific receptor proteins, mainly by immunocytochemical techniques, has presented us with very complex problems of understanding their functional significance in the mechanisms for control, communication, and information processing in cerebral cortex. A partial list is given in Table II. We are fortunate in being able to refer to two masterful reviews by Leo Renaud, one presented at a previous symposium of this series in May 1982 and as chairman of Section VI of the present volume (Renaud, 1983, this volume; but see also Bloom, 1980, 1986a,b; Hökfelt *et al.*, 1984; Gainer and Brownstein, 1981; Iversen, 1983; Kriger, 1983).

It is clear that many selected cortical nerve cells are very sensitive to the microiontophoretic application of small concentrations of numerous peptides, many of which are better known as hypophyseal and gastrointestinal hormones, as well as the family of endogenous opioids (enkephalins, dynorphins, and endorphins). Their actions upon cortical cells and CNS synapses are varied. Presynaptically, they may influence the release of other transmitter substances via the regulation of Ca^{2+} currents in nerve terminals. They may act in numerous ways upon postsynaptic membranes and the responsiveness of nerve cells to other transmitter substances and their modes of action includes depolarization or hyperpolarization, changes in voltage-dependent ionic conductances, or activation of membrane adenylate cyclases. Some peptide actions can only be manifested when interacting with another neurotransmitter. For example, vasoactive intestinal polypeptide (VIP) when tested by microiontophoresis on the spontaneous activity of cortical neurons in the sensorimotor area has varying effects, i.e., no effects on more than 50% of the cells and it excites or depresses the remaining units. However, when VIP was tested concurrently with a dose of NA that had no effect by itself, the inhibitory responses to VIP alone were enhanced, the excitations to VIP alone were converted to inhibitions, and cells nonresponsive to VIP alone now showed a slowing in firing (Ferron *et al.*, 1985). This interaction at the cortical cellular level can be explained by the synergistic activation of an adenylate cyclase, since both NA and VIP increase cAMP production (Magistretti and Schorderet, 1984).

Another example of peptide-neurotransmitter interaction is the enhancement of ACh effects by somatostatin (Mancillas *et al.*, 1986). The C-terminal tetradecapeptide (SS-14) of somatostatin when applied alone by iontophoresis depresses spontaneous firing. Moreover, when tested on the cholinergic responses either to brief pulses or to a continuous leak of ACh from the iontophoretic

Table II. Peptide Neurotransmitters and Neurohormones[a]

Adrenocorticotropin	Growth hormone (GH)	Neurokinin B (neuromedin)
Angiotensin I	GH-releasing factor	Neuropeptide Y
Angiotensin II	Insulin	Neurophysin(s)
Angiotensin III	Kassinin	Neurotensin
Avian pancreatic polypeptide	Kyotorphin	Oxytocin
Bombesin	Leucine-enkephalin	Pancreatic polypeptides
Bradykinin	α-Lipotropin	Physalaemin
Calcitonin	β-Lipotropin	Proctolin
Calcitonin gene-related peptide	Luteinizing hormone (LH)	Prolactin
L-Carnosine	LH-releasing hormone	Secretin
Cholecystokinin(s)	α-Melanocyte stimulating hormone	Sleep peptides
Corticotropin-releasing factor	β-Melanocyte stimulating hormone	Somatomedin
Dynorphin A	γ-Melanocyte stimulating hormone	Somatostatin
Dynorphin B	Melatonin	Substance P
β-Endorphin	Methionine-enkephalin	Thyrotropin
β-Ependymin	Motilin	Thyrotropin-releasing hormone
α-Ependymin	MSH-releasing hormone	Arginine-vasopressin
Gastrin	α-Neo-endorphin	Lysine-vasopressin
Gastrointestinal polypeptide	β-Neo-endorphin	Vasotocin
Glucagon	Neurokinin A (substance K)	Vasoactive intestinal peptide

[a]The putative neurotransmitter and neurohormone peptides have been arranged in alphabetical order, with the most frequently used nomenclature (Gainer and Brownstein, 1981; Hökfelt *et al.*, 1984; Iversen, 1983; Krieger, 1983; Nieuwenhuys, 1985; Schmitt, 1984; Takagi *et al.*, 1979).

pipette, SS-14 enhanced the excitatory responses in a dose-dependent manner. This effect appears to be a true interaction between SS-14 and ACh, since Glu-evoked excitations were unaffected, or rather depressed. A possible interpretation can be that SS-14 enables an underlying ACh-induced excitation. Therefore, although the primary effect of SS-14 is to inhibit spontaneous firing, in the presence of ACh it acts as an enabling neurotransmitter (Bloom, 1985). There may be many other actions not revealed by microelectrode studies or transient electrical properties of neurons and their synaptic circuits. The coexistence of peptides in axonal terminals containing other more classical transmitter substances would suggest a modulating role of interaction, still to be well understood.

Since peptides are far more complex molecules than are the classical neurotransmitters, they are capable of conveying information to widely distributed neuronal circuits containing key neurons with very specific receptors for a given peptide, perhaps acting in a hormonal fashion on nonjunctional portions of nerve membranes. This has been called a "parasynaptic action" by Schmitt (1984) in his interesting theoretical treatment entitled "Molecular regulators of brain function: A new view."

Schmitt has been one of the most persistent pioneers in the development of a molecular view of communication, information processing, and memory storage in the brain. This was the moving force behind the founding of the Neuroscience Research Program (NRP) in 1962 at the Massachusetts Institute of Technology. This was preceded by the organization of international interdisciplinary work sessions in 1960 on "Fast Fundamental Transfer Processes in Aqueous Biomolecular Systems" and "Macromolecular Specificity and Biological Memory" in 1961. At the same time, unbeknown to Frank Schmitt, there was being organized in Paris, with the help of UNESCO, an International Interdisciplinary Brain Research Organization known as IBRO with somewhat similar but more far-reaching objectives than were originally conceived for the NRP program led by Schmitt.

As a biophysicist, Frank has never lost sight of his primary objective in studying the "physics of the mind." This is shown by his recent important contributions to the significance of molecular messengers in the brain; the title of Schmitt's contribution to the Fourth Study Program of NRP is "The role of structural, electrical and chemical circuitry in brain function" (1979) and his chapter introducing the symposium on "Molecular Genetic Neuroscience" is entitled "A protocol for molecular genetic neuroscience." Floyd Bloom also contributed an important chapter to the NRP Fourth Study Program entitled "Chemical integrative processes in the central nervous system" (see also Bloom, 1984, 1985, 1986a,b; Bloom and Morrison, 1986).

In his most recent review in the IBRO journal *Neuroscience* entitled "Molecular regulators of brain function: A new view," Schmitt (1984) proposes the term "information substances" (ISs) for the many more complex neuroactive substances which may be delivered in a "para-synaptic" mode, not requiring the traditional specific synaptic junctions of the more classical synapses. This is acquired by their specificity of action upon neuronal nets by the selective binding to strategically located receptors on neuronal membranes throughout the brain. He points out that molecular communication of this form, without synaptic specialization, preceded the development of specific neuronal synapses in evolution. Of course, the view that humoral factors play an important role in determining mental attitudes and patterns of behavior is a very old view in the history of philosophical views of the mind and mind–body relationships.

2. Molecular Controls and Communication

2.1. The Importance of State-Dependent Reactions

The action of many neurotransmitters upon cortical function may be in establishing different states of reactivity, in form, intensity, and duration, to either internal or external stimuli. The response of cortical cells to a given constant sensory input may show a wide range of variability depending on its state of activity or reactivity which may be set by interaction with chemical substances other than those involved in the relatively stable transmission through the direct synaptic pathway. At the level of cerebral cortex, these "modulator" or reactive state-setting substances may include ACh, NA, DA, and 5-HT, as well as more complex peptide neurotransmitter substances such as enkephalins, endorphins, and dynorphins, the hypothalamic hormones (e.g., somatostatin, vasopressin), and the central representation of the gut hormones (e.g., VIP, cholecystokinins). Some of these substances may act as direct neurotransmitters in subcortical synaptic circuits, in brain stem, hypothalamus, or striatum, with indirect effects upon cortical function. The importance of these reactive states of sleeping or waking, hungry or satiated, sexually excited or satisfied, angry or afraid, happy or sad, interested or bored, and so on, in the determination of behavior and perceptual awareness is well known, and all probably exert their effects as neurotransmitters of the regulatory kind (neuromodulators, neurohormones) affecting both cortical and subcortical structures.

States of reactivity also depend upon past experience and anticipatory sets which have been learned from previous experience, or are a part of a conditioning paradigm. Tanji and Evarts (1976) have provided an elegant example of the effect of anticipatory set upon the response of single cells in motor cortex of the monkey, depending upon whether the animal had been exposed to a red or a green light prior to a constant stimulus (wrist flexion). The red light was a signal to pull, and the green a signal to push, opposite movements in response to the same stimulus depending upon motor set. This and other examples were discussed in the NRP colloquium on "Organization of the Cerebral Cortex" (Jasper, 1981). The neurotransmitters implicated in the establishment of such temporary states of reactivity of assemblies of cortical neurons, and the long-term reinforcement of synaptic circuits involved in conditioning and learning certainly call upon a combination of simultaneously active transmitter (or modulator) substances.

2.2. Behavioral States Dependent on NA and ACh

As we have gradually developed ways to study the temporary states of cortical function that depend on these neuromodulatory molecules, we have begun to develop hypotheses about their role in changing cortical neuronal excitability.

It seems likely that 5-HT, NA, and ACh are all released in greater quantities during consciousness than during either anesthesia or sleep (Celesia and Jasper, 1966; Jasper and Tessier, 1971; Hobson et al., 1986). The stimulating soup hypothesis, that the release of an elixir of these neuromodulators has an invigorating effect on cortical neurons, now appears naive.

Rather we must recognize the various lines of evidence presented here and elsewhere indicating that the effects of each of these substances are different, and further that some neurons remain unaffected by these substances. Clearly, neuromodulatory substances have different effects in different cells (see Marshall and Finlayson, this volume). Only about one-third of cortical neurons are overtly excited by ACh, but a greater proportion are inhibited by NA (Kolta et al., 1987; Olpe et al., 1980; Reader, 1978; Reader et al., 1979a, 1980). However, it may be just this specificity of effects that allows the cortex to perform complex functions.

It appears that the enhanced NA release during consciousness may cause an increased release of GABA from cortical interneurons (Moroni et al., 1983; Beani et al., 1986) through α_1 receptor-mediated stimulation and thus have an excitatory influence on some cells while inhibiting others. The release of ACh also has differential effects. Metherate et al. (1987) reported that the excitability of some neurons in somatosensory cortex was unchanged while others became more responsive in the presence of ACh and a few were less responsive. A similar range of effects to afferent stimulation has been reported in visual cortex (Sillito and Kemp, 1973). McCormick and Prince (1985) have shown that cortical neurons thought to be inhibitory interneurons have a very different response to iontophoretically administered ACh than do pyramidal cells. Consequently, the changes in release of ACh, NA, and 5-HT that accompany arousal may lead to rather different effects in different cells, thereby changing cortical circuitry in ways which we are unable to predict with current models of cortical function. It should also be recalled that in cerebral cortex the release (overflow) of endogenous DA and NA can be regulated by presynaptic ACh receptors of muscarinic and nicotinic nature localized on the catecholamineric nerve endings (Reader *et al.*, 1976, 1980). Other types of interacting mechanisms capable of regulating catecholamine and 5-HT release in the cortical terminal fields of innervation have been reviewed elsewhere (Reader and Jasper, 1984). In addition, there are postsynaptic interactions between ACh and the catecholamines such that NA and DA can modulate cholinoceptive responses (Reader, 1980, 1983; Reader *et al.*, 1979a, 1980; Stone *et al.*, 1975).

Some hints about the roles of these substances may come from studies of the factors which influence the aminergic and cholinergic cells which innervate the cortex. Catecholamine inputs have a tonic activity that is greatest during alertness and lowest during sleep. Most modalities of sensory stimulation can modulate their tonic activity. In the case of the cholinergic neurons of the basal forebrain, the neurons may remain silent until some motivationally charged event occurs. Thus, the release of ACh in cortex may be more selective than that of NA. DeLong (1971) recording from neurons in the region of the nucleus basalis of Meynert of macaque monkeys showed that the neurons discharged actively when the monkeys were rewarded for correct performance of a motor task.

More recently, based upon experiments in which monkeys were required to perform a delayed response task, Richardson and DeLong (1986) reported that neurons in the basal forebrain tended to respond to reward delivery and also to events that occur immediately before the reward, suggesting that the nucleus basalis of Meynert could play a role in the neural basis of positive reinforcement. In behavioral experiments on rats while recording in frontal cortex during conditioning, Rigdon and Pirch (1986) have shown changes in cortical neurons attributable to conditioning that are blocked by atropine or kainic acid lesions of the basal forebrain. From this they concluded that the cholinergic neurons of the nucleus basalis are involved in the generation of conditioned neuronal responses in frontal cortex. The cholinergic and aminergic inputs to cortex appear to have rather different functions.

The latter experiments take us to another class of effects that implicate the neuromodulatory substances in learning, and neuronal plasticity. During states of alertness or consciousness, a fraction of the ongoing neuronal processes can lead to long-term changes in neuronal excitability that are thought to be related to learning, memory, and other forms of cortical neuronal plasticity. All of these processes share two characteristics. The first is that the altered neuronal states do not return to their previous conditions; neuronal responses remain altered even though the animal subsequently sleeps or becomes unconscious thereby decreasing the levels of neuromodulators being released in cortex. Second, these changes require the participation of subcortical structures.

Singer (1983) has suggested that in the case of visual cortex the long-lasting changes require the contribution of subcortical structure as a permissive element or gate that allows the long-term changes to come about. In addition to the subcortical gate, long-term changes require that the cortical neurons be driven to discharge. This neural activity is often elicited by sensory inputs. NA and thus the locus coeruleus has been implicated in the neural plasticity of visual cortex of young kittens since the experiments of Pettigrew and coworkers (Kasamatsu and Pettigrew, 1976; Kasamatsu *et al.*, 1984). Cholinergic mechanisms have been implicated in long-term changes by many of the learning experiments. Metherate *et al.* (1987) have postulated that ACh, released by activity of the basal forebrain neurons, plays a permissive role in the long-term enhancement of receptive field properties they observed in cat somatosensory cortex when neurons were driven by somatic stimuli in the presence of ACh.

Bear and Singer (1986) have showed that both NA and ACh play roles in the experience-dependent neuronal plasticity seen in kitten cortex blocking the change in cortical neuronal function only when the afferent pathway for both neuromodulatory substances were transected. Kleinschmidt *et al.* (1987) suggested that these neuromodulatory substances express their effects and bring about long-term changes in neuronal excitability through the same cellular mechanism.

ACKNOWLEDGMENT. The authors gratefully acknowledge the collaboration of Helene Auzat throughout this symposium, as well as her assistance in the preparation of this manuscript.

References

Aprison, M. H., Davidoff, R. A., and Werman, R., 1970, Glycine: Its metabolic and possible role in nervous tissue, in: *Handbook of Neurochemistry*, Vol. 4 (A. Lajtha, ed.), Plenum Press, New York, pp. 62–75.

Bartolini, A., Weisenthal, L., and Domino, E. F., 1972, Effect of photic stimulation on acetylcholine release from cerebral cortex, *Neuropharmacology* **11**:113–122.

Beani, L., Tanganelli, S., Antonelli, T., and Bianchi, C., 1986, Noradrenergic modulation of cortical acetylcholine release is both direct and gamma-aminobutyric acid-mediated, *J. Pharmacol. Exp. Ther.* **236**:230–236.

Bear, M. F., and Singer, W., 1986, Modulation of visual cortical plasticity by acetylcholine and noradrenaline, *Nature* **320**:172–176.

Beaudet, A., and Descarries, L., 1978, The monoamine innervation of rat cerebral cortex: Synaptic and nonsynaptic axon terminals, *Neuroscience* **3**:851–860.

Bird, E. D., Spokes, E. G. S., and Iversen, L. L., 1979a, Increased dopamine concentration in limbic areas of brain from patients dying with schizophrenia, *Brain* **102**:347–360.

Bird, E. D., Spokes, E. G., and Iversen. L. L., 1979b, Brain norepinephrine and dopamine in schizophrenia, *Science* **204**:93–94.

Bloom, F. E., 1980, *Peptides: Integrators of Cell and Tissue Function*, Raven Press, New York.

Bloom, F. E., 1984, The functional significance of neurotransmitter diversity, *Am. J. Physiol.* **246**:C184–C194.

Bloom, F. E., 1985, Neurotransmitter diversity and its functional significance, *J. R. Soc. Med.* **78**:189–192.

Bloom, F. E., 1986a, Whither neuropeptides? in: *Neuropeptides in Neurologic and Psychiatric Disease* (J. B. Martin and J. D. Barchas, eds.), Raven Press, New York, pp. 335–349.

Bloom, F. E., 1986b, Genetic background for multiple messengers, *Prog. Brain Res.* **68**:149–159.

Bloom, F. E., and Morrison, J. H., 1986, Neurotransmitters of the human brain, *Hum. Neurobiol.* **5**:145–146.

Celesia, G., and Jasper, H. H., 1966, Acetylcholine released from cerebral cortex in relation to states of activation, *Neurology* **16**:1053–1064.

DeLong, M. R., 1971, Activity of pallidal neurons during movement, *J. Neurophysiol.* **34**:414–427.

Descarries, L., Reader, T. A., and Jasper, H. H. (eds.), 1984, *Monoamine Innervation of Cerebral Cortex*, Liss, New York.

Diop, L., Brière, R., Grondin, L., and Reader, T. A., 1987, Adrenergic receptor and catecholamine distribution in rat cerebral cortex: Binding studies with [³H]prazosin, [³H]idazoxan and [³H]dihydroalprenolol, *Brain Res.* **402**:403–408.

Elliott, K. A. C., 1958, γ-Aminobutyric acid and factor I, *Rev. Can. Biol.* **17**:367–388.

Elliott, K. A. C., and Jasper, H. H., 1959, Gamma-aminobutyric acid, *Physiol. Rev.* **39**:383–406.

Fahn, S., and Cote, L., 1986, Regional distribution of γ-aminobutyric acid (GABA) in brain of rhesus monkey, *J. Neurochem.* **15**:209–213.

Feldberg, W., 1945, Present views on the mode of action of acetylcholine in the central nervous system, *Physiol. Rev.* **25**:596–642.

Ferron, A., Siggins, G. R., and Bloom, F. E., 1985, Vasoactive intestinal polypeptide acts synergistically with norepinephrine to depress spontaneous discharge rate in cerebral cortical neurons, *Proc. Natl. Acad. Sci. USA* **82**:8810–8812.

Foote, S. L., Freedman, R., and Oliver, A. P., 1975, Effects of putative neurotransmitters on neuronal activity in monkey auditory cortex, *Brain Res.* **86**:229–242.

Gainer, H., and Brownstein, M. J., 1981, Neuropeptides, in: *Basic Neurochemistry,* (G. J. Siegel, R. W. Albers, B. W. Agranoff, and R. Katzman, eds.), Little, Brown, Boston, pp. 269–296.

Giarman, N. J., and Pepeu, G. C., 1964, The influence of centrally acting cholinolytic drugs on brain acetylcholine levels, *Br. J. Pharmacol. Chemother.* **23**:123–130.

Greengard, P., 1978, *Cyclic Nucleotides, Phosphorylated Proteins, and Neuronal Function*, Raven Press, New York.

Guidotti, A., Badiani, G., and Pepeu, G., 1972, Taurine distribution in cat brain, *J. Neurochem.* **19**:431–435.

Hobson, J. A., Lydic, R., and Baghdoyan, H. A., 1986, Evolving concepts of sleep cycle generation: From brain centers to neuronal populations, *Behav. Brain Sci.* **9**:371–448.

Hökfelt, T., Johansson, D., and Goldstein, M., 1984, Chemical anatomy of the brain, *Science* **225**:1326–1334.

Hong, J. S., Yang, H. Y. T., Fratta, W., and Costa, E., 1977, Determination of methionine enkephalin in discrete regions of rat brain, *Brain Res.* **134**:383–386.

Hoover, D. B., Muth, E. A., and Jacobowitz, D. M., 1978, A mapping of the distribution of acetylcholine, choline acetyltransferase and acetylcholinesterase in discrete areas of rat brain, *Brain Res.* **153**:295–306.

Iversen, L. L., 1975, Dopamine receptors in the brain, *Science* **188**:1084–1089.

Iversen, L. L., 1983, Nonopioid neuropeptides in mammalian CNS, *Annu. Rev. Pharmacol. Toxicol.* **23**:1–27.

Iversen, S. D., 1984, Cortical monoamines and behaviour, in: *Monoamine Innervation of Cerebral Cortex* (L. Descarries, T. A. Reader, and H. H. Jasper, eds.), Liss, New York, pp. 321–349.

Jasper, H. H., 1981, Problems of relating cellular or modular specificity to cognitive functions: Importance of state dependent reactions, in: *The Organization of the Cerebral Cortex* (F. O. Schmitt, F. G. Worden, G. Adelman, and S. Dennis, eds.), MIT Press, Cambridge, Mass., pp. 375–393.

Jasper, H. H., 1984, The saga of K. A. C. Elliott and GABA, *Neurochem. Res.* **9**:449–460.

Jasper, H. H., and Koyama, I., 1969, Rate of release of amino acids from the cerebral cortex in the cat as affected by brainstem and thalamic stimulation, *Can. J. Physiol. Pharmacol.* **47**:889–905.

Jasper, H. H., and Tessier, J., 1971, Acetylcholine liberation from cerebral cortex during paradoxical (REM) sleep, *Science* **172**:601–602.

Jasper, H. H., Khan, R. T., and Elliott, K. A. C., 1965, Amino acids released from the cerebral cortex in relation to the state of activation, *Science* **147**:1448–1449.

Kanazawa, I., and Jessell, T., 1976, Postmortem changes and regional distribution of substance P in the rat and mouse nervous system, *Brain Res.* **117**:362–367.

Kasamatsu, T., and Pettigrew, J. D., 1976, Depletion of brain catecholamines: Failure of ocular dominance shift after monocular occlusion in kittens, *Science* **194**:206–209.

Kasamatsu, T., Itakura, T., Jonnson, G., Heggelund, P., Pettigrew, J. D., Nakai, K., Kazushige, W., Kuppermann, B. D., and Ary, M., 1984, Neuronal plasticity in cat visual cortex: A proposed role for the central noradrenaline system, in: *Monoamine Innervation of Cerebral Cortex* (L. Descarries, T. A. Reader, and H. H. Jasper, eds.), Liss, New York, pp. 301–319.

Kety, S. S., 1970, The biogenic amines in the central nervous system: Their possible roles in arousal, emotion and learning, in: *The Neurosciences: Second Study Program* (F. O. Schmitt, ed.), Rockefeller University Press, New York, pp. 324–336.

Kleinschmidt, A., Bear, M. F., and Singer, W., 1987, Evidence that activation of NMDA receptors is necessary for experience-dependent modifications of kitten striate cortex, (manuscript).

Kolta, A., Diop, L., and Reader, T. A., 1987, Noradrenergic effects on rat visual cortex: Single-cell microiontophoretic studies of alpha-2 adrenergic receptors, *Life Sci.* **41**:281–289.

Krieger, D. T., 1983, Brain peptides: What, where, and why? *Science* **222**:975–985.

Krnjević, K., 1964, Microiontophoretic studies on cortical neurons, *Int. Rev. Neurobiol.* **7**:41–98.

Krnjević, K., 1974, Chemical nature of synaptic transmission in vertebrates, *Physiol. Rev.* **54**:418–540.

Krnjević, K., 1984, Monoamine receptors in cortex: An introduction, in: *Monoamine Innervation of Cerebral Cortex* (L. Descarries, T. A. Reader, and H. H. Jasper, eds.), Liss, New York, pp. 125–133.

Krnjević, K., and Schwartz, S., 1967, The action of γ-aminobutyric acid on cortical neurones, *Exp. Brain Res.* **3**:320–336.

Libet, B., Kobayashi, H., and Tanaka, T., 1975, Synaptic coupling into the production and storage of a neuronal memory trace, *Nature* **258**:155–157.

Lipinski, J. F., Schaumberg, H. H., and Baldessarini, R. J., 1973, Regional distribution of histamine in the human brain, *Brain Res.* **52**:403–408.

McCormick, D. A., and Prince, D. A., 1985, Two types of muscarinic response to acetylcholine in mammalian cortical neurons, *Proc. Natl. Acad. Sci. USA* **82**:6344–6348.

MacIntosh, F. C., 1941, The distribution of acetylcholine in the peripheral and the central nervous system, *J. Physiol. (London)* **99**:436–442.

MacIntosh, F. C., and Oborin, P. E., 1953, Release of acetylcholine from intact cerebral cortex, *Abstr. XIX Int. Physiol. Congr.* pp. 580–581.

Magistretti, P. J., and Schorderet, M., 1984, VIP and noradrenaline act synergistically to increase cyclic AMP in cerebral cortex, *Nature* **308**:280–282.

Mancillas, J. R., Siggins, G. R., and Bloom, F. E., 1986, Somatostatin selectively enhances acetylcholine-induced excitations in rat hippocampus and cortex, *Proc. Natl. Acad. Sci. USA* **83**:7518–7521.

Mesulam, M.-M., Mufson, E. J., Levey, A. I., and Wayner, B. H., 1983, Cholinergic innervation of cortex by the basal forebrain: Cytochemistry and cortical connections of the septal area, diagonal band nuclei, nucleus basalis (substantia innominata), and hypothalamus in the rhesus monkey, *J. Comp. Neurol.* **214**:170–197.

Metherate, R., Tremblay, N., and Dykes, R. W., 1987, Acetylcholine permits long-term enhancement of neuronal responsiveness in cat primary, somatosensory cortex, *Neuroscience* **22**:75–81.

Miller, F. R., Stavraky, G. W., and Woonton, G. A., 1940, Effects of eserine, acetylcholine and atropine on the electrocorticogram, *J. Neurophysiol.* **3**:131–138.

Mitchell, J. F., 1963, The spontaneous and evoked release of acetylcholine from the cerebral cortex, *J. Physiol. (London)* **165:**98–116.

Moroni, F., Tanganelli, S., Antonelli, T., Carla, V., Bianchi, C., and Beani, L., 1983, Modulation of cortical acetylcholine and gamma-aminobutyric acid release in freely moving guinea pigs: Effects of clonidine and other adrenergic drugs, *J. Pharmacol. Exp. Ther.* **227:**435–440.

Mullin, W. J., and Phillis, J. W., 1975, The effect of graded forelimb afferent volleys on acetylcholine release from cat sensorimotor cortex, *J. Physiol. (London)* **244:**741–756.

Nieuwenhuys, R., 1985, *Chemoarchitecture of the Brain,* Springer-Verlag, Berlin.

Olpe, H. R., Glatt, A., Lazlo, J., and Schellemberg, A., 1980, Some electrophysiological and pharmacological properties of the cortical noradrenergic projection of the locus coeruleus in the rat, *Brain Res.* **185:**9–19.

Pepeu, G., 1973, The release of acetylcholine from the brain: An approach to the study of the central cholinergic mechanisms, *Prog. Neurobiol.* **2:**257–288.

Perry, T. L., Berry, K., Diamond, S., and Mok, C., 1971, Regional distribution of amino acids in human brain obtained at autopsy, *J. Neurochem.* **18:**513–519.

Phillis, J. W., 1977, The role of cyclic nucleotides in the CNS, *Can. J. Neurol. Sci.* **4:**151–195.

Phillis, J. W., 1984, Microiontophoretic studies of cortical biogenic amines, in: *Monoamine Innervation of Cerebral Cortex* (L. Descarries, T. A. Reader, and H. H. Jasper, eds.), Liss, New York, pp. 175–194.

Reader, T. A., 1978, The effects of dopamine, noradrenaline and serotonin in the visual cortex of the cat, *Experientia* **34:**1586–1587.

Reader, T. A., 1980, Microiontophoresis of biogenic amines on cortical neurons: Amounts of NA, DA and 5-HT ejected, compared with tissue contents, *Acta Physiol. Lat. Am.* **30:**291–304.

Reader, T. A., 1983, The role of the catecholamines in neuronal excitability, in: *Basic Mechanisms of Neuronal Hyperexcitability* (H. H. Jasper and N. M. van Gelder, eds.), Liss, New York, pp. 281–321.

Reader, T. A., and Jasper, H. H., 1984, Interactions between monoamines and other transmitters in cerebral cortex, in: *Monoamine Innervation of Cerebral Cortex* (L. Descarries, T. A. Reader, and H. H. Jasper, eds.), Liss, New York, pp. 195–225.

Reader, T. A., and Quesney, L. F., 1986, Dopamine in the visual cortex of the cat, *Experientia* **42:**1242–1244.

Reader, T. A., de Champlain, J., and Jasper, H. H., 1976, Catecholamines released from cerebral cortex in the cat: Decrease during sensory stimulation, *Brain Res.* **111:**95–103.

Reader, T. A., Ferron, A., Descarries, L., and Jasper, H. H., 1979a, Modulatory role for biogenic amines in the cerebral cortex: Microiontophoretic studies, *Brain Res.* **160:**217–229.

Reader, T. A., Masse, P., and de Champlain, J., 1979b, The intracortical distribution of norepinephrine, dopamine and serotonin in the cerebral cortex of the cat, *Brain Res.* **177:**499–513.

Reader, T. A., de Champlain, J., and Jasper, H. H., 1980, Participation of presynaptic and postsynaptic receptors in acetylcholine–catecholamine interactions in cerebral cortex, in: *Presynaptic Receptors* (S. Z. Langer, K. Starke, and M. L. Dubocovich, eds.), Pergamon Press, New York, pp. 363–369.

Reader, T. A., Brière, R., Grondin, L., and Ferron, A., 1986, Effects of p-chlorophenylalanine on cortical monoamines and on the activity of noradrenergic neurons, *Neurochem. Res.* **11:**1025–1035.

Renaud, L., 1983, Role of neuropeptides in the regulation of neural excitability, in: *Basic Mechanisms of Neuronal Hyperexcitability* (H. H. Jasper and N. M. van Gelder, eds.), Liss, New York, pp. 323–360.

Ribak, C. E., Harris, A. B., Vaughn, J. E., and Roberts, E., 1979, Inhibitory, GABAergic nerve terminals decrease at sites of focal epilepsy, *Science* **205:**211–214.

Richardson, R. T., and DeLong, M. R., 1986, Nucleus basalis of Meynert neuronal activity during a delayed response task in monkey, *Brain Res.* **399:**364–368.

Rigdon, G. G., and Pirch, J. H., 1986, Nucleus basalis involvement in conditioned neuronal response in the rat frontal cortex, *J. Neurosci.* **6:**2535–2542.

Schmitt, F. O., 1984, Molecular regulators of brain function: A new view, *Neuroscience* **13:**991–1001.

Seeman, P., 1980, Brain dopamine receptors, *Pharmacol. Rev.* **32:**229–313.

Seeman, P., and Lee, T., 1975, Antipsychotic drugs: Direct correlation between clinical potency and presynaptic action on dopamine neurons, *Science* **188:**1217–1219.

Sie, G., Jasper, H. H., and Wolfe, L., 1965, Rate of ACh release from cortical surface in 'encephale' and ''cerveau isole'' cat preparations in relation to arousal and epileptic activation of the ECoG, *Electroencephalogr. Clin. Neurophysiol.* **18:**206.

Sillito, A. M., and Kemp, J. A., 1983, Cholinergic modulation of the functional organization of the cat visual cortex, *Brain Res.* **289:**143–155.

Singer, W., 1983, Neuronal mechanisms of experience-dependent self-organization of the mammalian visual cortex, *Acta Morphol. Hung.* **31:**235–260.

Stone, T. W., Taylor, T. W., and Bloom, F. E., 1975, Cyclic AMP and cyclic GMP may mediate opposite neuronal responses in the rat cerebral cortex, *Science* **187:**845–846.

Szerb, J. C., 1964, The effect of tertiary and quaternary atropine on cortical acetylcholine output and on the electroencephalogram in cats, *Can. J. Physiol. Pharmacol.* **42**:303–314.

Takagi, H., Shiomi, H., Veda, H., and Amano, H., 1979, Morphine-like analgesia by a new dipeptide, l-tyrosyl-l-arginine (Kyotorphin) and its analogue, *Eur. J. Pharmacol.* **55**:109–111.

Tanji, J., and Evarts, E. V., 1976, Anticipatory activity of motor cortex neurones in relation to direction of an intended movement, *J. Neurophysiol.* **39**:1062–1068.

von Euler, U. S., and Gaddum, J. H., 1931, An unidentified depressor substance in certain tissue extracts, *J. Physiol. (London)* **192**:74–87.

Wamsley, J. K., 1984, Autoradiographic localization of cortical biogenic amine receptors, in: *Monoamine Innervation of Cerebral Cortex* (L. Descarries, T. A. Reader, and H. H. Jasper, eds.), Liss, New York, pp. 153–174.

Whitehouse, P. J., Price, D. L., Clark, A. W., Coyle, J. T., and De Long, M. R., 1981, Alzheimer disease: Evidence for selective loss of cholinergic neurones in the nucleus basalis, *Ann. Neurol.* **10**:122–126.

39

Addendum of Appreciation

I would like to close the publication of this excellent symposium with an expression of most sincere thanks and profound appreciation to the organizers, Massimo Avoli, Tom Reader, Bob Dykes, and Pierre Gloor, in celebration of my 80th birthday. It was organized without my knowledge until the very last, when they had to be sure I would be present in Montreal, July 21–23, 1986, just following the International Congress of Physiological Sciences in Vancouver.

I was overwhelmed by the number of outstanding contributors and their carefully prepared and thoughtful presentations of many aspects of a most complex and rapidly expanding field of research on a subject which has been my own major research interest during the past 25 years at the Montreal Neurological Institute and in the Centre de Recherche en Sciences Neurologiques at the University of Montreal.

To have this symposium organized by colleagues from both universities is a special honor for which I am most grateful. It has provided many fond memories, which Mrs. Jasper and I shall long cherish.

This publication will be a landmark in current research into the most challenging of all scientific endeavors, as expressed in the subtitle "From Molecules to Mind." I have learned that this subtitle was suggested by the title of my chapter written for Frank Schmitt's 70th birthday party in Boston in 1974 (*The Neurosciences: Paths of Discovery*, MIT Press, 1975), i.e., "Philosophy or Physics—Mind or Molecules." I suspect that the genial organizing committee chose this subtitle as a kindly gesture, or perhaps a gentle jibe, to add to the many good stories, the kind remarks, and the good fellowship that were the outstanding features of this birthday party, adding a warm personal touch to the scientific celebrations.

Herbert H. Jasper

Contributors

Massimo Avoli • Montreal Neurological Institute and Department of Neurology and Neurosurgery, McGill University, Montreal, Quebec H3A 2B4, Canada

A. Beaudet • Montreal Neurological Institute, McGill University, Montreal, Quebec H3A 2B4, Canada

A. M. Benjamin • Department of Pharmacology and Therapeutics, Faculty of Medicine, The University of British Columbia, Vancouver, British Columbia V6T 1W5, Canada

Richard Brière • Centre de Recherche en Sciences Neurologiques, Département de Physiologie, Faculté de Médecine, Université de Montréal, Montreal, Quebec H3C 3J7, Canada

J.-W. Chen • Center for Biomedical Research and Departments of Human Development and Biochemistry, University of Kansas, Lawrence, Kansas 66045

M. Chrétien • Laboratory of Molecular Neuroendocrinology, Clinical Research Institute of Montreal, Montreal, Quebec H2W 1R7, Canada

B. Collier • Department of Pharmacology, McGill University, Montreal, Quebec H3G 1Y6, Canada

Laurent Descarries • Centre de Recherche en Sciences Neurologiques, Département de Physiologie, Faculté de Médecine, Université de Montréal, Montreal, Quebec H3C 3J7, Canada

Laurent Diop • Centre de Recherche en Sciences Neurologiques, Département de Physiologie, Faculté de Médecine, Université de Montréal, Montreal, Quebec H3C 3J7, Canada

Guy Doucet • Centre de Recherche en Sciences Neurologiques, Département de Physiologie, Faculté de Médecine, Université de Montréal, Montreal, Quebec H3C 3J7, Canada

Marianne Dunér-Engström • Farmakologiska Institutionen, Karolinska Institutet, S-104 01 Stockholm, Sweden

Robert W. Dykes • Departments of Physiology, Neurology, and Neurosurgery, McGill University, Montreal, Quebec H3A 1A1, Canada

Johan Fastbom • Farmakologiska Institutionen, Karolinska Institutet, S-104 01 Stockholm, Sweden

André Ferron • Centre de Recherche en Sciences Neurologiques, Département de Physiologie, Faculté de Médecine, Université de Montréal, Montreal, Quebec H3C 3J7, Canada

A. Ferroni • Department of General Physiology and Biochemistry, University of Milan, Milan, Italy

Paul G. Finlayson • Department of Physiology, Faculty of Health Sciences, University of Ottawa, Ottawa, Ontario K1H 8M5, Canada

Bertil B. Fredholm • Farmakologiska Institutionen, Karolinska Institutet, S-104 01 Stockholm, Sweden

Harold Gainer • Laboratory of Neurochemistry and Neuroimmunology, National Institute of Child Health and Human Development, National Institutes of Health, Bethesda, Maryland 20892   *Present address:* Laboratory of Neurochemistry, National Institute of Neurological and Communication Disorders and Stroke, National Institutes of Health, Bethesda, Maryland 20892

Pierre Gloor • Montreal Neurological Institute and Department of Neurology and Neurosurgery, McGill University, Montreal, Quebec H3A 2B4, Canada

R. W. Greene • Harvard Medical School, V.A. Medical Center, Brockton, Massachusetts 02401

E. Gruen • Mental Retardation Research Center, UCLA Medical Center, Los Angeles, California 90024

H. L. Haas • Department of Physiology, Johannes Gutenberg-University, D65 Mainz, Federal Republic of Germany.

E. Hamel • Montreal Neurological Institute, McGill University, Montreal, Quebec H3A 2B4, Canada

Herbert H. Jasper • Centre de Recherche en Sciences Neurologiques, Département de Physiologie, Faculté de Médicine, Université de Montréal, and Montreal Neurological Institute, McGill University, Montreal, Quebec H3A 2B4 Canada

L. H. Jensen • A/S Ferrosan Research Division, Sydmarken 5, 2860 Søborg, Denmark

M. S. Jensen • Institute of Physiology, Århus University, 8000 Århus C, Denmark

E. G. Jones • Department of Anatomy and Neurobiology, University of California, Irvine, California 92717

Bror Jonzon • Farmakologiska Institutionen, Karolinska Institutet, S-104 01 Stockholm, Sweden

P. Kitabgi • Centre de Biochimie du CNRS, Université de Nice, 06034 Nice Cedex, France

Arlette Kolta • Centre de Recherche en Sciences Neurologiques, Département de Physiologie, Faculté de Médicine, Université de Montréal, Montreal, Quebec H3C 3J7, Canada

George K. Kostopoulos • Department of Physiology, University of Patras Medical School, Patras 261 10, Greece

K. Krnjević • Departments of Anaesthesia Research and Physiology, McGill University, Montreal, Quebec H3G 1Y6, Canada

I. Kurcewicz • Unité de Recherches sur l'Epilepsie, INSERM U 97, 75014 Paris, France

J. D. C. Lambert • Institute of Physiology, Århus University, 8000 Århus C, Denmark

C. Lazure • Laboratory of Biochemical Neuroendocrinology, Clinical Research Institute of Montreal, Montreal, Quebec H2W 1R7, Canada

Benoît Lemay • Centre de Recherche en Sciences Neurologiques, Département de Physiologie, Faculté de Médicine, Université de Montréal, Montreal, Quebec H3C 3J7, Canada

K. Leonard • Montreal Neurological Institute, McGill University, Montreal, Quebec H3A 2B4, Canada

Benjamin Libet • Department of Physiology, School of Medicine, University of California, San Francisco, California 94143

Eva Lindgren • Farmakologiska Institutionen, Karolinska Institutet, S-104 01 Stockholm, Sweden

J. Louvel • Unité de Recherches sur l'Epilepsie, INSERM U 97, 75014 Paris, France

David A. McCormick • Department of Neurology, Stanford University School of Medicine, Stanford, California 94305   *Present address:* Section of Neuroanatomy, Yale University, School of Medicine, New Haven, Connecticut 06510

J. F. MacDonald • Playfair Neuroscience Unit, University of Toronto, The Toronto Hospital, Toronto, Ontario M5T 2S8, Canada

Daniel V. Madison • Department of Physiology, University of California, San Francisco, California 94143   *Present address:* Department of Physiology, Yale University School of Medicine, New Haven, Connecticut 06510

Kenneth C. Marshall • Department of Physiology, Faculty of Health Sciences, University of Ottawa, Ottawa, Ontario K1H 8M5, Canada

M.-Marsel Mesulam • Bullard and Denny-Brown Laboratories, Division of Neuroscience and Behavioral Neurology, Dana Research Institute, Harvard Neurology Department, Beth Israel Hospital, Boston, Massachusetts 02215

R. Metherate • Department of Physiology, McGill University, Montreal, Quebec H3A 1A1, Canada

E. K. Michaelis • Center for Biomedical Research and Departments of Human Development and Biochemistry, University of Kansas, Lawrence, Kansas 66045

Z. Miljkovic • Playfair Neuroscience Unit, University of Toronto, The Toronto Hospital, Toronto, Ontario M5T 2S8, Canada

E. Moyse • Montreal Neurological Institute, McGill University, Montreal, Quebec H3A 2B4, Canada

Penelope Clare Murphy • Department of Physiology, University College, Cardiff CF1 1XL, United Kingdom

Roger A. Nicoll • Department of Pharmacology, University of California, San Francisco, California 94143

A. Nistri • Department of Pharmacology, St. Bartholomew's Hospital Medical College, University of London, London EC1M 6BQ, United Kingdom

Christer Nordstedt • Farmakologiska Institutionen, Karolinska Institutet, S-104 01 Stockholm, Sweden

Ole Petter Ottersen • Anatomical Institute, University of Oslo, Karl Johansgate 47, N-0162 Oslo 1, Norway

Charles C. Ouimet • The Rockefeller University, New York, New York 10021

Hanna M. Pappius • The Goad Unit of the Donner Laboratory of Experimental Neurochemistry, Montreal Neurological Institute, McGill University, Montreal, Quebec H3A 2B4, Canada

E. N. Petersen • A/S Ferrosan Research Division, Sydmarken 5, 2860 Søborg, Denmark. *Present address:* Als Dumex, DK-2300, Copenhagen, Denmark

J. W. Phillis • Department of Physiology, School of Medicine, Wayne State University, Detroit, Michigan 48201

David A. Prince • Department of Neurology, Stanford University School of Medicine, Stanford, California 94305

E. Puil • Department of Pharmacology and Therapeutics, Faculty of Medicine, The University of British Columbia, Vancouver, British Columbia V6T 1W5, Canada

R. Pumain • Unité de Recherches sur l'Epilepsie, INSERM U 97, 75014 Paris, France

Remi Quirion • Douglas Hospital Research Centre and Department of Psychiatry, Faculty of Medicine, McGill University, Verdun, Quebec H4H 1R3, Canada

Tomás A. Reader • Centre de Recherche en Sciences Neurologiques, Département de Physiologie, Faculté de Médecine, Université de Montréal, Montreal, Quebec H3C 3J7, Canada

Leo P. Renaud • Neurosciences Unit, Montreal General Hospital and McGill University, Montreal, Quebec H3G 1A4, Canada

W. Rostène • INSERM U-55, Hôpital St. Antoine, 75012 Paris, France

S. Roy • Center for Biomedical Research and Departments of Human Development and Biochemistry, University of Kansas, Lawrence, Kansas 66045

J. H. Schneiderman • Wellesley Hospital, Toronto, Ontario M4Y 1J3, Canada

Peter Schubert • Department of Neuromorphology, Max Planck Institute for Psychiatry, 8033 Martinsried, West Germany

Philippe Séguéla • Centre de Recherche en Sciences Neurologiques, Département de Physiologie, Faculté de Médecine, Université de Montréal, Montreal, Quebec H3C 3J7, Canada

N. G. Seidah • Laboratory of Biochemical Neuroendocrinology, Clinical Research Institute of Montreal, Montreal, Quebec H2W 1R7, Canada

R. A. Sikstrom • Laboratory of Molecular Neuroendocrinology, Clinical Research Institute of Montreal, Montreal, Quebec H2W 1R7, Canada

Adam Murdin Sillito • Department of Physiology, University College, Cardiff, CF1 1XL, United Kingdom

T. M. Stormann • Center for Biomedical Research and Departments of Human Development and Biochemistry, University of Kansas, Lawrence, Kansas 66045

Jon Storm-Mathisen • Anatomical Institute, University of Oslo, Karl Johansgate 47, N-0162 Oslo 1, Norway

John C. Szerb • Department of Physiology and Biophysics, Dalhousie University, Halifax, Nova Scotia, B3H 4H7, Canada

N. Tremblay • Departments of Neurology and Neurosurgery, McGill University, Montreal, Quebec H3A 1A1, Canada

N. M. van Gelder • Centre de Recherche en Sciences Neurologiques, Faculté de Médecine, Université de Montréal, Montreal, Quebec H3C 3J7, Canada

M. Vial • INSERM U-55, Hôpital St. Antoine, 75012 Paris, France

J. P. Vincent • Centre de Biochimie du CNRS, Université de Nice, 06034 Nice Cedex, France

E. Wanke • Department of General Physiology and Biochemistry, University of Milan, Milan, Italy

Kenneth C. Watkins • Centre de Recherche en Sciences Neurologiques, Département de Physiologie, Faculté de Médecine, Université de Montréal, Montreal, Quebec H3C 3J7, Canada

C. D. Woody • Mental Retardation Research Center, UCLA Medical Center, Los Angeles, California 90024

Index